Cancer Care in Countries and Societies in Transition

Michael Silbermann
Editor

Cancer Care in Countries and Societies in Transition

Individualized Care in Focus

Springer

Editor
Michael Silbermann
Technion – Israel Institute of Technology
& Middle East Cancer Consortium
Haifa, Israel

ISBN 978-3-319-79435-8 ISBN 978-3-319-22912-6 (eBook)
DOI 10.1007/978-3-319-22912-6

Springer Cham Heidelberg New York Dordrecht London

Softcover reprint of the hardcover 1st edition 2016

Printed on acid-free paper

Springer International Publishing AG Switzerland is part of Springer Science+Business Media (www.springer.com)

This book is dedicated to Prof. Dr. A. Murat Tuncer, Rector of Hacettepe University and former Chairman of the Department of Cancer Control in the Ministry of Health, Ankara, Turkey, for his immense support, encouragement, and advice that enabled scientific and clinical collaborations in the Middle East.

Foreword

The English Renaissance poet John Donne wrote, “No man is an island, entire unto itself.” One could further extrapolate that when it comes to confronting the scourge of cancer, no nation is an island unto itself. Cancer knows no borders—geopolitical, racial, ethnic, or socioeconomic.

With this interconnectivity in mind, in 1996 an ambitious and innovative model for constructive collaboration was born that would reach beyond national borders to provide health and hope for thousands of cancer victims in the Middle East. Almost two decades after its launch, in which I played a part, the Middle East Cancer Consortium (MECC) has helped to build bridges of understanding and teamwork between healers and scientists working together to one day defeat one of our greatest common enemies—cancer.

The treatment of cancer is often erroneously, in my opinion, referred to as a “battle” fought by cancer patients, their families, and an army of healthcare professionals and researchers. Yet seen in the context of the MECC’s mission, cancer care is also akin to a diplomatic endeavor, with education, engagement, and understanding providing powerful tools that complement the traditional weapons of medicine, technology, and research.

The statistics are shocking—every year more than eight million citizens around the globe die from cancer, and according to the World Health Organization, more than 70 % of those deaths occur in low- and middle-income countries in Africa, Asia, and Central and South America. Considering that in many of these cases cancer is diagnosed in advanced stages when survival is less likely, the demand for prevention, early detection, and treatment becomes a humanitarian imperative, not just a privilege for those who can afford it.

Cancer Care in Countries and Societies in Transition—Individualized Care in Focus offers a much-needed account of the state of global cancer care—the good, the bad, and very much the hopeful. A quick glance at the table of contents reveals chapters that read like a roster of United Nations members and makes it abundantly evident that no corner of the Earth is untouched by the ravages of cancer. The thoughtful and illuminating work of the collected authors underscores that what is of concern in the Middle East is also of concern in Africa, Asia, and Latin America. Likewise, the advances available in North America and Europe provide a cautionary framework by which developing countries can better adapt and promote lifesaving care and treatments. From the wealthiest to the poorest of nations, they all grapple with defining what is the appropriate standard for care, which varies depending upon available resources, cultural sensibilities, and environmental risk factors, to name just a few.

Throughout this wide-ranging compendium, general themes emerge: the shortage of qualified personnel; limited technological capacity; the availability and expense of specialized drugs and treatment; the merits and shortcomings of hospital versus home versus hospice care settings; patients' personal responsibility, lifestyle choices, and prevention; and palliative care, quality of life, and end-of-life planning. And all nations, regardless of their relative affluence, struggle with balancing the cost of care versus the cost of illness—there are no easy answers.

There are also some common threads of real change and hope as they relate to healthcare providers becoming empowered advocates for their patients. The expectations are high that the role of nurses in providing patient-centered and cost-effective care will continue to grow. Also evident is a better, more open communication about a disease that has long been stigmatized as if a cancer diagnosis is somehow shameful. Educating and engaging patients and their families in their care is having a measurably positive impact on outcomes, and this includes honest discussions between patients and their physicians and caretakers about end-of-life care and advanced care planning.

What is abundantly clear is that our efforts will be successful only with the concerted and continuous commitments of governments, academia, the private sector, and multidimensional organizations across and within national boundaries. Clinical professionals, scientists, educators, and social workers all provide cancer patients and their families with the support—physical, mental, and spiritual—they require to face a terrible disease that does not care about the language one speaks or the color of one's skin. In this sense, cancer is an equal opportunity waster of life.

I applaud Professor Michael Silbermann, MECC executive director and editor of *Cancer Care in Countries and Societies in Transition: Individualized Care in Focus*, for this tangible accomplishment and commitment to saving lives and making the world stronger through healthier, more productive societies. I also want to acknowledge the leadership and contributions of the US Department of Health and Human Services and its National Institutes of Health; the US Department of State Bureau of Near Eastern Affairs, Office of Regional and Multilateral Affairs, and the Bureau of Oceans, Environment, and Science; the American Society of Clinical Oncology, Department of International Affairs; the American Oncology Nursing Society,

Department of International Leadership and Development; and the European Society for Medical Oncology Task Force for Emerging Countries, Department of International Affairs.

Donne goes on to proclaim in the same work, "For Whom the Bell Tolls," that "Each man's death diminishes me, For I am involved in mankind." Indeed. Not only is no one single man, woman, or child an island, we are all interconnected, and each death from cancer—no matter where in the world it occurs—diminishes us and our future potential as a whole.

Former Secretary of Health and Human Services Donna E. Shalala
New York, NY

Preface

Overview

The burden and complexities associated with cancer care are rapidly increasing globally, and the largest proportional increases are predicted in countries undergoing epidemiological-demographic transitions [1]. Among the causes for the rising cancer burden are the increasing longevity and gradual decline in fertility that lead to enhanced aging of the populations, particularly in low- and middle-income countries [2]. Whereas in developed countries the mortality rates from cancer are slowly declining, developing countries exhibit the highest age-standardized death rates.

Emerging countries in different regions over the globe are constantly struggling with the challenge of prioritizing achievable targets in the presentation and treatment of cancer, as high-priority medical interventions have to be feasible and reasonably cost-effective at the level of primary healthcare settings.

In almost all countries surveyed in this new book, it became apparent that cancer has its own epidemiological transition: With the increasing levels of human development, cancers associated with infections and poverty (e.g., cancers of the stomach, liver, and cervix) are surpassed by those more closely associated with affluence (e.g., cancers of the female breast, prostate, and colon) [2]. Moreover, cancers vary with respect to their geographic distribution, etiology, and treatment options [3].

Although there is no universal risk factor for cancer, the predictions of the future cancer burden suggest that the annual number of new cases of cancer will surpass 20 million as early as 2025, a 41% increase from 2012 [4]. The lung, breast, and colon have lower incidence and mortality in the lowest income countries, but they are increasing due to less favorable trends in smoking than in high-income countries. Further, the rapid changes in lifestyle, e.g., obesity and sedentary life, along with newly acquired reproductive habits, i.e., decrease and delay of childbearing, are considered to be linked to the increase in breast cancer [2].

The WHO Global Action Plan for Prevention and Control of Noncommunicable Diseases (adopted on May 27, 2013) endorsed the list of essential medicines for cancer patients that can be used in primary care settings, and the only clinical intervention included was that of palliative care [5]. The majority of countries included in this new book emphasized the lack of acceptable palliative care services in both the primary (communities) and tertiary healthcare levels (hospitals and cancer centers). In countries undergoing transition this issue becomes a cardinal one, as the majority of cancer patients are not screened and present themselves to the health system at a late stage of the disease, when the only treatment option available is that of palliation [6].

The current situation urgently calls for a much more global and regional coordination of cancer-care strategies. At present, individual countries try to implement their own cancer control plans with varying degrees of success [2].

The Middle East Cancer Consortium (MECC) is working closely with its partners in the Middle East and in other regions, worldwide, to draw attention to the increasing burden of cancer, highlighting the need to put forward the new challenges associated with cancer care in the upcoming decade. It is well recognized that there are still appreciable weaknesses in the ways that global health agencies address such challenges, fully realizing that the cancer community still has some way to go to ensure a realistic way to cope with the increasing cancer burden in the upcoming decade [7]. The current situation leads to an unacceptably low survival rate in some of the low- and middle-income countries (30–40%) as compared to those in developed countries which are today around 80% [8].

A burning issue in societies in transition refers to the unacceptable gap in adequate palliative care and access to pain relief for much of the world's population. The disparities in worldwide use of medical opioids are indeed of serious concern [8, 9]. Yet, updated reports that see light in this book reveal that considerable attempts are made to dispel the myth that effective, quality care is only achievable in high-income countries and that even in low resource settings, when appropriate programs are applied, acceptable solutions can be obtained. In order to further encourage and support such attempts, the cancer community needs to reach out to nontraditional partners via strong advocacy movement.

Recent developments have shown that by connecting the cancer community from the grassroots levels to national and regional cancer societies, opportunities can be created to see to it that more people with cancer will be treated in an acceptable manner.

Clinical cancer care plays a significant role in global cancer control. The European Society for Medical Oncology (ESMO) aims to play a pivotal role in the efforts to establish a global strategy. An important recommendation from the ESMO document on the WHO Global NCD Action Plan (GAP) at the 66th World Health Assembly in 2013 was to build upon the strengthening of primary care for NCDs as requested by GAP. ESMO experts also strongly emphasized the need and feasibility to prioritize the availability of a basic set of treatment options including palliative care interventions and improvement of access to morphine for pain relief. To achieve these goals, MECC joins ESMO, along with other global and regional agencies in leading a collaborative effort to help in the analysis and mapping of the current situation of the availability of cancer medicines globally [10].

This has resulted in the creation of an ESMO Global Cancer Task Force. The latter seeks to support the joint commitment to the regional and global cancer community and reinforce the belief that patients everywhere should have access to the best available treatment.

It should be emphasized that true knowledge brokering is not linear, but rather depends on network approaches that take advantage of what each focal point has to offer through multiple channels and intermediaries.

The populations in Middle Eastern countries, like those in other emerging countries, are expected to undergo demographic, economic, and social shifts, while their needs deserve high priority on both national and international health and political agendas. Demographic changes alone in emerging countries are projected to result in a substantial increase in cancer incidence and mortality in the two decades ahead of us.

The major obstacle to reducing the mortality from cancer is the limited socioeconomic development of these countries. Poor education of healthcare providers and the public gives rise to poor healthcare, while ill-health has an important impact on the ability to learn and to earn. Health and education are strongly influenced by poverty, which in turn reduces access to healthcare. Many factors influence access, including few primary care providers close to home. By and large, the community lacks nurses, physicians, and pharmacists and has remarkably few cancer specialists.

Therefore, even if drugs and equipment were available, they are of no value without knowledgeable health professionals, particularly oncologist who can make treatment decisions and work with a team comprised of pharmacists, oncology nurses, junior doctors, medical assistants, and social workers [11]. Thus, there is a need to increase practical responsibility for medical assistants, nurses, and community health workers. Further, there should be an incentive to practice in rural regions. It is clear that if cancer treatment were to be improved, training more oncologists must be one of the highest priorities [11].

The Critical Importance of Early Diagnosis

It is well documented that early detection generally leads to better results within the existing healthcare system at less cost and inconvenience. Hence, the education of the public and the medical community may be the single most important action to be taken if better survival rates are to be achieved. Moreover primary cancer prevention also requires public education.

Greater efficiency in detection and diagnosis should be feasible in all countries, but requires planning and individuals dedicated to developing the necessary educational tools [11].

Educating Oncologists

A partial and time-honored approach to the training of specialists is "learning by doing," e.g., gaining experience in the practice of oncology through working with a recognized oncologist. The primary focus would be on training and knowledge assessment strongly centered on clinical care. Training could be done in any cancer center or unit, and training in a cancer center would encourage the simultaneous development of interdisciplinary teams [11].

In the long run the training and employment of social workers in disciplines involved with rehabilitation and "trackers" who ascertain the status of patients who have completed therapy should increase efficiency as well as provide improved data on survival rates.

Management of the cancer burden in low-middle-income countries requires global partnerships between cancer-care mentors from high-income countries and community health workers familiar with the local circumstances [11].

Many countries in transition have been experiencing geopolitical conflicts, domestic political turmoil, and economic recessions which detracted attention from the "slow-motion disaster"—cancer. Such neglect invites future problems, since excessive cancer burdens contribute to social instability and intersocietal insecurity. Such trends will further intensify as the population ages and with the geographical movements of populations (see chapters on Jordan). In resource-rich countries, similar problems exist in rural underserved areas that merit attention [12].

Addressing the above challenges includes strengthening the functionality of the primary care health system. The latter, in most of the developing countries, is still disorganized, dysfunctional, and inadequate in size. Therefore, local-specific solutions are in great need in several countries in the Middle East, while Turkey, Lebanon, and Cyprus have started changing this situation.

Solutions must come from community participatory processes, and international mentors must serve not only as experts but also as facilitators and students of these processes [12].

It is suggested that the focus of global health programs will be enlarged from the current emphasis on the general training of students and practitioners to include attention on service and research that can be maintained throughout faculty careers similar to the laboratory, translational, and clinical research options while emphasizing social responsibility. The involvement of communities is cardinal for the long-term sustainability of development activities [12].

The concept of a long-term mentorship program is timely with a relative minor expense. Not only will it lessen cancer burden, but it will enhance the bridging of intercultural differences and put to better use the wisdom and expertise of resource-rich countries, which eventually can transform global health [12].

Communication

Going over the chapters from the different countries, one finds out that a common barrier to good cancer care refers to lack of communication between the caregivers, the patients, and their relatives. In North America hospital-based clinicians perceive family member-related and patient-related factors as the most important barriers to goals of care discussions [13].

The fact that family members and patients have difficulty accepting a poor prognosis emerged as a key barrier to goals of care discussions which highlights the sometimes high, but understandable, levels of anxiety and denial experienced by seriously ill hospitalized patients and their families. Effective communication skills are needed to navigate these strong feelings, and yet clinicians often report discomfort in responding to the emotional reactions of patients, and learners report insufficient training to have goals of care discussions [13].

The current situation underscores and supports the need for more and better training for all clinicians in having end-of-life discussions. Therefore, communication skills, training, and tools can enhance clinicians' ability to build rapport, listen with empathy, and discuss prognosis along with its inherent uncertainty—all these will help clinicians to better support patients and families through decisions about goals of care.

Also, very important are interventions aimed at improving patient and family preparedness to engage in goals of care discussions. Such interventions may include an expanded role for interprofessional team members in facilitating communication and decision making about goals of care [13].

Factors Interfering with Cancer Care

Cancer is becoming an emerging disease of public health importance in developing countries, and this situation is worsened by wars, poverty, and major demographic changes which are so characteristic of countries in transition. Socioeconomic and cultural factors often lead to late presentation and diagnosis, more mortality, and poor follow-up of cancer survivors. The above countries/societies are known to have rich and diverse cultures where religions, traditions, and family values greatly influence medical decision [14].

In many of the countries represented in this book, many afflicted with cancer live in rural areas and in poverty. As a consequence, delays in diagnosis and poor healthcare seeking behavior are common with these patients. The management of these patients is often fraught with socioeconomic, cultural, and ethical dilemmas. Among the ethical challenges are issues like: individuals' autonomy, family and community participation in care, and end-of-life issues. For the successful development of a viable and sustainable model of cancer care in resource-poor environments, these issues must be dealt with [14].

Culture and Religion

Diversity of cultural and religious beliefs of people in countries in transition, especially in Africa, Asia, and the Middle East, affects their views and perceptions of cancer care. Therefore, the healthcare systems in these regions have to take into consideration the cultural, traditional, and religious inclinations of their peoples. Unfortunately, in a large number of countries mentioned in this book, cancer is still considered to be a taboo, and many forbid the telling of a patient that he/she is dying. Also, because of the strong support provided by an extended family system, there seems to be reduced relevance for psychologists, social workers, and psychiatrists in cancer care [14].

Socioeconomic Issues

Poverty has a very serious implication for patients with cancer in the developing world. Further, many patients hide their diagnosis from family members because of financial burdens of hospital and medication payments [14].

Ethical Issues

These issues include the right to know, end-of-life decisions, death and dying, and health inequities.

The right to know. Issues related to management of information in patient receiving treatment for cancer are the center of literature on communication in cancer [15, 16]. Informing patients with cancer the truth about their diagnosis and progress, or otherwise, is still presumed harmful to the patient [6, p. vii–xiv]. The paternalistic concept in communication in which the physician was treated to act independently in the best interest of the patient is widely practiced [17]. Physicians in restrictive cultures such as those in Africa, the Middle East, and Southeast Asia remain unsupportive of full disclosure of information to patients, particularly of "bad news" [18]. This is in contrast to the attitude of physicians in more open West European and North American countries with high regard for patient's autonomy [19]. In most populations undergoing transition in the twenty-first century, the nuclear family is still very strong, and sentiments among family members influence a patient's choices and decisions [20].

Even in the absence of cultural restrictions, there are patients who prefer avoidance of bad news and delegate decision making to family members. The patient's religious conviction, educational attainment, age, and psychological maturity tend to influence this attribute.

End-of-life decisions. Dying is regarded in cancer care as a natural process which is neither to be hastened nor unduly prolonged while keeping the patient as active as possible until death [21]. The aim is a dignified death free of pain. Terminally ill patients tend to have varying degrees of depression.

Death and dying. Cultural attitude to death and dying is an important barrier to free communication with cancer patients [20]. Family dynamics and religious beliefs play major roles in shaping the concepts of death in a good number of societies in the emerging world. In a recent survey, it became apparent that many cancer patients throughout the Middle East seek complimentary therapies for a family member suffering from cancer [22]. Death and dying is a deeply emotional event in most African and Asian cultures.

Religion has dramatically different connotations in various cultures with prime drivers as history, politics, social events, and theological arguments [23]. Further, religion plays a vital role in determining patients' response to truth about their condition [24]. Also, religious, emotional, and psychological support ameliorate the impact of bad news and help patients to adjust to the reality of their situation [25].

Putting Palliative Care on the Global Health Agenda

Despite the lack of attention and investment, positive developments have occurred in promotion of palliative care in the past 15 years.

In May 2014, the World Health Assembly passed a landmark resolution urging member states to support access to essential medicines and to strengthen palliative care as an integrated component of universal health coverage throughout the life course, stating that palliative care is an ethical responsibility of health systems.

Cancer is a leading cause of morbidity and mortality worldwide; yet, despite the widespread need, only 20 countries (8.5%) have integrated palliative care adequately into their healthcare system [26].

In the greater Middle East region, a diagnosis of cancer is still mixed with social stigma, and physicians conserve a truth disclosure policy in which from one side they respect some of the historical and cultural misperceptions about cancer and, accordingly, tell the truth about cancer to one of the family members and, on the other hand, acknowledge the patient's right to know the truth and tend to disclose it for him (or her) when possible [27].

Education programs in breaking bad news are lacking in many countries. Thus, training programs are needed in this domain in Middle Eastern societies. In the Middle East, a legitimate conspiracy of silence regarding a cancer diagnosis often takes place with the aim of maintaining the patient's hope.

Iran—Anxiety and depression showed strong association with the knowledge of diagnosis of cancer [28]. And physicians disclose more frequently a cancer diagnosis to the patient's family members than to the patient himself. *There is insufficiency in communication skills* [27].

Israel—Only 63 % of physicians and 38 % of nurses stated that they always disclose bad news or negative prognosis to their patients. And patients may, on occasion, express dissatisfaction concerning their physicians' behaviors during truth disclosure of a cancer diagnosis. Family members, in Palestine, seem to be the most important interlocutor when disclosing a cancer diagnosis [29].

Jordan—It has been stated that the Islamic attitudes and beliefs about end-of-life issues should not deter physicians from discussing such matters with the patient's family [30].

Kuwait—More than 50% of patients want to know their cancer diagnosis [27].

Lebanon—A large majority of medical students prefer to disclose the cancer diagnosis directly to the patient [31], while patients highlight the importance of communication throughout the disease trajectory [32]. Patient-family communication and truth-telling are reported as major stressors. Further, patients emphasized the importance of wording during the communication and stress the need to *move from the paternalistic approach in care provision to patient-centered care* [27].

Pakistan—Irrespective of the city of residence, the social stigma attached to a cancer diagnosis in the Pakistani society seemed to have an important influence on women's psychological well-being [33].

Saudi Arabia—Most patients prefer a family-centered model of care. However, there is a slow but steady change in public education which leads to a more cultural openness [34]. Still, educational programs for medical students lack assessment as related to communication skills related to the breaking of bad news [27].

Turkey—Studies revealed that knowing the diagnosis of cancer has a positive correlation with anxiety and depression. About 30% of cancer patients suffer from psychiatric disorders [35].

Truthful disclosure to cancer patients is not a common practice despite the potential ethical problems associated with such an approach [36]. Turkish patients suffering from cancer clearly express their desire to be told about their diagnosis and prognosis; however, caregivers do not always respect this desire. *The high incidence of psychiatric morbidity in patients who are aware of their diagnosis could be related to the deficit in physicians' communication skills* [27].

Religiosity is one of the prominent features of daily life, and the social structure is based on the importance of the family bonds instead of the individual autonomy. To date, a diagnosis of cancer in many Middle Eastern countries is associated with a social stigma and misperceptions related to its incurability; and physicians, although many of them are trained in Western countries, still practice the truth disclosure policy that respects some of the historical and cultural misperceptions about cancer; and they frequently tell the truth about cancer to one of the family members and try to conceal it from the concerned patient. The most important explanation to this conduct is maintaining the patient's psychological well-being [27]. *One thing needs attention and that refers to the physician-patient communication, since the way of breaking bad news is as important as the news itself.* Of importance is the fact that additional healthcare professionals, such as nurses, are actively involved in communicating to patients their situation. That might also contribute to a faster openness about truth-telling to patients themselves [27].

Haifa, Israel Michael Silbermann, D.M.D., Ph.D.

References

1. Maule M, Merletti F. Cancer transition and priorities for cancer control. Lancet Oncol. 2012;13:745–6.
2. Franceschi S, Bray F. Cancer control 2014—cancer care in emerging health systems. Published in official association with the International Network for Cancer Treatment and Research. 2014. p. 17–23. http://www.cancercontrol.info.
3. Franceschi S, Wild CP. Meeting the global demands of epidemiologic transition—the indispensable role of cancer prevention. Mol Oncol. 2013;7:1–13.
4. Bray F. Transitions in human development and the global cancer burden. World Cancer Report 2014. Lyon: International Agency for Research on Cancer; 2014. p. 54–68.
5. Chestnov O, Mendis S, Bettcher D. A milestone in the response to non-communicable diseases. Lancet. 2013;382:481–2.
6. Silbermann M (ed.). Palliative care to the cancer patient. New York: Nova; 2014.
7. Adams C, Doherty RB. Cancer control 2014—cancer care in emerging health systems. Published in official association with the International Network for Cancer Treatment and Research. 2014. p. 26–30. http://www.cvancercontrol.info.
8. Pritchard-Jones K, Pieters R, Reaman GH, Hjorth L, Downie P, Calaminus G, Naafs-Wilstra MC, Steliarova-Foucher E. Sustaining innovation and improvement in the treatment of childhood cancer: lessons from high-income countries. www.thelancetoncology.com. Published online 20 Feb 2013.
9. Cherny NI, Cleary J, Scholten W, et al. The global opioid policy initiative (GOPI) project to evaluate the availability and accessibility of opioids for the management of cancer pain in Africa, Asia, Latin America and the Caribbean, and the Middle East. Introduction and methodology. Ann Oncol. 2013;24(11):xi7–xi13.
10. Martin-Moreno JM, Cazap E, Kerr D. Cancer control 2014. Cancer care in emerging health systems. Published in official association with the International Network for Cancer Treatment and Research. 2014. p. 31–35. www.cancercontrol.info.
11. Magrath I, Sutcliffe S. Building capacity for cancer treatment in low-income countries—cancer care in emerging health systems. Published in official association with the International Network for Cancer Treatment and Research. 2014. p. 60–66. www.cancercontrol.info.
12. Coleman CN, Love RR. Transforming science, service and society. Sci Transl Med. 2014;6:259fs42.
13. You JJ, Downar J, Fowler RA, Lamontagne F, et al. Barriers to goals of care discussions with seriously ill hospitalized patients and their families. A multicenter survey of clinicians. JAMA Intern Med. doi:10.1001/jamainternmed.2014.7732. Published online 2 Feb 2015.
14. Aniebu UU, Onyeka TC. Ethical, socioeconomic and cultural considerations in gynecologic cancer care in developing countries. Int J Palliat Care. http://dx.doi.org/10.1155/2014/141627.
15. Silbermann M, Epner DE, Charalambous H, Baider L, Puchalski CM, Balducci L, Gultekin M, Abdalla RF, Daher M, Al-Tarawneh MR, Smith TJ. Promoting new approaches for cancer care in the Middle East. Ann Oncol. 2013;24(vii):5–10.
16. Delgado-Guay MO, De La Cruz MG, Epner DE. I don't want to burden my family: handling communication challenges in geriatric oncology. Ann Oncol. 2013;24(vii):30–5.
17. Rassouli M, Sajjadi M. Palliative care in the Islamic Republic of Iran. In: Silbermann M, editor. New York: Nova; 2014. p. 39–51.
18. Nwankwo KC, Ezeome E. The perceptions of physicians in Southeast Nigeria on truth-telling for cancer diagnosis and prognosis. J Palliative Med. 2011;14:700–3.
19. Razzak R, Smith TJ. Palliative dare: a new and emerging paradigm. In: Silbermann M, editor. Palliative care to the cancer patient. New York: Nova; 2014. p. 223–38.
20. Baider L, Goldzweig G. Islamic culture in the Middle East: a glimpse into illness and death. In: Silbermann M, editor. Palliative care to the cancer patient. New York: Nova; 2014. p. 54–63.
21. Balducci L. Death and dying: what the patient wants. Ann Oncol. 2012;23(34):56–61.

22. Ben Arye D, Schiff E, Mutafoglu K, Omran S, Hajjar R, Charalambous H, Dweikat T, Ghrayeb I, Barsela G, Turker I, Hassan A, Hassan E, Popper-Giveon A, Saad B, Nimri O, Kebudi R, Dagash J, Silbermann M. Integration of complementary medicine in supportive cancer care: survey of health-care providers' perspectives from 16 countries in the Middle East. Support Care Cancer. doi:10.1007/s00520-015-2619-7.
23. Beyer P. Social forms of religion in a contemporary global society. In: Dollon M, editor. Handbook of the sociology of religion. Cambridge: Cambridge University Press; 2003. p. 45–60.
24. De Pentheny C, O'Kelly C, Brown EA. The impact of culture and religion on truth telling at the end of life. Nephrol Dialysis Transplant. 2011;26:3838–42.
25. Mystakidou K, Tsilika E, Parpa E, Katsouda E, Vlahos L. Patterns and barriers in information disclosure between health care professionals and relatives with cancer patients in Greek society. Eur J Cancer Care. 2005;14:175–81.
26. Powell RA, Mwangi-Powell FN, Radbruch L, Yamey CR, et al. Lancet Oncol. 2015;16:131–33.
27. Khalil RB. Attitudes, beliefs and perceptions regarding truth disclosure of cancer-related information in the Middle East, a review. Palliat Support Care. 2013;11:69–78.
28. Tavoli A, Mohagheghi MA, Montazeri A, et al. Anxiety and depression in patients with gastrointestinal cancer. J Cancer Educ. 2007;23:260–63.
29. Ben Natan M, Shahar I, Garfinkel D. Disclosing bad news to patients with life-threatening illness: differences in attitude between physicians and nurses in Israel. Int J Palliat Nurs. 2009;15:276–81.
30. Qaddoumi I, Ezam N, Swaidan M, et al. Diffuse pontine glioma in Jordan and Impact of upfront prognosis disclosure with parents and families. J Child Neurol. 2009;24:460–65.
31. Hamadeh GN, Adib SM. Changes in attitudes regarding cancer disclosure among medical students at the American University of Beirut. J Med Ethics. 2001;27:354.
32. Doumit MA, Abu Saad HH. Lebanese cancer patients: communication with truth telling preferences. Contemp Nurse. 2008;28:74–82.
33. Banning H, Hasson M, Faisal S, et al. Cultural interrelationships and the lived experience of Pakistani breast cancer patients. Eur J Oncol Nurs. 2010;14:304–9.
34. Al Amri AM. Cancer patients' desire for information: a study in a teaching hospital in Saudi Arabia. East Mediterr Health J. 2009;15:19–24.
35. Atesci FC, Baltalarli B, Oguzhanoglu NK, et al. Psychiatric morbidity among cancer patients and awareness of illness. Support Care Cancer. 2004;12:161–7.
36. Guven T. Truth-telling in cancer: examining the cultural incompatibility argument in Turkey. Nurs Ethics. 2010;17:159–166.

Contents

Contributors

Rania Y. Abu Seir, Ph.D. Department of Medical Laboratory Sciences, Faculty of Health Professions, Al-Quds University, Jerusalem, Palestine

Mohja Khair Allah, M.B.B.S. Radiation and Isotope Center, Khartoum, Sudan

Maha Arnaout, M.D. Department of Pediatrics, Istiklal Hospital, Amman, Jordan

Muhammad Shamvil Ashraf, M.B.B.S., D.C.H., M.C.P.S., M.R.C.P., F.C.P.S. Department of Pediatric Oncology, The Indus Hospital, Karachi, Pakistan

Lea Baider, Ph.D. Department of Psycho-Oncology, Institute of Clinical Oncology, Assuta Medical Center, Tel-Aviv, Israel

Lodovico Balducci, M.D. Moffitt Cancer Center, Tampa, FL, USA

University of South Florida College of Medicine, Tampa, FL, USA

Eran Ben-Arye, M.D. Integrative Oncology Program, The Oncology Service and Lin Medical Center, Clalit Health Services, Haifa and Western Galilee District, Haifa, Israel

Complementary and Traditional Medicine Unit, Department of Family Medicine, Faculty of Medicine, Technion-Israel Institute of Technology, Haifa, Israel

Stella Bialous, R.N., Dr.Ph.H., F.A.A.N. Social and Behavioral Sciences, School of Nursing, University of California, San Francisco, San Francisco, CA, USA

Joann Bodurtha, M.D. M.P.H. Departments of Pediatrics and Oncology, McKusick-Nathans Institute of Genetic Medicine, Johns Hopkins Medical Institutions, Baltimore, MD, USA

Saber Boutayeb, M.D. Department of Medical Oncology, National Institute of Oncology, Rabat, Morocco

Jeannine Brant, Ph.D., A.P.R.N., A.O.C.N., F.A.A.N. Department of Nursing, Billings Clinic, Billings, MT, USA

Fatma Betul Cakir, M.D. Bezmialem Vakif University Medical Faculty, Istanbul, Turkey

Barrie Cassileth, Ph.D. Integrative Medicine, Memorial Sloan Kettering Cancer Center, New York, NY, USA

Eduardo Cazap, M.D., Ph.D., F.A.S.C.O. Latin American and Caribbean Society of Medical Oncology (SLACOM), Buenos Aires, Argentina

Union for International Cancer Control (UICC), Geneva, Switzerland

National Cancer Institute (INC), Buenos Aires, Argentina

Haris Charalambous, B.M., M.R.C.P. (UK), F.R.C.R. (UK) Bank of Cyprus Oncology Centre, Nicosia, Cyprus

Jamal Dagash, M.D. Integrative Oncology Program, The Oncology Service and Lin Medical Center, Clalit Health Services, Haifa and Western Galilee District, Haifa, Israel

Complementary and Traditional Medicine Unit, Department of Family Medicine, Faculty of Medicine, Technion-Israel Institute of Technology, Haifa, Israel

Palliative Care—Home Care Hospice, Clalit Health Services, Haifa and Western Galilee District, Haifa, Israel

Michel Daher, M.D., F.A.C.S., F.E.B.S. Saint George Hospital University Medical Center, Achrafieh, Beirut, Lebanon

Dan Dumitraşcu, M.D. Center for Innovation in Medicine, Bucharest, Romania

Ali Elbaghir, M.D. Radiation and Isotope Center, Khartoum, Sudan

Haytham El-Salhat, M.D. Al Noor Hospital, Abu-Dhabi

Karima Elshamy, D.N.Sc. Medical Surgical Nursing Department, Faculty of Nursing, Mansoura University, Mansoura, Egypt

Alexandru Eniu, M.D., Ph.D. Department of Breast Tumors, Cancer Institute Ion Chiricuta, Cluj-Napoca, Romania

Daniel E. Epner, M.D., F.A.C.P. Department of Palliative Care and Rehabilitation Medicine, University of Texas MD Anderson Cancer Center, Houston, TX, USA

Mohammad Shafiq Faqeerzai, P.G.D., M.D. Cancer Control, Afghan Society Against Cancer, Kabul, Afghanistan

Jamie E. Flerlage, M.D., M.S. St. Jude Children's Research Hospital, Memphis, TN, USA

Nahla Gafer, M.D. Radiation and Isotope Center, Khartoum, Sudan

Marius Geanta, M.D. Centre for Innovation in Medicine, Bucharest, Romania

Gil Goldzweig Clinical Psychology Track, School of Behavioral Sciences, Academic College of Tel-Aviv-Yaffo, Tel-Aviv, Israel

Kate Shaughnessy Hankle, M.B.A. Oncology Nursing Society, Pittsburgh, PA, USA

Mohammed Jaloudi, M.D. Department of Oncology, Tawam Hospital, Abu Dhabi, UAE

David M. James, M.Sc. Department of Oncology, Tawam Hospital, Abu-Dhabi, UAE

Ahsan Jamil, M.B.B.S., M.Sc. Department of Pediatric Oncology, The Indus Hospital, Karachi, Pakistan

Aminah Jatoi, M.D. Department of Oncology, Mayo Clinic, Rochester, MN, USA

Bahar Javdan, B.A. Integrative Medicine, Memorial Sloan Kettering Cancer Center, New York, NY, USA

Dilyara Kaidarova, M.D., Ph.D. Almaty Oncology Center, Almaty, Republic of Kazakhstan

Jihad Kanbar, M.Sc. Department of Oncology, Tawam Hospital, Abu Dhabi, UAE

Rejin Kebudi, M.D. Istanbul University Cerrahpasa Medical Faculty, Istanbul, Turkey

Istanbul University Oncology Institute, Istanbul, Turkey

David Kerr, C.B.E., M.A., M.D., D.Sc., F.R.C.P. AfrOx Coordinating Office, Belsyre Court, Oxford, Oxfordshire, OX2 6HJ, UK

Radcliffe Department of Medicine, University of Oxford, Oxford, UK

Stewart Kerr, B.A. (Hon) AfrOx Coordinating Office, Belsyre Court, Oxford, Oxfordshire, OX2 6HJ, UK

Akram T. Kharroubi, Ph.D. Department of Medical Laboratory Sciences, Faculty of Health Professions, Al-Quds University, Jerusalem, Palestine

Suresh Kumar, M.B.B.S., D.A., M.A., Dip. Pall. Med. Institute of Palliative Medicine, Calicut, Kerala, India

Zakiya M.N. Al Lamki, F.R.C.P., F.R.C.P.C.H. Department of Child Health, Haematology/Oncology Unit, College of Medicine and Health Sciences, Sultan Qaboos University, Muscat, Sultanate of Oman

Barbara G. Lubejko, R.N., M.S. Oncology Nursing Society, Pittsburgh, PA, USA

Amos Deogratius Mwaka, M.B.Ch.B., M.Med. Department of Medicine, School of Medicine, College of Health Sciences, Makerere University, Kampala, Uganda

Mati Nejmi, M.D. Center of Pain and Palliative Care, Hôpital Cheikh Khalifa Ibn Zaid, Boulevard Mohamed Taieb Naciri, Hay El Hassani, Casablanca, BP, Rabat, Morocco

Phuong L. Nguyen, M.D. Department of Laboratory Medicine and Pathology, Mayo Clinic, Rochester, MN, USA

Omar Nimri, M.D. Jordan Cancer Registry, Ministry of Health, Amman, Jordan

Joseph F. O'Neill, M.D., M.P.H. Hospice and Palliative Medicine, Michaels, MD, USA

Christopher Orach Garimoi, M.B.Ch.B., M.P.H., Ph.D. Department of Community Health and Behavioural Sciences, School of Public Health, College of Health Sciences, Makerere University, Kampala, Uganda

Bhavana Pathak, M.D. Department of Medicine, Johns Hopkins Medical Institutions, Baltimore, MD, USA

Maryam Rassouli, Ph.D., R.N. Nursing Department, Nursing and Midwifery School, Shahid Beheshti University of Medical Sciences, Vali-e Asr Street, Niyayesh Cross, Tehran, Iran

Alberto Reggiori Varese General Hospital, Varese, Italy

Tamari Rukhadze, M.D., Ph.D. Oncology and Palliative Medicine, Faculty of Medicine of Iv. Javakhishvili Tbilisi State University, Tbilisi, Georgia

Moosa Sajjadi, Ph.D., R.N. Department of Medical-Surgical Nursing, Faculty of Nursing and Midwifery, Gonabad University of Medical Sciences, Beside Asian Road, Gonabad, Iran

Abdul Tawab Saljuqi, M.D., M.P.H., Ph. D. Public Health, Afghanistan National Public Health Association, Taimani, Kabul, Afghanistan

Massoud Samiei, M.B.A., M.Sc., D.I.C., Ph.D. Senior Consultant Nuclear Energy/Cancer Control, International Atomic Energy Agency, Vienna, Austria

Lidia Schapira, M.D. Department of Medicine, Massachusetts General Hospital, Harvard Medical School, Boston, MA, USA

Kathleen M. Schmeler, M.D. Department of Gynecological Oncology and Reproductive Medicine, University of Texas MD Anderson Cancer Center, Houston, TX, USA

Lisa Kennedy Sheldon, Ph.D., A.P.R.N., A.O.C.N.P. College of Nursing and Health Sciences, University of Massachusetts-Boston, Boston, MA, USA

Michael Silbermann, D.M.D., Ph.D. Technion – Israel Institute of Technology, Haifa, Israel

Thomas J. Smith, M.D., F.A.C.P., F.A.S.C.O., F.A.A.H.P.M. Departments of Medicine and Oncology, Sidney Kimmel Comprehensive Cancer Center of Johns Hopkins, Johns Hopkins Medical Institutions, Baltimore, MD, USA

Henry Wabinga, M.B.Ch.B., M.Med., M.D. Department of Pathology, Kampala Cancer Registry, School of Biomedical Sciences, College of Health Sciences, Makerere University, Kampala, Uganda

Esther Walker, M.B.E., B.S.C. St. Catherine Hospice, Crawley, West Sussex, UK

Chapter 1
Medical Care in Countries in Transition

Lodovico Balducci and Alberto Reggiori

Value of Health Care in Countries in Transition

Ethnic and political clashes between and within newly established nations emerged from the dissolution of colonial powers. Political and social instability is found especially, albeit not exclusively in Africa and the Middle East. Health care delivery is one of the casualties of perennial conflicts that also cause deaths, chronic disability, and family and social havoc. Existing demographic data suggests that life expectancy of populations living in war zones is lower than that of populations in stable countries even when adjusted for war-related mortality rate [1, 2]. This reasonable conclusion is supported by demographic data in stable countries where mortality risk is higher for the economically disadvantaged [3] and for those living in high crime rate areas, where family and social dissolution are also more common [4].

Seemingly health care rationing, war-related costs, and public health problems (care of the wounded, epidemics, chronic diseases of survivors, long-term disability, starvation, reduced caregiver pools for children, elderly, and disabled) conspire toward poor health outcomes. In addition, human suffering is itself a cause of more suffering. Crime and apathy are common consequences of human suffering [5]. In some countries, teen ager children are militarized as they don't know any other lifestyle but war [6, 7]. This experience predictably feeds a vicious cycle of perpetual and mounting violence.

Organized health care delivery may go a long way toward preventing diseases and deaths and assuaging human suffering. In addition, it may motivate people to

L. Balducci, M.D. (✉)
Moffitt Cancer Center, 12902 Magnolia Dr, Tampa, FL 33612, USA

University of South Florida College of Medicine, Tampa, FL, USA
e-mail: Lodovico.balducci@moffitt.org

A. Reggiori
Varese General Hospital, Varese, Italy

M. Silbermann (ed.), *Cancer Care in Countries and Societies in Transition*,
DOI 10.1007/978-3-319-22912-6_1

actively look for solutions to their problems, and it may promote human allegiance that by itself represents a containment for both crime and war. In his book, "When the gasoil is over" the Italian surgeon Alberto Reggiori narrates his experience in war-torn Uganda [8]. As he arrived there, the town hospital was inoperative and inoperable. War-worn and weary citizens did not have the strength, the initiative, or the motivation to manage the facility. When he asked for access to the operating room, the pharmacy, or the delivery room, the answer was always the same: "the man with the key is not here." When he left, 5 years later, the hospital had 20,000.00 yearly admissions, 1500.00 deliveries, and 2000.00 major surgical procedures. With his example, Reggiori demonstrated to the local people that effective health care could be delivered despite the uncertainties of war. This awareness awoke in the local people the desire to contribute to a beneficial and remunerative endeavor previously considered all but impossible.

For 20 years, the Middle East Cancer Consortium (MECC) promoted palliative cancer care in war-torn Middle Eastern countries. Through MECC, individuals from hostile countries could meet and cooperate toward the relief of human suffering caused by cancer [9]. Cancer, one of the worst health scourges of the modern world became a trait d'union for the MECC members and promoted a unity of intent that no political negotiations or compromise had been able to foster [10].

These examples indicate that health care may be effective in war-devastated countries and that the organization of health care delivery may promote a sense of justice as well as a common language of compassion and self-confidence. Justice and compassion may prove the most effective fundaments to a lasting peace, while self-reliance is the fundament of hope, a necessary condition for searching peace.

We will primarily deal with cancer care in the following discussion, as a model of medical care and health care delivery. Cancer management has been our area of expertise in the past three decades. Also, the management of cancer entails the whole gamut of health care interventions from prevention to palliative care, and cancer affects both the patient and his/her community. And the cancer is the disease for which there is the most reliable treatment record in war-torn countries, thanks to the MECC activities.

New Advances in Cancer Care

Undoubtedly, cancer prevention and cancer treatment have benefited tremendously from technological advances [11]. In Table 1.1, we list some of the major advances that have reduced cancer-related mortality, disability, and suffering. In general, one has observed the development of

- Ever more sensitive instruments to detect cancer in asymptomatic individuals
- Minimally invasive procedures that reduce the risk and the discomfort of surgical treatment and the time to postsurgical recovery
- New and more effective forms of locoregional treatment that may obviate the need for surgery for early disease (radiosurgery, cryosurgery, etc.) and may lead to better control of cancer metastases (radiofrequency and thermal ablation, regional infusional therapy)

Table 1.1 New advances in cancer care

Early cancer detection	Breast: mammogram, digital mammogram; MRI
	Lung: low radiation CT scan
	Prostate: PSA, multi-parametric MRI
	Large bowel: fecal occult blood, recto-sigmoidoscopy, colonoscopy, virtual colonoscopy
	Hepatocellular carcinoma: alfa fetoprotein; liver ultrasound
Surgery	Minimally invasive surgery
	Sentinel LN examination
Radiation therapy	Intensity modulated radiation therapy
	Image-guided radiation therapy
	Proton therapy
	Radiosurgery (brain, lung)
Interventional radiology	Image-guided biopsies
	Obliteration of metastasis with radiofrequency, heat, or cryosurgery
	Infusional therapy
	Radio and chemoembolization of liver metastases
Cytotoxic chemotherapy	New and more effective drugs
	Improved in supportive care (nausea and vomiting, myelosuppression, and mucositis)

- Targeted antineoplastic drugs that are both more effective and less toxic
- More effective palliation of symptoms related to cancer and its treatment

By and large, these advances imply a substantial increase in the cost of health care [12, 13] that cannot be afforded by developing countries, especially when the government and the economy of these countries have been made unstable by war. In some situations, modern technology may compensate for the scarcity of specialists in some areas of the world: for example, radiosurgery of lung cancer has been used in lieu of surgery in countries with a scarcity of thoracic surgeons [14]. Again, this type of technology is very expensive however and requires a well-organized medical and social infrastructure.

Perhaps the advances of major interest concern the delivery of palliative cancer care. In a seminal study, Temel et al. [15] demonstrated that early application of palliative care in patients with metastatic lung cancer resulted in improved quality of life, decreased cost, and kind of unexpectedly it led to improved survival. In this randomized controlled study, the scope of palliative care went beyond pure symptom management and included a discussion of treatment goals and treatment plans as well as the caregiver's support. This approach appears particularly appropriate for unstable countries for several reasons:

- Symptom palliation is the most basic medical need and should be assured prior to any other medical intervention [16].
- In face of limited resources, a discussion of patient's priorities and values may allow a more effective utilization of these resources congruent with individual patient's wishes.

- As demonstrated by the study of Temel as well as in previous studies [16], symptom palliation is effective in prolonging survival. Interestingly, Temel's study suggests that aggressive antineoplastic treatment may compromise the survival of these individuals in addition to increasing the treatment cost.
- Even in the absence of a cure, palliative care may be a source of healing [17]. Healing refers to the personal experience of the disease and is the ultimate goal of medical care. As death is unavoidable, the final task of the health professional is to help patients to deal with their deaths, to coopt death as a living experience.

Symptom management includes a wide array of symptoms such as pain, discomfort, nausea and vomiting, fatigue, and depression, just to mention a few. Though pain and suffering are mostly associated they need to be considered different symptoms [18]. You may have pain without suffering, as reported in the case of a catholic priest with metastatic prostate cancer [19]. The patient asked that only p.r.n. opioids be prescribed as he wanted to feel closer to the crucified Christ, when he experienced his pain. Likewise, a person with unresolved emotional burdens may experience suffering without pain [20]. Clearly, pain and suffering may need different approaches.

The distribution of medical resources should follow strict ethical principles [21]. These include autonomy, beneficence, non-maleficence, and justice. Justice holds that the treatment available should be offered to every patient irrespective of sex, age, ethnic origin, and beliefs. At the same time, the principle of autonomy holds that patients may refuse any medical intervention. That is when the discussion of patient's priorities and values [22] is important. An elderly patient with limited life expectancy may decide that the ordeal of cancer treatment is not worthy for him/her and choose a peaceful death, making more resources available for the treatment of young and healthier individuals. This decision should be made by the patient him/her and in no circumstances the provider is allowed to discriminate between patient and patient.

Healing is a spiritual experience that involves the discovery of one's life meaning even in the face of disease and death [20]. Palliative care is essential to healing [23]. Symptom controls allows a person to communicate with his/her loved ones, to proclaim and receive love, to ask for and concede forgiveness. In addition to these necessary healing steps, symptom control may allow a person enough thought concentration and depth that he/she becomes able to distillate from his/her own history those lifetime experiences that have been more meaningful [19]. Ideally, a spirituality professional should be available in the palliative management team. Spirituality professionals include but are not limited to religious ministers. In the USA, hospital chaplains maybe lay individuals trained to minister to patients of different religious belief and no belief at all [24].

Delivery Venues of Health Care in Countries in Transition

Any form of health care delivery requires a proper infrastructure that may be supported by the government, by private enterprise, or by philanthropic organizations. Jewish, Christian, and Moslem congregations have been on the forefront of health care delivery for centuries, until the eighteenth century [25].

A number of situations that jeopardize health care delivery may occur in countries in transitions:

- When the country is at war with another country, the national and local government are still empowered, but weakened from the tolls of war; in the case of occupation, the occupying government becomes responsible of health care.
- In the case of civilian conflicts, several different temporary governments may rule the same region in rapid succession and occasionally at the same time.
- Warlords and tribal leaders may dominate a certain area of the country and consider health care a commodity under their own full control. They may prevent the delivery of health care from philanthropic organizations not to lose their absolute control of the population.
- In any country at war, a medical black market may flourish [26]. Scalpers may hoard medications and medical supplies and sell them at increased price. Also they may dilute the doses of medications and sell it at full dose price. Both these phenomena had been observed in Europe after World War II. In addition, at the same time blood was diluted with normosaline and diluted blood was sold on the black market.
- In the majority of countries at war, different religious beliefs are professed. These beliefs may represent one of the very roots of the conflict, as currently is the case in Nigeria or in Syria and Iraq. Religious beliefs may influence the delivery of health care in different ways, including refusal of Western medicine in favor of traditional medicine, mistrust of the health care professional, and denial of the care of the enemy as a form of religious duty. When the Italian heretic Giordano Bruno was being burned at the stake in Rome's "Campo de Fiori" prior to losing his senses, he encouraged an old woman particularly eager to feed the pyre with more wood because he told her ironically "you are being a reliable and faithful servant of your God!" Things may not have changed that much since the inquisition executions of the sixteenth century.

In war-torn countries, health professionals will have to rely most of the time on philanthropic organizations for resources. Whenever possible, they need to assure the cooperation of the local government and law enforcement. In the meantime, they must try to avoid any activity or statement that may be constructed as an endorsement of the current regimen, as this may compromise their activity under a new regimen. Political neutrality appears as a must. Most of all, as the Reggiori experience suggests [8], health professional need to gain the trust of the local population to assure its support and cooperation. In the absence of an effective government and law enforcement, the local population, when adequately motivated, may assume the responsibility of health care management.

It is self-evident that health care professionals should avoid to step into religious conflicts. In the meantime, it may be wise in most circumstances to work with religious leaders to gain the trust of the population and to work with, rather than antagonizing, the practitioners of traditional medicine.

Finally, there may be situations where the delivery of health care may appear all but impossible, and the decision may have to be made to close the health care facilities not to jeopardize the life of the patients and of the health care workers, and to use the limited available resources in a place whether they may be more effective. The health care provider is responsible to take this difficult decision as he/she is responsible of the welfare of the staff and of the patients and of the proper management of the medical resources. Such situations might have occurred in Somalia few years ago, when battling warlords prevented free movements between different areas of the country and where stockpiling the country alimentary and medical supplies for military use and personal profit was common.

Health Care Priorities in Countries at War

As outlined in the previous section, the delivery of health care is influenced by a number of variables, most of which are outside the control of the health care professional. The professional in charge will have to establish the priority of health care delivery based on ethical principles and practical considerations. The ethical principles include [21]:

- Autonomy: no intervention may be performed without the patient consent, which includes disclosure of potential benefits and complications of the intervention and assessment of one's priorities and values. Clearly, in conditions of emergency when the patient cannot offer consent, one can presume that consent is present for life-saving procedures.
- Beneficence: the therapeutic index of the intervention (the ratio of benefits and risks) is positive.
- Non-maleficence: the intervention should not cause unnecessary damage. This principle needs to be emphasized in countries in transition and with limited resources, where the desire to do something may be the cause of hurt. My spouse and I, several years ago, visited an African country, and we were told by a local surgeon that the only procedure offered to men diagnosed with prostate cancer at that time was an orchiectomy. In patients asymptomatic and with early disease androgen deprivation may be the cause of discomfort and medical complications without any real influence on the course of the cancer and should be avoided [27]. Likewise, one may be tempted to use indiscriminately inexpensive antibiotics [28] in febrile patients with the triple risk of causing medication side-effects, antibiotic resistance, and reduced availability of drugs for the patients who need them.
- Justice: as already mentioned, it is not legitimate for a practitioner to discriminate among patients based on demographic variables. As an example, it is not legitimate to deny a life-saving procedure to an old man because with the money saved one can treat the life-threatening diarrhea of a 100 children. It is legitimate however for the patients to refuse the intervention if he/she feels that the potential benefits are not worthy the risks, the discomfort, and the cost. Unlike the practitioner in charge of the individual patient, the institution that manages health care resources (government, philanthropic organization) has the right and the duty to prioritize the use of these resources. It is legitimate, for example, to renounce expensive

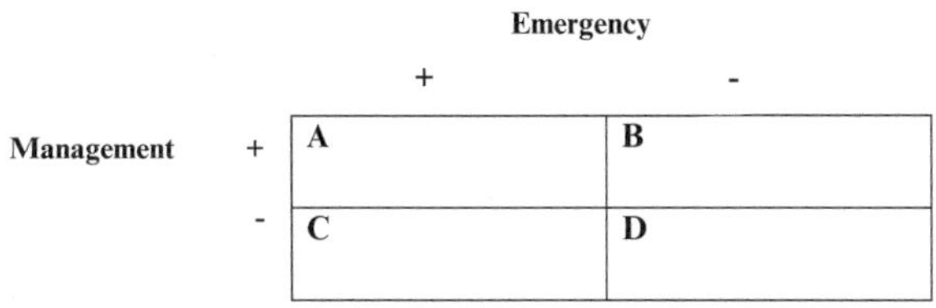

Fig. 1.1 Health care prioritization in countries in transition. Situations that are emergent and for which effective management is available (A) should have the highest priorities

chemotherapy treatment in favor of better maternal fetal care or prevention of malnutrition. To be consistent with the principle of justice, this decision must involve the whole population under the institution's jurisdiction.

Figure 1.1 shows a frame of reference on how a practitioner, a health organization, or a government may decide to apportion limited medical resources in countries in transition. The ability to manage an emergency situation depends on the practitioner's skill as well as on the infrastructures and the resources available. For example, appendectomy or cesarean sections should be feasible in almost every situation, whereas open heart surgery, though life saving, may rarely be available. In such case, the individual with the life-threatening emergency that cannot be managed should be provided adequate palliative and end-of-life care. As already emphasized, severe symptom management is always a priority and should be attended to the full extent at which resources are available. These may include just rubbing the body of an individual in pain as described by a physician working in Mother Theresa institution in Calcutta.

Among the situations in group B, maternal–fetal medicine should have the priority in our opinion because it may be associated almost always with a favorable outcome, requires relatively few resources, and portends the future health of the nation.

According to this framework, the management of cancer in unstable countries is seldom a priority, except for symptom management. However, some qualifications are in order.

Oncological emergencies are common [29] (Table 1.2). Those that are cancer related most often represent a terminal event, and in some case, such as hypercalcemia or renal failure, they may grant the patient a peaceful and comfortable death when the underlying disease cannot be treated. In other cases, such as organ obstructions, they may be a cause of extreme pain and discomfort and should be managed in the best possible ways under the circumstances. For example, in the absence of neurosurgical expertise or of radiation therapy equipment, steroids may still reduce the pain and the risk of paralysis and incontinence in patients with spinal cord compression.

For what concerns the treatment-related complications, the practitioner needs to use his/her best judgment in trying to avoid them. For example, aggressive adjuvant chemotherapy of breast cancer is best avoided in older women in the absence of myeloid growth factors, as the risk of neutropenic infections increases with age, but may still be indicated in a younger woman with advanced disease whose risk of neutropenic infection is minimal and for whom the treatment benefit is the greatest.

Table 1.2 Oncological emergencies

Cancer related
A. Organ compression or obstruction
• Spinal cord compression
• Upper airways obstruction
• Obstruction of the digestive tract
• Urinary tract obstruction
• Superior Vena Cava syndrome
B. Vascular emergencies
• Leukostasis (acute leukemia)
• Thromboembolic complications (hypercoagulable status, thrombocythemia)
• Hyperviscosity (Waldenstrom macroglobulinemia, multiple myeloma)
C. Metabolic emergencies
• Malignant hypercalcemia
• Hyponatremia
• Hypoglycemia
• Renal failure
Treatment related
A. Surgery
• Bleeding
• Organ perforation
• Would infection
• Dehiscence of anastomosis
B. Radiation therapy
• Mucositis
• Dermatitis
• Myelosuppression
• Organ perforation
C. Systemic treatment
• Neutropenic infection
• Bleeding
• Mucositis
• Renal failure
• Hypomagnesemia

Also, unattended cancer may be a cause of severe symptoms. For example, in the absence of surgery, breast cancer may grow into fungating and painful masses, and colorectal cancer may lead to intestinal obstruction and perforation. To prevent these late complications, these diseases should be managed to the full extent of the available resources.

Table 1.3 provides general suggestions on how to prioritize different steps of cancer management in countries in transition.

By and large, any form of cancer prevention in countries in transition is wishful thinking. Likewise, it is not reasonable to expect that individuals at risk of dying

Table 1.3 Cancer management in countries in transition

Steps in cancer management	Priority	Non-priority
Prevention	• Education	• Chemoprevention
	• Primary prevention	• Early diagnosis
Early disease	• Simple surgery • Simple radiation therapy	• Complex surgery (example debulking for ovarian cancer; Whipple resection)
	• Adjuvant treatment in selected cases	• Highly specialized radiation therapy
Metastatic disease	• Curative systemic treatment • Symptom relieving systemic treatment	• Life prolonging systemic treatment with little chance of cure or palliation
Palliative treatment	• Talk therapy • Pain medication • Pain relieving surgery • Emotional and religious support	• Complex interventions (example intrathecal medications)

every minute from a wandering bullet or random explosion may give up some habits that may cause cancer decades later such as smoking or alcohol. Yet education to prevent HPV infections (or vaccinations) may have some efficacy among sex workers. More in general education about recognizing early symptoms and signs of cancer (a new breast nodule, blood in the stools, a skin lesion that becomes larger, an ulcer that does not heal) may be life saving for some individuals and should be provided by health professionals.

As mentioned before, any form of early cancer that may be treated according to the resources available should be treated. For example, a mastectomy and an orchiectomy may be performed under local anesthesia and as outpatient procedures. Even if there are no expertise or resources for more complex interventions (such as abdominal perineal resections or debulking of stage III ovarian cancer), every effort should be made to prevent the most painful complications of these diseases. A diverting colostomy should be performed in all cases of intestinal obstruction.

In the case of systemic disease, it is reasonable to give priority to curative systemic treatment (chemotherapy for testicular cancer or lymphoma) or treatment that may reduce discomfort (androgen deprivation in men with painful bony metastases from prostate cancer).

Palliative treatment should be the priority for all cancer patients and every effort should be made to prevent terminal discomfort. If a blood transfusion is not available, opioids should be used to manage dyspnea and pain in dying anemic patients. Our recommendation is that basic palliative care be given the priority in countries in transition, and that adequate supply of pain medication be available before engaging the health care system in more complex forms of cancer treatment.

What Are the Developed Countries Supposed to Do?

We hold that developed and resourceful countries should help in any way countries in transition to provide basic health care to their citizens. We hold that this is a moral imperative. It is also a good investment for a twofold reason:

- In a global word, an epidemic that develops in a remote corner of Africa may easily reach the developed countries as the Ebola [30] infection showed recently. It is in the best interest of a developed country to stop an epidemic at its origin before it affects the whole world.
- As we repeatedly demonstrated in this chapter, health care may be a source of compassion and compassion is a powerful venue to peace. As the MECC experience demonstrated, health care may represent the most cost-effective investment toward peace, which is a universal goal.

In addition, the developed world may learn some important lessons from the delivery of health care in countries in transition.

First and foremost, it may learn the importance of personal contact in the comforting of the suffering. Personal contact is available to any goodwill person and can be delivered without the help of expensive technology and infrastructure.

Second, it can learn alternative pathways of care in conditions of emergency. It is not farfetched to expect the health infrastructure of a major city or a state may become temporarily disrupted by a cyber or a terrorist attack as well as from some natural disaster. In this situation, the care in a country in transition may represent the best available care even in a developed country.

At the end it is appropriate to quote John Donne (meditation XVII):

> *All mankind is of one author, and is one volume; when one man dies, one chapter is not torn out of the book, but translated into a better language; and every chapter must be so translated...As therefore the bell that rings to a sermon, calls not upon the preacher only, but upon the congregation to come: so this bell calls us all: but how much more me, who am brought so near the door by this sickness....No man is an island, entire of itself...any man's death diminishes me, because I am involved in mankind; and therefore never send to know for whom the bell tolls; it tolls for thee.*

References

1. Adetunji A, Boss ER. Levels and trends in mortality in sub-Saharan Africa: an overview. In: Jamison DT, Feachem RG, Makgoba MW, Bos ER, Baingana FK, Hofman KJ, Rogo KO, editors. Disease and mortality in Sub-Saharan Africa. 2nd ed. Washington, DC: World Bank; 2006 (Chapter 2).
2. Gillespie DO, Trotter MV, Tuljapurkar SD. Divergence in age patterns of mortality change drives international development in lifespan inequality. Demography. 2014;51:1003–17.
3. Nelson K, Fritzell J. Welfare states and population health: the role of minimal income benefits for mortality. Soc Sci Med. 2014;112:63–71.
4. Avendano M, Kawachi I. Invited commentary: the search for explanations of the American health disadvantage relative to the English. Am J Epidemiol. 2011;173:866–9.

5. Ritchie EC. Psychiatry in the Korean war: perils, PIES, and prisoners of war. Mil Med. 2002;167:898–903.
6. Song SJ, Told W, de Jong J. Indero: intergenerational trauma and resilience between Burundian former child soldiers and their children. Fam Process. 2014;53:239–51.
7. Johannessen S, Holgersen H. Former child soldiers' problems and needs: the concolese experience. Qual Health Res. 2014;24:55–66.
8. Reggiori A. Dottore, e' finito il diesel. Milan: Eidzioni Marietti; 2005.
9. Silbermann M, Arnaut M, Daher M, et al. Palliative care in Middle Eastern countries: accomplishments and challenges. Ann Oncol. 2012;23 Suppl 3:15–28.
10. Silbermann M, Dweib Khleif A, Balducci L. Healed by cancer. J Clin Oncol. 2010; 28:1436–7.
11. Hoffe S, Balducci L. Cancer and age: general considerations. Clin Geriatr Med. 2012; 28:1–18.
12. Khera N. Reporting and grading financial toxicity. J Clin Oncol. 2014;32:3337–8.
13. Zafar SY, Abernethy AP. Financial toxicity Part I: a new name for a growing problem. Oncology. 2013;27:253–4.
14. Padda SK, Burt BM, Trakul N, et al. Early stage non-small Cell lung cancer: surgery, stereotactic radiosurgery, and individualized adjuvant therapy. Semin Oncol. 2014;41:40–56.
15. Temel JS, Greer JA, Muzikanski A, et al. Early palliative care for patients with metastatic non small cell lung cancer. N Engl J Med. 2010;363:733–42.
16. Bauman GR, Temel JS. The integration of early palliative care in oncology care: the time has come for a new tradition. J Natl Compr Canc Netw. 2014;12:1763–71.
17. Byock IR. To life: reflections on spirituality, palliative practice, and politics. Am J Hosp Palliat Care. 2007;23:436–8.
18. Balducci L. Suffering and spirituality: analysis of living experiences. J Pain Symptom Manage. 2011;42:479–86.
19. Balducci L. And a time to die. J Med Person. 2008;6:99–103.
20. Otis-green S, Ferrell B, Borneman T, et al. Integrating spiritual care with palliative care: an overview of nine demonstration projects. J Palliat Med. 2012;15:154–62.
21. Richardson HS. Specifying, balancing and interpreting bioethical principles. J Med Philos. 2000;25:285–307.
22. Balducci L. Active listening, effective communication: the pillar of personalized medicine. J Med Person. 2014;12:35–6.
23. Estle K. Healing: the spiritual work of palliative care. J Palliat Med. 2013;16:106–7.
24. Cadge W, Freese J, Christakis NA. The provision of hospital chaplaincy in the United States: a national overview. South Med J. 2008;101:626–30.
25. Anonymous: history of hospitals Enc Britannica online.
26. Shama G. Antibiotics, the BBC, penicillin and the second world war. BMJ. 2008;337:a2746. doi:10.1136/bmj.a2746.
27. Allan CA, Collins VR, Fryndenberg M, et al. Androgen deprivation therapy complications. Endocr Relat Cancer. 2014;21:T119–29.
28. Niederman MS. Principles of appropriate antibiotic use. Int J Antimicrob Agents. 2005;26 Suppl 3:S170–5.
29. Shiber JR. Oncologic emergencies. Crit Care Med. 2013;40:2212–22.
30. Helleringer S, Grepin KA, Noymer A. Ebola virus disease in West Africa: the first nine months. N Engl J Med. 2015;372:188–9.

Chapter 2
How to Prioritize Cancer Care for Countries in Transition

Stewart Kerr and David Kerr

Introduction

As cancer increasingly becomes a global health problem, WHO predicts 22 million new cases of cancer a year by 2030 60 % of which will be in low to middle income countries [1].

Developing countries face great challenges in addressing the ever-growing burden of cancer in their countries, there is a growing view that a global response is needed to achieve significant success in cancer control and prevention throughout the developing world. This view has been backed up by:

The UICC in 2009 launched The World Cancer Declaration [2]. The declaration brings the growing cancer crisis to the attention of government leaders and health policymakers across the globe. To those who sign up to it, it represents a consensus among government officials, public health experts, and cancer advocates from around the world who are committed to eliminating cancer. So far, the declaration has collected over 500,000 signatures.

In September 2011, the adoption of the Political Declaration of the High-Level Meeting on the Prevention and Control of Non-Communicable Diseases (NCDs) by the 193 member states of the United Nations (UN) provided the global cancer community with a robust platform to launch the next phase of advocacy to ensure the following World Cancer Declaration targets are met by 2020:

S. Kerr, B.A. (Hon)
AfrOx Coordinating Office, Belsyre Court, 57 Woodstock Road,
Oxford, Oxfordshire, OX2 6HJ, UK
e-mail: stewart.kerr@afrox.org

D. Kerr, C.B.E., M.A., M.D., D.Sc., F.R.C.P. (✉)
AfrOx Coordinating Office, Belsyre Court, 57 Woodstock Road,
Oxford, Oxfordshire, OX2 6HJ, UK

Radcliffe Department of Medicine, University of Oxford, Oxford, UK
e-mail: david.kerr@ndcls.ox.ac.uk

M. Silbermann (ed.), *Cancer Care in Countries and Societies in Transition*,
DOI 10.1007/978-3-319-22912-6_2

1. Ensure effective delivery systems in all countries
2. Significantly improve measurement of the cancer burden
3. Decrease tobacco, alcohol consumption and obesity
4. Ensure universal coverage of the HPV/HBV vaccine
5. Dispel damaging myths and misconceptions surrounding cancer
6. Diagnose more cancers via screening and early detection
7. Improve access to diagnosis, treatment, rehabilitation and palliative care
8. Provide universal availability of effective pain control
9. Improve training opportunities for cancer control professionals
10. Reduce emigration of health care workers specialized in cancer
11. Through all of the above, significantly improve global cancer survival rates

Members of the UN have a responsibility to respond to and work towards these targets [3].

Before considering how cancer care should be prioritized in transition countries, there is a case to be made for jointly tackling NCDs (diabetes, cardiovascular/strokes and respiratory disease) as a whole rather than focusing on improving just one of them, as it could be argued that an integrated approach will do more to strengthen individual Nation's health systems, than taking a vertical, disease-specific programme.

Although all NCDs require different treatment and specialist clinics are needed in each field to treat the different conditions, when it comes to prevention and awareness of NCDs there are a number of overlapping risks that make increase the chance of people developing an NCD like diet, usage of tobacco, fitness and amount of alcohol you consume (see Fig. 2.1 poster being used in Ghana). It is likely that there will be a movement towards more generic NCD planning in developing nations, but in the short and medium term, there is momentum behind Cancer Control, driven by need and mobilization of the global oncology community.

National Cancer Control Plan

A National Cancer Control Plan (NCCP) defines a nation's strategy for preventing, detecting, treating and providing palliative care for cancer. There are a number of steps needed to begin developing an NCCP:

- Establish a National Cancer Control Committee of Oncology experts, Health Ministry Officials and NGOs
- Use the committee to research the actual burden of cancer within the country and the current resources the country has
- From this assessment establish what resources will be needed to help reduce the burden of cancer within the country and which cancers and care models should be prioritized
- Write the national cancer plan based on these assessments, prioritizing steps that the National Health service needs to take to reduce the burden of disease

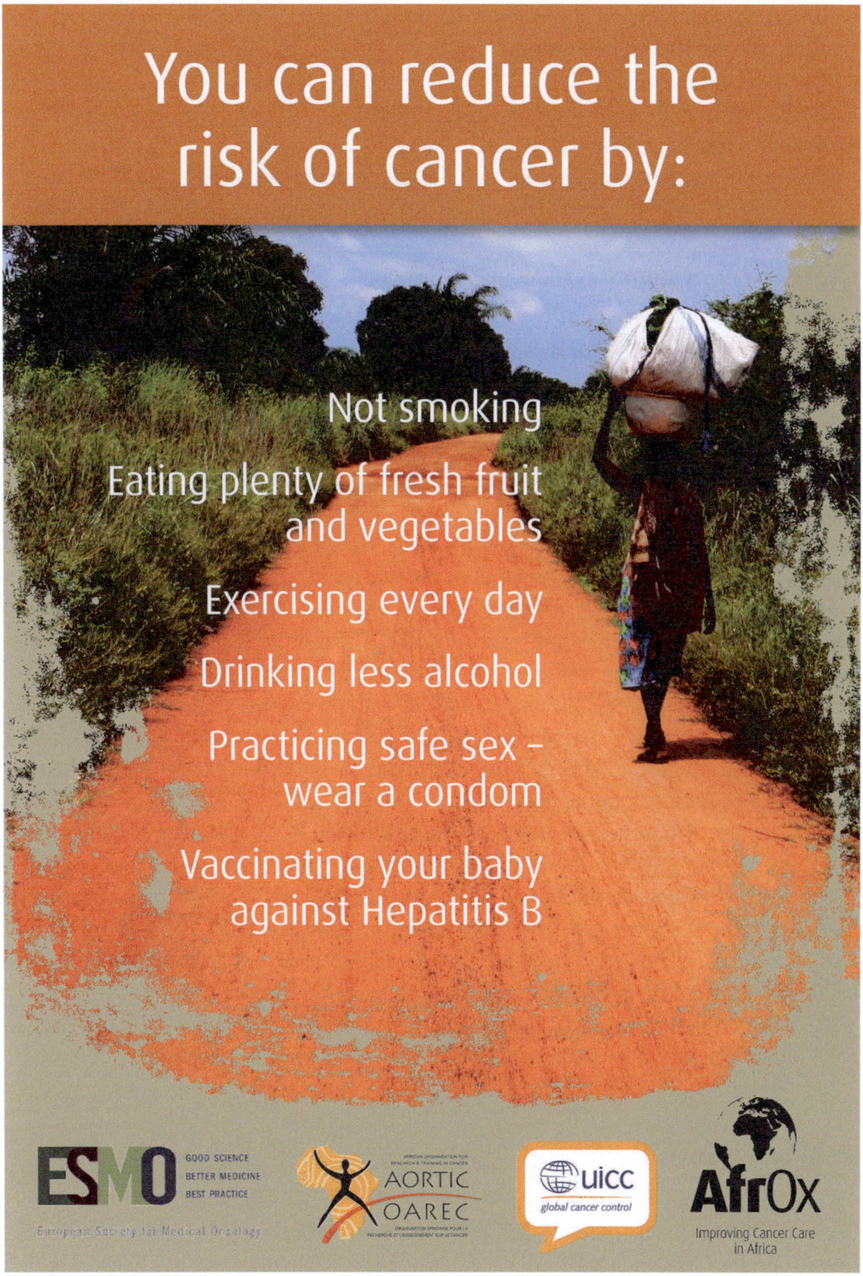

Fig. 2.1 A cancer awareness poster designed for use in African Health Centres

All NCCPs should) include the seven elements of cancer control:

- Cancer intelligence units
- Tobacco control

- Awareness raising and advocacy from civil society
- Early diagnosis and prevention
- Cure the curable
- Palliative care
- Training and education
- Health economy and budgeting individual elements of the plan

Cancer Intelligence Units

A cancer intelligence unit or registry is a vehicle to enable the systematic collection of regionally relevant data on cancer incidence, making it possible to assess reliably the types and prevalence of cancers experienced by populations in low to middle income countries, assess changes in these patterns over time and, therefore, assess the effect of any interventions associated with the cancer control programme.

There are two different types of cancer intelligence unit:

Hospital-Based Registries (HBR), collect data on all patients diagnosed and treated for cancer within that hospital or collection of hospitals.

Population-Based Registries (PBR), collect data on new incidences of cancer in a geographical region with a population of 100,000 or more to meaningfully extrapolate data on cancer for an entire population of their country.

PBRs are the most reliable way to collect data on cancers that are effecting.

Cancer registries also form a useful framework for evidence-based cancer research and, therefore, the lack of provision is undermining research capacity within low to middle income countries.

In common with all other areas of cancer control, there is a need for infrastructure, appropriate software and hardware, human resources and training, together with incentives for sustainability. The obvious partner to drive this programme forward is the International Agency for Research on Cancer (IARC)—the world leader in this field. IARC has developed a cost-effective training programme with scalable capacity to accommodate more trainees from low to middle income countries.

The World Health Organization (WHO), IARC has created the Global Initiative for Cancer Registry Development (GICR).

Tobacco Control

Tobacco-related illness already kills 5.4 million people globally a year if current trends continue smoking will kill more than eight million a year by 2030 of which 80 % [4] will be in low and middle income countries, in relation to cancer smoking is liked linked to cancers of the lung, throat, mouth, pancreas, bladder, stomach, liver and kidney.

Further, decreasing markets for the tobacco industry in high income countries cause the industry to seek new markets, such as in sub-Saharan Africa, where it sees enormous potential for growth.

Use of chewed tobacco is high in some nations, especially in villages in rural areas. Efforts must be made to control this more traditional use of tobacco in order to avert cancers of the mouth and throat.

It is possible to avert the epidemic of tobacco-related morbidity and mortality manifest, we need to educate civil society about the dangers of tobacco use and the benefits of cessation, special efforts are needed to educate young people, health care practitioners and policymakers. It is necessary to adopt effective policies such as tax and price increases on tobacco, which will not only lower prevalence but also increase government revenues, which can be used to pay for tobacco control measures and other health and social programmes. Other required policy changes include the placing of effective warning labels on tobacco products, banning advertising and promotion of tobacco use, prohibiting smoking in public places, banning sales of single cigarettes and prohibiting the sales of tobacco to the young. In order to implement effective tobacco control policies and programmes, civil society must be mobilized in support of this issue. A key to this is the nomination of champions who will promote the cause of tobacco control. Such individual champions throughout the world have proved to be essential in influencing policymakers, educating civil society and exposing and fighting the tactics of the tobacco industry.

In countries where farmers rely on growing tobacco for income, support needs to be provided to farmers to encourage planting of alternative crops, and to establish the infrastructure for distribution of the alternative crops.

Surveillance data are needed to track tobacco use and related behaviours, knowledge and attitudes. Without such data evaluations of tobacco control programmes are not possible.

Most importantly with tobacco control, we need to educate and raise awareness about populations, the damage smoking does to your health and how it affects you and others around you.

Early Diagnosis and Prevention

Liver cancer [predominantly hepatocellular carcinoma (HCC)] has one of the highest mortality rates of cancer in low to middle income countries. The main aetiological agents are chronic infections by hepatitis viruses, mainly hepatitis B (HBV), which is endemic throughout these countries and present in 8–10 % of the general population. The effect of HBV is compounded by widespread exposure to a potent carcinogen, aflatoxin and a mycotoxin that contaminates staple diets.

Thus, the two main risk factors for HCC are relatively well known and effective strategies are at hand to reduce their effect. A safe and efficient HBV vaccine has been available since the early 1982. Simple, behavioural methods to reduce aflatoxin exposure have been tested in the field, with significant improvements on individual contamination.

HBV is available in)116 countries worldwide with the Global Alliance for Vaccines (GAVI) ensuring it is available to all poorer nations by the end of 2015.

Worldwide there are more than 273,000 deaths from cervical cancer each year, and it accounts for 9 % of female cancer deaths. Mortality rates vary 17-fold between the different regions of the world. Cervical cancer contributes over 2.7 million years of life lost among women between the ages of 25 and 64 worldwide, of which, tellingly, some 2.4 million occur in developing areas and only 300,000 in developed countries. Cervical cancer incidence and mortality rates have decreased substantially in high income countries following the introduction of screening; however, such programmes are either rudimentary or non-existent in low to middle income countries. The vast majority of women who suffer cervical cancer in these countries present with disease advanced far beyond the capacity of surgery or other treatment modalities to offer cure. Palliative care services are poorly developed and, therefore, these unfortunate women are often sentenced to a miserable end of life.

Human papillomavirus (HPV) types 16 and 18 cause 70 % of cervical cancer cases and two vaccines that guard against these HPV types have been developed by the pharmaceutical industry. There is a large, international trials database that suggests that these vaccines can offer 100 % protection against infection by these HPV types (given as three injections over 6 months). The data are sufficiently compelling that the UK recently announced its commitment to a national vaccination programme for all 12–13-year-old girls. These remarkable vaccines give us the opportunity to eradicate 70 % of all known cervical cancer within a generation, saving almost 200,000 lives per annum, the vast majority in the developing world. GAVI is also helping to introduce HPV vaccinations to low income countries.

High income countries have reduced the burden of cancer in their populations by the screening of vulnerable groups, identified through their cancer surveillance programmes, for example, in the UK all women over 25 are invited to cervical cancer screening to check for precancerous lesions. In low to middle income countries, these programmes are in their infancy, using techniques such as Visual Inspection by Acetic Acid (VIA) and new DNA marker tests.

Cure the Curable

Although treatment is often considered to be overemphasized relative to primary prevention, it has been estimated that between that between 2012 and 2030 that cancer annual cancer cases will increase to 22 million a year (from 14 million in 2012) 13.2 million of these cases will be in low to middle income countries. Although it is crucially important to institute primary preventive measures, even if all such measures were fully implemented today they would have little effect on cancer mortality in the next 10–15 years. Mortality: incidence ratios are much higher in low to middle income countries than in more affluent world regions, and therefore improved access to proven, cost-effective therapy, efficiently delivered, would save many lives. However, as the majority of poorer patients present with advanced disease, when cure is unlikely, treatment programmes must be undertaken in concert with attempts to diagnose cancer earlier; it is essential, if such programmes are to be successful, that patients diagnosed with early-stage cancer have immediate access to care, with a preliminary focus on childhood cancer.

Cancer treatment should be included in NCCP and afforded a proportion of the available resources. Treatment programmes will need to be built in the context of the available human resources and infrastructure and supported to the degree feasible by in-country resources as well as by external assistance. Ideally, countries should have at least one National Cancer Centre with access to surgery, radiation and chemotherapy. Radiation programmes might be built on models provided by the International Atomic Energy Agency (IAEA), and their excellent Programme for Action on Cancer Treatment [5] and chemotherapy regimens based on simplified regimens using drugs from the WHO Essential Drugs List.

Cytotoxic and Adjuvant Medicine from WHO Essential Drugs List:

Complementary list	
Allopurinol	Tablet: 100, 300 mg
Asparaginase	Powder for injection: 10,000 IU in vial
Bleomycin	Powder for injection: 15 mg (as sulphate) in vial
Calcium Folinate	Injection: 3 mg/mL in 10-mL ampoule
	Tablet 15 mg
Carboplatin	Injection: 50 mg/5 mL; 150 mg/15 mL; 450 mg/45 mL; 600 mg/60 mL
Chlorambucil	Tablet: 2 mg
Cyclophosphamide	Powder for injection: 500 mg in vial
	Tablet: 25 mg
Cytarabine	Powder for injection: 100 mg in vial
Dacarbazine	Powder for injection: 100 mg in vial
Dactinomycin	Powder for injection: 500 μg in vial
Daunorubicin	Powder for injection: 50 mg (hydrochloride) in vial
Docetaxel	Injection: 20, 40 mg/mL
Doxorubicin	Powder for injection: 10, 50 mg (hydrochloride) in vial
Etoposide	Capsule: 100 mg
	Injection: 20 mg/mL in 5-mL ampoule
Fluorouracil	Injection: 50 mg/mL in 5-mL ampoule
Hydroxycarbamide	Solid oral dosage form: 200, 250, 300, 400, 500 mg; 1 g
Ifosfamide	Powder for injection: 1 g vial; 2 g vial
Mercaptopurine	Tablet: 50 mg
Mesna	Injection: 100 mg/mL in 4-mL and 10-mL ampoules
	Tablet: 400 mg; 600 mg
Methotrexate	Powder for injection: 50 mg (as sodium salt) in vial
	Tablet: 2.5 mg (as sodium salt)
Paclitaxel	Powder for injection: 6 mg/mL
Procarbazine	Capsule: 50 mg (as hydrochloride)
Thioguanine	Solid oral dosage form: 40 mg
Vinblastine	Powder for injection: 10 mg (sulphate) in vial
Vincristine	Powder for injection: 1 mg; 5 mg (sulphate) in vial

Regional or transnational networks could be built on a hub-and-spoke model, integrating vertically with existing AIDS programmes, and would greatly benefit from the sort of teleconferencing or telemedicine being pioneered in India by the Tata Memorial Centre and its associate centres [6].

In addition, it is important to exploit modern innovations in delivering chemotherapy in a predominantly out-patient setting. It should prove possible to design effective treatment regimes that do not require access to costly in-patient beds and seek to use oral agents when available [7, 8].

One other aspect of such an approach is to consider carefully the clinical pharmacology and therapeutic window for each antineoplastic drug so as to widen the safety margin as effectively as possible. For example, there are several trials suggesting that low dose is as effective as high dose folinic acid, with the potential to reduce drug costs tenfold. Conventional cytotoxic drugs have steep dose–response curves, but if we aim to generalize drug usage and widen access then we must think how we might train paramedical personnel to deliver cancer therapeutics with a simplified dosing algorithm that minimizes toxicity. Clearly, we must not carry this utilitarian approach too far, especially when considering treatment of childhood cancer, but this could be the subject of important research in low to middle income countries.

All oncologist use treatment guidelines to best treat their patients, unfortunately these guidelines have been written by high income countries using the newest treatment options they use available to them, so even though they are useful in low to middle income countries they sometimes are not fit for purpose. Therefore, we need to work with partners in Low to Middle Income Countries (LMICs) to develop setting appropriate guidelines.

Palliative Care

Palliative care must be a priority component of affordable and effective cancer care. It should be provided as early as possible after diagnosis as it provides pain and symptom control, terminal care and bereavement support.

Palliative care greatly improves the quality of life of patients and their families facing problems associated with cancer. It is ideally suited to home-based care, where it supports people during illness, enabling them to die with dignity.

The best palliation drugs are opiates like morphine, unfortunately 90 % of the world's morphine is used by the USA, Canada, Britain, Japan, France and Germany reducing the amount of morphine available to LMICs. Also due to strong anti-drugs laws in most LMICs, there is a legislative barrier to access the morphine making it difficult for doctors and their patients to access it.

Training and Education

There need to be an emphasis on training and education in all NCCPs. Most importantly to reduce the prevalent lack of cancer awareness, to improve knowledge and capacity throughout countries and to ensure that education and training programmes cover specialist and generic requirements, from specialist clinical disciplines to research training to health care management and operational/logistical health care disciplines, as well as initial and continuing needs.

Successfully tackling each of these identified priorities could be considered a major project in its own right, but, of course, sustainable and comprehensive integration of the clinical and public health systems requires a parallel approach. The key to cost-effective and successful implementation of the fit-for-purpose training, mentorship and public and professional education programmes that are required to meet the priority objectives is connectivity.

Connectivity at all levels, namely in a country, across regions and internationally, is needed to achieve strong collaborative leadership and effective sharing of existing and newly created resources. With the rapidly rising number of cancers in low to middle income countries, partnerships between existing bodies, health care organizations and consortia in high income countries and low to middle income countries (including local health care delivery systems, research institutions, international organizations, NGOs, national governments and the pharmaceutical industry) will be essential [9].

Moreover, AfrOx will seek to collaborate with the UK National Health Service, which is well placed to provide resources to underpin the cancer care training, education and partnership objectives for Africa [10].

Prioritization of Elements of Cancer Control Plans

In 2011 the WHO along with the World Economic Forum published a report,'Reducing the Economic Impact of Non-Communicable Diseases in Low to Middle Income Countries', which estimated that between 2011 and 2025 that the cumulative economic losses from cancer, cardiovascular disease, diabetes and chronic respiratory diseases will surpass 7 trillion US dollars, an average annual economic loss of around 500 billion US dollars which is equivalent to an estimated 4 % of these countries annual economic output.

By contrast, the findings from a WHO research into "best buys," population-based measures for reducing tobacco, harmful alcohol consumption, trying to reduce unhealthy diets, informing people to do more physical activity are estimated to cost $2 billion a year to reducc the burden of NCDs in LMICs.

In health terms, these "best buys" would help many millions of people to avoid an early death.

The best buys recommended in this report are:

Risk factor/disease	Interventions
Tobacco use	• Tax increases
	• Smoke-free indoor workplaces and public places
	• Health information and warnings
	• Bans on tobacco advertising, promotion and sponsorship
Harmful alcohol use	• Tax increases
	• Restricted access to retailed alcohol
	• Bans on alcohol advertising
Unhealthy diet and physical inactivity	• Reduced salt intake in food
	• Replacement of trans fat with polyunsaturated fat
	• Public awareness through mass media on diet and physical activity
Cardiovascular disease (CVD) and diabetes	• Counselling and multi-drug therapy for people with a high risk of developing heart attacks and strokes (including those with established CVD)
	• Treatment of heart attack with aspirin
Cancer	• Hepatitis B immunization to prevent liver cancer
	• Screening and treatment of precancerous lesions to prevent cervical cancer

This is not to say that improving treatment facilities, training health care workers and developing clinical pathways for the management of patients with cancer should be ignored. This clearly depends on the fraction of a Nation's GDP is allocated to the Health Ministry, and how much of that would be devoted to cancer. It is essential to have an estimate for the cost and likely impact of any intervention in the NCCP and to use these data to prioritize which programmes will be funded from existing resources [11, 12].

Funding NCCP

While any foreign funds would be welcome, the financing of cancer care requires money from the national budget. This needs to be supplemented by a system of health insurance which covers basic care for the common tumour types. This "investment" will be offset against the negative economic impact of cancer on society by loss of workforce, skills and key family members.

References

1. http://www.who.int/mediacentre/factsheets/fs297/en
2. www.uicc.org/decleration
3. http://www.un.org/en/ga/ncdmeeting2011

4. http://www.smokefreepartnership.eu/news/tobacco-low-and-middle-income-countries
5. http://cancer.iaea.org/
6. http://indox.org.uk
7. Midgley RS, Middleton MR, Dickman AR, Kerr DJ. Oncology drugs handbook. Oxford: Oxford University Press; 2013.
8. Kerr DJ, Midgley R. Can we treat cancer for a dollar a day. N Engl J Med. 2010;363:801–3.
9. Adewole I, et al. Building capacity for sustainable research programmes for cancer in Africa. Nat Rev Clin. 2014;11(5):251–9.
10. Kerr DJ, Scott M. British lessons on health care reform. N Engl J Med. 2009;361(13), e21.
11. Lingwood R, Boyle P, Milburn A, Ngoma T, Arbuthnott J, McCaffrey R, Kerr S, Kerr D. The challenge of cancer control in Africa. Nat Rev Cancer. 2008;8:298–403.
12. Gray M, Kerr DJ. How to get better value cancer care. Oxford: OffOx Press; 2013.

Chapter 3
Cancer Trends and Risk Factors in Morocco

Mati Nejmi and Saber Boutayeb

Introduction

Morocco (population 32.52 million people) is a country in Northern Africa that covers an area of 700,000 km^2. Its boundaries border the North Atlantic Ocean and the Mediterranean Sea, between Algeria and Mauritania. The capital of Morocco is Rabat (Fig. 3.1).

According to the United Nations human development index (HDI), Morocco is ranked 125/177 countries worldwide (value 0.620) and 6/45 African countries for which an index is available [1].

This places Morocco in the group of countries with medium human development.

The age distribution of the Moroccan population is as follows: 0–15 years, 27.85 %; 16–59 years, 64.54 %; and 60 years and above, 7.61 %.

Population living in urban areas 57 % and 43 % lives in rural Morocco. The estimated life expectancy at birth is 72 years (for males, 70 years and for females, 74 years). Literacy rate among adults aged 15 years or more is 56.10 %. GDP per capita is $3082.4 [2].

Morocco is currently in an epidemiological transition marked by a double burden due to the coexistence of infection and chronic diseases. While the prevalence of infectious diseases and the malnutrition is progressively declining, there is an increase in the prevalence of noncommunicable diseases, such as cardiovascular diseases, chronic diseases, and cancers, accountable for 56 % of total

M. Nejmi, M.D. (✉)
Center of Pain and Palliative Care, Hôpital Cheikh Khalifa Ibn Zaid, Boulevard Mohamed Taieb Naciri, Hay El Hassani, Casablanca, BP, 82403, Rabat, Morocco
e-mail: mati.nejmi@gmail.com

S. Boutayeb, M.D.
Department of Medical Oncology, National Institute of Oncology, Rabat, Morocco

M. Silbermann (ed.), *Cancer Care in Countries and Societies in Transition*, DOI 10.1007/978-3-319-22912-6_3

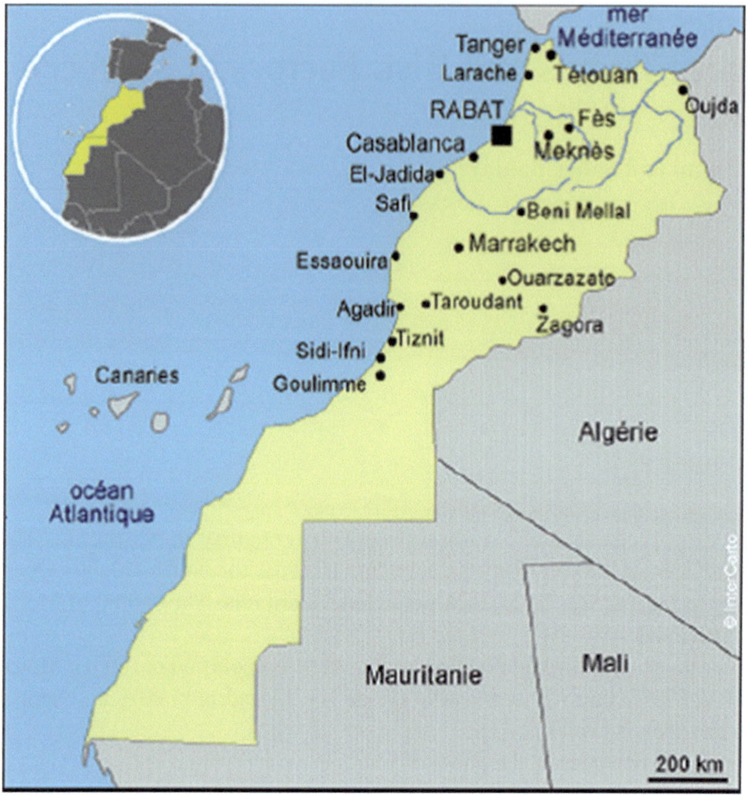

Fig. 3.1 Map of Morocco

morbidity. In particular, cancer burden is getting more and more overwhelming for the health system.

The main factors contributing to these changes are

- The increasing live expectancy which rose from 47 years in 1962 to 72 years in 2008
- The rapid socioeconomic development
- The environmental change
- The lifestyle changes: sedentary lifestyle, greater and quicker adoption of western diet, and high prevalence of smoking

The situation of cancer in Morocco is alarming. There are about 35,000 new cases of cancer each year. Cancer is responsible for 7.2 % of death. The cost of the management of cancer is very high and the situation is all the more worrying that more than two-thirds of the population has no medical coverage. The results of impact studies on the costs related to cancer care are sufficient proof of the heavy burden incurred by households as well as the severe social and economic repercussions of a cancer disease; up to 90 % of the cost of certain cancers are incurred by patients. The result being that cancer contributes inevitably to making its patients even poorer.

Major Oncology Hospitals and Medical Oncology

In Morocco, there is a lack in sufficient numbers of Medical Oncologists. Medical Oncology (MO) is a relatively new specialty. MO was recognized as a separate specialty in 1994 but the real taking-off was done only since the 2000s after the creation of the chair of medical oncology in the University of Rabat. The AMFROM (Moroccan Association for training and research in medical oncology) was created in 2008 to assure a high level of qualification for young oncologists and to improve the recognition of medical oncology. In the same way, the GRIOMM (Moroccan group of trialist in medical oncology) was created in 2011. Its first study is Eva-onco which is a national survey about the practice of medical oncology in the public health centers across Morocco [3].

The cancer health system in Morocco includes (2011) seven public hospitals (four university clinics) and seven private centers. In 2011, the AMFROM listed 28 medical oncologists in Morocco. There were more medical oncology positions in public (18) than private practices (6). Few medical oncology positions were located in military hospitals (4).

This first data provided by Eva-onco survey could be used by the Moroccan health authorities aiming to reduce the inequalities between regions and centers concerning medical oncology workforce.

The calculated density of MOs (MOs per 100,000) in Morocco is 0.09/100,000 habitant and is still low compared to the European and North-American countries [4, 5]. The average of 718 new patients per oncologist is very high compared with the national recommendations as defined in the cancer plan against cancer (one medical oncologist for 300 new cases). Using these recommendations, the shortfall of MOs in Morocco in 2011 is about a minimum of 26 oncologists. To our knowledge, there are no international recommendations concerning the number of MOs/habitants even if such countries like UK recommend a density of 1.1 MOs/100,000 habitants [6]. The pipeline of potential medical oncologists depends on the number of residents who complete training in medical oncology. Currently, there are approximately 50 residents who are in training in three university (Rabat, Fes, and Casablanca) so the current shortfall of MO is expected to disappear in the future.

The healthcare financing in oncology is characterized by inequity, the medical insurance covers only 35 % of the population. But demand for medical oncology services is expected to rise rapidly, driven by a medical assistance plan launched in 2010 for the benefit of the low-income populations in aim to give them a free access to all healthcare services provided by the public hospitals. Also, recently, a very active Moroccan NGO (Princess Lalla Salma Foundation for Prevention and Care of Cancer) is providing anticancer drugs to all government-run oncology centers [7].

Cancer Epidemiology

In Morocco, two cancer registries have been implemented in the greater areas of Rabat [8] and Casablanca [9]. In 2004, the preliminary epidemiologic result of the RCRC (Registre des Cancers de la Region du grand Casablanca), based on a population sample accounting for 10 % of the Moroccan population [1], has reported a global 35,000 new cases of cancer each year. Unfortunately, treatment reaches only 15,000 of those, leaving many with no treatment at the time of diagnosis. Cancer is responsible for nearly 8 % of death each year.

The most common cancers are breast (36.1 %), lung (31.5 %), cervix (13.3 %), colorectal (12.2 %), and prostate (3.7 %) (Table 3.1).

In a recent study conducted by Tazi et al. [8], 39.9 % of cancer cases are breast cancer patients, this study included all new cases of cancer diagnosed in the resident population of the Rabat area between 2005 until 2008.

Worldwide breast cancer is the most common malignancy in women with nearly a half million deaths each year (IARC Globocan, 2008). In Morocco, breast cancer represents serious public health problem. It's the first cancer among women and the third one of all registered cancer cases. The interest of studying breast cancer has clearly increased during the last decade in Morocco, and different studies were

Table 3.1 Number of cancer cases by localization and by gender for the Grand-Casablanca (2004)

	Female	%	Male	%	Total	%
Breast	662	36.1	–	–	662	19.8
Lung	31	1.7	358	23.8	389	11.7
Cervix	235	12.8	–	–	235	7.0
NHL	73	4.0	92	6.1	165	4.9
Prostate	–	–	125	8.3	125	3.7
Stomach	46	2.5	62	4.1	107	3.2
Rectum	51	2.8	47	3.1	98	2.9
Thyroid	97	5.3	–	–	97	2.9
Colon	40	2.2	56	3.7	96	2.9
Ovarian	92	5.0	–	–	92	2.7
Larynx	–	–	84	5.6	84	2.5
Bladder	–	–	84	5.6	84	2.5
Skin	42	2.3	41	2.7	83	2.5
Primitive loc. inc.	–	–	68	4.6	68	2.0
Nasopharynx	–	–	65	4.3	65	1.9
Uterine body	49	2.7	–	–	49	1.5
Brain	–	–	42	2.8	42	1.3
Pancreas	–	–	32	2.1	32	0.9
HL	29	1.6	–	–	29	0.9
Gallbladder	22	1.2	–	–	22	0.7
Oesophagus	20	1.1	–	–	20	0.6
Others	343	18.7	350	23.3	693	20.8
Total	1833	55	1503	45	3336	100

conducted to characterize breast cancer at epidemiological, molecular, and genetic levels [10]. It's widely accepted that establishment of the epidemiological profile of breast cancer is essential to provide hypothesis for understanding the etiology of the disease. Overall, the incidence of breast cancer in Morocco have clearly increased during the last decade, the 2012 updated versions of the RCRC (Registre des Cancers de la Region du grand Casablanca) and RCR (Registre des Cancers de Rabat) have reported a standardized incidence of 39.9 and 49.2 per 100,000 women, respectively (RCRC, 2012; RCR, 2012). Overall, the mean age at diagnosis in Morocco is less than in Western countries where the average age onset of breast cancer is 55 years old [11].

Regarding cancer in children, estimated crude incidence according to the RCRC is 11.34 for 100,000 children. In children, each year, approximately 1000 new cases of cancer are registered. This figure accounts for 3.2 % of all cancer cases collated. Girls are greater in numbers with a proportion of about 53.8 % versus 46.2 % for boys. The most frequent cancers in children are malignant hemopathy (19.8 %), followed by tumors of the brain and meninges (17.1 %), then cancers of bones (12.33 %), adrenal glands (11.3 %), and eye (10.4 %).

The situation studies has showed the deficiency of healthcare structures and specialized human resources; thus patients have to travel long distances for very belated appointments. The huge difficulty to access to healthcare causes patients to be more often diagnosed at very advanced stage of the disease: for breast cancers the diagnosis is made at stage I in only 6 % of cases versus 57 % of cases in stages III and IV; as for lung cancers, their diagnosis is made at stages I or II only in 4 % of cases, whilst 96 % of the cases are diagnosed at the stages III and IV.

The time length between the onset of the first symptoms and the first medical examination exceeds 1 month in 36 % of cases, this period is even greater than 6 months in 14 % of cases. Furthermore, the period between the first medical examination and the diagnosis of cancer is greater than 3 months in 52 % of cases and greater than 6 months in 27 % of cases.

The absence of standardized protocols for diagnosis and treatment is the cause of the poor quality and the high cost of patient management.

The follow-up period of cancer patients is very low with a high number of lost-to-follow-up. In fact, the follow-up period is below 2 years in 74 % of cases.

Besides, about half of the patients are lost to follow-up after 1 year and almost seven of ten patients are lost to follow-up the second year, 83 % are lost the third year, and 96 % of patients are lost to follow-up at 5 years. Therefore, there is no reliable data to estimate the patient survival at 5 years, which is an essential indicator of the quality of cancer patients' management.

Palliative Care [12]

Pain is an important concern in patients with cancer who are receiving active treatment and in long-term cancer survivors. It is one of the most feared aspects of cancer, and it can have a major adverse impact on quality of life. It has long been recognized that untreated or undertreated pain is common in patients with cancer, with little evidence of recent improvement. Before 1994, end-of-life care in Morocco was non-existent. Dozen thousands of cancer patients were leaving to suffer needlessly because of the failure to ensure adequate access to pain-relieving drugs. Despite published guidelines by the WHO in 1986, most deaths occurred at home with the dying suffering great pain. The first data released during 1994 about the management of cancer pain paints a shocking picture of unnecessary pain on a national scale. This survey suggests that cancer-related pain may be a major issue of the Moroccan healthcare system where training for palliative care is not included in healthcare education curricula. Even in medical circles, many doctors and other healthcare providers remain unaware of not only pain control but also what palliative care provides more generally. Medical services have all too often focused on preventing death rather than helping people meet death without suffering pain, discomfort, and stress. Patients are stymied by regulatory barriers at multiple steps along this process; the end result being that dozen thousands of patients don't have access to essential pain-relieving medications. The issue was complicated by the perception that palliative care was often associated with "giving up." Since that, we were determined to tackle this problem at every level because the quality and availability of care was often absent and policy coordination lacking. Deeper integration of palliative care into our national healthcare was also vital. Palliative care need not mean institutional care, but more training is needed.

The World Health Assembly in May 2014 endorsed a resolution calling for palliative care to be fully integrated into healthcare in every setting, specifically highlighting community settings, and throughout the course of advances illnesses [13]. The Prague Charter also calls for universal access to palliative care [14]. Palliative care at the end of life is realized when strong networks exist between specialist palliative providers, primary generalists, primary specialists and support care providers and the community working together to meet the needs of all people. Palliative care must be available regardless of location, age, income, diagnosis or prognosis, social and cultural background.

A recent 2012 report from the Pain and Policy Studies Group at the University of Wisconsin, and Human Rights Watch pointed this failure. In 2009, a total of 14.278 cancer and 708 HIV patients died. The opioids quota was at this time only sufficient to relieve pain from 31.6 % of these patients. The result was that 11.777 patients died in unnecessary moderate-to-severe pain. The morphine necessary to meet the minimum demand of deaths due to HIV and cancer is 73 kg annually [15], which means that Morocco's 7.7 kg quota provides for only a tenth of those in need. Clearly, this is an insufficient amount. The main barriers to necessary availability and accessibility are the fear of addiction and the high cost of opioids.

This dramatic situation must be evaluated by the Governmental Division of Medicine and Pharmacy as soon as possible. WHO guidelines could help formulate a national drug control policy, estimate annual requirements, report consumption statistics to be submitted to the International Narcotics Control Board (INCB), and administer an effective distribution system to patients.

Despite the launching of the National Plan of Cancer Prevention and Control (NPCPC), the Moroccan government's recognition of palliative care as a policy priority and the model care offered by the Moroccan Society of PC as well as dealing with clinically complex patients, specialist palliative care has a role to support and train generalists and to help develop palliative care in the community. Such care nonetheless remains out-of-reach to the majority of Moroccans in need. The most relevant act recently is the amendment in last July 2014 of the obsolete law of 1952 about the number of 7 days of prescription of morphine. Recently, this prescription is for 28 days as needed. Nonetheless, the major reason discouraging the generalization of palliative care across all the country is the lack of government funding for end-of-life care. Actually, advocates of end-of-life care point to evidence that palliative care can be cheaper than traditional medical treatment for patients at the end of their lives. Certainly, by increasing the proportion of community and homecare, end-of-life care can reduce costs associated with hospital stays and emergency admissions.

Knowledge, Attitudes, Perceptions, and Practices [7]

Moroccan's population generally has a poor understanding of cancer and end-of-life issues.

A survey was conducted to identify perceptions of cancer and its treatment among the general public, patients, and caregivers in Morocco in 2008.

This population-based survey on knowledge, perceptions, and attitudes toward cancer shows many misconceptions and that the terms mostly used to refer to cancer are "Li makaytssamach" (unnamed), "Al mard el khaib" (bad ill), and "Laâdou" (the enemy).

Some evocations linked to the term "cancer" and the symbolic associated to the disease are fear, isolation, divine punishment, curse, death, a)disease that causes havoc in the family, family disintegration, incurable disease, very costly disease with death at the end even when treated. In rural areas, the disease gives rise to the following comments: "it is better to save one's property and one's cattle and leave them to one's children, since the patient is going to die anyway."

The most widely known cancers are those of breast, uterus, throat, lung, and prostate. Symptoms are often mixed up with treatment side effects (hair loss, nausea, and browning of skin). The main disincentives for early detection are lack of financial resources and absence of health insurance, ignorance of early signs of the most frequent cancer forms, ignorance of the fact that early diagnosis can increase the possibilities of remission and finally ignorance of where to turn for advice and support.

Among the reasons for the more or less significant hesitation period between the discovery of the first signs, the first examination, even after the diagnosis and the start of treatment, there is the fact that the formulation of the disease by the physician is often felt with strong resentment by the patient because of its ambiguity.

This medical behavior does not seem to contribute to the mobilization of the patient. Certain patients declared to have "preferred to know the reality of their disease so that they can become psychologically armed with a strong will to fight it."

Cancer Charity Organization

Since 2005, date of the creation of the Foundation Lalla Salma of Prevention and Control of Cancer (FLSPCC), cancer care in Morocco has improved and became a public health priority. This national NGO works hand in hand with all its partners, to make of the fight against cancer a public health priority in Morocco and the region.

The FLSPCC aims at setting up a national plan dedicated to fight cancer which will apply the best clinical practices, by implementing a strategy using an innovative and participative approach adapted to the specificities of the country.

Created at the initiative of Her Royal Highness Princess Lalla Salma, the FLSPCC is working ceaseless to improve the patients' care, to promote the prevention and to make of the fight of cancer a public health priority in Morocco. Furthermore, the FLSPCC made a commitment in terms of scientific research, hence multiplying partnerships in Morocco and worldwide.

The FLSPCC adopted a participative and multidimensional approach to figure out the cancer issue. The Foundation Lalla Salma is officially recognized as a non-profit organization and pretends not to replace any public, private, nor foundation institution. The FLSPCC acts in concert with all its partners, working together at implementing a)national health-system dedicated at fighting cancer that would be modeled on the best international practices.

The FLSPCC has always been privileging the well-being and the comfort of the patient, who is at the center of all its concerns. The FLSPCC is fortunate to rely on the never-ending and active implication of all and every one of the private and corporate partners, working out to meet the cancer challenge in Morocco.

In less than 3 years since its founding, the FLSPCC has mobilized efforts to raise public cancer awareness throughout Morocco launched an ambitious building campaign, organized the first national cancer registry, and linked arms with an array of international partners in the fight against cancer. Inspired by the vision and leadership of HRH Princess Lalla Salma, the NGO is already making significant inroads in improving the quality of cancer management and the ensuring that all Moroccan patients have access to a high standard of cancer care. Early detection projects in breast and cervical cancer are underway, and the Foundation oversees a program of tobacco control is partnership with the Ministry of Health and business and education leaders. In 2006 the Foundation became associate UICC member.

A number of "Houses of life" were built near the different center of oncology by the FLSPCC with many humanitarian objectives:

- To host the patients and family for the ambulatory treatment period
- To ensure the patients have a regular follow-up of their treatment

- To assist patients by providing them moral and psychological support
- To organize their social and cultural activities

The residents of "Houses of life" are taken care by a multidisciplinary team consisted of healthcare professionals, psychologists, and social workers working together to ensure their well-being during their stay. Groups of volunteers provide a wide range of social and cultural activities, by organizing outings, dinners, musical evenings, as well as educational sessions for diet and hygiene.

Up to date, five houses of life opened in the main big Moroccan cities.

An increasing number of volunteers join the teams working in the "Houses of life" and make a personal and effective commitment to the patients, as they operate in a polyvalent way and take care of their welcoming, orientation, support and follow-up, raising awareness, hygiene education, and organization of recreational and educational activities.

Assisting the children affected by cancer is one of the Foundation Lalla Salma's major concerns, and the Foundation brings a quite particular care to the follow-up and support of the youngest patients, thus helping them to better live despite their unfair disease.

As a matter of fact, a lot of organizations in Morocco do fight against this plague that is cancer, some of which existing for more than 20 years. The domains of intervention are split between the Foundation Lalla Salma focusing on women and breast cancer, others mobilizing efforts to help out the children or yet all those promoting prevention first and foremost. Many operations are carried out by all the community sectors acting jointly.

The National Plan for Prevention and Care the Cancer [7]

Several findings vindicate the implementation of a National Plan for the Prevention and Control of Cancer (NPPCC) in Morocco:

- Importance of the cancer morbidity burden, with more than 35,000 new cases each year
- Inadequate primary prevention activities
- Lack of structured programs for early detection
- Inadequate specialized infrastructures and human resources
- Poor management of available resources: absence of standards for the diagnosis and treatment management, no policy regulating generic drugs, etc.
- Unavailability of palliative care and psychological support
- The costs of treatment exceeds the financial capabilities of the majority of patients, and less than one-third of the population has medical insurance
- Lack of communication strategy on and about cancer
- The applicable legislation and regulation have become inadequate for an efficient prevention and management of the disease

Furthermore, this situation being common to the majority of countries, the World Health Assembly has adopted in 2005 a resolution (WHA 5822) recommending to all members states to strengthen the actions against, by developing or strengthening the existing cancer control program. Improving against cancer has therefore become an issue of global concern for all public powers, private sector, NGOs, professional associations, etc. All must contribute to the implementation of the global concern cancer control strategy, which aims at reducing the incidence, mortality, and risk factors of the disease, and improving the quality of life of the patients and their families.

Hence, under the guidance of Her Royal Highness Princess Lalla Salma, President of the FLSPCC and WHO Goodwill Ambassador for Promotion of Cancer Prevention and Care, Morocco, has adopted the international strategic approach and rallied efforts of the Ministry of Health (MoH), civil society organizations and other stakeholders, particularly for the design of the NPCPC in the line with the Global Strategy.

The NPPCC development project was prepared by the FLSPCC and validated by a steering committee and a joint panel made up of FLSPCC and the Ministry of Health (joint committee). An ad hoc commission was created for the follow-up and monitoring of the project.

The NPCPC development began by situation analysis, carrying out 15 studies creating and collecting of data in all fields associated with cancer: incidence data, behavioral and professional factors, demographics, healthcare, information on prevention and early detection activities, diagnosis and therapeutic practices, information on applicable legislation and regulations, information on the needs of patients and their families, the needs of healthcare practitioners and individuals exposed to risk, population perceptions, knowledge, attitudes, and practice toward cancer.

Taking into account the situation analysis results, six workshops were organized by the FLSPCC and the MoH in order to develop a specific strategy of the different areas of the plan: prevention, early detection, diagnosis and treatment management, palliative care, communication, and legislation. These workshops were facilitated by national and international experts with the participation of the relevant departments and organizations in each component of the plan, along with the resource persons concerned by the specific themes of each workshop.

Officially launched on March 24, 2010, the NPPCC listed up 78 operational measures that are modeled according to the targeted goals to be applied in strategic domains such as prevention, early detection, therapeutic coverage, palliative care, and patients' follow-up conditions. This program is the result of a strategic partnership between the Foundation Lalla Salma and the Ministry of Health, with the active participation of many national and international specialists.

Conveying the community spirit as a national humanitarian project, the NPPCC will certainly boost the whole chain of the healthcare system through a complementary combination of actions led by the professionals together with the patients and their relatives.

Real keystone of the Moroccan modern public-health policy, the NPPCC planned out a strategic program for the next decade.

The ambition of the NPPCC is to prevent and control all types of cancers through a multi-sectoral approach suggesting concrete and long-lasting concerted measures, to be readjusted if needed according to the priorities, and adapted to the socioeconomic and cultural contexts of the country.

The objective of this ambitious plan is to reduce the cancer prevalence and the mortality rate, and to improve the patients' quality of life as well as that of their relatives.

The Plan will pilot a rational and relevant use of the existing resources and will find out moreover the means to fill the gaps so as to better meet the patients' needs.

Early Detection

According to the WHO, the screening operation is defined as being a collective measure of public health, watchfully worked out so as to lead at identifying should the case occur, a disease or an anomaly yet ignored by persons considered as totally healthy till they passed through screening. Thus the early detection as an operation covering all of the population, people who can at random present a risky anomaly due to a hidden disease.

The aim of this cancer screening campaign is to identify premature cases prior to cancer development and even precancerous lesions at a curable stage, by using affordable and reliable screening tests presenting no danger and accepted by the largest number of persons. The outcome of these tests is to separate the healthy persons from those who could possibly be developing a cancer and who need more detailed examinations.

The early diagnosis consists in diagnosing cancer forerunners and first symptoms to ease the diagnosis before the malady is at an advanced stage, so that a lighter and more effective treatment can be applied. In other words, the aim of the early screening is to detect cancers at a curability stage to decrease their mortality rate by using means of diagnosis apt to cover the largest number of persons with a much less aggressive therapy.

The early detection is a very important prevention measure in the reduction of certain cancer's incidence. Thanks to a battery of efficient programs of information, screening, early diagnosis and to the therapeutic care, the mortality rate and the proportion of people affected by cancer can be reduced by the third.

In Morocco, the NPPCC set up as a strategic priority the early detection of the breast and cervix cancers.

To be effective, the activities of early detection of the breast and cervix cancers must be integrated into the national health system, which is split in three levels of intervention:

Level 1: health centers, general practitioners' offices.

Level 2: district and province hospitals, diagnostic centers, specialists' offices, and private hospitals.

Level 3: university hospitals, regional centers on oncology, private ward cancer hospitals.

Importance of the Screening

In Morocco, breast and cervix cancers constitute a burning issue for the public health. They are the most frequent as they represent approximately half of the cancers affecting the women and are in general diagnosed in very late stages, thus delaying their therapeutic care and complicating their cure.

Since the implementation of the NPPCC in 2010, national-scale operations of breast cancer screening are regularly carried out everywhere throughout the Kingdom, whilst that of the cervix cancer is fully operational in six regions but will be widened to all the Basic Health Centers by 5 years at the very latest.

Furthermore, early diagnosis services for these two cancers are already available in all the reference centers of reproductive health.

To date, all the types of treatments (chemotherapy, radiotherapy, and surgery) have been standardized by formal procedures and are equally provided in the different oncology centers.

The Moroccan programs of early screening set up the clinical breast examination and. the cervical visual inspection with acetic acid as the screening tests to be used in breast and cervix cancers early detection. They are receivable, reliable, and not that expensive.

The catchment population for the breast cancer screening is the group of women between 45 and 69 years old, as well as the women having breast cancer cases in their family history (grandmother, mother, aunt, sister). Are excluded from the program the women who already passed through breast cancer. T.o be totally safe and protected against cancer, every woman should redo the breast screening every year, or at least every other year if the result of the previous test is negative.

The target population for the cervix cancer screening concerns all the 30-year-old women till at least over 49 years old. The pregnant women from the 8th week as well as those who already passed through cervix cancer are prohibited from screening. The aim of such screening is to detect the precancerous lesions if any, to treat these lesions as soon as possible and to eliminate hence the risk of a cervix cancer appearance. To be totally safe and protected against cervix cancer, women must redo the cervical screening every 3 years provided that the result of the previous test was negative.

Carcinogenic Environmental Risk Factors

Many environmental factors have been associated with cancer development including smoking, diet, alcohol, various viruses, asbestos, radon, radiation, water and air pollution, and medical conditions whose development is influenced by the environment, such as diabetes and the metabolic syndrome. The way these factors may interact with another as well as with genetic factors is not fully understood. In Morocco, even though some of these factors are quite prevalent, their association with cancer has not been investigated. In the subsequent paragraphs the presence of such environmental cancer risk factors in Morocco is described.

Breast Cancer

Social Determinants and Risk Factors

All the Moroccan studies found that the risk of breast cancer was clearly associated with a high socioeconomic level [9, 16]. This is consistent with published literature [17, 18]. The difference in incidence may be seen as a direct consequence of the gradient in risk factors between social classes (such as parity, age at first menstruation and menopause). Indeed, women with high socioeconomic status have generally low parity, breastfeed only rarely, little, or not at all [19].

According to the INCA (Institut National du Cancer) [20], breastfeeding exclusively and ideally until the age of 6 months remains one of the absolute recommendations for primary prevention of cancer. This recommendation is consistent with Maamri data [16] since he found a statistically significant difference between non-breastfeeding and breastfeeding woman regarding breast cancer.

Kato also found that in countries with low incidence, increased incidence of breast cancer is the result of westernization of lifestyle on women's reproductive life, diet, physical activity, and other factors [21]. It should be recalled that, researchers recognized long ago that early puberty and/or a first pregnancy at a late age and/or absence of breastfeeding are the main risk factors associated with the reproductive life of woman. Usually in developing countries, women are protected by a delayed puberty, an early first birth and high parity which causes often a long period of lactation. But the new generations, the behaviors of the reproductive life have evolved in a rapid and significant way: first birth later, often not breastfeeding [17].

Taking into account the sociocultural context of our country, it appears that the age of marriage becoming increasingly late and the first pregnancy increasingly postponed. Consequently, births are delayed and periods of breastfeeding shortened, putting women at a higher risk of cancer [22]. Moreover, the age of puberty is being reached earlier and earlier over the years [23].

In Morocco, according to RCRC and RCR, women diagnosed with breast cancer are aged between 18 and 80 years old, and the mean age at diagnosis is 49.5 and 50 years, respectively (RCRC, 2012; RCR, 2012). On the other side, Abbas et al. showed in a cohort of 265 women with breast cancer in the Fez region that the median age is 45 years [24]. Overall, the mean age at diagnosis in Morocco is less than in western countries where the average age of onset of breast cancer is 55 years old [11].

In a comparative clinical study, Chalabi et al. have clearly demonstrated that South Mediterranean breast cancer patients are younger than French patients. In this study, including Moroccan, Tunisian, and Lebanese patients, authors found that South Mediterranean patients were 10 years younger than French breast cancer patients, with more aggressive parameters; more SBRIII grade (Scarff Bloom and Richardson histological grade) and positive lymph node invasion [25].

Interestingly, large tumor size and high histological grade were found in a Moroccan series, which was explained by the lack of awareness of breast cancer risks [24].

As the average of onset of breast cancer in Morocco is young, many authors were interested to investigate the epidemiological, clinical, and treatment characteristics in patients under 35 years old. In Morocco, reported data showed that 8–25.4 % of women with breast cancer are young [26–28]. While worldwide studies have reported that approximately 2–24 % of patients with breast carcinoma are under 35 years old at the time of diagnosis [29, 30]. The results obtained in Morocco by Boufettal et al. [26] are the highest level published so far.

The family history of breast cancer seems to affect young women as it was described by Tazzite et al. [31]. The findings of this study that was conducted on 570 cases of breast cancer were significant. 18.4 % of the cases had a family history of breast cancer and presented high SBR grade tumors, positive lymph node status, and absence of progesterone receptors. These results must be more investigated to be used as predictor markers in this subtype group.

Inflammatory Breast Cancer (IBC) is the most aggressive subtype of breast cancer. It was reported that IBC is more common in North Africa than Europe and North America [32]. In Morocco, only one study was published on IBC and showed that IBC cases represent 6.3 % of total breast cancer cases [33]. However, this study was based on data from 2003 and has to be updated to evaluate the evolution of IBC cases in Morocco. Similarly, IBC cases represent 5.7 % of total breast cancer in Tunisia [34], whereas in Europe and North America, IBC represents 2–5 % of breast cancer cases [32, 35]. No explanations could be given for these high frequencies in North Africa; further investigations are needed to identify the probable impact of genetical, virological, and immunological factors in IBC development in this area.

Genetic Effect

Breast cancer is a complicated disease characterized by the accumulation of multiple molecular alterations that give each tumor a specific phenotype that can be used as a molecular signature to reach a personalized therapy.

During the last decade, molecular genetics have known a great evolution at both conceptual and methodological levels and has made an outstanding contribution to our understanding of genetic disease etiology. Molecular genetics highlighted the partly involvement of predisposition and genetic mutations in breast carcinogenesis.

The genetic component may be responsible for breast cancer in one part of the population. For instance, in European populations, approximately 2 % of breast cancer may be due to gene mutations, but the proportion of breast cancer is higher among young people around 10 % below the age of 40 years [36, 37].

According to Sasco [38], the most remarkable discoveries of the past 20 years, in terms of etiology of breast cancer, were made in the field of genetics.

Worldwide, genetic predisposition is observed in about 5–10 % of cancers [39]. Two genes with high penetrance susceptibility to breast cancer have been identified,

BRCA1 (Breast Cancer 1) in 1994 and BRCA2 (Breast Cancer 2) in 1995 [40, 41]. Germline mutations in BRCA1 and BRCA2 have been shown to play an important role in genetic predisposition to breast/ovarian cancer, and are responsible for 3–5 % of breast cancers [42].

In Morocco, three studies have focused on the study of BRCA1/2 mutations. The first study was conducted and interested in the study of BRCA1/2 mutations in five healthy women belonging to three families with an elevated risk of breast cancer. As results of this study, three asymptomatic women were carriers of BRCA1/2 mutations [43].

The second study is a Moroccan cohort with 40 women diagnosed with breast cancer with a familial history of breast/ovarian cancer or aged less than 40 years old. Tazzite et al. [44] showed that 25.64 % of patients carried BRCA1/2 mutations. This prevalence is higher compared to Tunisia and Algeria with, respectively, 19.4 % and 11.4 % of breast cancer patients carrying BRCA1/2 mutations [45, 46].

The last study was conducted on 121 Moroccan women diagnosed with breast cancer, only BRCA1 status was investigated. BRCA1 mutations were found in 36.1 % of familial cases and 1 % (1/102) of early-onset sporadic [47].

Overall, 14 BRCA1/2 point mutations have been reported: nine in BRCA1 and five in BRCA2 [43, 44, 47].

Cervix Cancer and Human Papillomavirus

Human Papillomavirus (HPV) is the most common sexually transmitted infection. HPV is so common that nearly all sexually active men and women get it at some point in their lives. In most cases, HPV goes away on its own and does not cause any health problems. But when HPV does not go away, it can cause health problems like genital warts and cancer.

There are many different types of HPV. Some types can cause health problems including genital warts and cancers.

In Morocco, as in other developing countries, the lower social conditions, the average age at first intercourse, the high rate of parity, and the lack of primary care in the health systems are important risk factors for the rate of cervical cancer. In 1998, the prevalence of HPV-16 in invasive carcinomas from northern Morocco represented 49 % of the HPV-positives specimens [48]. This value is somewhat lower than the results found in other developing countries: Latin America (54 %), Thailand (59.3 %), and India (64 %). In some European countries, the HPV-16 prevalence was higher, such as 78.3 % in Poland and 76.5 % in Germany [49]. In 2003, HPV-18 was found in 22 % of HPV-positive specimens, which is more than twice the previously in Moroccan samples [50]. The relative proportion of HPV-16/HPV-18 in this study is similar to that for Africa and other countries such Algeria, but is different from that in other countries in Europe, which have a higher proportion of HPV-16 cases [49]. The persistence of HPV DNA is an indicator of possible cervical cancer development in the future. Thus the detection of high-risk HPV types in women is an important risk factor that allows identification of those women who should be monitored more closely, rather than concentrating limited medical resources on patients with lesions that will spontaneously regress. The magnitude of the public health problem represented by cervical carcinoma in developing countries might be even bigger in the future, considering that the population of these countries is relatively young compared to that of developed countries. This means that if public health measures are not taken in order to identify the high-risk subpopulation, the burden of cervical carcinoma in these countries will increase considerably. HPV is currently the target of many vaccine development projects for prevention and therapy of cervical carcinoma. The knowledge of HPV types circulating in developing countries is an essential component for the future application of prophylactic vaccines that aim to reduce the burden of cervical carcinoma. In developing countries the control of HPV by vaccination is likely to be a more effective and practical approach than the implementation of regular and periodic cytological screening. Currently prophylactic vaccines are based on HPV-16 [HPV vaccines: Promise and challenges on World Wide Web URL http://www.path.org//files/isrp1370.pdf].

Tobacco

Tobacco smoking has been associated with the development of many malignancies, such as lung, urinary bladder, oral, pharyngeal, head and neck, and laryngeal cancers [51]. Lung cancer incidence and mortality exceeds that of any other cancer in the world, with approximately 1.2 million new cases and 1.1 million deaths estimated globally for the year 2000. A case-control study of cancer in Casablanca [52] was conducted to evaluate etiologic factors for lung cancer and demonstrate that the active tobacco smoking was the strongest risk factors for lung cancer. In addition to tobacco smoking, respiratory diseases such as chronic bronchitis, occupational exposures, and indoor air pollution have been associated with increased risk of lung cancer.

In 2009, the MARTA survey (MAROC TABAC) [53] has revealed that the smoking prevalence among the Moroccan population was 17 % (31.5 % for males and 3.3 % for females). Among nonsmokers, passive smoking is also high: 32 % are exposed in their close family circle, 17 % are exposed in their professional environment, and 60 % are exposed in public places. There is a lag time of a few decades between smoking and the development of cancer; therefore, data on lung cancer in the coming decades and better evaluation of smoking trends a few decades ago will resolve this question. This study revealed that cigarette smoking remains an important public health problem and that a comprehensive strategy for tobacco control was needed.

In line with the international approach in terms of fighting tobacco strategies, the Foundation Lalla Salma set as a priority the fight against smoking, to prove the tobacco's misdeeds and its direct link with cancer. This antismoking strategy is mainly based on the CLE Program (Collèges, Lycées, Entreprises), besides the large-scale antismoking campaign carried out in 2009, a national campaign which covered a very wide public all over Morocco. This antismoking program was implemented for the benefit of middle and high schools teenagers, adults in their working and private environment, and healthcare professionals. The CLE program goals are the prevention against the first cigarette, the protection of the nonsmokers, and the support and the follow-up to quit smoking.

Nutrition

Nutrition has been associated with the development of many cancer types [54]. Regarding food-related factors, 63 % of the Moroccan population eat five types or more of fruits and vegetables per day, 11 % of the population eat poultry more than three times per week and only 3 % of the population eat fish three times or more a week. Among the general population, the prevalence of obesity is 14 % (BMI 30) and 30 % of the population are on overweight ($25<BMI<30$).

A case-control study of Cypriot women with breast cancer has shown that a Mediterranean diet rich in vegetables, fish, legumes, and olive oil may favorably influence the risk of breast cancer [55].

In Morocco, 400 overweight Breast cancer patients were compared to a group of 400 healthy controls at the National Institute of Oncology of Rabat. This 2 years case control study shows very interesting and significant results. Hypertriglyceridemia and obesity are connected to breast cancer risk while physical activity have protective role on breast cancer risk [56].

By using the findings of this study, overweight women in Morocco should be alarmed about this situation through public awareness campaigns encouraging them to adopt a healthy lifestyle and frequent sports activity.

It would be interesting, considering the worsening of dietary habits in Morocco, to see how cancer dynamics will change in the next two decades when the effects of dietary changes and deviations from the Mediterranean diet would exert their effect.

Ultraviolet radiation (UVR) has been linked to the development of skin cancer [20]. Morocco has year-round sunshine and therefore UVR levels are on the high end. Sixty-four percent of the Moroccan population are usually exposed to sun during hot time of the day (1 a.m.–4 p.m.), one-third of them is not using any protection from the sun.

In occupational environments, some exposures to carcinogenic substances or products are frequent, and use of protective means is quite weak. In the wood-made handicraft objects, exposure to wood dust is 100 % and to paint fuel is 62 %. In the leather-made handicraft, the prevalence of exposure to salt and paint is, respectively, 100 % and 55 %. In the copperware handicraft, the most frequent exposures are those to wood dust (20.5 %), ethanol (18.1 %), and sulfuric acid (17.3 %). In the pottery sector, the main exposures are wood dust (54 %), paint (44 %), and lead (21 %). Finally, in the sector of building and public works, wood dust is the main exposure (11.3 %), followed by paint (9.7 %). Asbestos is also believed to be prevalent in certain constructions.

Alcohol has been associated with .cancer and is actually one of the major aetiologies of liver cancer. Among males in Morocco, 6.8 % drink alcoholic beverages, and two out of 1000 drink on a daily basis. However, data on the incidence of alcohol-related disease is not available.

Specific Objectives of the NPPCC

- Reduce active and passive smoking
- Increase the number of persons with healthy lifestyle
- Reduce prevalence of obesity
- Reduce the number of people drinking alcohol
- Prevent infections
- Improve protective measures and practices in occupational environments
- Formulate specific measures against environmental pollution
- Implement a strategy for the surveillance of cancers and risk factors

Expected Results

Some of the most significant prerequisites of a successful implementation of the NCPCP are

- The Ministry of Health must assume leadership
- Social mobilization and partnership at all levels
- Phased in implementation, on the basis of scientifically verifiable models
- The approach must be realistic and feasible in our social and cultural context
- The overriding objective of the plan must remain patient oriented.

The expected outcomes of NCPCP implementation for the period 2010–2019 are

- Prevention: Reduce by 30 % the prevalence of behavioral and environmental risks
- Early detection: Have a screening program expanded on a nationwide scale. Screen for breast and cervical cancers a minimum of 50 % of women representing the target population.

Diagnosis and Therapeutic Management

- Have available infrastructures complying with the standards, and skilled and motivated human resources, throughout the Kingdom
- Take care of 100 % of the patients according to international standards
- Cure 50 % of treated cancer patients

Palliative Care

- Have a nationwide palliative care network
- Support 100 % of patients requiring palliative care

Monitoring and Evaluation Indicators

For the evaluation of outcomes, several indicators will be defined and monitored throughout the implementation of the plan:

- Reduction by 30 % of risk factors prevalence
- Number of women screened for breast and cervical cancer
- Number of functional screening structures operating nationwide
- Number of patients managed
- Number of patients cured
- Number of operating structures of diagnosis and treatment
- Number of patients managed under palliative care

These global indicators will be detailed in the actions' plan specific to each component of the NPPCC and must be subjected to continuous monitoring.

References

1. Report of the United Nations Development program 2004 (HDI 2002). http://hdr.undp.org/statistics/data/indic_8_1_1.html
2. WHO. http://www.who.int/chp/chrnic_disease_report
3. Saber B, et al. The practice of Medical Oncology in Morocco: The National Study of the Moroccan Group of Trialist in Medical Oncology (EVA-Onco). ISRN Oncol. 2013;2013:341565. doi:10.1155/2013/341565.
4. Hortobagyi GN, et al. A shortage of oncologists? The American Society of Clinical Oncology workforce study. J Clin Oncol. 2007;25(12):1468–9.
5. Blinman PL, et al. The shortage of medical oncologists: the Australian Medical Oncologist Workforce Study. Med J Aust. 2012;196(1):58–61.
6. The Royal College of Radiologists. Clinical oncology UK workforce in 2010. London: The Royal College of Radiologists; 2011. http://www.rcr.ac.uk/docs/oncology/pdf
7. Foundation Lalla Salma against cancer. The National Plan for Prevention and Cancer Care (2010–2019). http://www.contrelecancer.ma/en/
8. Tazi MA, et al. Cancer incidence in Rabat. Morocco: 2006–2008. Cancer. 2013;7:33851.
9. Benidder A et al. Le Registre des cancers de la Région du Grand Casablanca 2005–2006–2007. Edition 2012.
10. Slaoui M, et al. Breast cancer in Morocco: a literature review. Asian Pac J Cancer Prev. 2014;15:1067–74. http://dx.doi.org/107314/APJCP.2014.15.3.1067
11. Blamey RW, et al. ONCOPOOL—a European database for 16,944 cases of breast cancer. Eur J Cancer. 2010;46:56–71.

12. Nejmi M, et al. Moroccan experience in palliative care. In: Silbermann M, editor. Palliative care to the cancer patient: the Middle East as model to emerging countries. Hauppaugu: Nova Science; 2014. ISBN 978-1-63117-709-5.
13. WHA resolution: strengthening palliative care as a component of comprehensive care. WHO Executive Board. WHO global action 2013–2020. WHO Department of Communications.
14. The Prague Charter "Palliative Care: a human right". European Association of Palliative Care (EAPC 2013). 2013.
15. Report 2012 WHO Collaboration Center. Pain and Policy Studies Group. University of Wisconsin. Carbone Cancer Center (USA). 2012.
16. Maamri A, et al. Cervix and breast cancers in Oujda city in Eastern Morocco: determinants and risk factors. Open J Prev Med. 2012;2(1):9–15.
17. BenAbdallah M, et al. Cancer du sein en Tunisie: Caractéristiques épidémiologiques et tendance évolutive de l'incidence. Tunis-Med Industrie. 2009;87:417–25.
18. Shapiro S, et al. Risk of breast cancer. Am J Epidemiol. 2000;151:396–403.
19. Kogevinas M, et al. Social inequalities and cancer. Lyon: IARC Scientific Publications; 1997.
20. INCA. la situation du cancer en France en 2009. Collection rapport, synthèses. Ouvrage collectif édité par l'INCA. Boulogne Billancourt. 2009.
21. Kato I, et al. A case-control study of breast cancer among Japanese women: with special reference to family history and reproductive and dietary factors. Breast Cancer Res Treat. 1992;24:51–9.
22. Boutayeb A. Social determinants of reproductive health in Morocco. Afr J Reprod Health. 2011;15:57–66.
23. Sakka F, et al. Age et vécu de la puberté chez la jeune femme Tunisienne. Tunis-Medindustrie. 2000;78:191–4.
24. Abbass F, et al. Epidemiological and biological profile of breast cancer in Fez-Boulmane, Morocco. East Mediterr Health J. 2011;17:12.
25. Chalabi N, et al. Comparative clinical and transcriptomal profiles of breast cancer between French and South Mediterranean patients show minor but significative biological differences. Cancer Genomics Proteomics. 2008;5:253–61.
26. Boufettal H, et al. Cancer du sein chez la femme jeune au Maroc. Cancer Radiother. 2010;14:698–703.
27. Abahssain H, et al. Breast cancer in Moroccan young women: a retrospective study. BMC Res Note. 2010;3:286–94.
28. Znati K, et al. Cancer du sein chez la femme jeune dans le Nord-Est du Maroc. Gynecol Obstet Fertil. 2014;42(3):149–54.
29. Merill RM, et al. Cancer prevalence estimates based on tumor registry data the Surveillance, Epidemiology and End Results (SEER) program. Int J Epidemiol. 2000;29:197–207.
30. Agarwal G, et al. Spectrum of breast cancer in Asian women. World J Surg. 2007;31: 1031–40.
31. Tazzite A, et al. Relationship between family history of breast cancer and clinicopathological features in Moroccan patients. Ethiop J Health Sci. 2013;23:2.
32. Sutherland S, et al. Inflammatory breast cancer: the Royal Marsden hospital experience. Cancer. 2010;116:2815–20.
33. Errihani H, et al. The inflammatory breast cancer-Moroccan experience. Eur J Cancer Suppl. 2008;6:76.
34. Boussen H, et al. Inflammatory breast cancer in Tunisia. Cancer. 2010;116:2730–5.
35. Nokes BT, et al. In vitro assessment of the inflammatory breast cancer cell line SUM 149: discovery of 2 single nucleotide polymorphisms in the RNase L gene. J Cancer. 2013;4:104–16.
36. The breast cancer linkage consortium. Cancer risks in BRCA2 mutation carriers. J Natl Cancer Inst. 1999;91:1310–6.
37. Collaborative Group on Hormonal Factors in Breast Cancer. Familial breast cancer: collaborative reanalysis of individual data from 52 epidemiological studies including 58209 women without the disease. Lancet. 2001;27:1389–99.

38. Sasco AJ. Breast cancer and the environment. Horm Res. 2003;60:50–9.
39. Yoshida K, et al. Role of BRCA1 and BRCA2 as regulators of DNA repair, transcription and cell cycle in response to DNA damage. Cancer Sci. 2004;95:866–71.
40. Miki Y, et al. A strong candidate for the breast cancer and ovarian cancer susceptibility gene BRCA1. Science. 1994;266:66–71.
41. Wooster R, et al. Identification of the breast cancer gene BRCA2. Nature. 1995;378:789–91.
42. Rishch HA, et al. Population BRCA1 and BRCA2 mutation frequencies and cancer penetrances: a kin-cohort study in Ontario, Canada. J Natl Cancer Inst. 2006;98:1694–706.
43. Laarabi FZ, et al. Genetic testing and first presymptomatic diagnosis in Moroccan families at high risk for breast/ovarian cancer. Oncol Lett. 2011;2:389–93.
44. Tazzite A, et al. BRCA1 and BRCA2 germline mutations in Moroccan breast/ovarian cancer families: novel mutations and unclassified variants. Gynecol Oncol. 2012;125:687–92.
45. Troudi W, et al. Contribution of the BRCA1 and BRCA2 mutations to breast cancer in Tunisia. J Hum Genet. 2007;52:915–20.
46. Cherbal F, et al. BRCA1 and BRCA2 germline mutations screening in Algerian breast/ovarian cancer families. Dis Markers. 2010;28:377–84.
47. Laraqui A, et al. Mutation screening of the BRCA1 gene in early onset and familial breast/ovarian cancer in Moroccan population. Int J Med Sci. 2013;10:60–7.
48. Chaouki N, et al. The viral origin of cervical cancer in Rabat, Morocco. Int J Cancer. 1998;75:546–54.
49. Bosch FX, et al. Prevalence of human papillomavirus in cervical cancer: a worldwide perspective. J Natl Cancer Inst. 1995;87:796–802.
50. Lalaoui K, et al. HPV DNA in cervical lesions from Morocco and its implication for cancer control. Clin Micobiol Infect. 2003;9:144–8.
51. IARC monographs on the evaluation of carcinogenic risk to humans. WHO vol. 83. 2004.
52. Sasco AJ, et al. A case-control study of lung cancer in Casablanca, Morocco. Cancer Causes Control. 2002;13:609–16.
53. Nejjari C, et al. Prevalence and demographic factors of smoking in Morocco. Int J Public Health. 2009;54:447–51.
54. Byers T, et al. American Cancer Society guidelines on nutrition and physical activity for cancer prevention: reducing the risk of cancer with healthy food choices and physical activity. CA Cancer J Clin. 2002;52:92–119.
55. Demetriou C, et al. The Mediterranean dietary pattern and breast cancer risk in Greek-Cypriot women: a case-control study. BMC Cancer. 2012;12:113.
56. Laamiri FZ, et al. Lipid profile among Moroccan overweight women and breast cancer: a case-control study. Int J Gen Med. 2013;6:439–45.

Chapter 4
The Magic of Dreams: Conflicts and Quandaries Within Multicultural Societies in Transition

Lea Baider and Gil Goldzweig

The Story of Mira and Ramzi

> He whose face gives no light, shall never become a star.
>
> —William Blake [1]

Patient: Mira—Jewish female, 36 years old, student
Husband: Ramzi—Muslim male Arab, 37 years old, religious

Background

Mira was in her first year of an M.A. program in English and Arabic Literature. She was an exceptionally bright student, and had worked as a research coordinator on several projects. She came from a middle-class background—her mother worked as a teacher and her father was a computer programmer. Her nuclear family included two teenaged sisters and a younger brother, all living in Jerusalem. Although the family was not strictly religious, a traditional atmosphere was maintained at home.

Ramzi worked as a car mechanic. His extended family, including his two older, unmarried sisters and three brothers with their families, lived together in his

L. Baider, Ph.D. (✉)
Department of Psycho-Oncology, Institute of Clinical Oncology, Assuta Medical Center, Habarzel 20, Tel-Aviv, Israel
e-mail: baider@mail.huji.ac.il

G. Goldzweig, Ph.D.
Clinical Psychology Track, School of Behavioral Sciences, Academic College of Tel-Aviv-Yaffo, Tel-Aviv, Israel
e-mail: giligold@mta.ac.il

M. Silbermann (ed.), *Cancer Care in Countries and Societies in Transition*,
DOI 10.1007/978-3-319-22912-6_4

grandfather's house in the north. They owned a restaurant in the center of the village where the family worked. The entire family professed to be religious Muslims and adhered strictly to the Quran.

Mira and Ramzi met more than 8 years earlier in an open forum focusing on equal rights, which was accessible to both Arabs and Jews. They found a common language and a common dream for an integrated Utopian society. At first they lived together. Later, they were married in a Muslim ceremony despite the blunt disapproval and resentment of both families. In keeping with Ramzi's family tradition, Mira became part of the *hamula* (Arabic term for extended family). Mira wanted to continue her studies but her wishes met with opposition from Ramzi's family, who felt she should become pregnant, produce male progeny, and take part in running the large household. Ramzi promised Mira that in just a few years, after children would be born to them, she would be able to resume her studies. Due to geographical distance, Mira seldom saw her own family but regardless of her sense of guilt for abandoning them, she stayed in telephone contact, especially with her mother.

Medical History

In December 2012, after having visited a number of family physicians in the north, Mira went for a consultation at a cancer center in a centrally located hospital, accompanied by Ramzi, her mother and her sisters. She complained of severe pain, excessive tiredness, swelling in her breast, and difficulty breathing. She was 4 months pregnant after countless miscarriages. Owing to her physical condition and the long distance from her home, she was admitted to the oncology department to facilitate a total physical examination for a clearer prognosis. According to her medical history, Mira had felt ill for more than 2 years. Upon admission to the hospital, she was weak, without an appetite and in extreme pain. Ramzi's family and Mira had assumed that her symptoms were a result of accumulated stress, pressure to become pregnant, and her sense of alienation for not providing what was expected of her. Mira referred to several instances when she had wanted to visit a family physician because of her difficulties in becoming pregnant. Ramzi's family agreed that she see the *imam* (Muslim religious leader) and the nurse of the community who had delivered all the babies in the family. Their recommendations included various medicines and herbs for her "confused soul" as well as for her pain. During the past year, Mira had felt a growth in her breast, but dismissed the possibility of a malignancy, thinking and hoping it would disappear.

Diagnosis

Stage IV, metastatic breast cancer with metastasis to spine, liver, and brain.

Medical Recommendations

Radiation therapy as a palliative measure for localized symptomatic metastasis, hormone therapy (Tamoxifen), an immediate abortion, and strong opiates for pain control.

Outcome

Ramzi and his family were fretful about the abortion procedure and distraught about losing the baby. Mira agreed to the abortion as she believed that the baby was already infected by the cancer. Ramzi's family, however, felt that the baby was their redemption for Ramzi's disobedience in marrying a non-Muslim. They met with the local *kalifa* (leader of the Muslim community, who has political and religious authority), until an agreement was reached allowing the operation. Afterwards, it was revealed that the fetus had been a boy. Ramzi was desperate, guilty, and broken in his mourning. He felt that he had killed his only son. Ramzi's family was reluctant for Mira to take strong pain medication, especially morphine.

Mira died in May in her husband's home. Her mother and two sisters were with her throughout the final week. Ramzi fasted, prayed, and cried just outside the wall of Mira's room.

I had several meetings with Mira while she was hospitalized, at which time she seemed to be living inside herself. She communicated in words of self-reflection interwoven with drowsy silences.

> Why do I have this punishment? Why did I kill my only son?… because I transgressed the religious boundaries?….I believed in co-existence and mutual understanding…I dreamed that love could surface and endure a dialogue of reconciliation and connection…My dreams have been overturned and become a punishment, my death… Why is death so total, so invincible, so powerful that it strips away every shred of human kindness and human hope?… Dying is like evaporating forever, like a wind that guides the flames of destruction without any compassion…My family and friends could not grasp my radical change of being with Ramzi…Their non-acceptance was reduced to a simple thought: "It will pass." It is like my illness that has become dormant inside my skin, and if there is no reconciliation it will destroy my body. I love Ramzi. He is a dreamer, he is kind and generous. He believes in our being together, but it was very hard and strange for his family. I remained a stranger, the outsider without an identity. Now, my illness is their premonition of shame and dishonor. My body has been punished by not bearing Ramzi's children, by not perpetuating their generations of males… Anger and frustration infiltrated his family's landscape along with their prayers, their moans and their whispers of unspoken words about my death…

Ramzi's family was obedient to their father and the male elders' judgments and decisions. To the women of the household, Mira was "different" and had learned to speak Arabic with her tongue, but not with her soul. She was not a devoted Muslim, and her prayers were not accepted by Allah. Her illness was Allah's demonstration of infinite compassion and wisdom for her mind and body.

Ramzi soothed his anguish of death through his unconditional belief in the afterlife and Paradise. Death was Allah's gift to purify Mira's life. But shadows of grief and mourning emerged from this backdrop of tapestries, painted walls, and the scent of incense. Dreading his own death and impending punishment, Ramzi became silent and withdrawn. His silence was the scream of his pain, his despair, and his loss of a thousand dreams. His prayer evolved into a doleful wail of anger, despair, and guilt. Allah had punished him for his disobedient actions, and now his mantra would forever be a credo of unconditional submission to Him, His truth, and His omnipresent wisdom.

In her wail of whispers before death, Mira begged forgiveness for the shame inflicted on Ramzi's and her own families. She hadn't fulfilled the norms of behavior according to Ramzi's family—refusing to convert to Islam, not bearing children, not reading the Quran and had also dismissed the roots of her Jewish tradition.

Mira implored her family and was granted her final wish to be buried in the old Jewish cemetery in Jerusalem, alongside her grandparents. During her childhood Mira had spent hours visiting these tombs, speaking to the souls of her grandparents and discovering the secrets of the trees. To Mira, that eternal garden of silence had belonged to her in her short life, as it did now in the infinitude of her death. She dreamt of the smell of the earth following the cries of the raindrops, the sound of water being consumed by dormant trees. As she glimpsed at an endless sky, Mira died, her face radiating the brightness of her inner life.

Now Mira had become a radiant star.

(Permission was granted by both of Mira's families to use her story. Names and identities have been completely altered to maintain privacy. Translated from the patient records of L. Baider.)

Intercultural Realities in a Transforming World

Due to globalization, there is an ever-increasing number of countries and societies which can be described as multiethnic or multicultural. Modern societies are characterized as pluralistic, open, and diverse. People from dissimilar origins, cultures, and languages live together or in distinct communities within the same geographic area. A multicultural society poses challenges relevant to every aspect of human life notwithstanding health and health care services, such as overcoming differences in cultural beliefs concerning health, illness, and medication compliance as well as language barriers. Health care practitioners and policy makers face an enormous task in providing effective health care in any multiethnic environment [2].

Given these challenges we propose three fundamental guidelines for health care professionals:

1. Cultural diversity should be respected.
   Respecting cultural diversity implies more than treating individuals as equals, it encourages health care professionals to strive for a fuller understanding of cultural and ethnic differences. Health care providers must understand that the basic values of Western medicine, such as patient autonomy, are not necessarily shared

by patient-families of all cultural backgrounds [3]. Health care providers should seek knowledge about the communities they serve ("cultural competence") while being reflective about their own values and cultural beliefs, and how these shape the care they provide ("cultural humility") [4]. In the last decade, a substantial number of epidemiological cancer studies have been categorized as Cross-Cultural Collaborative Epidemiological (CCCE) studies [5], in addition to those studies which address epidemiological issues from a cultural perspective [6, 7]. In view of these trends, it is clear that every analysis of data—individual data deriving from a patient interview or epidemiological data resulting from large community surveys—would not be considered complete without allowing for the full cultural context.

2. Proper balance between respect for diversity and "common ground" (i.e., equivalent treatment for all) should be achieved.
   Generally speaking, medical treatment is moving in the direction of individually tailored therapies. This personalized approach takes into account the biological, behavioral, and genetic factors influencing the interindividual variability in drug response. Proponents of this approach point to its potential for maximizing drug efficacy and minimizing toxicity [8]. Nonetheless, there are limitations to this approach in the area of psychosocial interventions. Individual manuals for each problem area and patient may result in difficulties in researching, integrating, and implementing therapy protocols [9]. It is desirable to achieve a proper balance between diversity and "common ground." Race or ethnicity may no longer serve as a reliable base for common ground and for studying variation in health, as there are more genetic variations within racial groups than between races and many persons undeniably belong to multiple race categories. Then again, the concept of culture may have positive explanatory power for the differences in health behavior and health outcomes than race and ethnicity [10]. In the context of health behavior, Pasick and D'Onofrio (cited Egede, L.E. 2006) [10] define culture as "unique shared values, beliefs and practices that are directly associated with a health-related behavior, indirectly associated with a behavior, or influence acceptance and adoption of the health education message." This definition may set the scale for balancing individually tailored therapy and respect for diversity with a "common ground" approach. Both practitioners and researchers may then be able to seek the common beliefs and values concerning health, sickness, and disease that influence personal health behavior.
3. Conflicting cultural backgrounds and beliefs may be used as leverage for achieving better quality of life.
   Conflict may carry the potential for positive development [11] and similarly, cultural conflict doesn't necessarily lead to devastating results. A well-managed conflict resolution may lead to reconciliation, mutual understanding and more pluralistic views and beliefs by conflicting parties [12]. Societies with "built-in" mechanisms (political and religious institutions or rules and norms) for managing conflicts are possibly better able to accommodate cultural conflicts and resolutions. Societies with conflicts between population subgroups, extreme norms of religious behavior, unstable demographic outcomes and conflicts

regarding values and family traditions are more likely to live in fragile stability with an ever-present threat of unresolved conflicts (as in the clinical vignette about Mira and Ramzi, where resolution was only possible in the aftermath).

Israel as an Example

Israel can be described as an amalgamation of cultures, religions, and people from different origins spread over an area of 21,643 km^2 with a density of 353.1 people per km^2 [13]. In fact, Israel can serve as a laboratory for studying cultural conflicts.

At the beginning of 2013, the total population of Israel was 7,984,500 people, with 91.4 % considered "urban," as almost half the population is concentrated in 14 large cities. The population is relatively young when compared to other Western countries, with a relatively high number of children per family (the 0–14 age group constitutes 28.2 % of the population; the 65+ age group constitutes 10.4 % of the population; while the average number of individuals per family is 3.72). Age at first marriage is relatively low (27.5 for men; 24.7 for women) and the total fertility rate is 3.05, i.e., higher than the world average [14].

The data presented above draws a complex picture of Israeli society. On the one hand, it is similar in many respects to traditional societies (higher rates of children per family, lower age at first marriage, etc.). On the other hand, according to many standard rankings, Israel is more comparable to developed Western countries. The standard of living in Israel is considered relatively high: ranking 19th among 187 nations on the United Nation's Human Development Index, with high rankings in education and health and low (3.5) infant mortality rates [15].

Looking at population subgroups in Israel, the picture becomes more complex: The Israeli Central Bureau of Statistics [13] reports that Jews (including small percentages of non-Arab Christians and undefined groups) make up 79.4 % of the Israeli population and Arabs total 20.6 %. The Arab population is subdivided into Muslims (84.3 %), Druze (8 %), and Christians (7.7 %). More than three million immigrants of Jewish origin arrived in Israel since its establishment in 1948. Roughly one-third of these immigrants were born in Africa or Asia (approximately half were born in the former USSR), while two-thirds were born in Europe or America [13].

Muslim Arab families are larger than Jewish families (34 % of Arab families number six persons or more in comparison to only 9 % of Jewish families). The majority of the Arab population lives in the northern regions of Israel in Arab villages and cities, in close proximity to extended family.

Among Jews aged 20+, 9.4 % define themselves as Ultra-Orthodox, 9.9 % as Orthodox, 36.2 as traditional, and 43.9 % as secular. Among Muslims and Christians, 8.5 % defined themselves as very religious, 47.3 % as religious, 25.6 % as not so religious, and 18.4 % as not religious at all [16].

Relating the Israeli Demographic Data to Cultural Conflict

The mixture of countries of origin, religions, and levels of religiosity is fertile soil for cultural conflict revolving around diverse aspects of life, from everyday differences and restrictions (regarding food, music, dress code, and literary topics), to lifecycle events (marriage, birth, and death) and traditional practices and customs. For example, formal marriage in Israel can only be performed under the auspices of the religious community to which the couple belongs, as civil marriage does not exist in Israel. The religious authority for Jewish marriage is the Chief Rabbinate of Israel and the rabbinical courts, while Muslim marriages are conducted in accordance with Islamic law and customs. Couples who choose to marry outside of Israel are registered as officially married upon their return to Israel.

Given the tense and unstable situation between Israel and the Palestinian population, the neighboring Arab countries and the threat of terror and war, the Israeli population finds itself constantly exposed to death threats. The Terror Management Theory predicts that under such circumstances individuals will identify more with their cultural worldview which serves as a buffer against the perceived threat [17–19]. Thus, in Israel groups may live within walking distance of each other and even speak the same language, yet maintain very high cultural barriers between themselves. Under these conditions, even a simple physician–patient encounter is a prospective cultural conflict, for example, in the case of an Ultra-Orthodox Jewish male patient, who normally avoids being alone with a woman, who finds himself alone with an Arab female physician in the general practitioner's room.

Percentagewise, the demographic data may offer insight into the complexity and cultural diversity of the Israeli population, but it is only through the lens of Mira and Ramzi's story, that the true nature and consequences of cultural conflicts can be discerned. Mira and Ramzi shared a common dream of an idealistic and integrated society. The first crack to appear in their dream was their marriage, which due to the complex religious-legal situation in Israel, was a religious. Muslim ceremony, predictably resented by both families. Mira became physically and culturally separated from her family by crossing the line from traditional Jewish culture into traditional-religious Muslim culture. As part of her new culture she was expected to live with the extended family and bear children. (As mentioned above, many Arab families live in Arab cities and villages in northern Israel, many with an average younger age of first marriage and with more children per family than Jewish families.) Yet when facing a life-threatening illness such as cancer, Mira found herself isolated from any social support, one of the most salient predictors of lower distress rates among cancer patients [20]. Living in constant pain and at-risk for death, she dismissed any strong extra-cultural worldview as a lost dream. Towards the end of her life, Mira seemed ambivalent about Ramzi's culture and values. On the one hand, she was labeled a "bad wife" for her inability to produce male children; nonetheless she desired the acceptance and recognition of Ramzi's family. The chasm between these perceptions caused her desperation and total frustration.

Israel: Cancer Epidemiology

Cancer: According to the last update of the Israeli National Cancer Registry [21], the age-standardized incidence per 100,000 for all invasive cancers were higher among Jews (250.9 for men; 255.3 for women) than for Arabs (218.9 for men; 175.8 for women). The rates for Jewish men were lower than the rates for Jewish women, while the rates for Arab men were higher than those for Arab women. The standardized death rates per 100,000 were higher among men (114 for Arab men; 97.9 for Jewish men) than for women (81.8 for Jewish women; 60.2 for Arab women). Among men, higher death rates were found for Arab men and among women, higher rates were found among Jewish women.

Smoking: According to the Secretary of Health's 2012 Report on Smoking in Israel [22], there are higher standardized smoking rates (for adults 21+) among Israeli Arabs (24.9 %) than among Israeli Jews (19.8 %). The gender specific smoking rates are 23.7 % for Jewish men, 15.9 % for Jewish women, 43.8 % for Arab men and 6.7 % for Arab women.

Breast Cancer: Although the last decade has seen a decrease in incidence of breast cancer among Jewish and Arab women, according to the 2011 Israeli National Cancer Registry [21], breast cancer constitutes 31 % of cancer incidence among women in Israel. Eighty-seven percent of newly diagnosed women were Jewish, while 8 % were Arab. In 2011, age-standardized incidents per 100,000 were 90.1 for Jewish women and 57.1 for Arab women. The risk for very young women (up to age 34) is similar for both Arab and Jewish women, but in all other age categories the risk is lower for Arab women. The 5-year survival rate for Jewish women with breast cancer was 87.2 % and 78.4 % for Arab women.

Israeli Data and Culture

Understanding the epidemiological data regarding cancer vis-à-vis cultural diversity calls for very cautious interpretations based on relating the epidemiological data to the demographic data as well as to cultural norms. The cancer data presented above leaves room for more questions than answers. For example, the fact that breast cancer incidences among Muslim Arab women are lower than those of Jewish women, but survival rates are higher for Jewish women, may point to problems in screening and treatment of Arab women. Are Arab women screened any less or at different stages for cancer? To what extent is this due to the concentration of Arab families in the north, while centralized health centers are less accessible? To what extent is it related to the cultural attitude toward cancer? Behavior observed among our own patients, for example, indicates that Ultra-Orthodox Jews consider cancer a curse which should not be named nor spoken of. Is this likewise true of traditional Arab women? Answers to these questions must be sought so that the relationship between cultural norms and behavior towards cancer can be better comprehended.

Given the disparity in cancer rates between Jewish and Arab women it may have been difficult for Ramzi's family to acknowledge that Mira was sick. His family was less familiar with cancer symptoms and less receptive to the possibility of screening and therapy, all of which accentuated Mira's feelings of isolation.

In order to fully understand the statistics of the epidemiological and demographic data in relation to cultural diversity, it is vital that data collection be designed to take cultural diversity into account. Items relating to cultural values and beliefs concerning health must be included in any health care survey. With these three components in place—demographic data, epidemiological data, and data concerning cultural health behavior—the delicate work of correlating these three outcomes to each other can begin. A fully reliable picture can only be achieved with cultural openness and sensitivity to all systems of belief, norms, and behaviors.

Constraints and Opportunities in the Changing Middle East

When the disease has advanced to the point where the patient's condition has worsened despite massive amounts of medical and spiritual support, the challenge for the physician will be to predict futility while at the same time decreasing the patient's and their caregiver's suffering. In order to minimize potential conflicts, health care professionals should become aware of the complex attitudes and the perception process of terminal illness and end-of-life issues [23].

The Institute of Medicine's yearly seminal report, "Unequal Treatment," cites prior experiences of discrimination, bias, prejudice, and mistrust in the health care system as specific factors which influence patient health and family health care behaviors. The report posits that these mechanisms play a role in health care disparities across all multicultural populations. Health care providers note that families and social groups who undergo medical care which is incongruent with their beliefs and values show signs of cultural conflict and ethical concern, with subsequent nonadherence to medical recommendations [24, 25].

The American Medical Association Council of Ethics and Judicial Affairs [26] recommends that all involved professionals collaborate in the following paradigm:

- Establish boundaries for futility, usually in the early stages of illness and throughout prognosis and death
- Establish goals for treatment according to need, expectations, and cultural acceptance
- Involve consultants and patient–family representatives holding divergent views with the goal of facilitating and clarifying discussion about diagnosis and prognosis
- Mediate via institutional medical committees and families to make recommendations when disagreements or conflicts are irresolvable

Von Gunten et al. [27] provide a conceptual model of communication process with five basic factor analyses:

- Prepare for the discussion with relevant family and community groups
- Establish what the patient–family knows and is prepared to know
- Clarify how information will be handled and disseminated within the patient–family—prioritize by whom, to whom, and when
- Respond to emotions, fears, doubts; show compassion to the patients and families and respect their silences
- Discuss goals for care and treatment priorities corresponding to mutual cultural understandings of all partners

As is the case with the Middle East, many societies are becoming increasingly multiethnic and multicultural. The patient's system of beliefs and health rituals may appear "unscientific" and contradictory in comparison to Western medicine. There is a risk of misunderstanding and conflict, particularly, when medical systems have ingrained and inconsistent values which collide with the family's traditional cultural background [28, 29].

Studies found that patient–family caregivers have a high demand for information during all stages of the disease. Thus, delivering clear and truthful information to patient-families concerning health care is a relevant component in preventing conflicts [30]. Not only is it important to communicate knowledge effectively to patients, but health care professionals must understand that the very concept of knowledge varies across cultures [31].

Furthermore, Carey and Cosgrove [28] discuss cultural issues surrounding end-of-life care and urge medical providers to be aware of the variations and differences in patient–family cultural values throughout the process of illness and health.

A more recent systematic review on the topic of perception looked at 51 studies which described significant discord between patients, families, and health care professionals, in regard to their perception of information provided to them. More importantly, there was a significant discrepancy between the patient's stated understanding and awareness of his medical condition and the health care professionals' perceptions of the patient's perspective. The same study found that health care professionals often underestimated the patient–family need for information [32, 33].

Grace et al. [34] compared Asians with Western populations and found that Asians were more likely to externalize responsibility for the disease, reporting general life circumstances as the principal cause in comparison to internalized responsibility by Western groups. Nonetheless, both groups cited an internal belief that it was their destiny to suffer cancer. Magical and religious beliefs influencing the incidence of disease are possibly common among patients with a terminal prognosis; however, such beliefs have often been strongly fuelled by an irrational fatalism. Fatalism was often portrayed as just and congruent with cultural beliefs, attributing illness to specific events or agents beyond the physical condition of the body. Interestingly, even patients with a family and genetic history of cancer and an appreciation for the biological mechanisms of the disease often mentioned God and fate as being ultimately responsible for their illness and death [35].

Ludwig et al. [36] described the female participants who expressed a strong sense of fatalism concerning personal health risks and early ageing, as normal and inevitable. Causal attributions were influenced by fatalistic approaches to health and the uptake of health behaviors, always strictly defined by cultural or religious beliefs. Patients with a distinct intergenerational family history of cancer tended to view their diagnosis as "inevitable fate," and were convinced they could do nothing to avoid the onset of their condition, diagnosis, and prognosis [37].

A relevant summary of views encompassing terminal illness has been presented in *The Lancet* [38–42], where Buddhist, Christian, Hindu, Islamic, and Jewish viewpoints are represented. The article examines how families can integrate their systems of beliefs, taboos, and rituals within the framework of secular and religious health care initiatives.

Systems of belief assume a very relevant status affecting and influencing the individual's private and social life. The individual is enmeshed within his own family group, sect, or community, as religion continues to dictate a crucial role in collective lives [43]. The Middle East, birthplace of the three monotheistic faiths—Judaism, Christianity, and Islam—plays a crucial, symbiotic, and unconditional role in the behavior of generations of families and community life [44]. Significant issues in the Middle East, such as the authority of patrilineal families, the question of ethnicity, the relevance of identity, the nature of tribal and clan solidarity, the key role of family relationships, and the salience of norms concerning honor and shame, are embedded within the geographical and sociocultural context.

According to Jewish tradition, the land, the people, and the *Torah* (the totality of Jewish teaching, culture, and practice) are inseparable. The Torah advocates respect for all of humanity and educates in favor of free-will rather than submission and hope rather than fatalism. None of these values can be isolated. In Islam, the Quran dictates—both temporally and spiritually—a total reverence and submission to God and to the people within the Islamic *ummah* (nation). The centrality of these systems of belief can ideally be tapped for conflict resolution as well as for policymaking.

There is a correlative relationship and cohesion between a system of authority and its doctrine. The system of authority infers and sometimes distances the rulings from the doctrine. In Islam, the essential chore of religious authority is to demonstrate belief in the divine laws of the Quran. The prophet substantiates the intention of "Allah, the Exalted." The divine doctrine determines the boundaries of the words, deeds, life and death, goals and means of attaining these goals [42].

In contrast to the Western notion of free choice and freedom from constraints ("freedom to do"), Islam accentuates existential freedom ("freedom to be"). The dignity of the individual is actualized through his service to the family, within the broader context of human solidarity [45]. The Islamic perspective affirms cultural pluralism, communal obedience, social justice, and unconditional faith. Strong emphasis is placed on linkages between personal and group identity, between the individual and the collective and the achievement of restorative justice within the context of utter submission to family and religious norms of conduct [46].

Family in Islam is dominated by the powerful authority retained by patriarchy in the sphere of decision-making. The father's authority in the family is an integral part of the overall authoritative system. Patriarchal authority maintains the genealogical cohesiveness of the family and of the social system of life [47].

Health care is rife with cultural differences and potential for conflict. The most intimate events of our lives—reproduction, birth, and death—draw us into the health care system and expose our most fundamental attitudes, values, and beliefs. More generally, concepts of health and disease and expectations regarding the behavior of families with an ill or suffering member are suffused with assumptions and values reflecting culturally distinct views of relationships with others, with the world and with a "transcendent order." Health care ethics now face the increasingly important challenge of determining how to handle conflicts that may be deeply embedded in diverse cultural and religious outlooks on life and the world [48].

Cultural factors also determine how people describe their illness and symptoms, resulting in diverse accounts and possibly divergent treatments for the same disease. As religious values and beliefs are intricately linked to cultural norms and practices, they definitively shape a patient's ideas about health and illness, influence expectations of encounters with health care providers, affect adherence to doctors' recommendations, guide medical decision-making, and influence health outcomes. Religion and spirituality also directly affect psychological and physical health, for they influence coping strategies, health behaviors, and health care-seeking attitudes [49].

Systems of Belief in the Middle East

An unfamiliar, imposed cultural environment has as much influence over individual perception of threat as quantitative outcomes of demographic-racial disparities. Given the relationship of threat and tolerance, the general expectation is that high levels of threat will contribute to lower overall tolerance levels. In their groundbreaking work, Coser [50] and Simmel [51] argue that social groups respond with hostility to "alien" conditions, especially those threatening group cohesion. Simmel [51] describes the traditional group reactions to intended threats as the perception of internal danger by the remainder group, aggravated by the existence of a new situation. Internal threats, particularly those posing a danger to social order, foster internal cohesion within the family group [52]. The mere existence of other social groups with similar systems of belief validates one's identity as projected onto one's cultural worldview [53].

When confronted with emotionally laden values and beliefs, individuals and families, Jews, Muslims, and Christians perceive and react differently in situations of terminal illness and death. Recognizing the differences in values and behaviors can generate a deeper understanding of why the overlap of moral and religious areas creates conflict. One group's fundamental and cherished assumptions about their norm of conduct may differ radically from the values held by another group.

Likewise, families may have differing standards of truth and integrity and will question opposing answers to fundamental moral and ethical dilemmas [54].

Family emotions, e.g., shame, anger, and distrust, and taboo subjects which are not open for discussion, exploration, or mutual resolution are often the cause of "covert" conflict [55]. A determinant of social perceptions of reality is a socially inherited and shared culture as well as learned ways of living, as retained by families and subgroups. Conflict across cultural boundaries also appears across cognitive and perceptual boundaries, and is especially susceptible to problems of intercultural and interfaith miscommunication and misunderstanding [56].

In the Middle East, rigidity, fear, and rejection of flexibility among extremely religious families have the potential to destroy any new encounter, system of communication, or dialogue. Families may differ as to the meaning of their beliefs and their normative behaviors, however imposing artificial homogeneity, is to insist that only our culture-specific truths are authentic, while all others are deviations [57].

The Pursuit of Visionary Dreams

> The darkest places in life are reserved for those who maintain their neutrality in times of moral crisis.
>
> –Dante Alighieri, The Divine Comedy [58]

Is our devotion and attachment to our beliefs so vulnerable that they need to be protected? In most families our beliefs provide powerful meaning to our existence. They may be regarded as religious credos or eclectic ideological worldviews. They provide a path and a breadth of scope illuminating what is relevant in life. What were the expectations of Ramzi's family regarding Mira's pursuit of enduring support? Cultural identity provides a conception of what is true, valued, and accepted within the diverging social groups. It encompasses our central beliefs and attitudes about the world and what is most important in our inter- and intra-family relations. It imbues the universe with meaning and stability [59].

Cultural identity could be described as the norms, beliefs, rituals, and traditions by means of which one engages with one's environment. Self-perception underlies the notion of identity, a pivotal component of the social-cultural model. Mira's self-perception provides the lens through which she viewed others and interpreted their views about her.

Culture minimizes anxiety and provides an orderly conception of the universe that imbues the world with coherence and permanence. This familiar world provides a reservoir of shared norms congruent with the collective family identity. Culture links individual and collective identities, binding them together emotionally and defining clear boundaries between diverse social groups [60].

Mira didn't belong. Her dual identities were blurred with ambivalence, fears, and the frustration building bridges supported by pillars of vanishing sand. Mira didn't belong and Ramzi could not accept their deteriorating dreams of family reconciliation and integration.

As people from diverse cultural and ethnic backgrounds attempt to relate, opportunities for conflict proliferate concerning their beliefs, values, and perceptions of reality.

If respect and adherence for cultural diversity is the proper response, what are the limits of this tolerance or cultural sensitivity? If, on the contrary, deference to the views of the majority may legitimately be demanded, what justifies a "cultural imposition"?

End or Beginning? Open Dialogue in the Middle East

> Whatever occurs between these beginnings and ending is the narrative of people lives, the events that can offer up meaning only when configured out of their chaos into some kind of temporal and familiar order.
>
> –A. Makarenko, Road to Life, 1955 [61]

We do not live in this world as isolated fragments, but as parts of a larger, dynamic, and mutable universal culture. Culture, as a shifting and dynamic set, has oriented us to particular ways of thought and action. The ethics of palliative care in the Middle East is a moral imperative for interactive dialogue [62].

Society has a multiplicity of cultures, each imposing and commanding what is considered normal and acceptable according to their distinct criteria. When others do not meet the expected social behavior of care within their society, it confirms that their individual cultures and beliefs are different from and alien to the expected norms [63].

Cultural diversity is an essential part of conflict and conflict-resolution, and is a powerful and piercing influence on our perceptions and behavior. Cultural diversity operates as a series of lenses that shape our perception, interpretation, cognitions, and values [64].

Conflict is often perceived as a symptom of the need for change. While conflict can lead to separation, hostility, civil strife, and terrorism, it can also stimulate dialogue and fairer and socially just solutions, i.e., the pursuit of a more moral, pluralistic, and free society. It can lead to stronger and compassionate relationships and open interactive encounters [65].

Schartz and Hage [66] described an interconnected model concerning the perception of moral dilemmas:

- Clarify the values and ethical norms of behavior and how they might conflict with each other. It is useful to understand what values, principles, or guidelines are involved and how they may have been violated or misunderstood by any of the interacting persons.
- Identify the primary interacting people to be affected by the conflict or dilemma. Before rendering a decision it is crucial to understand who is affected by the situation, and who will be affected by any behavioral action.
- Consider the needs and moral values of the most vulnerable family groups. Some groups require more protection than others due to their isolation, fragility, and vulnerability.

- Recognize the multiple constructions of reality involved in the conflict. Be flexible to the diversity of perceived reality by all the interacting people.
- Give all involved parties an opportunity to express their views despite disagreements. Talk to each other, do not withdraw.

Diversity of cultural and religious interactions could become an open tapestry of unfolding views in which there is deep respect for differences and equally intentional openness to the possibility of connection with the other. This connection embodies an encounter that Chapman [67] has called "sacred encounters." It is making a meaningful connection where a person feels accepted, valued, respected, and honored [68]. Creating and developing sacred encounters between patients and health care professionals does not require more science, but it does require the knowledge and feeling of empathy, flexibility, respect, and unconditional presence! Your presence of care!

References

1. Blake W. Proverbs of hell. The Marriage of Heaven and Hell. 1757–1827.
2. Bhopal RS. Ethnicity, race, and health in multicultural societies: foundations for better epidemiology, public health and health care. Oxford: Oxford University Press; 2007.
3. Deiss R. Ethics and multiculturalism in the patient-physician encounter. Virtual Mentor. 2007;9:523–6.
4. Tervalon M, Murray-Garcia J. Cultural humility versus cultural competence: a critical distinction in defining physician-training outcomes in multicultural education. J Health Care Poor Underserved. 1998;9:117–25.
5. Lam TH, Leung GM. Geoethnic-sensitive and cross-cultural collaborative epidemiological studies. Int J Epidemiol. 2003;32(2):178–80.
6. Zeeb H, Spallek J, Razum O. Epidemiological perspectives of migration research: the example of cancer. Psychother Psychosom Med Psychol. 2008;58:130–5.
7. Sighoko D. Ethnic and geographic variations in corpus uteri cancer burden: evidence based on data from 29 states and the District of Columbia. C15 IX, X and SEER data (1998–2010). Cancer Causes Control. 2014;25:1197–209.
8. Ross S, Anand SS, Joseph P, Pare G. Promises and challenges of pharmacogenetics: an overview of study design, methodological and statistical issues. JRSM Cardiovasc Dis. 2012;1(1):5.
9. Garland AF, Hawley KM, Brookman-Frazee L, Hurlburt MS. Identifying common elements of evidence-based psychosocial treatments for children's disruptive behavior problems. J Am Acad Child Adolesc Psychiatry. 2008;47:505–14.
10. Egede LE. Race, ethnicity, culture, and disparities in health care. J Gen Intern Med. 2006; 2:667–9.
11. Calhoun LG, Tedeschi RG., editors. Handbook of posttraumatic growth: research & practice. Mahwah: Lawrence Erlbaum Associates; 2006.
12. Dessel AB, Dessel NB. Arab/Jewish intergroup dialogue courses: building communication skills, relationships, and social justice. Small Group Res. 2012;43:559–86.
13. Israeli Central Bureau of Statistics. Israel in figures. Tel-Aviv-Yafo, Israel. 2013.
14. United Nations, Department of Economics and Social Affairs, Population Division. Population estimates and projections sections. http://esa.in.org/unpd/wpp/Excel-Data/fertility.htm. Accessed Nov 2014.
15. United Nations Human Development Programme. Human development reports. http://hdr.undp.org/en/content/exporting-data-and-understanding-api. Accessed Nov 2014.

16. The Central Bureau of Statistics. Statistical Abstracts of Israel. No. 65. Tel-Aviv-Yafo, Israel. 2014.
17. Asbrock F, Fritsche I. Authoritarian reactions to terrorist threat: who is being threatened, the me or the we? Int J Psychol. 2013;48:35–49.
18. Bassett JF, Connelly JN. Terror management and reactions to undocumented immigrants: mortality salience increases aversion to culturally dissimilar others. J Soc Psychol. 2011;15:117–20.
19. Burke BL, Martens A, Faucher EH. Two decades of terror management theory: a meta-analysis of mortality salience research. Pers Soc Psychol Rev. 2010;14:155–95.
20. Goldzweig G, Hasson-Ohayon I, Meirovitz A, et al. Agents of support: psychometric properties of the Cancer Perceived Agents of Social Support (CPASS) questionnaire. Psychooncology. 2010;19:1179–86.
21. State of Israel Ministry of Health. Update of incidence and mortality data for 2011 and presentation of relative cancer survival data in Israel 1991–2010, International cancer day 2011, National Cancer Registry. 2011. http://www.health.gov.il/PublicationsFiles/ICR_18032014.pdf
22. State of Israel Ministry of Health. Secretary of Health Report on Smoking in Israel (in Hebrew). 2012. http://www.health.gov.il/PublicationsFiles/smoking-2012.pdf
23. Campinha-Bacote JC. Delivering patient-centered care in the midst of a cultural conflict. Online J Issues Nurs. 2001;16(5):1–11.
24. NSW (New South Wales) Health Department. Guidelines for end-of-life care and decision-making. Gladesville: Better Health Centre—Publications Warehouse; 2005. ISBN: 0 7347. http://advancecareplanning.org.au/library/uploads/documents/nsw/NSW_end_of_life_care.pdf
25. Wehbe-Alamah H. Bridging generic and professional care practices for Muslim patients through use of Lenninger's culture care modes. Contemp Nurse. 2008;28(1–2):83–97.
26. American Medical Association Council on Ethical and Judicial Affairs. Medical futility in end-of-life care. Report of the Council on Ethical and Judicial affairs. J Am Med Assoc. 1999;281(10):937–41.
27. Von Gunten CF, Ferris FD, Emanuel LL. Ensuring competency in end-of-life care: communication and relational skills. JAMA. 2000;284(23):3051–7.
28. Carey SM, Cosgrove JF. Cultural issues surrounding end-of-life care. Curr Anesth Crit Care. 2006;17(5):263–70.
29. Rao AS, Desphande OM, Jamoona C, Reid CM. Elderly Indo-Caribbean Hindus and end-of-life care: a community-based exploratory study. J Am Geriatr Soc. 2008;56(6):1129–33.
30. Parker SM, Clayton JM, Hancock K, Walder S, Butow PN, Carrick S, et al. A systemic review of prognostic/end-of-life communication with adults in the advanced stages of a life-limiting illness: patient/caregiver preferences for the content, style, and timing of information. J Pain Symptom Manage. 2007;34(1):81–93.
31. Baider L, Goldzweig G. Islamic culture in the Middle East: a glimpse into illness and death. In: Silbermann M, editor. Palliative care to the cancer patients: the Middle East as a model to emerging countries. New York: Nova; 2014. p. 53–64.
32. Hancock K, Clayton JM, Parker SM, Walder S, Butow PN, Carrick S. Discrepant perceptions about end-of-life communication: a systematic review. J Pain Symptom Manage. 2007;34(2):190–200.
33. Baider L, Surbone A. Cancer and the family: the silent words of truth. J Clin Oncol. 2010;28:1269–72.
34. Grace C, Begum R, Subhani S, Kopelman P, Greenhalgh T. Prevention of disease in Bangladeshis: qualitative study of community, religious, and professional perspectives. Br Med J. 2008;337:1094–7.
35. Farooqi A, Nagra T, Khunti K, Edgar T. Attitudes to lifestyle risk factors for coronary heart disease amongst South Asians. Fam Pract. 2000;17:293–7.
36. Ludwig AF, Cox P, Elahi B. Social and cultural construction among Muslim women in North West England. Public Health Nutr. 2011;4:1–9.

37. Baider L. My illness, myself: on the secrecy of shame. Asian Pac J Cancer Prev. 2010;11:59–62.
38. Dorff EN. End-of-life: a Jewish perspective. Lancet. 2005;366:862–5.
39. Englehardt Jr HT, Ilitos AS. End-of-life: the traditional Christian view. Lancet. 2005;366:1045–9.
40. Keown D. End-of-life: the Buddhist view. Lancet. 2005;36:952–5.
41. Markwell H. End-of-life: a Catholic view. Lancet. 2005;366:1132–5.
42. Sachedina A. End-of-life: the Islamic view. Lancet. 2005;36:774–1132.
43. Giddens A. Modernity and self-identity: self and society in the modern age. Palo Alto: Stanford University Press; 1991. p. 204.
44. King-Irani LE. Kinship, class and ethnicity; strategies for survival in the contemporary Middle East. In: Gerner D, editor. Understanding the contemporary Middle East. Boulder: Lynne Rienner; 1999. p. 309–44.
45. Irani GE, Funk NC. Ritual of reconciliation: Arab Islamic perspectives. Arab Stud Q. 1998;20(4):53–73.
46. Dallmayar FR, editor. Border crossings: toward a comparative political theory. New York: Lexington Books; 2000.
47. Sharabi H. Neopatriarchy: a theory of distorted change in the Arab society. New York: Oxford University Press; 1998.
48. Larson DB, Larson SS, Koenig HG. Mortality and religion/spirituality: a brief review of the research. Ann Pharmocother. 2002;36(6):1090–8.
49. Koenig HG. Research on religion, spirituality, and mental health: a review. Can J Psychiatry. 2009;54(5):283–91.
50. Coser LA. The functions of social conflict. Glencoe: The Free Press; 1956.
51. Simmel, G. Conflict. Translated by K. H. Wolff. Glencoe: The Free Press; 1955. p. 97.
52. Kafka F. The metamorphosis. 2nd ed. New York: Schocken Books; 1969.
53. Howard, G. Speaking of difference: reflections on the possibility of culturally competent conversation. New Horizons Learn Online J. 2003:9(2). http://www.ghequityinstitute.com/gh_articles/speaking_of_difference.pdf. Accessed 28 Nov 2014.
54. Bartos O, Wehr, P. Using conflict theory, vol. 41. New York: Cambridge University Press; 2000. p. 40–6.
55. Satish M. Formulating a new tree energy framework of personality for conflict analysis. J Hum Values. 2014;20:153–65.
56. Docherty JS. Learning lessons from Waco: when the parties bring their gods to the negotiation table. Syracuse: Syracuse University Press; 2001. p. 310.
57. Drury S. Response to Right Rev. Peter Short and Dr. Bisson. Religion is about life. SIPP. 2008. Briefing Note May 14 2006, 9. http://www.schoolofpublicpolicy.sk.ca/_documents/outreach_event_announcements/SIPP_archived_publications/SIPP_briefing_notes/BN14.pdf. Accessed 29 Nov 2014.
58. Alighieri D. The divine comedy of Dante Alighieri (Borders Leatherbound Classics. New York: Borders Classics; 2004.
59. Cushman F, Young L. The psychology of dilemmas and the philosophy of morality. Ethical Theory Moral Pract. 2009;12(1):9–24.
60. Ross MH. Culture and identity in comparative political analysis. In: Burgess G, Bergess H, editors. Comparative politics: rationality, culture, and structure. New York: Cambridge University Press; 1997. p. 42–80.
61. Makarenko A. Road to life, vol. 1, 2nd ed. Moscow: Foreign Language Publishing House; 1955. p. 56
62. Salzburg S. Lovingkindness: the revolutionary art of happiness. Boston: Shambhala; 1995.
63. Hutchison ML. Tolerating threat. J Confl Resolut. 2014;58(5):796–824.
64. Malek, C. A family's journey from Armenia to Syria and back again. Guernica: Magazine of Art and Politics; 2013. https://www.guernicamag.com/features/enduring-exile/
65. Bar-Tal D. Socio-psychological foundations of intractable conflicts. Am Behav Sci. 2007;50:1430–53.

66. Schartz J, Hage S. Prevention: ethics, responsibility, and commitment. In: Kenny M, Horne A, Orpinas P, Reese L, editors. Realizing social justice: the challenge of preventative interventions. Washington, DC: American Psychological Association; 2009. p. 123–40.
67. Chapman E. Radical loving care. Nashville: Baptist Healing Hospital Trust; 2005.
68. O'Grady L, Jadad A. A shifting from shared to collaborative decision-making: a change in thinking and doing. J Particip Med. 2010;8:2–13.

Chapter 5
Modeling Integrative Oncology for the Arab Population in Northern Israel

Eran Ben-Arye and Jamal Dagash

Sociocultural and Lifestyle Challenges in the Israeli Arab Population

The Arab population in Israel is characterized by a rich mosaic of communities distinguished by religious, social, and cultural elements. Arabic-speaking Israeli citizens include Muslims, Christians, and Druze who together constitute the largest minority group in Israel (according to the 2014 Census, about 1.7 million), comprising roughly 20.7 % of the country's total population [1]. This large and diverse population is often defined by the Israeli political establishment as "Israeli-Arabs" based on their right to Israeli citizenship, as opposed to Palestinian communities residing outside the sovereign borders of Israel (e.g., about 77 % of the world's population of Palestinians are residing in the West Bank, Gaza Strip, Arab, and non-Arab countries) [2]. There is considerable agreement that Arabs in Israel represent a distinctive population group compared with both the Jewish Israeli

E. Ben-Arye, M.D. (✉)
Integrative Oncology Program, The Oncology Service and Lin Medical Center, Clalit Health Services, Haifa and Western Galilee District, 35 Rothschild St., Haifa 35152, Israel

Complementary and Traditional Medicine Unit, Department of Family Medicine, Faculty of Medicine, Technion-Israel Institute of Technology, Haifa, Israel
e-mail: eranben@netvision.net.il

J. Dagash, M.D.
Integrative Oncology Program, The Oncology Service and Lin Medical Center, Clalit Health Services, Haifa and Western Galilee District, 35 Rothschild St., Haifa 35152, Israel

Complementary and Traditional Medicine Unit, Department of Family Medicine, Faculty of Medicine, Technion-Israel Institute of Technology, Haifa, Israel

Palliative Care—Home Care Hospice, Clalit Health Services, Haifa and Western Galilee District, Haifa, Israel

M. Silbermann (ed.), *Cancer Care in Countries and Societies in Transition*,
DOI 10.1007/978-3-319-22912-6_5

population and the Palestinian population outside Israel and other Arab countries. This unique social-cultural identity, which originated as a result of the 1948 War, has generated an impressive sociocultural and lifestyle transition, manifested in population morbidity, health outcomes and life expectancy [3], including the arena of oncology.

In 2006, the Middle East Cancer Consortium (MECC) published a comprehensive monograph of its Cancer Registration Project concerning cancer incidence during the period of 1996–2001 in four of its six member countries (Cyprus, Egypt, Israel, and Jordan) [4]. The authors reported that overall incidence of cancer was substantially higher in the Jewish-Israeli and the US Surveillance, Epidemiology, and End Results Program populations, compared with the Israeli-Arab population (assessed with intermediate rates) and with Cypriots, Egyptians, and Jordanians. Overall age-standardized incidence rates per 100,000 population was 274 in Israeli Jews compared with 149 in Israeli-Arabs, 143 in Egyptians, and 113 in Jordanians. Nevertheless, studies published in the last decade in Israel indicate a dramatic surge in cancer incidence of Israeli-Arabs who had until recently been regarded, along other Arab communities, as having a lower cancer risk. Keinan-Boker and her colleagues (2013) examined breast cancer trends in Israeli Jewish and Arab women and reported that from 1996 to 2007, the incidence of invasive breast cancer increased by 98 % for Arab women while simultaneously decreasing by 3 % for Jewish women [5]. The authors observed that breast cancer mortality rates remained stable in Israeli-Arab women while significantly decreasing in Jewish women. In the past decade, a similar trend of increased cancer incidence in the Israeli-Arab population, compared with the Jewish population, has been reported in left-sided colorectal [6] and gastric [7] cancer.

Aiming to explain the increase in cancer prevalence among the Israeli-Arab population, researchers hypothesized a correlation with environmental factors, particularly lifestyle changes characterizing the sociocultural metamorphosis the Arab community has been experiencing between traditional and westernized lifestyles and health models. Although evidence for the linkage between lifestyle and cancer incidence in the Israeli Arab population is limited, several studies suggest a probable correlation. A case control study conducted in northern Israel revealed a significant inverse association between a Mediterranean diet and cancer prevalence in Arab participants [8]. Probable lifestyle changes were also hypothesized by researchers reporting on altered incidence and sites of colorectal cancer in the Israeli Arab population [6] and of an increase in lung cancer incidence among Israeli Arab men without evidence of increased smoking prevalence [9]. Other potential cancer-associated lifestyle changes yet to be probed in the Arab community in Israel include stress-related modernized settings, a tendency towards distancing from traditional codes and familial bonding, and gender-associated elements (e.g., attenuation of protective factors in breast cancer such as younger age of motherhood and breastfeeding).

Traditional and Complementary Medicine in the Israeli Arab Population

Complementary medicine use among Arabs in Israel is predominantly related to traditional medicine, mostly herbs used for centuries with the aim of healing and ameliorating acute as well as chronic diseases. Traditional Muslim medicine, at times regarded as Greco-Islamic medicine [10], is rooted in historical Middle-Eastern schools of medical practice (ancient Egyptian, Mesopotamian, Greek, and Persian medicine) and influenced by the great East Asian medical schools of Chinese and Ayurvedic medicine in India. In the Middle Ages, Islamic medicine mediated between the Western and Eastern medical cultures and integrated hundreds of indigenous Mediterranean and Middle-Eastern herbs within a medical practice enriched by remedies brought from Europe and the Far East. The use of herbs was complemented by spiritual practices and manual techniques including massage and cupping.

Although complementary and traditional medicine (CTM) use is highly prevalent in the Israeli-Arab population as well as in other Middle Eastern Arab and Muslim societies, the line between **traditional** (*al tibb al-taklidi*), **alternative** (*al tibb al-badil*), and **complementary** (*al tibb al-mukamel*) concepts of medical care is often indistinct. In practice, many herbs are used in the Arab diet or regarded as an integral part of the Arab culture. Thus, a common herb like sage (Salvia fruticosa mill) is frequently used throughout the year as a beverage but may also be applied to cure specific ailments such as abdominal pain. Aiming to explore the prevalence of CTM use (for medicinal purposes) in the Israeli-Arab population, researchers studied perspectives of 2184 Arabic-speaking patients (Muslims, Christians, and Druze) attending primary care clinics in northern Israel. Arab and Jewish respondents reported comparable overall CTM use during the previous year (above 40 %), but Arab respondents reported greater use of herbs and traditional medicine [11]. This high prevalence of CTM use reported in primary care was also documented among Arab patients confronted with cancer diagnosis and treatment. A study of 324 Arab patients in the oncology setting revealed that nearly 40 % of patients reported CTM for cancer-related outcomes [12]. Moreover, CTM use was correlated with active chemo/radiotherapy treatment and a higher degree of spiritual quest. As in the primary care setting, herbal medicine was the prominent CTM modality of choice (reported by nearly 90 % of CTM users). In the present study, more than 80 % of respondents supported integration of a complementary medicine consultant within the oncology department mainly to improve their quality of life (QOL) including gastrointestinal symptoms, fatigue, and pain, alleviating chemotherapy's side effects and enhancing their coping with the disease.

Challenges of CTM Integration in Arab Patients with Cancer in Israel

Patients' expectation to integrate complementary medicine within their conventional supportive cancer care is shared by many patients worldwide in various phases of cancer treatment, be it active treatment for local disease (e.g., surgery, chemotherapy, radiotherapy, hormonal, and biological treatments), during surveillance, or palliative care for widespread metastatic cancer. In the past decade, leading oncology centers in the US and Europe have integrated complementary medicine services within conventional care settings aiming to provide evidence-based consultation and treatments to improve patients' QOL [13, 14]. A new paradigm of integrative oncology has been introduced calling for improved patient-doctor dialogue on CTM use, a nonjudgmental patient-centered approach, and the need to ensure the safety of complementary practices (e.g., avoiding risk of detrimental herbal supplement/chemotherapy interactions) [15, 16].

In 2008, an Integrative Oncology Program (IOP) was launched as a free-of-charge clinical service within the Clalit Health Organization's oncology service at the Lin Medical Center (Haifa, Israel) aspiring to improve patients' QOL during chemotherapy and advanced disease state [17]. Patients are referred by their oncology care practitioners (oncologist, oncology nurse, or psycho-oncologist) to an initial consultation with integrative physicians (IPs) dually trained in conventional care and CTM. Typical IP assessment includes evaluation of patient's expectations regarding CTM, previous CTM experience, and QOL status. The session concludes with an outlining of the treatment goals followed by construction of a treatment plan tailored to the patient's expectations, concerns, and health belief model, level of scientific evidence (efficacy, safety, possible interactions with chemotherapy, etc.), and feedback of the patients' oncologist, family physician, nurse, and psycho-oncologist. Patients are typically scheduled for weekly integrative treatments that may include herbal medicine and nutritional counseling, mind-body and manual therapies, spiritual care, acupuncture, Anthroposophic medicine, and other CTM modalities. Prior to therapeutic sessions, an additional clinical assessment is conducted, aimed to modify, if necessary, the treatment goals and plan. Concluding QOL assessments are performed during initial and follow-up visits aiming to monitor patients' concerns, changes, and impact of the integrative treatment on their well-being.

In the first years of the IOP's activity, more than 500 patients were referred to IP consultations. Yet, compared with Jewish patients, the number of referred Arab patients was significantly smaller and continuity of integrative care was achieved more rarely. Attempting to identify barriers to optimal integrative care in Arab patients, the IOP practitioners analyzed a cohort of 15 patients monitored through a registry protocol [18]. The main barriers identified included the following: (1) limited oncology care practitioners' referral to IP consultation; (2) patient-related factors (e.g., patients expecting CTM to "cure" them rather than "just" improve their QOL); (3) factors determined by the medical institution (e.g., geographical factors that limit Arab patients' access to the IOP service; limited patient–practitioner communication due to the small number of Arabic-speaking practitioners within the oncology service and the IOP team).

Aiming to identify better potential barriers to optimal integrative treatment for Arab patients with cancer, IOP researchers initiated additional studies targeting three stakeholders: (1) patients (compared cohorts of Israeli-Arab cancer patients from northern Israel and Palestinian cancer patients from the town of Nablus, in the Palestinian Authority) [19]; (2) oncology practitioners and researchers from seven Middle Eastern countries [20, 21]; and (3) Israeli-Arab CTM providers experienced in treatment of Arab patients with cancer [22–24]. The three angles of exploration suggested repeatedly an inevitable need to base an integrative oncology model for Arab patients on a cross-cultural perspective. In contrast to the individual-oriented perspective emphasized in integrative oncology centers in the West (patient-centered approach), we perceived a need for a supplementary community-oriented approach that would also address the unique bio-psycho-cultural-religious-spiritual dimension of patients from distinct Arab communities. In the following sections, we wish to illustrate the daily challenges we confront with Arab patients in our integrative oncology setting in Haifa and to suggest strategies to integrate a patient-tailored approach attuned with the patient's and caregivers' cultural, community, and health care model.

Manal: Between Individual and Collective Values in the Christian-Arab Society

Manal, a 56-year-old married woman, was referred by a nurse oncologist to an integrative oncology consultation aiming to alleviate emotional distress prior to administration of chemotherapy (Adriamycin and Cytoxan) scheduled the same morning in the oncology department. Manal had been recently diagnosed with local breast cancer but was advised to receive neo-adjuvant chemotherapy prior to surgical lumpectomy. The initial consultation was provided by an IP, a family physician trained in complementary/integrative medicine, and a spiritual care provider who assessed Manal's expectations and concerns, seeking to co-identify treatment goals and construct a preliminary treatment program. Assessment of the patient's narrative and health belief model revealed a sense of transformational experience. Manal, who until recently had experienced good health and a promising career as a senior academic lecturer, felt that the new cancer diagnosis did not only challenge her well-being but also focused her attention inwardly to "my body that now demands attention." During the following appointments, the IP reassessed Manal's concerns, focusing on chemotherapy-induced fatigue, nausea, and the metallic taste in her mouth. Integrative treatment included consultations on herbal medicine and nutrition, some of which were familiar to Manal as an Arab-Christian from traditional Arab medicine and the Palestinian cuisine (e.g., Carob paste to alleviate mouth sores), and weekly acupuncture sessions combined with manual therapy and discussions with the spiritual care provider. Following 6 weeks, an interim IP assessment documented a moderate aggravation of pain, fatigue, nausea, and sleep, possibly related to the increasing impact of the third chemotherapy cycle on the patient's well-being. In contrast to her seemingly deteriorating well-being, Manal regarded her situation as "*the best thing in life*" and characterized the integrative treatment as "*medical support that gives me energy and hope.*" The gap between the formal QOL questionnaires based on visual analogue scales and Manal's documented narrative illustrates one of the important challenges in the integrative clinical setting: a need for a bio-psycho-social-cultural approach enabling better assessment of the therapeutic process. The interaction between Manal, the IP, and the spiritual care provider reflects, on the one hand, a patient-practitioner dialogue focusing on Manal's individuality and striving to tailor the treatment plan to the patient's concerns. However, on the other hand, Manal is an individual active in a broader society of an Arab minority in Israel encountering the tension between traditional collective identity and a more Western call for individuality. In this context, Manal does not represent merely herself as an individual but also carries collective values that may impact her expectations towards integrative treatment as well as her readiness and openness to assess her physical and emotional concerns during the first IP evaluation. A qualitative assessment tool is highly essential in this cross-cultural context, in addition to quantitative questionnaires aiming to expose the subtextual realm of therapy. With this in mind, Manal's main expectation along the weekly integrative treatments was "*to strengthen myself*" rather than merely alleviate cancer-related fatigue. The integrative treatment supported Manal in her quest for healing through the vale of "*death that encircles me*," by acknowledging her journey as an individual, woman, mother, and academic leader in a transforming Arab society where she encounters an interplay of collective and individual values. In this context, Manal represents a group of independent, highly educated Arab women who can quite easily relate to integrative medicine of the kind that is offered within the oncology service at the Lin Medical Center in Haifa.

Salwa Facing Compliance and Adherence to Integrative Care

Salwa is a 54-year-old Muslim woman, residing in a remote Jewish town following her divorce, although recently she was spending more and more time with her daughter and grandchildren who live in a large Arab village. Similar to Manal, Salwa was diagnosed with localized breast cancer but received chemotherapy in an adjuvant setting following breast surgery. Despite similarities in oncological status, initial IP assessment revealed a dissimilar picture of the two women's symptoms. Salwa is unemployed, with poor socioeconomic status and a mere elementary school education. Her main concerns following chemotherapy included severe fatigue, nausea, insomnia, and decreased appetite but, additionally, she suffered from severe emotional turmoil. Following cancer diagnosis, she felt that "*if it is cancer I would gladly rid myself of this life.*" Despite declaring non-religiosity,

Salwa started "wearing a wig instead of a hijab [traditional Muslim woman's headscarf]" and disclosed, "I believe that what has happened to me, with the cancer, is God's will and that I need to handle the challenge He has given me." Unlike many other Muslim patients, Salwa reported no previous or current experience with herbs or alternative and traditional medicine. Although she was willing to listen to IP consultation on herbal and nutritional use and to experience acupuncture, a follow-up assessment documents low to no compliance to herbal supplement intake and non-optimal continuity of care (every 3–4 weeks instead of recommended weekly sessions). Six weeks following initial assessment most QOL parameters were deteriorating and debilitating, with no change for the better. Summarizing her impression (through qualitative narrative assessment), Salwa stated, "*I cannot say if the treatments have helped me, but still I expect some physical and emotional improvement as a result of these treatments.*" Hoping to identify the barriers for optimal continuity of care, the IP asked Salwa what might encourage her to attend regular, more frequent appointments and suggested a complete makeover of the therapeutic program. During the next 6 weeks, Salwa attended weekly acupuncture sessions combined with manual and breathing techniques and spiritual care consultations. The next IP assessment documented an improvement in pain, fatigue, drowsiness, depression, anxiety, sleep, and well-being. The dramatic shift in the therapeutic relationship of Salwa with the integrative practitioners surrounds not only the theme of compliance. Adherence to integrative care is a better way of conceptualizing Salwa's compliance. As opposed to compliance that focuses on the individual's willingness to experience a remedy or to attend regular visits, adherence of patients like Salwa depends also on external factors (remote geographical distance, limited accessibility due to financial restraints or non-availability of caregivers) and psychological resistance to therapy that may be related to Salwa's lack of familiarity with "peculiar modalities" (e.g., acupuncture in this particular cultural setting) or an integrative approach incongruent with Salwa's health-belief model. Recognizing these barriers provided the key to improving the patient's compliance and adherence to integrative care leading eventually to her improved QOL, despite the progressive schedule of ongoing chemotherapy cycles. In her struggle to achieve continuity of integrative care, Salwa shares the challenges of many other Palestinian Arab women from traditional, low socioeconomic status in Israel who have limited accessibility to health care as a result of residing in outlying areas, having economic limitations and/or non-availability of caregivers.

Amal and Her Caregiver: Facing Irritability Following Chemotherapy

Amal is a 46-year-old Druze woman living with her husband and their three children in a rural Druze village in northern Israel. Amal continues working as a bank clerk despite chemotherapy cycles prescribed every 3 weeks for locally advanced breast cancer. At the beginning of the IP consultation, Amal described her rich experience with CTM including acupuncture, reflexology, and massage. Following cancer diagnosis, she began drinking pomegranate juice and honey, a lemon-based bitter juice to improve nausea, and an herbal decoction of Ephedra foeminea recommended by other cancer patients in her village. Although Amal reported moderate nausea and fatigue, her leading concern was the irritability she experienced during the week following chemotherapy. She said, "*I have 'a short fuse,' every word someone utters bothers me. Please explain the situation to my husband.*" The integrative treatment plan suggested by the IP included herbal consultation (e.g., augmenting the anti-nausea effect of the lemon juice by adding freshly ground ginger), recommendations for moderate physical activity, and a variety of weekly integrative treatments including acupuncture, massage, and music therapy. Additionally, the IP recommended discontinuing the Ephedra use, which not only lacks scientific evidence for effectiveness in cancer care, but was also found, in an in-vitro study conducted by the IP and colleagues, to inhibit the specific chemotherapy Amal was being treated with. Amal's adherence to integrative care was excellent and included 8 sessions in the first 6 weeks of treatments. In a follow-up IP assessment, Amal reported significant improvement in symptoms that included headache, irritability, depression, anxiety, fatigue, and nausea. The patient-IP rapport was successful, despite the geographical barrier, and intensified through the active support of the patient's caregiver. Amal viewed her personal involvement in the therapeutic process as a "*struggle to expel the chemical substances from my body without relating to the cancerous lumps*; *to think rationally rather than emotionally.*" Amal illustrates in this case the role of an assertive and decisive woman, supported by her caregiver and family; she is well versed and experienced in CTM use and can benefit from nonjudgmental integrative consultation aimed towards "separating the wheat from the chaff" based on updated research and listening openly to her expectations and narrative.

Mustafa Challenged with Palliative Integrative Care

Mustafa, a 60-year-old married man, had been facing life-threatening medical deterioration along the previous 10 years that included CVA, myocardial infarction, and lately a grave diagnosis of stage IV gastric cancer with liver metastasis. Mustafa was referred to IP consultation by his nurse oncologist who indicated severe hiccups and constipation following palliative chemotherapy of cisplatin and gemcitabine. Though never having used CTM before, Mustafa began exploring any and every available venue to find CTM remedies that would hopefully provide cure. Alarmed by thoughts of his two brothers who had died of cancer in recent years and of his sister who had just been diagnosed with cancer, Mustafa purchased 15 expensive nutritional supplements recommended by a Jewish alternative healer who also advised him on major nutritional changes. In addition, he travelled to the outskirts of his neighborhood to pick fresh leaves recommended for cancer cure by patients from the Palestinian Authority, in order to prepare a fresh potion of this herbal remedy daily.

Along the first 6 weeks of integrative care, including IP consultations on nutritional aspects and informed use of herbal supplements, Mustafa received nine integrative treatments, often three times a week. At first, he reported a significant improvement in nausea and constipation for the 24 h following acupuncture. In some of the sessions, acupuncture was combined with music therapy, guided imagery, and spiritual counseling, allowing Mustafa to shed a tear and share his emotional concerns including anger and frustration: "*Settling accounts with God: first CVA, then MI, and now cancer. Why*?!" In a follow-up assessment, Mustafa reported, "*I leave the room calmer and feeling less pain; feeling better mentally and also in terms of fatigue, but the improvement lasts only two days at the most and then the pain and the feelings gradually intensify*." Following the first weeks of integrative treatments, Mustafa's condition deteriorated despite palliative chemotherapy and overwhelming supportive care. Adherence to integrative treatments declined and the "magic touch" of the integrative effort lost its charm. Mustafa suspected that some of the prescribed supportive remedies, conventional and herbal alike, were in fact increasing his fatigue and pain. On one occasion he associated deterioration in kidney function with acupuncture needles that had been inserted in previous sessions. Attempting to gain an additional perspective on Mustafa's condition, the IP gave a feedback questionnaire to the nurse oncologist who had first initiated Mustafa's referral to integrative care. The nurse wrote, "Mustafa is in a state of great anxiety and repeatedly speaks of his symptoms. Undoubtedly, with your help it is easier to treat him and address his needs; he is making fewer demands on me, and he seems to be calmer."

Mustafa's case illustrates some challenging barriers to optimal integrative treatment during palliative care when physical, emotional, and spiritual concerns are intensified and existential fear floods the daily encounter with QOL issues. Mustafa represents archetypal communicational challenges with an Arab male undergoing palliative care who cannot guarantee continuous adherence to integrative care and faces significant difficulty in voicing his anxiety when confronted by an existential threat. Therapeutic success in this setting is a multi-dimensional concept that enlightens and enhances patients' and caregivers' quality of life from a rich bio-psycho-social-familial-cultural-spiritual prism of supportive care.

Concluding Remarks and Recommendations

Modeling an integrative oncology approach for the Arab population in northern Israel is a challenging task requiring a cross-cultural perspective and nonjudgmental approach. Integrative physicians and practitioners need to approach Arab patients from an individual perspective aspiring to tailor patient-centered therapy based on the patients' expectation, needs, and concerns. At the same time, the patient-centered approach should be complemented by acknowledging the patient's sense of connectedness to his/her sociocultural community. The interplay of individual and collective identity forms the patient's health belief model which also entails affinity towards traditional and complementary medicine. The dramatic transition from traditional to modern Western lifestyle and values impacts patients from different communities (Muslim, Christian-Arab, or Druze) and specifically determines the quest for CTM in patients facing cancer diagnosis and treatment. Thus, we recommend viewing the integrative oncology approach with Arab patients as a continuum of care rather than one single IP consultation. Along this continuous process, integrative physicians and practitioners need to consider their patients' needs and co-define treatment goals with the patient, caregiver, and the entire team of care providers in the oncology department. Next, modeling of the integrative treatment plan should address the patient's perspective with research-based knowledge on the effectiveness of specific CTM modalities pertaining to QOL improvement and safety issues, mainly concerning potential interactions of herbal and non-herbal nutritional supplements with chemotherapy.

We recommend that IPs and cancer care practitioners specifically relate to the following aspects in the treatment of an Arab patient facing active oncology treatment:

- Focusing anamnesis on CTM use for cancer-related outcomes (including intent to enhance QOL and alleviate specific chemotherapy side effects) as well as for general CTM use for non-cancer indications. CTM-use screening should specifically deal with herbal use.
- Exploring the patient's perspective on the role of CTM in cancer care (alternative, complementary, or integrative context) and their expectations of integrative care
- Use of culturally valid assessment questionnaires concerning QOL status and psycho-spiritual well-being echoing Arab health-belief models (rather than translated questionnaires lacking sociocultural validation)
- Tailoring of the integrative treatment plan should include not only evidence-based research, effectiveness, safety, and cost issues but also compliance and adherence considerations. The therapeutic plan may be modeled as a multi-step intervention that starts with more acceptable CTM interventions (e.g., herbal and nutritional counseling) and progresses, as therapeutic trust grows, to less familiar modalities (e.g., acupuncture, guided imagery, and spiritual counseling).
- Modeling an integrative care program should also take into account personnel considerations as to the composition of the integrative practitioners' team (e.g., gender, MD vs. non-MD professional background, Arabic vs. non-Arabic speaking practitioners).
- Integrative treatment should also focus on the patient's caregiver, the family's needs, and the patient's social-cultural-spiritual aspects in the context of his/her community)
- Integrative physician communication with the patient's entire team of health care providers (oncologist, family physician, nurse oncologist, psycho-oncologist, etc.) is essential through the entire process of integrative care provision, from providers' referrals to therapeutic plan construction and feedback.

Last but not least, we do not purport having optimal skills which enable us to overcome barriers to integrative care with Arab patients with cancer. Recognizing the existence of barriers in everyday common practice may inspire and lead us to better attend to our patients' needs. At the end of day, the interplay of recognizing the barriers and making sincere nonjudgmental efforts to overcome them is not only gratifying but also empowering to our own resilience as attentive practitioners privileged to accompany our patients along their journey.

Acknowledgment Thanks to Marianne Steinmetz for editing the chapter.

References

1. Central Bureau of Statistics, Government of the State of Israel. 2014. http://www.cbs.gov.il/publications14/yarhon0914/pdf/b1.pdf. Accessed 15 Oct 2014.
2. Kanaaneh AR. Birthing the nation: strategies of Palestinian women in Israel. Oakland: University of California Press; 2002.
3. Na'amnih W, Muhsen K, Tarabeia J, Saabneh A, Green MS. Trends in the gap in life expectancy between Arabs and Jews in Israel between 1975 and 2004. Int J Epidemiol. 2010;39(5):1324–32.
4. Freedman LS, Edwards BK, Ries LAG, Young JL, editors. Cancer incidence in four member countries (Cyprus, Egypt, Israel, and Jordan) of the Middle East Cancer Consortium (MECC) compared with US SEER. NIH Pub. No. 06-5873. Bethesda: National Cancer Institute; 2006.
5. Keinan-Boker L, Baron-Epel O, Fishler Y, Liphshitz I, Barchana M, Dichtiar R, Goodman M. Breast cancer trends in Israeli Jewish and Arab women, 1996–2007. Eur J Cancer Prev. 2013;22(2):112–20.
6. Rozen P, Rosner G, Liphshitz I, Barchana M. The changing incidence and sites of colorectal cancer in the Israeli Arab population and their clinical implications. Int J Cancer. 2007;120(1):147–51.
7. Lavy R, Kapiev A, Poluksht N, Halevy A, Keinan-Boker L. Incidence trends and mortality rates of gastric cancer in Israel. Gastric Cancer. 2013;16(2):121–5.
8. Idilbi NM, Barchana M, Milman U, Carel RS. [Mediterranean diet in cancer patients and cancer free adult Arabs in Israel—a case-control study]. Harefuah. 2013;152(7):385–8, 435.
9. Tarabeia J, Green MS, Barchana M, Baron-Epel O, Ifrah A, Fishler Y, Nitzan-Kaluski D. Increasing lung cancer incidence among Israeli Arab men reflects a change in the earlier paradox of low incidence and high smoking prevalence. Eur J Cancer Prev. 2008;17(4):291–6.
10. Zaid H, Silbermann M, Ben-Arye E, Saad B. Greco-arab and islamic herbal-derived anticancer modalities: from tradition to molecular mechanisms. Evid Based Complement Alternat Med. 2012;2012:349040.
11. Ben-Arye E, Karkabi K, Karkabi S, Keshet Y, Haddad M, Frenkel M. Attitudes of Arab and Jewish patients toward integration of complementary medicine in primary care clinics in Israel: a cross-cultural study. Soc Sci Med. 2009;68(1):177–82.
12. Ben-Arye E, Massalha E, Bar-Sela G, Silbermann M, Agbarya A, Saad B, Lev E, Schiff E. Stepping from traditional to integrative medicine: perspectives of Israeli-Arab patients on complementary medicine's role in cancer care. Ann Oncol. 2014;25(2):476–80.
13. Deng G. Integrative cancer care in a US academic cancer centre: the Memorial Sloan-Kettering Experience. Curr Oncol. 2008;Suppl 2:s108.es68–71.
14. Frenkel M, Cohen L, Peterson N, et al. Integrative medicine consultation service in a comprehensive cancer center: findings and outcomes. Integr Cancer Ther. 2010;9(3):276–83.
15. Deng GE, Cassileth BR, Cohen L, Gubili J, Johnstone PA, Kumar N, Vickers A; Society for Integrative Oncology Executive Committee, Abrams D, Rosenthal D, Sagar S, Tripathy D .Integrative oncology practice guidelines. J Soc Integr Oncol. 2007;5(2):65–84.
16. Ben-Arye E, Schiff E, Zollman C, Heusser P, Mountford P, Frenkel M, Bar-Sela G, Lavie O. Integrating complementary medicine in supportive cancer care models across four continents. Med Oncol. 2013;30(2):511.

17. Ben-Arye E, Schiff E, Shapira C, Frenkel M, Shalom T, Steiner M. Modeling an integrative oncology program within a community-centered oncology service in Israel. Patient Educ Couns. 2012;89(3):423–9.
18. Ben-Arye E, Steiner M, Karkabi K, Shalom T, Levy L, Popper-Giveon A, Schiff E. Barriers to integration of traditional and complementary medicine in supportive cancer care of Arab patients in northern Israel. Evid Based Complement Alternat Med. 2012;2012:401867.
19. Ben-Arye E, Hamadeh A, Schiff E, Jamous RM, Dagash J, Jamous R, Agbarya A, Bar-Sela G, Massalha E, Silbermann M, Ali-Shtayeh MS. Compared perspectives of Arab patients in the Palestinian Authority and Israel on the role of complementary medicine in cancer care. J Pain Symptom Manage. 2015;49(5):878–84.
20. Ben-Arye E, Schiff E, Hassan E, Mutafoglu K, Lev-Ari S, Steiner M, Lavie O, Polliack A, Silbermann M, Lev E. Integrative oncology in the Middle East: from traditional herbal knowledge to contemporary cancer care. Ann Oncol. 2012;23(1):211–21.
21. Ben-Arye E, Ali-Shtayeh MS, Nejmi M, Schiff E, Hassan E, Mutafoglu K, Afifi FU, Jamous RM, Lev E, Silbermman M. Integrative oncology research in the Middle East: weaving traditional and complementary medicine in supportive care. Support Care Cancer. 2012;20(3):557–64.
22. Popper-Giveon A, Schiff E, Hatem D, Samuels N, Ben-Arye E. One hand cannot clap-a study of Arab Practitioners of traditional and complementary medicine in Israel: identifying barriers to integrative oncology care. Explore (NY). 2014;10(6):364–71. pii: S1550-8307(14)00151-7.
23. Popper-Giveon A, Schiff E, Samuels N, Ben-Arye E. Women supporting patients, men curing cancer: gender-related variations among Israeli arab practitioners of traditional medicine in their treatment of patients with cancer. J Immigr Minor Health. 2015;17(3):737–45.
24. Popper-Giveon A, Schiff E, Ben-Arye E. We and they in the house of healing: debate among Arab complementary medicine practitioners on an integrative versus alternative approach to supportive cancer care. Integr Cancer Ther. 2013;12(6):488–95.

Chapter 6
Cancer Care in Palestine

Akram T. Kharroubi and Rania Y. Abu Seir

and when I am sick, then He restores me to health

Ash-Shu'araa, Sura 26 Verse 80

Introduction

In this chapter, the current status of cancer care describes the care provided for the Palestinians living in the West Bank and Gaza. The Palestinians living in East Jerusalem are usually treated in Israeli hospitals and not in Palestinian hospitals located in East Jerusalem because they are covered by the Israeli health insurance. Therefore, the statistics are somehow misleading because the population of the Palestinians living in East Jerusalem is accounted for, but the number of cancer patients in that area is not. Therefore, the term "Palestinians" in this chapter refers to the Arab population in the West Bank and Gaza and "cancer in Palestine" refers to cancer in this Palestinian sector excluding Palestinians living in East Jerusalem who are treated routinely in Israeli hospitals. Data about cancer care in Gaza is limited and most of the data was acquired from the study of Abed [1], and information about cancer care facilities is coming from Abou Amer [2] and interviews of head of oncology departments of Gaza hospitals.

Epidemiology

Over the last century and like many other developing countries, Palestinians have been undergoing a demographic and epidemiologic transition characterized by rapid urbanization and changing lifestyles and further by a persistent burden of

Dedication
To Jerusalem, my beloved home town.
To Palestinian cancer patients who died because they had no access to treatment.

A.T. Kharroubi, Ph.D. (✉) • R.Y. Abu Seir, Ph.D.
Department of Medical Laboratory Sciences, Faculty of Health Professions, Al-Quds University, Jerusalem, Palestine
e-mail: akram.kharroubi@gmail.com; abusear@staff.alquds.edu

M. Silbermann (ed.), *Cancer Care in Countries and Societies in Transition*,
DOI 10.1007/978-3-319-22912-6_6

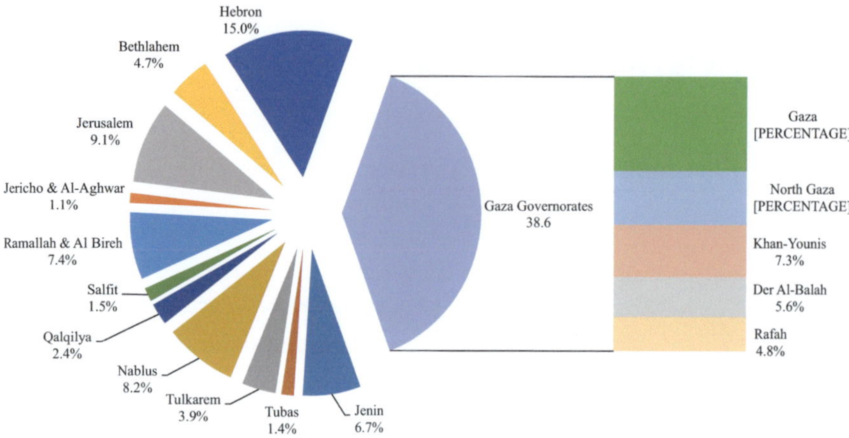

Fig. 6.1 Distribution of the Palestinian Population by governorates, Palestine, 2013. *Source*: Data from Ministry of Health Report, Palestine, 2013

infectious diseases and an increase in noncommunicable (chronic) diseases such as cancer [3].

In 2013, the Palestinian population was approximately 4.5 million distributed between the West Bank (61.4 %) and Gaza (38.6 %). The regional distribution of the population was 24.1 %, 17.6 %, and 19.7 % in the north, middle, and south of the West Bank, respectively (Fig. 6.1). Males accounted for 50.8 % of the population and female accounted for 49.2 % with approximately 39.9 % of the population was under the age of 15 years and 2.9 % aged above 65 years indicating a young population in comparison to the western countries. According to the Palestinian Central Bureau of Statistics (PCBS), in 2013, 26 % of West Bank residents were predicted to live in rural areas compared with 40 % in the year 2006 and 62 % in the early 1990s confirming the demographic transition in the Palestinian society [4].

Cancer in the West Bank and Gaza is considered to be the second most common cause of mortality in 2013 and is increasingly becoming a public health concern. A total of 2189 new cancer cases were reported in 2013 in the eleven governorates in the West Bank (Fig. 6.2), with 51 % of all cases were females and 49 % were males. Most of the incident cases were reported in the Northern regions (87.9 cases per 100,000) followed by the southern (85.7) and then the middle regions (61.0) [5].

Figure 6.3 shows the increase in cancer incidence rates with increasing age among both males and females as people in age groups of 50 years and older had much higher risk of cancer compared to the age group of less than 50 years [5].

Furthermore, the available data from the Ministry of Health reports showed high but fluctuating incidence rates between 2000 and 2011 (Fig. 6.4) but a sharper increase in the trend was observed after 2011. This increase was noticed among both genders and in most regions.

Lung cancer is reported to be the most commonly diagnosed cancer among men with an incidence rate of 13.2 cases per 100,000 men, followed by colon cancer

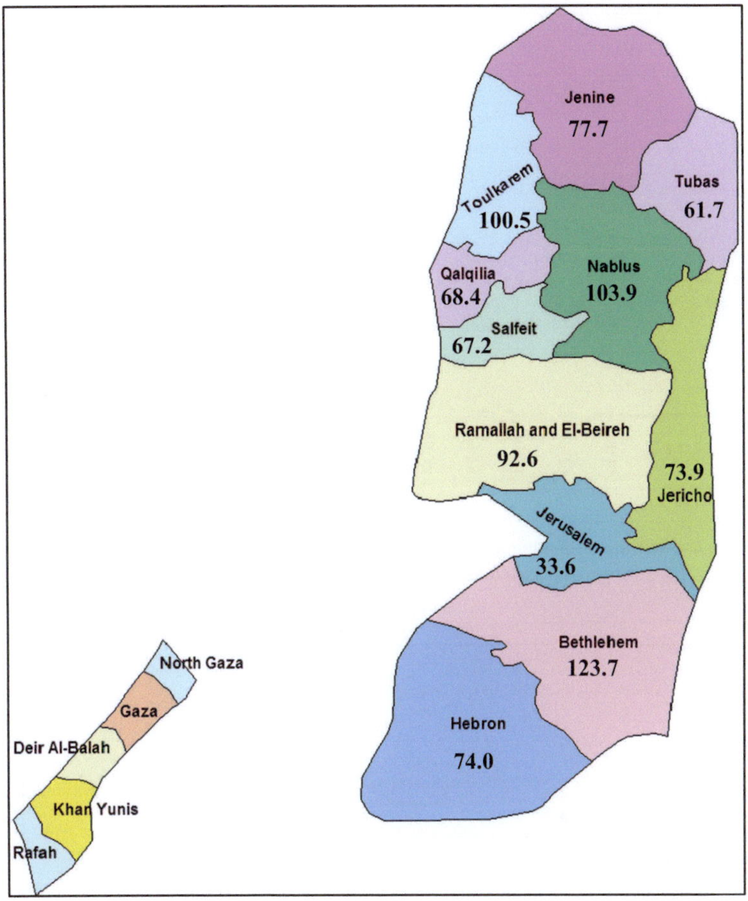

Fig. 6.2 Incidence rates of cancer (per 100,000) in the West Bank governorates in 2013. *Source*: Data extracted from the Ministry of Health Report, Palestine, 2013

(8.9), leukemia (5.8), bladder cancer (5.6) and brain cancer (4.9). Breast cancer is the most commonly diagnosed cancer among women with an incidence rate of 29.4 cases per 100,000 women, followed by colon cancer (8.3), leukemia (4.0), brain cancer (3.4) and thyroid cancer (3.3). Among children less than 15 years old, leukemia is the most common cancer with an incidence rate of 2.6 cases per 100,000 children, followed by brain and nervous system cancers (1.3) and then bone cancer (0.6) (Fig. 6.5) [5].

A total of 6879 deaths were recorded in the death registry in the West Bank in 2013 with cancer mortality accounted for 13.3 % of total deaths. Cancer mortality pattern in the West Bank showed a slight decrease between 2000 and 2006 then a slight increase with fluctuations between 2006 and 2013 (Fig. 6.6). Lung cancer was the most common cause of cancer deaths (17.9 % from total cancer deaths) in 2013, followed by colon cancer (15.2 %) and then breast cancer (9.1 %) (Fig. 6.7) with

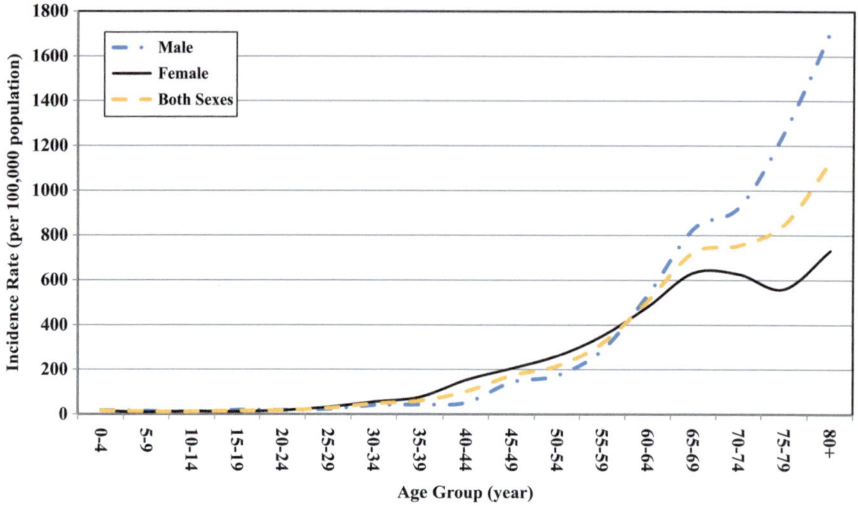

Fig. 6.3 Distribution of incidence rates by age for both sexes, males and females, West Bank, Palestine, 2013. *Source*: Data extracted from the Ministry of Health Report, Palestine, 2013

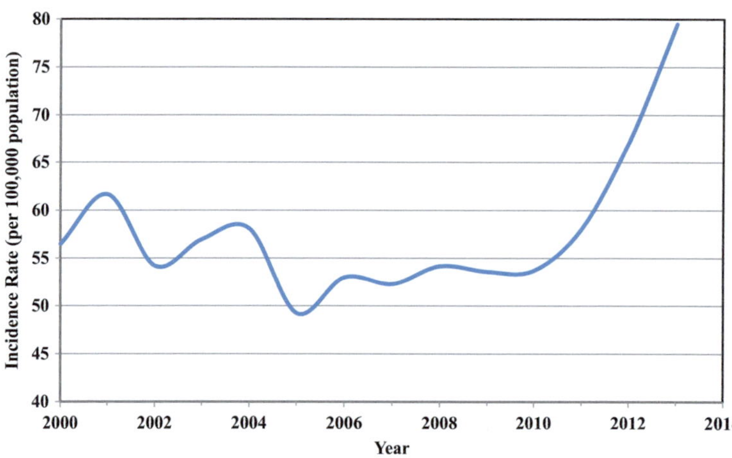

Fig. 6.4 Cancer incidence rates (per 100,000), West Bank, Palestine, 2000–2013. *Source*: Data extracted from Ministry of Health Reports, Palestine, 2009–2013

cancer related mortality reported mostly in the northern regions of the West Bank followed by the southern and then the middle regions [5].

Regarding Gaza little data is available on cancer. In a study performed by Yehia Abed about the incidence of cancer in Gaza between 1998 and 2008 which was based on data from the cancer registry in Gaza, it was shown that a total of 7412 cancer cases were reported with 48 % of them were males and 52 % were females with an average incidence rate of 49.2 cases per 100,000. Gaza governorate reported

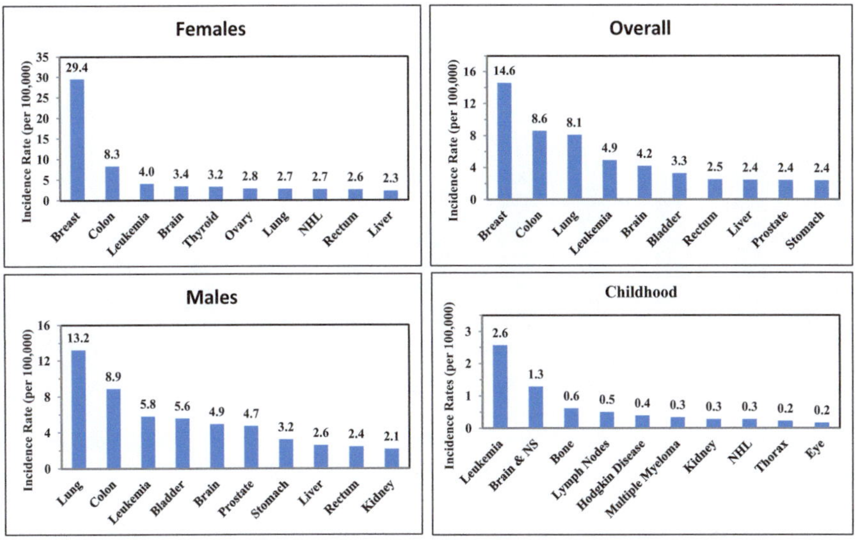

Fig. 6.5 Top ten cancers in the West Bank, Palestine, in 2013. *Source*: Data extracted from the Ministry of Health Report, Palestine, 2013

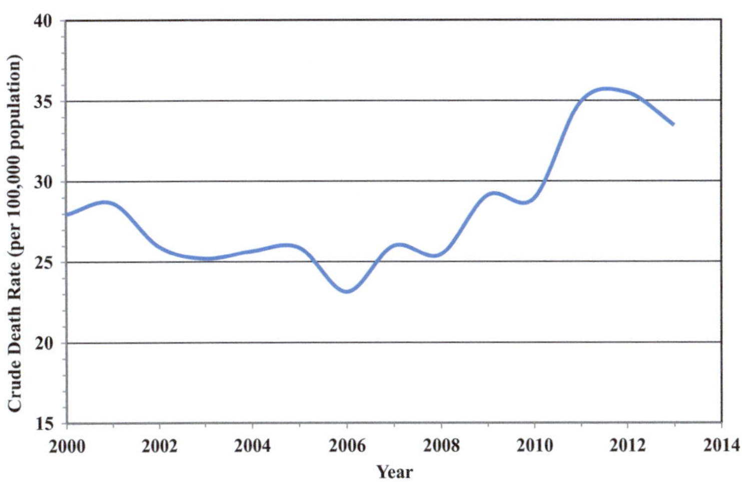

Fig. 6.6 Cancer crude death rates (per 100,000), West Bank, Palestine, 2000–2013. *Source*: Data extracted from the Ministry of Health Reports, Palestine

the highest incidence rate (67 cases per 100,000) during the period from 1998 till 2008. Breast cancer was the most diagnosed cancer in Gaza with an incidence rate of 7.8 cases per 100,000, followed by colorectal cancer (4.7), leukemia (4.1), and lung cancer (3.7). Lung cancer was the most common cancer among males with an incidence rate of 5.8 case per 100,000 men, followed by colorectal (4.6), leukemia (4.5) and prostate and bladder cancers. In females, breast cancer had an incidence

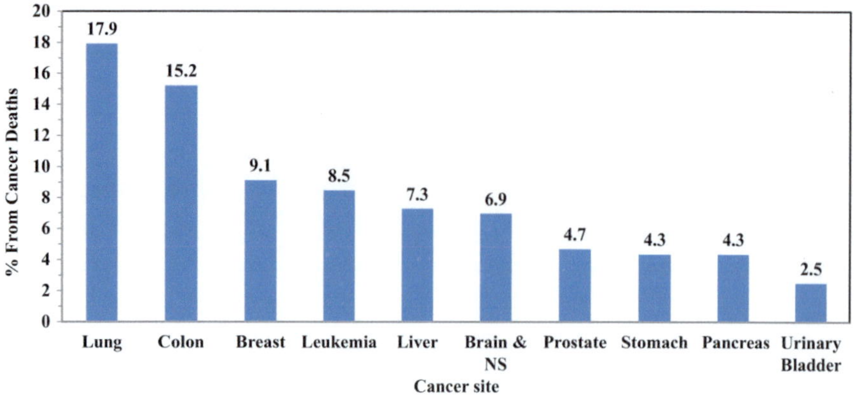

Fig. 6.7 Cancer mortality by site (top ten) in the West Bank, Palestine, in 2013. *Source*: Data extracted from the Ministry of Health Report, Palestine, 2013

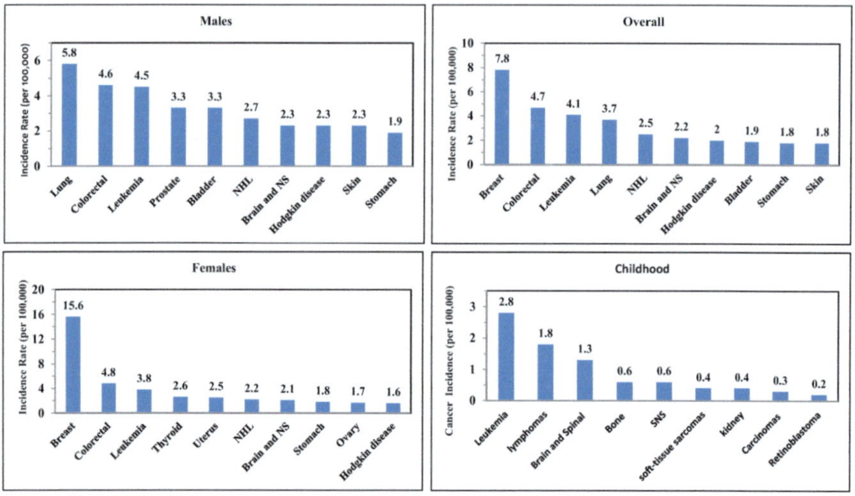

Fig. 6.8 Top ten cancers in the Gaza, Palestine, between 1998 and 2008. *Source*: Data extracted from Abed, Y. (2014), personal communication. *NHL* Non-Hodgkin Lymphoma, *SNS* Sympathetic Nervous System, *NS* Nervous System

rate of 15.6 cases per 100,000 females and ranked the first most common cancer among them, the second most common cancer among females was colorectal cancer (4.8), then leukemia (3.8) and thyroid (2.6). Among children younger than 15 years, leukemia was the first most common cancer comprising 30.3 % from all childhood cancers between 1998 and 2008, followed by lymphomas (19.4), and brain and spinal neoplasms (13.9) (Fig. 6.8). Similar to the West Bank, cancer was the second leading cause of death in Gaza with mortality rate of 36.5 per 100,000, comprising 11.8 % of total deaths, with lung cancer being the most common cause of cancer deaths followed by breast cancer and colon cancer [1].

Current Status of Cancer Care

The Palestinians are facing a cancer crisis represented by the noticed increase in cancer incidence and its contribution to the mortality as now it is considered to be the second leading cause of death. Despite that, poor medical facilities, shortage of medicines and primitive approaches that are far away from the currently used advanced multimodality diagnostics and therapeutics are the features of cancer care in this region. In addition, radiation therapy, which is a crucial therapy in cancer treatment, is completely unavailable in the West Bank and Gaza except for the radiotherapy provided by Augusta Victoria Hospital in East Jerusalem for the Palestinians referred from the West Bank and Gaza. Adding to this, the insufficient numbers of specialized doctors and other health professionals in all fields related to cancer care and the very limited and ineffective cancer-prevention strategy. Moreover, the majority of Palestinian cancer patients have late stage incurable disease when first diagnosed and further unavailability of palliative care.

Despite the inadequate health care infrastructure and political and economic instability, governmental health insurance is the only one that covers the treatment of cancer in the country in the governmental hospitals or in referring the patients to other hospitals in the neighboring countries. Cancer registry as one of the governmental institutions is also affected despite the achieved progress during the recent years. The lack of accurate population-based data and the weakness of health information systems are the hallmark of cancer registry. Augusta Victoria Hospital (a nonprofit nongovernmental organization, NGO) is considered to be a leading oncology center both in the infrastructure and the advanced technology used compared to other Palestinian hospitals. Unfortunately, at the academic level, universities are not well integrated in the health care system and there are no invested efforts to capacity build the insufficiency in the human resources in the oncology field except for few training workshops in palliative and cancer care that were organized by universities like a workshop on palliative care held in 2014 by Al-Quds University in collaboration with Middle East Cancer Consortium (MECC) for 40 health professionals from the West Bank and Gaza.

Interrelationships Between Cancer Care and Local Culture

Culture is defined as a set of shared and socially transmitted ideas about the world that are passed down from generation to generation. Local culture has both a negative impact leading to late diagnosis and a positive impact of family providing a warm incubator in addition to religion providing serenity for Palestinian cancer patients. The Interaction between culture, religion, and traditions is one reason that might have contributed to the increase in the cancer incidence in the Middle East, leading cancer to be diagnosed at more advanced stages of the disease. In the West Bank and Gaza, 42 % of cancer cases were not caught until they had spread locally (Stage III) and 18 % until they had spread throughout the body (Stage IV).

Most cancer types, like other diseases, such as diabetes and hypertension, have no symptoms for years after onset. Screening tests are not common because of the high cost in low-economic countries. Personal medical checkup is not part of the culture of the Palestinians. On the contrary, people are afraid to go to doctors to be diagnosed with a disease and they prefer to stay away as long as symptoms are absent. Even with symptoms, traditional medicine using herbs and other traditional prescriptions are preferred. Many breast cancer women and colon cancer in men and women can be easily detected at early stages by simple testing like mammography and colonoscopy, respectively. However, these tests are rarely done by undiagnosed Palestinian women and men. So culture is the most significant factor that influences individuals not to seek cancer diagnosis and treatment. The lack of knowledge about cancer also contributed to diagnosing cancer at more advanced stages.

The impact of culture on the individual and on the family is one of great resistance to being diagnosed with cancer. In some Palestinian families, a married women is afraid to be diagnosed with cancer because this will have a negative impact on her personal status in the family and may also affect negatively the reputation of her children especially daughters to get married. Therefore, getting involved in screening tests and going to a family doctor are not in the dictionary of most Palestinians. In fact, there are no such "family doctors" in Palestinian culture.

The family is considered as a significant social organization system in the Palestinian culture. Families in the Palestinian culture are very supportive for their members. Support comes also from the extended family, friends, and neighbors. Regardless of the age of the patient, old people, sick or healthy, stay with the family structure which has a great psychological comfort and is reflected on the healing process of the patient. Families in general have great fear of cancer and cancer is not looked at like other diseases. Cancer is known to be a stigma and most people call cancer "that disease" and are afraid to say "cancer" which inflicts a great psychological stress from the disease and this is reflected on the extra care that cancer patients get from the family and the community in general.

Religious beliefs play an important role at the level of the patient and health care. Islam and Christianity are the primary religions in the West Bank and Gaza. Most patients, like the community in general, have faith in Allah (GOD) which is reflected on how they perceive sickness. Religion imparts more perseverance on cancer patients because of the belief that a person is rewarded in the hereafter and on this life for his/her tolerance to pain and disease. Families and people in general also believe that they are rewarded for taking care of sick people. On the other hand, one study in Gaza revealed that religion and culture were not a barrier to conduct mammography, however, limited resources, lack of awareness and of access to medical facilities were identified as the major barriers.

Many people have little experience with cancer patients and they don't know what to say to them or how to act. This can be difficult especially when the patient is part of a married couple. The disease often changes hopes and dreams that the couple shares, so, some of their friends or family members may not be able to offer the support that the patient expects.

The Palestinian society sympathizes greatly with cancer patients, and it provides psychological support for them by means of care and giving them strength to face the disease and cope with it. For this we note that friends and relatives visit them frequently because they think that they will not live for a long time, and that they should support and help them as much as they can.

Many families do not like the fact that their ill relatives and loved ones stay at the hospital, especially in the last stages of their disease and they consider it disrespectful, so they are more accepting of home care, this is reflected positively on the cancer patients and families and friends provide some type of support groups.

Individualized Oncology in Focus

In a recent review by Kalia [6], the importance of personalized oncology has been discussed, shedding the light on the importance of genomic analysis, targeted drugs, cancer therapeutics and molecular diagnostics on personalized medicine. The use of biomarkers is the essence of individualized oncology which has already proven to result in more effective treatment protocols. The review highlighted the definition of personalized medicine by the US President's Council of Advisors on Science and Technology as referring to "*…the tailoring of medical treatment to the individual characteristics of each patient; to classify individuals into subpopulations that differ in their susceptibility to a particular disease or their response to a specific treatment so that preventive or therapeutic interventions can then be concentrated on those who will benefit, sparing expense and side effects for those who will not.*" To this definition, the Personalized Medicine Coalition has added, "*…the molecular methods that make personalized medicine possible include testing for variations in genes, gene expression, proteins, and metabolites, as well as new treatments that target molecular mechanisms. Test results are correlated with clinical factors—such as disease state, prediction of future disease states, drug response, and treatment prognosis—to help physicians individualize treatment for each patient.*"

The use of personalized medicine assays requires coordination between a highly qualified team of molecular biologists and clinical staff. In the West Bank, Augusta Victoria is the only hospital that offers individualized oncology genomic-based treatment but it is still limited to certain molecular testing. In breast cancer genetic testing for some genes particularly BRCA (breast cancer) 1 and 2, guides preventive and treatment strategies based on susceptibility risk for breast and ovarian cancers. This screening is performed as part of research collaboration between Augusta Victoria Hospital and Bethlehem University. Colon cancer therapy selection is assessed by genetic assays of *KRAS* (v-Ki-ras2 Kirsten rat sarcoma viral oncogene homolog) and *EGFR* (Epidermal growth factor receptor) which are used to check for response to tyrosine kinase inhibitors (TKI) and consequently to provide information for the selection of various therapies. In leukemias and lymphomas individualized medicine also plays a role in Augusta Victoria. In chronic myeloid leukemia or acute lymphoblastic leukemia, Philadelphia chromosome is detected through the quantification of the *BCR/ABL* (breakpoint cluster region/c-abl oncogene 1, non-receptor tyrosine kinase) and is used to indicate certain therapies like with Imatinib for patients with *BCR/ABL* and the disease should be followed up by serial quantitative measures of the BCR/ABL. In promyelocytic leukemia which is characterized by the presence of t (15;17) translocation, molecular detection of *PML/RARA* is used to indicate arsenic trioxide and tretinoin for patients for induction of remission and consolidation. FMS-like tyrosine kinase-3 (*FLT3*) is used for acute myeloid leukemia treatment. CD20 expression is used to indicate rituximab for the treatment of patients with non-Hodgkin lymphoma. There are several genes involved in the selection of the most appropriate therapies for lung cancer in Augusta Victoria Hospital including *EGFR*, *RRM1* (ribonucleotide reductase M1), and *KRAS* in addition to several other tests that are used for therapy guidance of different types of cancer.

Critical Clinical Issues

In the West Bank, chronic diseases have become the biggest medical concern and have replaced communicable diseases. The specialized health care professionals and infrastructure needed to diagnose and treat cancer have not caught up. Currently, cancer is the second leading cause of death in the West Bank and Gaza, trailing only cardiovascular diseases, and accounts for 13.3 % of all deaths.

A number of critical clinical issues need to be addressed here. The shortage of specialized physicians including oncologists, hemato-oncologists, surgeons, pathologists, and radiologists is considered the biggest problem that faces proper diagnosis and treatment of cancer patients. In addition, the methodologies that are used in cancer diagnosis are not precise and need to be improved. For example, pathology diagnosis is not based on the state of the art immunostaining, molecular and genetic tools are still not introduced into our hospitals and laboratories except at a limited level in Augusta Victoria Hospital. Consequently, efforts should be invested to improve the diagnostic levels.

Lack of implementation for an effective preventive policy is another challenge facing the Palestinian cancer care system. There is a limited availability of governmental services for colonoscopy and bronchoscopy. Despite the free availability of mammography screening in 13 governmental primary health care centers distributed all over the West Bank in addition to some other mammography screenings provided by religious and social welfare organizations for a symbolic cost, still late diagnosis of breast cancer as well as other types of cancer is another critical issue revealed by cancer statistics in the West Bank. It was shown that 60 % of total cases are incurably ill at the time of diagnosis, most likely at the late stage of the disease (Stage III or IV). This could be attributed to the lack of awareness and the absence of educational resources and preventive policies that obligate the people to perform regular screening.

Treating cancer requires more than just chemotherapy, most cancers requires multimodality therapy including surgery, chemotherapy, and radiation therapy. This means that a comprehensive system with multidisciplinary team should provide these services under one roof. In the West Bank and Gaza, not only chemotherapy is not available in many cases and consequently the patients have to wait or to be referred to other hospitals, but also radiation therapy is not available in any of the West Bank and Gaza health facilities and is only limited to Augusta Victoria Hospital. Surgical oncology requires surgeons to work closely with oncologists as teams for cancer patients, which is hardly the case. The Ministry of Health is taking the responsibility of covering most of the health expenses of cancer patients in terms of diagnosis and treatment. With the economic crisis of the Palestinian Authority, the health care system is suffering at all levels including the health care of cancer patients. Moreover, infrastructure facilities such as proper rooms for cancer patients and isolation rooms are limited with the increasing number of cancer patients.

From diagnosis and treatment to follow-up of cancer, the use of the new technology in this field is highly limited. PET-CT as one of the mostly used scanning equipment is lacking in the West Bank and Gaza; cancer patients are usually referred to Israeli hospitals to perform this test. In addition, the use of biomarkers in the follow-up is also very limited. Despite the fact that most patients are diagnosed at late stages and they can only benefit from palliative care rather than curative treatment, palliative care for the Palestinians is a new concept and is not applied yet. Bone-marrow transplantation and personalized medicine are lagging behind and require not only specialists but also the right facilities. One of the solutions is for Augusta Victoria Hospital in Jerusalem to specialize only in oncology to diagnose and treat cancer patients and get the permission for obtaining a PET-CT scan.

Insights on Palliative Care

Palliative care is an important part of cancer care that is supposed to reduce patient's symptoms, improve quality of life, and support patients and their families. It is defined by the World Health Organization (WHO) as: *"an approach that improves the quality of life of patients and their families facing the problem associated with life-threatening illness, through the prevention and relief of suffering by means of early identification and impeccable assessment and treatment of pain and other problems, physical, psychosocial and spiritual.*" People with cancer often receive treatment for cancer and treatment to ease the symptoms at the same time. Palliative care is best given in the cancer treatment process and continues through all stages of illness, regardless of whether complete remission of cancer is possible or not. Health care providers must evaluate and alleviate a patient's physical, psychological, and social distress. While palliative care was first introduced to Arabs in the Middle Eastern countries in the early 1990s, its development process has been slow.

The typology that defines different stages of palliative care and hospice development are divided into four categories: "no services identified," "capacity building," "localized provision," and "approaching integration," the West Bank and Gaza are on the border between "no services" and some limited "capacity building." Palliative care is not yet integrated into the Palestinian health care system, just like most of Middle Eastern countries, and it is not considered one of the basic concerns of the governmental policies that must be provided to cancer patients and is not covered by health insurance inside Palestinian governmental hospitals.

Although palliative care remains an undeveloped and an under resourced area in the Palestinian health care system, there are a few nongovernmental organizations (NGOs) that provide palliative care in the West Bank. Al-Sadeel Society, an NGO in the West Bank, is the first and only registered palliative care society in Palestine. It is located in Bethlehem and was established in November 2008 to provide palliative care for patients with cancer and chronic diseases. The society's vision is that "life is a gift from God," and therefore, it should be kept pain free as much as possible, using updated knowledge and skills.

Al-Sadeel provides free services for patients and their families through activities, fun days, and scientific days by means of medical, social, emotional, and psychological approaches. This institution is cooperating with MECC to provide training programs for medical staff as well as for patients and their families. In November 2008, this institution organized a Scientific Day in Bethlehem for a group of health workers from the governmental and nongovernmental sectors as a first step to introduce the idea of palliative care to the Palestinian community.

In addition, another NGO center, the Patients Friends Society (PFS) located in Augusta Victoria Hospital in East Jerusalem was established in the early 1980s by some Palestinian academics and health professionals. This society has held some activities that support palliative care for cancer patients, and currently offers palliative care and psychological support to women with breast cancer during their treatment. The society conducted a workshop in collaboration with the College of Nursing at the University of Al-Najah and the United Nations in which palliative care for cancer patients issue was well introduced and presented to the participants that included doctors, pharmacists, and nurses.

Moreover, Dunya Women's Cancer Center in Ramallah provides high quality complementary health services to women with breast and gynecological cancers from different areas in the West Bank according to international standards. The center also provides palliative care to chronic cases and psychological help to the patients and their families.

There are also some informal services supported by other NGOs, UNRWA organization and health teams inside the Palestinian hospitals which offer palliative care services for chronic diseases and cancer patients provided by the medical teams.

In an overall evaluation of the current status of palliative care for cancer patients in the West Bank, Thweib [7] showed that the quality of life (QOL) of Palestinian cancer patients is lower than the international quality due to the absence of palliative care service in the Palestinian oncology care system. Furthermore, a triangulated study about palliative care for cancer patients in the West Bank was conducted at Al-Quds University in 2012 and included three Palestinian hospitals: Beit Jala Hospital, Al-Watani Hospital, and Augusta Victoria Hospital. The study showed that cancer patients need palliative care to improve their quality of life and to reduce their pain and the suffering of their families and their friends. In addition, the study reported the huge difficulties facing Palestinian cancer patients in terms of quality of life and emphasized the urgent need to integrate palliative care for cancer patients in their medical care system [8].

The Palestinian government efforts are directed towards curing rather than palliating late stages cancer patients. Providing morphine for patients is still in argument, since the current regulations in the Palestinian Authority regarding opioid use and consumption are difficult and requires a long routine procedure. Most health care providers in the West Bank and Gaza need training and education concerning palliative care for cancer patients. In addition, the staff with a high work load and limited time available to assess the needs and pain of the patients is considered an obstacle in developing palliative care. The public tend to believe that bearing pain is part of the human well-being. People also tend to fear addiction on opioids; they believe that they shouldn't take opioids for mild or moderate pain because they will not find anything for their pain if it gets worse. People also relate the use of morphine with death and end of life.

In summary, palliative care suffers at all levels; there is no service for patients or their families; no organizational strategic planning; absence of educational resources; absence of communication or consultation; no sadness support groups; no follow-up for patient or family; no standards or training programs; and no community awareness for palliative care.

Local Innovations

Similar to the Western care systems, a multidisciplinary cancer center should be established with an infrastructure and personnel to meet the goals for providing comprehensive cancer care needs and improving cancer prevention, early diagnosis, curative and palliative therapy. To this aim, a professional team should be well trained on global standards in cancer care including oncologists, hemato-oncologists, radiologists, pathologists, surgeons, palliative care professionals, nurses, psychologists, social workers, health care educators, and laboratory practitioners. This team will formulate the core of cancer control strategy and will empower the capability and the capacity of cancer care.

Our transformation should not be limited to the human resources, but also expands to include the advanced methodology used in accurate diagnosis and cure of different types of cancers in addition to experts capable to mentor the introduction of these new techniques. On top of these are radio-imaging, accurate pathology diagnosis based on immunostaining, flow cytometry for the leukemias and lymphomas diagnosis, molecular and genetic diagnosis.

In this context, there is an urgent need to work on broadening the use of radiation therapy which is a key component in its efficacy to cure even in the advanced stages of diseases. Chemotherapy still remains the cornerstone of optimal cancer care. The Palestinian Ministry of Health should take on the lead to ensure the continuous availability of drugs. Moreover, personalized medicine assays should be implemented to provide the best possible cancer care in terms of treatment, prediction of prognosis of patient, and finally to introduce prevention policies in mutations that are well characterized to be inherited as in breast cancer, ovarian and colon cancer where these preventive approaches are expected to make a huge difference. Hopefully in the near future we would reach to the level of using microarrays to detect specific single nucleotide polymorphisms (SNPs) or to perform a genome wide association studies or using new generation sequencing methodologies to detect nucleic acid polymorphisms especially when several different polymorphisms might be relevant to predict a disease, response to treatment or prognosis.

To improve the cancer care scenario in the West Bank and Gaza, academic institutions should play an integral part in the process by conducting extensive persuasive health education programs. People at all levels should be educated to change their behavior to avoid preventable cancers and to increase the public awareness of regular screening and checkup approaches. Partnerships and collaborations with international health programs and institutions will support and enforce the transformation process. Furthermore, efforts should be invested to introduce clinical research into our hospitals and universities, both should work cooperatively to bring this into life.

A step further should be taken in palliative care since the core concepts of palliative care are not well understood. Awareness should be increased among patients and families in terms of palliation, as well as among the medical staff and policy makers in terms of the role of different therapies and care models used in palliative care. Opioids should be made available and covered by the government in all cancer care centers as it is well known that 60 % of cancer patients die of the disease in developed countries, while in developing countries, 80 % of cancer victims die since they already have late-stage incurable tumors when they are diagnosed. In addition, home care services for cancer patients, integrated psychosocial support programs, spiritual care programs, administration support, medication, and financial resources should be all made available.

Governmental and Institutional Involvement in Cancer Care

In the West Bank there are four hospitals that provide health care to cancer patients, two of them are governmental and two are private. The two governmental hospitals are *Beit-Jala Hospital* in Beit Jala, Bethlehem governorate, and *Al-Watani Hospital* in Nablus, Nablus governorate. The two private hospitals are *Augusta Victoria Hospital* in East Jerusalem and *An-Najah National University Hospital* in Nablus. In addition to hospitals, there is one small cancer care provider called *Dunya Women Cancer Center* in Ramallah, Ramallah governorate. In Gaza governorates there are three governmental medical centers and two histopathology laboratories. The three medical centers providing care for cancer patients are: *Al-Shifa Hospital* in Gaza city, *the European Gaza Hospital* in Khan Younis, and *Al-Rantissi Specialized Pediatric Hospital* in Gaza city. The two histopathology laboratories are located at Al-Shifa Hospital and at the European Gaza hospital. Most cancer patients from Gaza are referred to Egyptian, West Bank, and Israeli hospitals.

Augusta Victoria Hospital, Jerusalem

Augusta Victoria Hospital has created the most advanced oncology department, which houses medical oncology, radiation oncology, and surgical oncology units both for pediatrics and adults. Each year, the hospital performs more than 25,000 sessions of radiation oncology and at least 15,000 chemotherapy sessions. The hospital has 6 pediatric and 18 adult ambulatories; the pediatric ambulatories include 12 beds while the adult ambulatories include 16 beds for solid tumor and 12 beds for liquid tumor. Augusta Victoria Hospital has four isolation rooms for BMT, well equipped and ready to be opened in 2016.

Augusta Victoria Hospital has CT scan to detect cancer. Bronchoscopy is also available for lung cancer detection and mammography for breast cancer. Surgical pathology testing is carried out for the diagnosis and evaluation of stage and metastasis of cancer. Flow cytometry was recently introduced for the diagnosis of lymphomas and leukemias. The methodology is well known and the role it plays in clinical hematology is vital. It is becoming critical for the clinical assessment of hematological malignancies particularly with the substantial increasing burden of leukemias and lymphomas among Palestinians. Its role is not limited to initial diagnosis but extends further to follow up the patient response to treatment and to detect relapses or transformations. Initial panels for differentiating lymphoid from myeloid malignances are used and advanced panels for further precise diagnosis of the subtypes of lymphomas and leukemias. In addition, the hospital houses a well-equipped molecular-biology laboratory which is used for several purposes including oncological diagnosis and individualized medicine for colon cancer, breast cancer, lung cancer, and hematological malignancies. It also performs karyotyping for fresh biopsies and for blood samples. Furthermore, tumor-marker tests (CA-19-9, CEA, CA15-3, and AFP) are frequently performed to support the diagnosis and the follow-up of the patients.

Augusta Victoria Hospital, by purchasing two medical linear accelerators, is the first and only Palestinian hospital to provide radiation therapy for the West Bank and Gaza cancer patients. More than 40 % of all cancer treatments are for patients from Gaza especially after the difficulty of traveling to Egypt for treatment. Gaza patients are housed in a hospital-rented hotel rooms for the duration of their treatment. Augusta Victoria Hospital has the highest number of oncologists compared with other hospitals in the West Bank and Gaza. The hospital has six oncologists, several pathologists, surgeons, and nutritionists. Surgeons are available to carry out surgeries for cancer patients and nutritionists to customize food for different patients. Treatment of cancer by chemotherapy and radiation is up to the highest standard, yet the hospital lacks PET-CT scanning technology which is important for diagnosis and follow-up, but the hospital is planning to provide this service in the future. Furthermore, recently the hospital finished installing a highly advanced laboratory setup for bone marrow and stem cell transplant.

Beit-Jala Hospital, Beit Jala

There are two oncology departments at Beit-Jala Hospital specialized in cancer treatment, one for pediatrics and the other for adults. The pediatric department, Huda Al-Masri Pediatric Cancer Department, is a facility with fourteen beds, including two isolation rooms. It was launched in 2011 by the head social worker and the founding members of the Palestinian Children's Relief Fund (PCRF) to honor Huda Al-Masri who passed away after a 6-month battle with leukemia. It was opened in 2013 and it currently provides care for the hundreds of Palestinian children diagnosed each year with cancer. The department has one hemato-oncologist, six pediatricians, eight nurses, one pharmacist, and one social worker. The department offers chemotherapy for children patients as prescribed by the specialized oncologist. Annually, the pediatric department receives around 100 new cases from all Palestinian governorates; most of them come from Hebron, Bethlehem, and Ramallah.

The adult department contains 24 beds with no isolation rooms. The department has four oncologists, two hematologists, two residential oncologists, and 17 nurses. Cancer patients who require BMT are usually referred to An-Najah National University Hospital and nearby countries.

At Beit-Jala Hospital cancer detection is facilitated by the presence of mammography and CT scan. The hospital houses a pathology department where oncological diagnosis and staging is based on biopsy stains and immunostaining for selected primary antigens. In addition, chemotherapy and surgical treatment are offered in this hospital. Both radiation therapy and BMT are not available and patients who are in need for these treatments are referred to Augusta Victoria for radiotherapy, to Al-Hussein center in Jordan or to Israeli hospitals for radiotherapy or BMT.

The hospital lacks scanning technologies that are needed for detection and precise diagnosis of cancer type and stage such as PET-CT Scan, MRI, and breast ultrasound. In addition medical procedures such as gastroscopy and colonoscopy are not performed. Tumor-marker tests and personalized oncology treatment are also not available.

Al-Watani Hospital, Nablus

Al-Watani Hospital in Nablus has only an adult department with 23 beds, four for women and 19 for men and it has one hematologist, one oncologist, eight nurses, one pharmacist, and one social worker. Monthly, Al-Watani Hospital receives around 300–330 cases of solid-mass cancer, mainly colon and lung cancer in males, breast cancer in females. Some tumor markers are measured to help diagnosis and follow-up of cancer patients. Pathology tests are referred to the nearby Rafidia Hospital; mammography, CT scan, and MRI are referred to other Palestinian hospitals. Patients who require BMT are referred to An-Najah University Hospital and nearby countries.

An-Najah National University Hospital, Nablus

Al-Najah National University Hospital was established in April 2013 with only an oncology department and it started to treat adult and pediatric hematological cancer cases in June 2013. The hospital receives all cancer cases from different regions of the West Bank and Gaza that are referred from governmental hospitals. It includes outpatient and inpatient departments, the outpatient department is divided into oncology and hematology; the oncology department has 15 beds and the hematology department has nine beds for leukemia, lymphoma cases, and pediatric hematology. Inpatient oncology department started in September 2013 and it includes 13 beds for adult hematology–oncology cancer cases. An-Najah National University Hospital is the first hospital in West Bank that performs BMT. The BMT unit has six beds and it is totally isolated and equipped with HEPA filter. The pediatric hemato-oncology department treats 6–10 cases daily, with an average of 30 admissions per month and more than 75 % of the cases are acute lymphocytic leukemia. The staff at the hospital includes three physicians one for adult medical oncology, one for adult hematology, and one for both pediatric hematology and oncology and 30 nurses. The bone marrow aspiration and biopsy are done in the adult hematology department without anesthesia in a special-procedure room, but the pediatric cases are done under anesthesia. The chemotherapy is distributed for both outpatient and inpatient units. The hospital has also a pathologist for the diagnosis of all oncology and hematology cases. A flow cytometry is available for diagnosis of leukemia and lymphoma cases. Oncology surgeries, CT scan, MRI, breast ultrasound, and an advanced endoscopy unit are available, but radiotherapy, PET-CT scan, and mammography are not available. A specialized laboratory carries out clinical testing as well as offers all routine and tumor marker tests. The hospital is provided with pneumatic tube system which incorporates variable speed delivery of drugs, specimens, and documents. Patients' information and medical files are computerized. Monthly, the hospital receives 450 visits of hematology adult patients, only 60–70 cases are proved to have hematology disorders whereas the oncology adult department receives 400 visits.

Dunya Women Cancer Center, Ramallah

Dunya Women Cancer Center is the first center in providing diagnostic services for breast and gynecological cancers. Dunya Center was established in 2011 through partnership between Palestinian NGOs, Health Work Committees and Medipalestine-Switzerland. This center provides high quality diagnostic services according to international standards for early detection of breast and cervical cancers including clinical and laboratory examinations, regular checkup by mammography, breast ultrasound, and Papanicolaou test (pap-smear). Advanced tests are also available like ultrasound-guided Tru-cut biopsy guided, wire localization, breast tissue marker, colposcopy and cervical biopsy, cytology and oncology consultation, nutritionist, physiotherapy, and psychotherapist consultations who support cancer patient and their families and the follow-up of the patients after treatment for 5 years. Annually, Dunya center receives approximately 1110 cases, out of which 110 cases are diagnosed with cancer. The medical team consists of professional medical specialists in oncology and gynecology, in addition to professional nurses and technicians. Health work committees also offer continuous training opportunities for the staff to guarantee quality services according to international standards. The center contributes in raising awareness in the community and focuses on the early detection of cancer through conducting lectures and training workshops at different locations in the West Bank. They constantly raise funds to cover the diagnostic medical examination costs for poor patients.

Al-Shifa Hospital, Gaza

Oncology Department has three foundations: surgical treatment, which consists of eradicating the tumor and is mostly carried out in Gaza; chemotherapy, a type of treatment that is not always available; and radiation, which is not available at all, despite that a device was set up in the hospital 6 years ago for this purpose but is now damaged. This delays treatment and leads to a deterioration in the patients' condition, not to mention the physical and mental suffering that patients endure due to the trips they have to make. The number of rooms are seven in the inpatient services (three of which are isolation rooms) with a total of 19 beds, and one hall for day care that contains six beds and five chairs. The number of oncologists is eight.

European Gaza Hospital, Rafah

The oncology department was established in the year 2000. The number of beds is 27 and 10 for the outpatient. Cancer care is provided for adults and only two oncologists supervise the cancer patients. Mammography and CT are available for diagnosis, tumor markers are done at hospital and private laboratories and research laboratories at the Islamic University in Gaza help in carrying out genetic testing. Pathological tests are available at hospital laboratories. The hospital receives about 500 cancer patients every month with 40–50 new cases being diagnosed with cancer. The availability of cancer treatment by oncology departments is suffering, like Gaza hospitals and Gaza in general, from the siege of Gaza. Chemotherapy is not available all the time and radiology and targeted therapy are usually referred to Augusta Victoria Hospital and An-Najah National University Hospital in the West Bank. Ninety per cent of referred cases are to the West Bank hospitals for treatment and only 10 % to Israeli hospitals whereas all cancer cases are referred to Israeli hospitals for PET-CT.

Al-Rantissi Specialized Pediatric Hospital, Gaza

The hemato-oncology department was established in 2008 with 15 beds. There are three isolation rooms and two halls with a total of 15 beds. Three specialists work in this department and ten nurses. Approximately 50 new cases of cancer patients are diagnosed in this hospital each year.

Cancer Registry

Population-based cancer registries (PBCR) are important for cancer control and treatment. Designing and monitoring of cancer control activities and policies are based on cancer-registry data, which is the main source of information. Cancer registry aims to collect data to classify cancer types in order to produce statistics on the incidence of cancer within a population; to provide the basis to asses and control the impact of cancer on the community and the deficiencies in the health care system; and to plan nationally and internationally for cancer control and treatment. High quality cancer registry is difficult to achieve in low- and middle-income countries due to political and economic instability and the low funding of health care systems.

The West Bank Cancer Registry was established by the Palestinian Ministry of Health in 1996 in conjunction with the MECC. In 2009, two branches of Palestinian Cancer Registry (PCR) were established, one in Gaza and the other one in the West Bank. The PCR had cooperated with the International Agency for Research on Cancer (IARC), Lyon, France, that had sent first a cancer registry system and then a new version of the CanReg3. The system was used to perform all the tasks needed for the management of a good quality cancer registry which made it easier to analyze information. The main purpose of the PCR was to define the size of the cancer problem and the pattern of its occurrence. Palestinian Health Information Center (PHIC) is a department within the Palestinian Ministry of Health which is responsible for health management information system in the West Bank and Gaza. The mission of PHIC is to produce and disseminate health related data and information for the Palestinian health providers and other relevant agencies, as well as to all interested personnel. The most important PHIC activities include daily editing, supervision of population file through data entry of birth notifications and death certificates, cancer information and preparing a quarter, midyear, and annual reports about the health status in the West Bank.

Financial coverage for cancer diagnosis and treatment is almost fully covered by the governmental health care system of the Palestinian Authority despite its financial crisis. Cancer cases that require facilities not available locally are referred mainly to Jordanian, Egyptian, and Israeli hospitals. A referral committee is responsible for evaluating the applications of cancer patients. In 2013, the number of referred oncology cases was 9577 compared to 9898 in 2012; this includes referrals to nongovernmental Arab Hospitals like Augusta Victoria Hospital in East Jerusalem and An-Najah National University Hospital in Nablus. However, the number of referred cases concerning diagnostic tests like isotope scans (like PET-CT) increased from 2103 cases in 2012 to 2374 cases in 2013. There are no specific data from the Ministry of Health concerning the transfer of oncology cases to different countries. However, total referrals in general decreased dramatically to Jordan from 3219 cases in 2010 to 256 in 2013 and approximately 34 % decrease in 2013 compared to 2010 to Egypt. The referrals to East Jerusalem increased from 23,186 cases in 2010 to 26,850 cases in 2013. The total referrals to Israeli hospitals increased from 3870 cases in 2010 to 8118 cases in 2013. The data seems to indicate that the number of referred cancer cases to other countries is decreasing with time and this is probably due to the improvement of the local cancer care services provided to patients in terms of diagnosis and treatment.

Summary

Cancer care in the West Bank and Gaza, like health care in general, is suffering from a low allocated budget, which is reflected on the delay in early diagnosis, scarcity of facilities, lack of sophisticated equipment used in diagnosis and treatment, shortage of drugs and specialized well-trained health care professionals. Despite these obstacles, cancer diagnosis and treatment have improved dramatically in the past few years and referred cases to neighboring countries are gradually decreasing.

Recommendations

A coherent national cancer policy should be formulated by the Palestinian Ministry of Health and then be approved, implemented, and followed up in all cancer care providing facilities, whether private or public. The policy should emphasize early detection of cancer in order to decrease the rate of remission and consequently to reduce the financial burden on the government. To this aim, it is recommended to health educate and to increase awareness among the society for the importance of regular checkup and the recognition of the symptoms of cancer by various means. In inherited types of cancers like breast, cervical, and colorectal cancers, screening and preventive programs for the high risk groups should be developed and implemented with prevention policies be given a high priority.

More attention should be also paid in the policy to invest in the human resources necessary to provide proper cancer care according to the international standards. Collaborations and partnership should be established to build a comprehensive multidisciplinary cancer care teams, well trained and capable of performing definitive diagnosis of cancer based on advanced methodologies. Then treatment should be available, evidence-based, and individualized.

Recommendations for improving the understanding and introduction of palliative care in the West Bank and Gaza includes the need for national policy and standards for palliative care and opioids regulations, and the need for interdisciplinary team work in the issue of cancer, to involve palliative care education within the programs of schools of health professions.

References

1. Abed Y. Cancer incidence in the Gaza Strip, Palestine 1998–2008 based on the population-based cancer registry Gaza. 2014.
2. Abou Amer W. Cancer prevention and control. Evaluation of the strategy in Gaza Governorates. Jerusalem: Al-Quds University; 2012.
3. Rionda ZaC, A. The burden of disease in the West Bank and Gaza: an assessment report the United States Agency for international Development in the West Bank and Gaza, Ramallah. 2000.
4. Statistics PCBo. Palestine in Figures 2013. Ramallah, Palestine. 2014.
5. Ministry of Health P. Annual Health Reports, Palestine (2000–2013).
6. Kalia M. Personalized oncology: recent advances and future challenges. Metab Clin Exp. 2013;62 Suppl 1:S11–4.
7. Thweib N. Quality of life of Palestinian cancer patients. J Pediatr Hematol Oncol. 2011;33 Suppl 1:S68–9.
8. Khleif M. Quality of life for Palestinian patients with cancer in the absence of a palliative-care service: a triangulated study. Lancet. 2013;382:S23.

Chapter 7
Influx of Foreign Refugees to Jordan and Its Overall Burden on Cancer Care

Omar Nimri

The Syrian refugees, and before that, the Iraqis, earlier the Lebanon crisis too and previously the Palestinians; all these human crowds are like a succession of individuals running in a funnel-like path to the safe land, Jordan, in the mutinies and uprisings areas around it. Jordan is a small country with very limited resources and those huge floods of people who are clear-presented true composites, fusions, which is very difficult to separate from the Jordanian community nowadays. Those humans are displaced to Jordan; they are of different ages, genders, ethnicity, and religions.

Each person, each one of those humans is a story. Mostly it will be hard one, sad, and inhuman. This severe humanitarian disaster recently in Iraq and Syria had been outlined by many international organizations and it had been estimated that more than seven million Syrian have been displaced inside the country Syria and to the surrounding countries like Turkey, Lebanon, and mostly to Jordan with less numbers in other countries in the region as well as remotely.

Those became refugees, and more have been left displaced in unsafe, poor living conditions with shortage of clean water to drink or any water at all, food and shelters in cold or hot; frightening panic moments round the clock with unclear future ahead. Children missed going to school, playing, learning, and their right to live taken away in many inhuman manners and miserable occasions.

Those who fled to the neighboring countries are forced to do so running out for their lives; small, big, young or old, male or female, those unexpected visitors are welcomed and the peoples of those neighboring countries share with them the homes, food and water, sympathy, and tender feelings.

Nevertheless, the numbers went increasing on and on which can no longer be ignored and countries should deal with it and face the inevitable. These unavoidable conditions and situations made this difficult circumstance to deal with on a country

O. Nimri, M.D. (✉)
Jordan Cancer Registry, Ministry of Health, Amman, Jordan
e-mail: onimri@gmail.com

M. Silbermann (ed.), *Cancer Care in Countries and Societies in Transition*,
DOI 10.1007/978-3-319-22912-6_7

level and the global assistance was much required and obligatory to face this tragedy and demanding conditions of Syrian refugees fleeing the escalating violence in their country.

Hundreds of thousands of refugees are currently in Jordan. Almost all have fled the ongoing violence and unrest in neighboring Syria and Iraq. Many are poor, unable to legally obtain a job, and struggle to meet their daily needs. Women and children in those groups of peoples are more particular vulnerable to exploitation and violence conditions.

Jordan agreed to create camps to house the swelling numbers of refugees and began construction refugee camp in northern Jordan. Jordan currently hosts beyond one and a half million Syrians; the majority of them being absorbed in the homeland of Jordan communities, less of them living in a number of refugee camps in the provinces of the northern part of the country, Jordan. While the majority are now inhabitants (more than a million) among natives who live their life on own financial support, one way or another. The International rescue committee and some other humanitarian NGOs are providing assistance, medical care, and other support to those refugees in Jordan.

Approximately 80 % of Syrian refugees in Jordan live in urban areas in Amman and the northern part of Jordan, while the remaining 20 % live in the camps. Jordanians have experienced the conflict via the thousands who have crossed into the country. When Syrian conflict first began, many Syrians went to Jordan to stay with relatives; they did not consider themselves "refugees." Many Syrian residents of northern Jordan feel, as they are Jordanian—they have lived and married together same families and crossing the border was easy. Nevertheless, as the war escalated, the situation became critical: Syrians without relatives in Jordan began to cross the border too and in huge numbers.

Syrians opted to stay and work in Northern Jordan mostly, housing refugees and assisting those whose savings were dwindling. Yet the Jordanian government did not officially recognize the growing refugee crisis until 2012, when increased fighting yield an average of more than 1000 people a day crossing the border. To cope with that, Za'atari refugee camp was set up in July 2012 in a windswept desert.

The economics behind Jordan's refugee program has also been a subject of significant domestic contention and anxiety? The Jordanian Ministry of Planning estimated the cost of refugee accommodation to be around $850 million, or roughly 2 % of the country's $40 billion GDP. According to the Jordanian response plan for the crisis of Syrian refugee government needs about $850 million in support of the goals to enable them to continue to provide essential services and materials backed for Syrian refugees in Jordanian cities and towns and some of the camps' needs, which was allocated 371.8 million dollars to enable the Syrian refugees to take advantage of commodity support for energy and cost of health and security, education, water and municipal services. It had been estimated according to neutral studies; of the cost per refugee, hosting is about 2500 dinars per year of the United Nations and donor countries.

Jordan has absorbed more than 600,000 Syrian refugees, as the numbers registered by High Commissioner for Refugees (UNHCR). The presence of Syrian refugees, although stimulate economic activity in the retail, but also cause strain on resources, not to mention higher wages for housing on the Jordanians and the worsening of unemployment among young people and an increase in demand for water, health, and education. Moreover, congestion hospitals and schools endure mainly citizens of Jordan not the state treasury. There is a need to study the economic and social effects of Syrian refugees in Jordan, an objective manner, a scientific clear methodology.

Globally the non-communicable diseases and sickness have received little attention in spite of their overall burden. In refugees, such diseases present specific challenges, including continuity of care and avoidance of treatment interruptions due to displacement, the need for expensive and regular treatments, and the dependence on specialty physician skills, multi-morbidities, and harm reduction through regular screening and lifestyle modifications. In some patients, chronic disorders become emergent or evolve into acute presentations if the disease is unaddressed or their treatment suddenly stops.

Syrian refugees who have become a heavy burden on the health and education sectors of Jordan, not to mention the burden on the infrastructure and the labor market, and the pressure on the state's limited resources. Moreover, Jordan will not close the border (North with Syria) in front of the refugees from the humanitarian dimension of the crisis (Syrian) stemming from the national obligations and constants of Jordan. Health consequences of the ongoing war in the Arab world are much more than the collateral damage inflicted on civilians, infrastructure, environment, and health systems not in the country itself but much more in the countries hosting those refugees displaced population.

The Syrian refugees in Jordan have the same demographic and health, fashion, the character of that of a middle-income country, which is characterized by the high proportion of chronic diseases (NCDs), which is always costly and difficult to manage. These diseases put a lot of pressure on the limited health care resources available for secondary and tertiary care in the country. Common diseases among Syrians includes bronchial asthma, diabetes, high blood pressure, cardiovascular conditions, renal failure, and to some extent cancer diseases.

The Ministry of Health (MoH) in Jordan has maintained its policy of free access to primary and secondary care in health facilities for registered Syrians living outside of camps. Most refugees, therefore, have the right to access MoH services, which was a huge burden to the health system in Jordan; by the end of 2014 and the begging of 2015, this privilege recently is not anymore available and attending to such services are to be paid for.

Primary health care and essential secondary care continued to be provided for Syrians through a network of UN agencies, local and international NGOs, private businesses, embassies as well the Jordanian government.

According to the UNHCR the distribution of the registered Syrian refugees in Jordan is shown in Table 7.1 where most of those refugees are living in Amman the

Table 7.1 UNHCR, distribution of the registered Syrian refugees in Jordan

Percentage	Governorate name	Rank
28	Amman	Max
25	Mafraq	
23	Irbid	
11.3	Zarqa	
3.2	Balqa	
1.8	Jarash	
1.7	Madaba	
1.6	Ajlon and Karak	
1.2	Ma'an	
0.5	Tafelah and Aqaba	Min

capital and this increase of the inhabitants of about 170,000–200,000 people who need shelter, food and water, medication, and sanitary life even at the minimum levels to keep human dignity, beside the teaching services. All these are burdens and more demands and challenges to the providers and mainly the government, which eventually all will be affecting the common man's daily life in the Jordanian street.

Cancer among the Syrians in Jordan, based on the cases registered with the Jordan Cancer Registry, which shows the number of those patients who have been diagnosed and treated in Jordan in a particular period of time/one year. So Syrian's cancer registered by the Jordan Cancer Registry (as shown in the latest official cancer data published for the cases of the year 2011 and the previous 2 years of 2010 and 2009):

The year 2009—male 78 cancer cases, female 67 cancer cases, =total of 145 cases (19 cases are under the age 20 years).
2010—male 87 cancer case, female 47 cancer case, =total of 134 cases (13 cases are under the 20 years).
2011—male 88 cancer cases, female 67 cancer cases, =total of 155 cases (29 cases are under the 20 years).

Other numbers of the cancer cases for more recent data, a Non-JCR Figures but these are from the governmental hospitals, mainly and some other health sectors who are treating Syrian cancer patients and these numbers as totals which are as

2012—188 cancer case
2013—169 cancer case
2014—245 cancer case

Data for cancer in refugees were derived from the UNHCR's records that included registered refugees in Jordan showed the types of cancers among them as: breast cancer was the most common cancer noted in refugees in Jordan in 2011 and 2012, breast cancer accounted for 65 (23.5 %), colorectal cancer for 33 (12.0 %), and soft-tissue cancers for 27 (9.8 %).

It is estimated that there is around 600–700 cancer cases of different types and different age groups of the Syrian refugees currently under treatment which can cost a figure from 10 to 12 million JDs (15–20 M $) per year, this beside the strain and the demand on hospital beds and physicians and other services. This compared to the total Jordanian cancer cases/year, the Syrian refugee cancer load represents an about 14 % increase in Jordan's total cancer disease burden to already difficult economic conditions; therefore, the Jordanian Ministry of Health has limited capacity to cover additional costs due to existing huge debt.

This significant number of refugees and non-refugee Syrians and unregistered refugees contribute to the demographic alteration and burdens. The negative impact is across multiple sectors, high burden on health, water, sanitation, shelter, jobs, and education. There is often a disproportionate focus on camps as 75–80 % of Jordan's Syrian refugees are outside camps.

The economic and social burden of the Syrian conflict has significantly affected Jordan and the region, but Jordan remains committed to provide timely and relevant humanitarian assistance to Syrian refugees without any discrimination. Jordan remains a preferred destination for Syrians seeking refuge. According to the numbers, Jordan hosts most of the displaced Syrian refugees outside their homeland, which constitutes about 15 % of the total Jordan population.

It is evidenced by many studies that Jordan and its people bear the biggest burden of the regional humanitarian crisis. It is also evidenced that Jordan health system may no longer be able to sustain the pressure that the Syrian regional crisis are posing on MOH fiscal and health systems. Credible studies have shown that the entire Jordan's public health system is dangerously overstretched. Lack of sustainable and ongoing funding for Jordan's health sector poses increasingly grave risks to health status and social stability. The Jordan health sector remains committed to sustaining positive health indicators for all.

Based on that one can note the Refugees Impact on Jordan Health System as an overstretched health system capacity and functionality as in 2013, over 45,000 Syrians utilized MOH Health Care services on a monthly basis. Overcrowded facilities, bed capacity. Increased pressure and workload on health professionals across all levels of health services. Significant pressure on Health Information System and capacity to properly evaluate and plan. Significant budgetary/financial burden and resource allocation. Significant shortage of medicines and medical supplies, Syrian patients with chronic diseases use over 30 % of annul supply of chronic disease medications. Challenges while dealing with a high number of cancer patients among Syrians in Jordan. Increased burden of communicable disease patients and high risk of disease outbreaks. Increased tensions between Jordanian and Syrian patients sharing health services. High financial costs and uncertainty about Jordan ability to continue provision of timely and quality services may pose a social instability and risk.

This huge burden is not dealt with the Jordanian government and its health system alone, as many national and international NGOs, and other community sites did have their contributions in helping those unfortunate Syrian refugees and still do.

Catastrophic crisis brings humans back to be one family and have feelings and caring so it was astonishing to see variety humanitarian groups are present in Turkey, Lebanon, and Jordan to assist Syrian refugees who are fleeing their country's civil war.

Cancers including other many non-communicable diseases are increasingly recognized as an important disease burden that needs to be addressed in humanitarian emergencies and prevention, diagnosis, and treatment as it is a major public health issue in crises especially in middle-income countries.

Finally hope for a better healthier future for our region, where everyone can enjoy tranquility, peace, and life.

Chapter 8
Caring for Children with Cancer in a Country Conflicted with Massive Refugee Migration: Jordan as an Example

Maha Arnaout

Abbreviations

ASR	Age Standardized Incidence Rate
CIA	Central Intelligence Agency
CIR	Crude Incidence Rate
ECC	Exceptional Care Committee
GDP	Gross Domestic Product
JCR	Jordan Cancer Registry
JUH	Jordan University Hospital
KAUH	King Abdullah University Hospital
KHCC	King Hussein Cancer Center
MOH	Ministry of Health
NCD	Noncommunicable Diseases
NGOs	Nongovernmental Agencies
RC	Royal Court
RMS	Royal Medical Services
UNHCR	United Nations High Commissioner for Refugees

Introduction

Armed conflicts in Iraq and Syria have led people from these countries to forcibly migrate to neighboring countries such as Jordan, Lebanon, and Turkey.

Jordan, because of its geographical position and stability, continues to be a safe country for refugees since the Palestinian migration in 1948. In addition to receiving

M. Arnaout, M.D. (✉)
Department of Pediatrics, Istiklal Hospital, Amman, Jordan
e-mail: mahaarnaout@gmail.com

M. Silbermann (ed.), *Cancer Care in Countries and Societies in Transition*,
DOI 10.1007/978-3-319-22912-6_8

Palestinians, Jordan has also accommodated forced migrants from other countries in the Middle East, such as Lebanon during the 1975–1991 civil wars, and Iraq since the 1991 Gulf War and after 2003. Since the beginning of the war in Syria, Jordan has accommodated different forced migration waves from Iraq and Syria [1].

Refugees were usually formed of the lower income classes in undeveloped countries. In the twentieth century, infectious and nutritional diseases were the main problems and were managed by health interventions such as vaccinations, antibiotics, and nutritional support. The demographics of refugees in the twenty-first century are changing and now include low-income and middle-income economy classes and both communicable and noncommunicable and chronic diseases are becoming of importance. The need of providing both primary health care, secondary as well as tertiary care is becoming of greater importance in order to manage and fund such situations at times of crisis.

Geography

Jordan is a small country in the Middle East with the geographical coordinates of 31 00 N, 36 00 E. The area of Jordan is 89,342 km^2. It is bounded in the north by Syria, in the east by Iraq and Saudi Arabia, in the south by Saudi Arabia, and in the west by Israel and the Palestinian authority (Fig. 8.1).

The climate of the country is mostly moderate to dry desert; temperature on average ranges from 4 to 31 °C. Natural resources in Jordan include phosphates, potash, and shale oil. Natural freshwater resources are limited [2].

People and Society

The population of Jordan is estimated at 7,930,491 (July 2014). Ninety-eight percent of the population is Arab, while Circassian and Armenian account for the other 2 %; 97.2 % are Muslim, and Christians account for 2.2 % [2].

The population of Jordan age structure is mostly young with the age group of 0–14 years accounting for 35.8 % (2014 estimate). Population growth rate is estimated in 2014 to be 3.86 %, leaving Jordan at the fourth position in comparison to the world (Fig. 8.2).

Health System in Jordan

The country's health care system is divided between the public and private sectors. The Ministry of Health (MOH) operates 1245 primary health care systems and 31 hospitals accounting for 37 % of all hospital beds in the country [3].

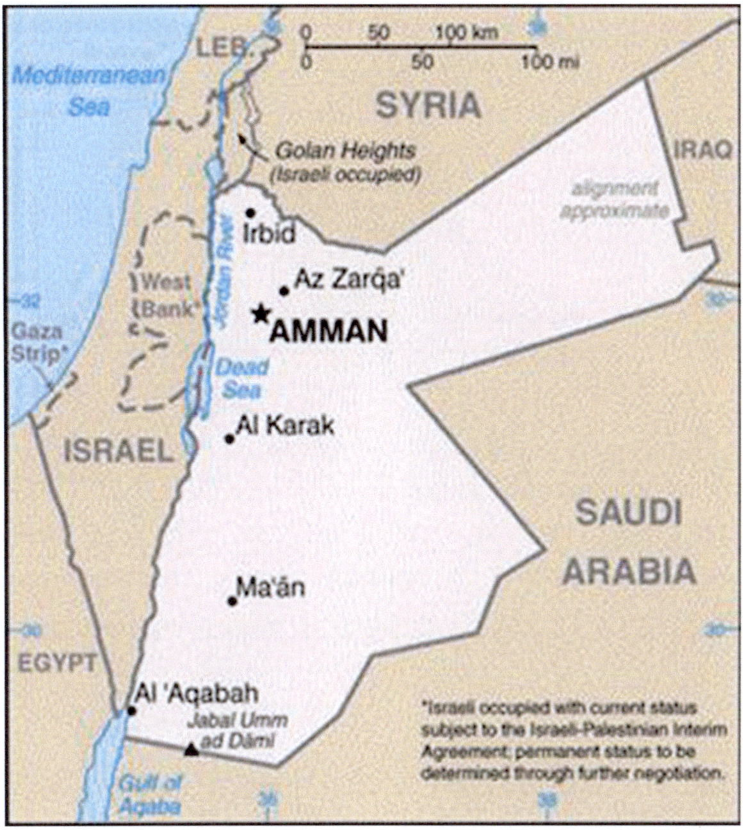

Fig. 8.1 Map of Jordan (CIA World Factbook)

The Royal Medical Services (RMS) runs 12 hospitals providing 24 % of all beds. RMS provides comprehensive insurance for around 25 % of the population [3].

Jordan has two university hospitals, the Jordan University Hospital (JUH) in Amman and the King Abdullah University Hospital (KAUH) in Irbid, both account for 3 % of total beds. The private sector provides 38 % of all hospital beds distributed among 61 hospitals [3].

As a percentage of Gross Domestic Product (GDP), total expenditures on the health sector amounted to 8.4 %, around $483 per capita (2012). The physicians' density was 2.56 physicians/1000 population and hospital bed density was 1.8 beds/1000 population (2011) [2, 3].

Refugees in Jordan

Beginning from 2011 the civil war in Syria resulted in large numbers of Syrians to seek refuge in Jordan. Jordan has received the second highest number of Syrian refuges, relative to its population (8 %). According to United Nations High

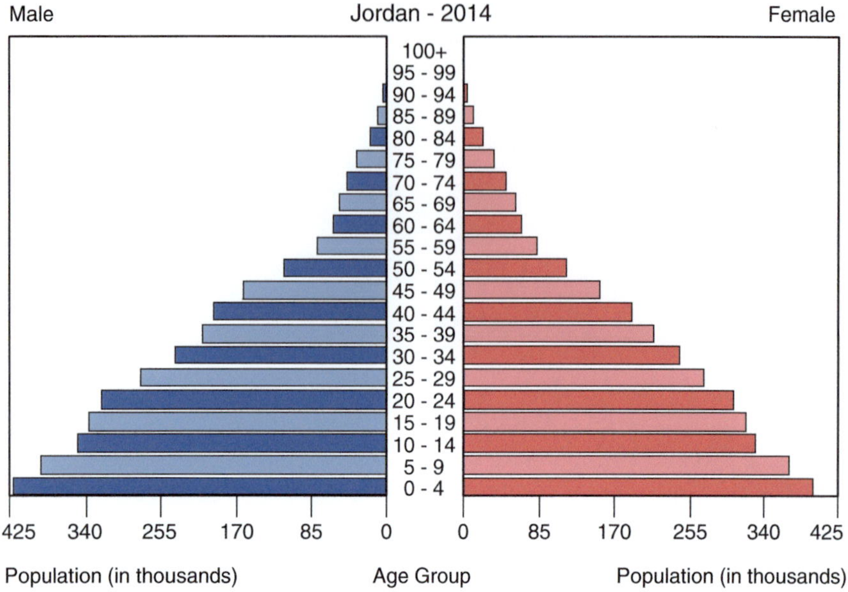

Fig. 8.2 Age structure of Jordanian population of August 2014 (CIA World Factbook)

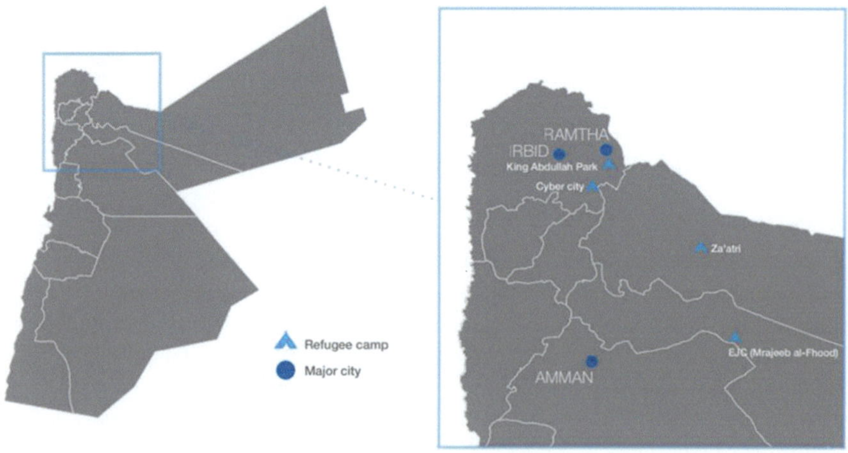

Fig. 8.3 Map of refugees camps in Jordan (UNHCR 2014)

Commissioner for Refugees (UNHCR), 618,515 Syrians reached Jordan as of November 2014, of those 53 % are children [4, 5]. These refugees are distributed at Zaatari camp and Mrajeeb Al Fhood refugee camps (Fig. 8.3). About 70 % of Jordan's refugees are outside of the refugee camps [4].

Other Refugees and internally displaced persons to Jordan include 63,037 from Iraq (2012), thus resulting in a net migration rate of 17.22 migrant(s)/1000 populations (2014 estimate), leaving Jordan in the fifth position as compared to the world [1].

Cancer in Jordan

Cancer is the second most common cause of death after cardiovascular diseases in Jordan. Both cancer incidence and prevalence have been increasing in the last decades and cancer patterns are changing quickly in Jordan. The progression of cancer is an important cause of morbidity and mortality in the country; therefore, the MOH became aware of the urgent need to develop appropriate policies to control this increasing problem [6].

In Jordan, cancer burden continues to grow, which is similar to growth trends in low to middle income countries. Additionally, the population in Jordan is growing and aging, yet, has not fully adopted healthy lifestyles that may help prevent many noncommunicable diseases (NCD) including cancer. The incidence and burden of cancer in Jordan are overwhelming especially with the burden of the refugee crisis.

In the 2010 report of the Jordanian Cancer Registry (JCR) [6] on cancer incidence and epidemiology in Jordan, the total number of reported new cancer cases was 6820, of those 4921 were Jordanians (72.2 %) and 1899 were non-Jordanian (27.8 %). In 2010, the number of new cases among Jordanians increased by 123 cases compared to 4798 cases in 2009 [6].

The number of new cancer cases diagnosed among Jordanians has increased by 46% in the past 10 years, from 3362 cases in 2000 to 4921 in 2010. The Crude Incidence Rate (CIR) of all cancers among Jordanians was 79.4 per 100,000 (74 for males and 85.1 for females). The Age Standardized Incidence Rate (ASR) adjusted to the world standard population was 135.1 per 100,000 population (132.8 for males and 138.4 for females). Overall, 32.4 % of new cancer cases in 2010 were diagnosed among people aged 65 and older, who account 3.3 % of Jordanian population [6].

Distribution of new cancer cases by age group showed that 4 % of the cases were below 15 years and 25 % in the age group 15–44 years, and 38.4 % in the age group 45–64 years.

Among Jordanian males, the top five cancer types were colorectal 332 (14.2 %), lung 311 (13.3 %), prostate 218 (9.4 %), urinary bladder 186 (8 %), and leukemia 127 (5.5 %) [6].

Among Jordanian females, the top five cancers were breast 941 (37.4 %), colorectal 226 (9 %), thyroid 136 (5.4 %), non-Hodgkin Lymphoma 130 (5.2 %), and uterine 113 (3.6 %) [6].

Cancer in Children in Jordan

The age structure of Jordanians is mostly of younger age group, where 35.8 % of Jordanians are below the age of 14 years, 56.2 % are below 24 years (median age 21.8 years) (Fig. 8.4).

According to the Jordanian cancer registry of 2010 [6], there were 194 children in the age group 0–14 years diagnosed with a new cancer in Jordan which constitutes 4 % of all registered malignant tumors in the year 2010. The distribution of cases by

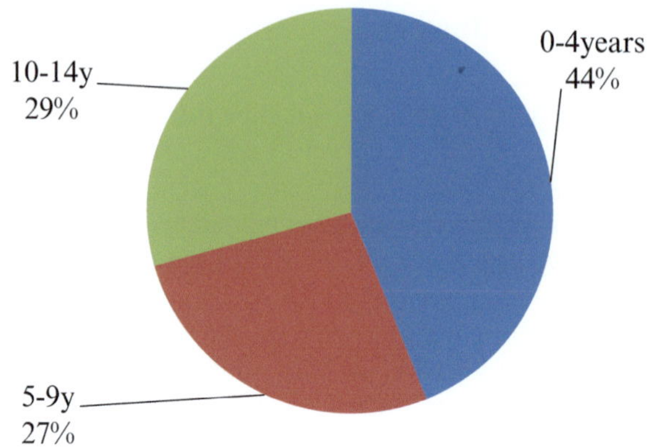

Fig. 8.4 Percentage distribution of pediatric cancer case by age group, 2010—Jordan, Cancer Incidence in Jordan-2010

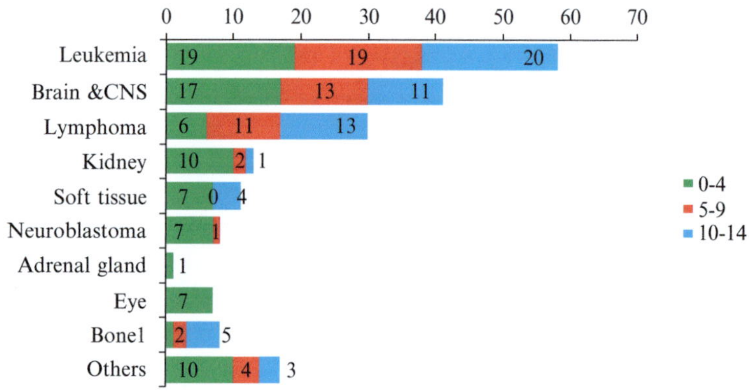

Fig. 8.5 Distribution of childhood cancer by age group and site of tumor, 2010—Jordan, Cancer Incidence in Jordan-2010

sex shows that there were 110 cancer cases in males (56.7 %) and 84 cases in females (43.3 %). The male-to-female ratio was 1.3:1 [6].

The CIR for all cancers in this age group was 85 per million (94 per million for boys and 76 per million for girls). Mean age at diagnosis was 6.5 years. About 44 % of registered cases were under the age 5 years [6, 7].

The top five cancer types in the pediatric age group were leukemia 31 %, brain and CNS 26 %, lymphoma 18 %, kidney 10 %, and soft tissue cancers 9 % (Figs. 8.5 and 8.6). The five year survival and ten year survival rates in children are 79.8 % and 76.7 %, respectively. The best survival rates were best seen in Acute Lymphoblastic Leukemia and lymphoma (may reach up to 90 % in certain types) and the worst rates were seen in bone tumors and adrenal tumors (70 %) [7]. The pattern of childhood cancer in Jordan appears similar to other countries in the region but the survival rates are better in Jordan than in other countries in the region [7, 8].

Children with cancer receive treatment in pediatric oncology wards in the King Hussein Cancer Center (KHCC) and in the RMS hospital in the capital Amman or

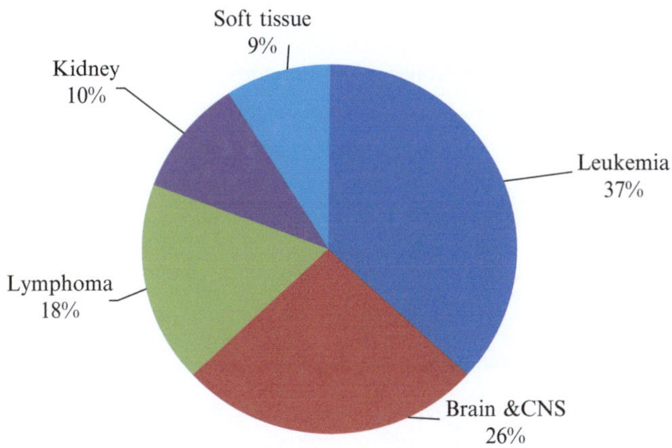

Fig. 8.6 Percentage of top five cancers in pediatric age group (both sex), 2010—Jordan, Cancer Incidence in Jordan-2010

in the pediatric departments in KAUH and Princess Rahma Hospital in Irbid with full government coverage [8–10]. Pediatric cancer treatment in Jordan follows the most recent treatment protocols from the USA or the UK, and Europe. Most chemotherapeutic agents are available but may be expensive; radiotherapy is available and modern. Pediatric oncologists are available and well experienced; most are trained in the USA or the UK [10].

Currently pediatric palliative care is very limited. There is a program limited to KHCC which provides inpatient care, outpatient clinics, emergency room, counseling, home care coverage, and other services. The lack of palliative care other than in KHCC stresses the need to develop a special plan to initiate these services in other hospitals in the country [8–10].

Cancer in Non-Jordanians

The total number of cancer cases among non-Jordanians was 1899 accounting for 27.8 % of all cancers reported and registered by the JCR in 2010 [5], of these, 1875 cases were invasive cancer. The distribution of cases by sex shows that: males were 987 (52.6 %) while females were 888 (47.4 %). The median age at diagnosis for non-Jordanians was 52 years. The most common types of cancer among non-Jordanians are breast, colorectal, and lung cancer [5] (Fig 8.7).

Cancer in Syrian Children

According to UNHCR, 618,515 Syrians reached Jordan as of November 2014, of those 53 % are children [4, 5]. In the year 2010, 108 cases below the age of 15 years were reported to JCR which amounted to 5.8 % of all non-Jordanians registered [5].

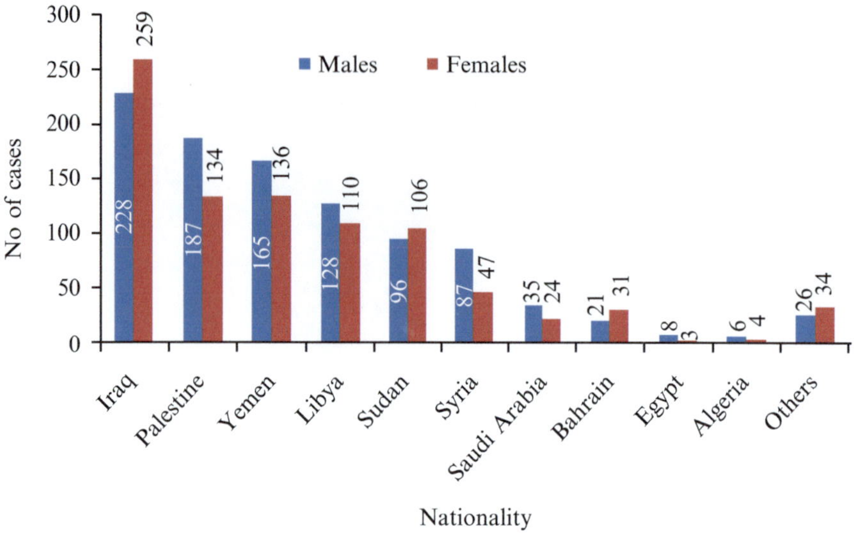

Fig. 8.7 Number of cancers among non-Jordanians by nationality, 2010, Cancer Incidence in Jordan-2010

The estimated number among Syrian children for the first half of 2014 is 48. The number of cancers in children recorded in the Azraq and Zaatari camps between January and June 2014 was 24 cases [4].

Cancer Treatment in Jordan

Treatment of cancer is distributed among KHCC, RMS, MOH, and the private sector. KHCC is the only comprehensive cancer center in Jordan and treats the bulk of cancer cases. In 2008, 250,000 patients sought treatment in the Kingdom including Iraqis, Palestinians, Sudanese, Syrians, and Gulf Cooperation Council citizens, and Egyptians.

The cost of cancer treatment in Jordan is very high. Cancer treatment costs are covered by the government (MOH), military (RMS), and the Royal Court (RC). All Jordanians who have a social security number are treated for free. Non-Jordanians who need treatment for cancer will have to pay for it themselves, at very high cost. Most non-Jordanians will not be able to afford such treatment without a sponsor whether it is through international agencies, nongovernmental agencies (NGOs), charities, or governmental support [10].

Health for Syrian Refugees

Access to health care is one of the biggest concerns for Syrian refugees. The United Nations High Commission for Refugees (UNHCR) and other agencies are prioritizing provision of primary health care and emergency and lifesaving interventions, primarily in cases of emergency obstetric care. Primary health care covers 90 % of the refugees in the camp and 75 % are covered by free health care for community access. Services beyond primary health care are not free [11].

While providing high coverage rate, health facilities for both the local population and the refugees are strained due to the ongoing growing demand. In Jordan's northern governorates, the hospitals and health centers are under the auspices of the MOH; yet one out of ten patients' visits is by Syrians, totaling 35,200 visits per month. There are instances of shortage of medicines for common illnesses and chronic conditions.

The government of Jordan estimated that it incurred additional costs of about $250 million during 2012 and the first quarter of 2013 to meet the increased demands for services. For health care services the MOH has already spent 53 million to accommodate the needs of the Syrian refugees.

The MOH predicts that the work capacity of health staff (number of doctors, nurses, dentists, and pharmacists per population) was reduced by 15 % by the end of 2013, due to the high refugee influx compared to June 2012, while the bed capacity in public hospitals is expected to decrease by over 10 % [11]. Even in the private sector some treatments, medical equipment, medical supplies, and medical technologies cannot cope with the increasing number of patients.

Communicable diseases among Syrian children refugees taken care at the MOH facilities include Tuberculosis, Measles, and Leishmaniasis. Further, the demand for pediatric care has doubled. Common morbidities among Syrian children include acute respiratory illnesses, diarrheal diseases, vaccine-preventable illnesses, skin diseases, and genetic disorders. The MOH's purchases of vaccines almost doubled from 2012 to 2013 ($12–$20 million), whereas the secondary and tertiary level cares need a continued increase of funding to ensure access to essential care [11, 12]. Syrian refugees have a high proportion of chronic or NCD, which are costly and complex to manage. Common diseases among Syrians include asthma, diabetes, hypertension, cardiovascular diseases, renal failure, and autoimmune diseases, while one-third of the families having chronic disease or disability [13]. Cancer treatments are complex and costly, and certain types of cancer cannot be supported with the available resources which require difficult choices in allocating the available resources. Several of the major cancers that were recorded are amenable to prevention and early detection and such programs need to be developed for refugees [13].

Cancer Treatment for Syrian Refugees

Cancer treatment in Syrian patients has a low priority in the list of treatments for medical conditions; cancer treatment requires not only expensive care, but also expensive medications and investigations, and requires close health provider care.

UNHCR's Exceptional Care Committee (ECC) receives applications from cases with serious medical problems that require costs beyond the maximum allocated per person, which ranged between $1000 and $2000 per person per year from 2009 to 2012 [13, 14].

Refugees with serious medical illness that require treatment beyond these amounts are referred to ECC. The ECC reviews such cases to decide whether to support or reject treatment and the level of treatment provision [13, 14].

The decision criteria for the ECC to accept or reject treatment for a refugee and the level of treatment are transparent and include:

1. Necessity and adequacy of the recommended treatment.
2. Need of assistance (financial vulnerability).
3. Feasibility of treatment plan.
4. Disease prognosis.
5. Cost of care.
6. Eligibility as a registered refugee.

The following are treatments that are not usually approved by UNHCR:

1. High cost treatment when less costly alternative is equally effective and available.
2. Organ transplant, kidney, liver, heart, bone marrow, etc.
3. In vitro fertilization.
4. Cosmetic treatment and surgery.
5. Elective procedures.
6. High cost complex treatment of chronic illnesses not available to the average Jordanian.
7. Thalassemia, multiple sclerosis treatment.

Five hundred eleven cancer cases among refugees were registered from 2010 to 2012. The average amount requested from the ECC for cancer treatment for a refugee in Jordan was $11,250 in 2011 and $5151 in 2012; the actual amounts that were approved were $4626 in 2011 and $3501 in 2012 [13, 15–17]. In comparison, in 2012, the average approved costs by the ECC were $4458 for cardiovascular diseases, $2061 for respiratory diseases, $2788 for renal diseases, $1746 for eye disorders, and $1628 for trauma. Unfortunately children with cancer are also evaluated according the above criteria and don't receive adequate treatment, although they have a better prognosis than adult cancers [13].

In 2011 the MOH treated 134 Syrians with cancer; in 2012 this number increased to 188 cases and is expected to further increase to more than 600 cases. This represent about 14 % rise in the number of patients treated. This increase represents an additional burden on the MOH in cancer control efforts in Jordan [13].

Conclusion

Cancer treatment is expensive for both adults and children. The increasing number of refugees is an additional burden on UNHCR, and Jordan. Therefore capacities of the health system for incoming refugees need to be improved. The needs for primary and emergency health care should be balanced with those of secondary and tertiary care.

A uniform reporting mechanism for cancer cases among the refugees must be developed by UNHCR, as well as the hosting countries. Efficient data management systems and cancer registries need to be developed.

For preventable or early detection cancer, programs need to be developed, such as mammography. Education of refugees about the early detection and prevention techniques need to be actively approached. Several major cancers that were recorded were amenable to prevention and early detection, the most prominent being breast cancer.

Sustainable financing for international agencies such as UNHCR must be secured for both communicable and noncommunicable diseases for children and adults.

References

1. Chatelard G. Jordan: a refugee haven. The Online Journal of the Migration Policy Institute. http://www.migrationpolicy.org/artile/Jordan-refugee-haven. Accessed 23 Apr 2014.
2. Central Intelligence Agency (US). The world fact book 2014. https://www.cia.gov/library/publications/the-world-factbook/geos/jo.html. Accessed 30 Mar 2014.
3. Khammash T. The Jordanian Health Sector. Jordan Investment Trust P.L.C. http://jordinvest.com.jo/uploads/documents/health-sector-report-09-09-2012.pdf. Accessed 27 Sept 2014.
4. UNHCR. UNHCR global appeal 2015 Update—Jordan. http://www.unhcr.org/528a092c13.html. Accessed 1 Nov 2014.
5. United Nations Office for the Coordination of Humanitarian Affairs (UNOCHA). Country Overview: Jordan. The evaluation of the refugee influx; Comprehensive Regional Strategic Framework. http://syria.unocha.org/content/comprehensive-regional-strategic-framework-syria-crisis-framework. Accessed 8 July 2014.
6. Arqowb K, Nimri O, Tarawneh M, Al Zaghal M. Cancer incidence in Jordan-2010. Jordan Cancer Registry. 15th ed. http://www.moh.gov.jo/Annual%Incidence%20of%20cancer%20in%20Jo. Accessed 12 Feb 2014.
7. Arqowb A, Nimri O, Tarawneh M, Zuraikat R. Pediatric cancer incidence & survival 2000–2009 for Jordanian population. http://conference.ncri.org.uk/abstracts/2014/abstracts/A220.html. Accessed 12 Feb 2014.
8. Al-Rimawi H. Pediatric oncology situation analysis. J Pediatr Hematol Oncol. 2012;34:S15–8.
9. Silbermann M, et al. Pediatric palliative care in the Middle East. In: Knapp C, Madden V, Fowler-Kerry S, editors. Pediatric palliative care: global perspectives. Dordrecht: Springer; 2012. p. 127–59.
10. Arnaout M. Pediatric oncologist and palliative care. Personal experience. 22 Dec 2014.
11. UNHCR, UNICEF, WFP. Joint assessment review of the Syrian refugee response in Jordan. January 2014. https://data.unhcr.org/syrianrefugees/download.php?id=4309. Accessed 9 Mar 2014.
12. Ministry of Planning and International Cooperation, Jordan. Brief on the Impact of the Syrian Crisis by Sector. National Resilience Plan 2014–2016. 1 June 2014. http://un.org.jo/sites/default/files/NRP.pdf. Accessed 12 Oct 2014.

13. Spiegel P, Khalifa A, Mateen F. Cancer in refugees in Jordan and Syria between 2009 and 2012: challenges and the way forward in humanitarian emergencies. Lancet. 2014;15(7):e290–7. http://www.thelancet.com. Accessed 20 July 2014.
14. Guide to UNHCR Supported Health Care Services in Jordan. UNHCR. http://data.unhcr.org/syrianrefugees/. Accessed 14 Aug 2014.
15. The Lancet. Refugees struggling to access cancer treatment, experts warn. Sciencedaily. 25 May 2014. www.sciencedaily.com/releases/2014/05/140525204409.htm. Accessed 14 Aug 2014.
16. Mhailan M, Hijawi M, Jreisat S, Eltom A. Syrian refugees and Jordan's health sector. Correspondence. The Lancet. 2013;382:206. www.thelancet.com. Accessed 25 Apr 2014.
17. Syrian refugees and Jordan's health sector. Editorial. The Lancet. 2013;382:2056. www.thelancet.com. Accessed 16 Aug 2014.

Chapter 9
Challenges and Future Trends for Cancer Care in Egypt

Karima Elshamy

Introduction

Cancer is an increasing problem in Egypt. The commonest sites were liver (23.8 %), breast (15.4 %), and bladder (6.9 %) (both sexes): liver (33.6 %) and bladder (10.7 %) among men, and breast (32.0 %) and liver (13.5 %) among women. By 2050, a threefold increase in incident cancer relative to 2013 was estimated, these results based upon results of National Cancer Registry Program (NCRP) [1]. Egypt is expected to experience the highest increase in the coming two decades. Cancer is already an important health problem and will become increasingly important not only in terms of rank order, as infections are better controlled, but also in terms of incidence and mortality, which will both increase as populations continue to grow and age, and as risk factors for cancer associated with greater affluence continue to increase. At present, resources for cancer control in Egypt are not only inadequate but directed almost exclusively to treatment. This strategy, although successful to a degree, is suboptimal because the impact of preventive measures on incidence is not taken full advantage of, while the lack of approaches to earlier diagnosis reduces the value of therapy. The curability of cancer is directly related to its stage at the time of diagnosis, and in the majority of cancer is generally diagnosed when at a relatively advanced stage. According to WHO, 40 % of cancers could be avoided (prevention), 40 % could be cured (if detected early), and the rest should be managed with palliation. Prevention therefore offers the greatest public health potential and the most cost-effective long-term approach for cancer control [2].

K. Elshamy, D.N.Sc. (✉)
Medical Surgical Nursing Department, Faculty of Nursing,
Mansoura University, Mansoura, Egypt
e-mail: karima_elshamy2002@yahoo.com

M. Silbermann (ed.), *Cancer Care in Countries and Societies in Transition*,
DOI 10.1007/978-3-319-22912-6_9

Egypt: Background Information

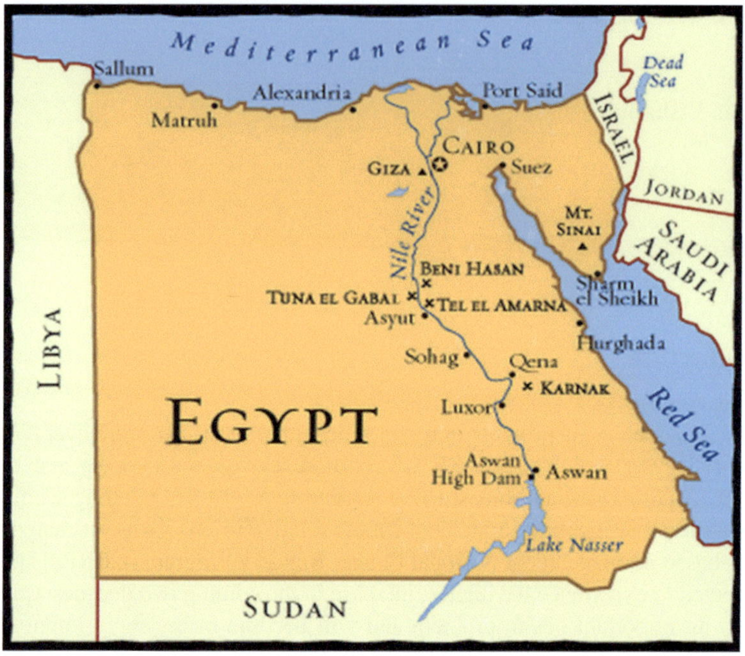

The Land and Geography: Egypt is located in the northeastern corner of Africa. Rectangular in shape, it covers an area of 386,000 mile^2. To the West lie the Western Desert and Libya, and the East is bordered by a desert plateau, Red Sea, Sinai, and Israel. The Sudan is on Egypt's southern border and to the North lies the Mediterranean. Egypt can be divided into The Eastern Desert, The Western Desert, and The Nile Valley.

The people: Population (2012 est.): 83,688,164 (growth rate: 1.92 %. Cairo, 10,902,000, Alexandria, 4,387,000; Giza, 2,597,600 and the country is divided into 26 governorates. Poverty has declined over the past few decades; however, there is disparity—poverty in Upper Egypt increased from 29 to 34 % in rural areas and from 11 to 19 % in urban areas. Although Egypt has experienced a rapid transition to lower fertility, Egypt is the second most populous country in the WHO Eastern Mediterranean Region, with 43 % of the population living in urban areas and overcrowded conditions. The Egyptians are outgoing, warm, and have a distinct sense of humor. They have respect and a liking for foreigners, and a deep sense of tolerance for other races, religions, and nationalities [3].

Language: Arabic is Egypt's official language. However, most Egyptians understand and speak English and French. In larger towns, the foreign visitor will encounter no difficulty in communicating with the people [4].

Religion: Approximately 85 % of the populations of Egypt are Moslems. Most of the balance, about nine million, is Christian Orthodox who belongs to the Coptic Church. In most cities in Egypt, mosques and churches can be found next to each other. There are also some synagogues since a small Jewish community still lives in Egypt [4].

Economy: Egypt is classified as a lower-middle-income country; however, characteristics of high-income, middle-income, and low-income countries coexist. Poverty has declined over the past few decades; however, there is disparity—poverty in Upper Egypt increased from 29 to 34 % in rural areas and from 11 to 19 % in urban areas [4].

The structure of the Egyptian Government is a democracy in transition, having recently elected a president; with all political authority is vested in the Government in Cairo [4].

The Egyptian health system: The health care system in Egypt is quite complex with a large number of public entities involved in the management, financing, and provision of care. Egypt's wide network of public (several ministries beside the military and police), NGO, faith-based charity organizations, and private health facilities allow good geographic accessibility and coverage. The Ministry of Health and Population is responsible for overall health and population policy as well as the provision of public health services, and is responsible for health insurance organization that provides services too. The Ministry of higher education is however responsible for health profession education (medical, nursing, dentistry, and pharmacy) and also runs university teaching hospitals. Public health expenditure is low and has pluralistic and complex financing mechanisms: tax-based financing, health insurance, and fee for service through out-of-pocket expenditures. To achieve universal coverage, Egypt is rolling out a new insurance scheme, currently being piloted in Suez Governorate, based on a "family physician model" which will separate financing from service provision. Despite Government's efforts for universal coverage, about half of total health expenditure comes from out-of-pocket (50 %) at the point of service in public and private facilities. Egypt produces over 90 % of the pharmaceuticals it consumes. Pharmaceuticals account for just over one-third of all health spending, of which approximately 85 % is private expenditure. Publicly produced medicines are heavily subsidized, which to a considerable extent accounts for their overuse [4, 5].

The Egyptian constitution enshrines free medical care as a basic right for all citizens, and though access to primary health care is fairly widespread, this ideal has yet to be fully realized. Vaccination rates, a good indicator of the access to basic health services, are high, and Egypt has also achieved some success in controlling communicable diseases. However, access to even basic services varies widely according to gender, region of residence, and socioeconomic status [4, 5].

The organization of the Egyptian health system is fairly complex. Public health care is highly centralized within the Ministry of Health and Population (MOHP), though a number of other public entities are involved in managing and financing health care services. The most important of these are the Health Insurance Organization (HIO), which finances and provides services to almost half the population, and the Ministry of Higher Education (MOHE), which is responsible for medical education and some service delivery (i.e., in university hospitals). There is no overarching institutional oversight of all public entities involved in providing health services, limiting coordination between the various branches [4, 5].

Expenditure on health: is divided in the following manner: 36 % goes to pharmaceuticals, 19 % to services provided by the MOHP, 18 % to the private sector, 10 % to university hospitals, 8 % to services provided by the insurance system, 6 % to NGOs, and 3 % to other public institutions. Private insurance is fairly limited in Egypt, as premiums are low and companies find it hard to turn a profit. Recent reforms have de-regulated premiums, making the regulatory environment somewhat less restrictive, but still difficult to operate in [4, 5].

Magnitude of Cancer Care in Egypt

The Demographic Profile of Egypt

1. Population trends

   (a) *The population size of Egypt*
   Currently, Egypt is experiencing significant size, age structure changes that will have major implications for its socioeconomic development. The population size of Egypt increased from 44.9 million in 1980 to approximately 78.1 million in 2010. It is projected that in 2050, the population size of Egypt will reach approximately 121.8 million.

   (b) *Population growth in Egypt*
   The growth rate of the population of Egypt has been decreasing since the period 1980–1985, where it stood at 2.28 %. It reached 1.56 % in the period 1995–2000 and slightly increased afterwards to 1.68 % in the period 2005–2010. The population growth rate is expected to continue declining and will reach 0.69 % in the period 2045–2050.

2. Indicators of demographic transition

   (a) *Mortality transition in Egypt*

- Life expectancy
- Life expectancy at birth in Egypt gained 10 years from the period 1980–1985 to the period 2005–2010, increasing from 59.9 to 69.9 years. It is expected to reach 77.3 years in 2045–2050.

Table 9.1 The most frequent cancers in Egypt estimated using the results of the National Population-Based Registry Program of Egypt 2008–2011

Sex	The most frequent cancer site	%	Crude rate	ASR
Male	Liver	33.63	39.5	61.8
	Bladder	10.71	12.6	21.1
	Lung[a]	5.69	6.7	10.4
	Non-Hodgkin lymphoma	5.48	6.4	8.8
	Brain[b]	5.48	6.4	8.8
	Prostate	4.27	5.0	9.3
Female	Breast	32.04	35.8	48.8
	Liver	13.54	15.1	24.4
	Brain[b]	5.18	5.8	8.0
	Ovary	4.12	4.6	6.3
	Non-Hodgkin lymphoma	3.80	4.2	6.1
	Thyroid	3.28	3.7	4.3
Both sexes	Liver	23.81	27.5	43.6
	Breast	15.41	17.8	24.3
	Bladder	6.94	8.0	13.5
	Brain[b]	5.29	6.1	8.5
	Non-Hodgkin lymphoma	4.64	5.4	7.5
	Lung[a]	4.22	4.9	7.5

[a]Includes trachea, bronchus, and lung tumors
[b]Includes brain and nervous system tumors
Amal S. Ibrahim et al. [1]

3. The population structure

   (a) *Egypt's population age composition*
   The proportion of the population under 15 years of age has been decreasing since 1980 and is estimated to continue declining to 2050. At the same time, the proportion of the working-age population (15–64) has been increasing since 1980. It is projected to reach 66.9 % in 2040 then it will decline to 65.9 % in 2050. The proportion of the elderly population (65+) has also been increasing and is expected to reach 12.3 % in 2050.

   The age distributions in Egypt vary widely with major differences in the percentage of young and old as seen in Table 9.1. Hence, currently there is less cancer, but the expected change in demographics over the next 20–30 years is likely to result in an explosive increase in noncommunicable diseases such as cancer and heart disease [6].

   (b) *Changing age structure*
   In 1950, the pyramid had a wide base signaling the structure of a young population. In 2050, the pyramid is expected to narrow down [6].

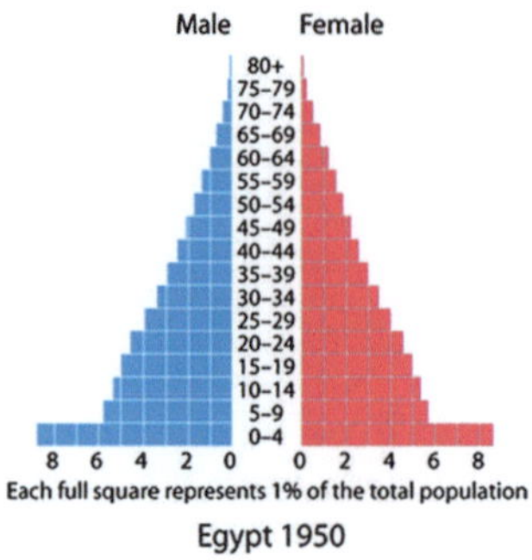

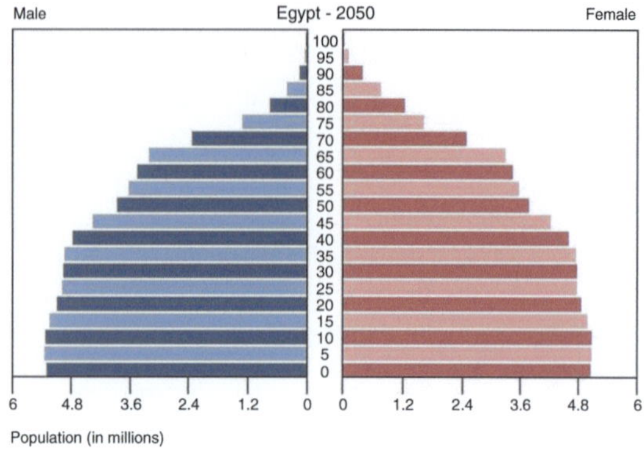

(c) *Egypt's youth population*
In 1980, youth aged 15–24 years constituted 19.4 % of the total population and 35.16 % of the working-age population. In 2005, the percentage of youth increased to reach 21.1 % of the total population then started decreasing and is projected to reach 14.5 % in 2050 [6].

(d) *Egypt's elderly population*
The percentage of the elderly population (65+) in Egypt increased from 3.0 % in 1950 to 5.5 % in 2005 and remained as such in 2010. It is projected to continue increasing to reach 12.3 % in 2050 [6].

Current Status of Cancer Care in Egypt

An Overview and Profile of Frequent Cancers in Egypt

In men, liver and bladder cancers represented approximately 44 % of cancer in males.

In females, breast cancer occupied the top ranks accounting for 32.4 % of all cancers, followed by liver that accounting 13.54 %.

In both sexes, the proportions and rates of the most frequent cancer sites by gender, there was predominance of liver, breast, and bladder cancer that represented approximately 46 % of all cancers (Table 9.1).

During the period 2013–2050, population of Egypt is expected to increase to approximately 160 % the 2013 population size (Table 9.2). Applying the current age-specific incidence rates to successive populations would lead to a progressive increase in number of incident cases from 114,985 in 2013 to 331,169 in 2050, approximately 290 % of 2013 incidence (Table 9.3). This increase reflected both population growth and demographic change mainly due to aging of population. Population growth alone would increase the number of incident cases by 55.2 % in 2015. This fraction progressively decreased to become 32.8 % in 2050. The fraction due to aging gradually increased to reach 67.2 % in 2050 (Figs. 9.1, 9.2, 9.3, and 9.4).

Table 9.2 Incidence rates of cancer in Egypt (/100,000 populations) classified by region and sex for all cancer sites with and without nonmelanoma skin cancer (C44)

	Male		Female		All		Male:female ratio	
	Crude rate	ASR	Crude rate	ASR	Crude rate	ASR		
	(95 % CI)	(95 % CI)	(95 % CI)	(95 % CI)	(95 % CI)	(95 % CI)	Crude rate	ASR
All sites								
(i) Upper Egypt	97.1	142.8	116.9	167.1	107.0	155.0	0.8:1	0.9:1
	(89.1–105.8)	(133.1–153.2)	(108.1–126.5)	(156.5–178.4)	(101.0–113.3)	(147.7–162.6)		
(ii) Middle Egypt	109.7	170.0	95.9	132.1	102.9	151.1	11:1	13:1
	(105.4–114.1)	(164.7–175.5)	(91.1–100.2)	(127.4–137.0)	(100.0–106.0)	(147.5–154.8)		
(iii) Lower Egypt	138.5	191.8	131.7	173.3	135.2	182.6	11:1	11:1
	(133.2–144.0)	(185.6–198.2)	(126.5–137.2)	(167.3–179.6)	(131.4–139.1)	(178.2–187.1)		
(iv) Calculated rates of Egypt	117.3	178.5	111.7	159.1	114.5	169.0	11:1	11:1
	(116.0–118.6)	(176.9–180.2)	(110.4–113.0)	(157.6–160.7)	(113.6–115.5)	(167.9–170.2)		
All sites (excluding nonmelanoma skin cancer C44)								
(i) Upper Egypt	96.0	141.0	115.1	163.9	105.5	152.5	0.8:1	0.9:1
	(88.1–1104.6)	(131.4–151.4)	(106.3–124.5)	(153.4–175.1)	(99.5–111.8)	(145.5–160.1)		
(ii) Middle Egypt	108.0	167.2	94.9	130.7	101.6	149.0	11:1	13:1
	(103.8–112.3)	(162.0–172.6)	(90.9–99.1)	(126.0–135.6)	98.7–104.6)	(145.5–152.6)		
(iii) Lower Egypt	136.7	189.1	130.1	170.9	133.5	180.0	11:1	11:1
	(131.5–142.2)	(182.9–195.5)	(124.8–135.5)	(164.9–177.1)	(129.7–137.3)	(175.7–184.4)		
(iv) Calculated rates of Egypt	115.7	175.9	110.3	157.0	113.1	166.6	11:1	11:1
	(114.4–117.0)	(174.3–177.5)	(109.0–111.6)	(155.4–158.5)	(112.2–114.0)	(165.5–167.8)		

Cancer Care Facilities in Egypt

Egypt has more facilities for cancer treatment than any other country in Africa; however, many elements of cancer control strategy still need to be implemented or improved [7]. Cancer treatment facilities, in fact, include the biggest and more specialized center. In the Middle East is the National Cancer Institute (NCI) which is affiliated to Cairo University. NCI is carrying research, education, and clinical responsibilities and is considered the main reference in Egypt regarding cancer. Also, South Egypt Cancer Institute, Assiut University, Assiut, Egypt, 14 clinical

Table 9.3 Estimated cancer incidence in the period 2013–2050 and causes of increase

	2013	2015	2020	2025	2050
Estimated population	85,294,388 (100 %)	88,487,396 (103.7 %)	96,260,017 (112.9 %)	103,742,157 (121.6 %)	137,872,522 (161.6 %)
Number of cases[a]	114,985	122,783 (106.8 %)	144,255 (125.5 %)	168,723 (146.7 %)	331,169 (288.0 %)
Increased cases from 2013[b]		7798 (6.8 %)	29,270 (25.5 %)	53,738 (46.7 %)	216,184 (188.0 %)
Increased cases due to population growth[c]		4303	14,783	24,869	70,880
Increased cases due to population structure change[d]		3494	14,487	28,869	145,304
% increase due to population growth[e]		55.20 %	50.50 %	46.28 %	32.79 %

[a]Number of expected cases depending on 2013 rates of incidence
[b]Number of increased cases from 2013 number of cases
[c]Number of increased cases (from 2013) that is attributed to increase in population number (population growth)
[d]Number of increased cases (from 2013) that is attributed to change in population structure (aging of population) and not to population growth
[e]Percentage of increased number of cases (from 2013) that can be attributed to population growth only (not due to change in population structure)
Amal S. Ibrahim et al. [1]

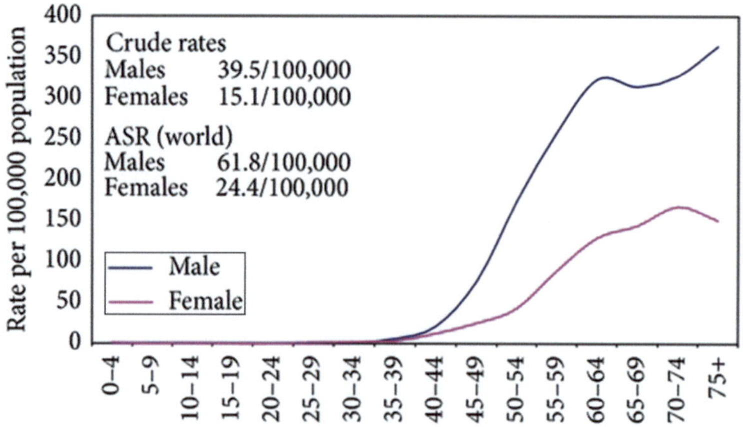

Fig. 9.1 Calculated age-specific incidence rates for liver cancer in Egypt 2008–2011

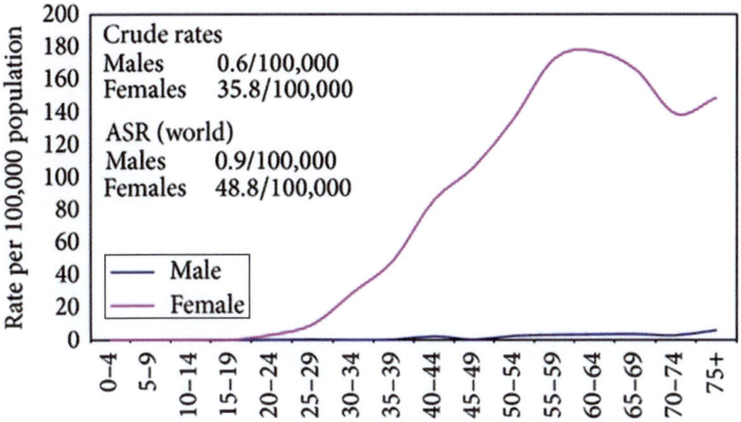

Fig. 9.2 Calculated age-specific incidence rates for breast cancer in Egypt 2008–2011

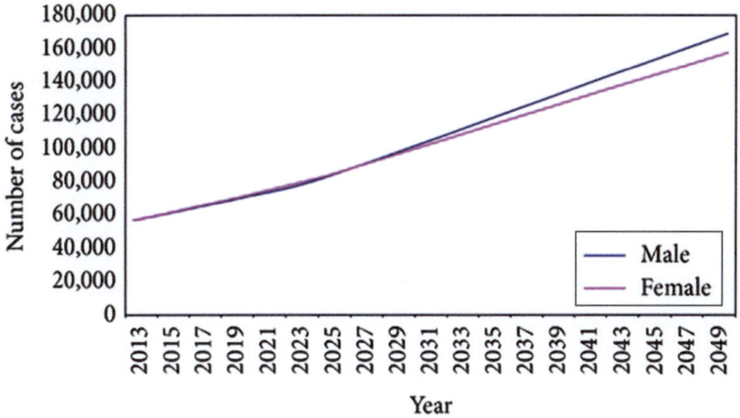

Fig. 9.3 Estimated number of cases in Egypt (2013–2050)

oncology departments in the other public universities; ten cancer centers affiliated to the Ministry of Health in 12 governorates; 11 military cancer units that treat both civilian and military patients; oncology clinics at the hospitals run by the Egyptian Health Insurance Organization in most major cities; semi-private, NGO-operated cancer facilities; a charity-run Centre of Excellence of Pediatric Oncology in Cairo; and private-sector clinics and centers. In addition to surgery, most of these facilities have chemotherapy and radiotherapy capabilities (either linear accelerators or cobalt-60 units). Most centers have CT scanners and MRI machines, and the country has five PET-CT scanners [8].

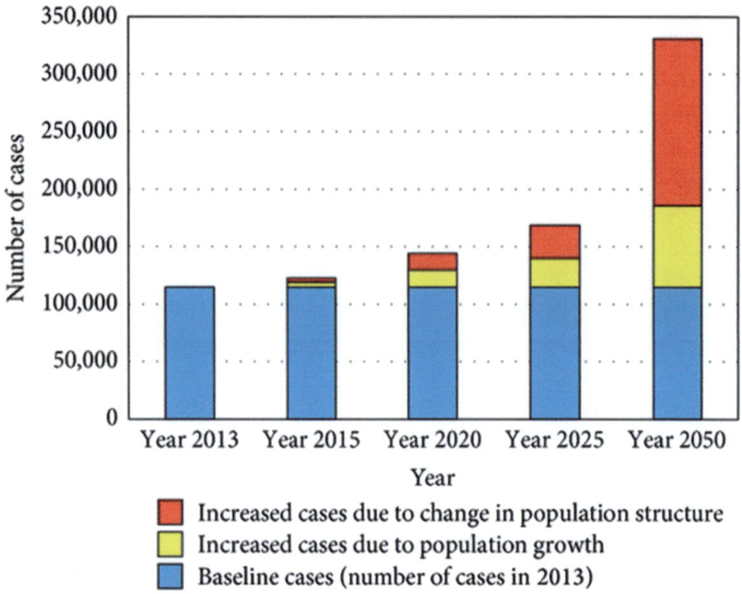

Fig. 9.4 Estimated number of cases in Egypt (2013–2050) and causes of the increase in cases

According to the WHO survey, Egypt had an operational policy, strategy, or action plan for cancer in 2010. However, no structured national cancer control program as recommended by WHO is in place. Practical measures are needed for the optimum allocation of available resources to reduce the numbers of cancer cases and deaths and to improve quality of life for patients with cancer, through adoption of WHO recommendations [9].

Approaches to Cancer Control

Prevention and Early Detection of Cancer

Although screening by mammography has been accepted as the gold-standard to ensure early detection of BC, its cost–benefit ratio is still debated in the scientific community. It is important to keep in mind that even in the best screening settings, most deaths from breast cancer are not currently prevented by mammography screening. The latest reviews indicate a reduction of no more than 15 % in BC mortality rate after introduction of mammography screening in western countries. Recent studies suggest that screening by CBE could achieve a reduction of 52–88 % of this magnitude with a better cost-effectiveness ratio.

Whatever screening tool is used, screening programs are resource-demanding and heavy-to-implement health interventions. Downstaging programs are an appealing alternative when resources are scarce, and should be considered as the first option in regions where a majority of BC is diagnosed at late stage.

In Egypt, most cancers present at an advanced stage when cure is improbable even with the best treatments. Where still a vast majority of tumors diagnosed are above 2 cm, there is room for improvement by a downstaging approach. Screening by CBE would be relevant to regions/groups where stage distribution is good enough that downstaging has no potential for major improvement. Early detection can result from both downstaging in some part of the country and screening in other parts. However, Egypt should follow the WHO and BHGI guidelines which call for countries to conduct research and pilot projects prior to establishment of national programs, as neither benefit of screening nor benefit of downstaging programs have been formally demonstrated to date in any developing country. A major element in improving survival rates in many cancers has to be the much earlier stage of disease at diagnosis and this could be brought about by public education and, in some cases, screening for premalignant lesions or early cancer [10].

In Egypt, primary health care workers are rarely provided with sufficient education about the early signs of cancer or where to refer suspected cases. This could be remedied by short training courses (ideally coupled to continuing education programs), brochures or posters, and by establishing links between those who deliver primary health care and referral centers. Population-based registries disease data are recorded. These data for breast cancers are 25.5 % of cases present at an early stage. It is clear that a high fraction of patients reaching these centers predominantly have advanced stage (stage III and IV) [11].

The Ministry of Health and Population Pilot Screening Program

The MOHP of Egypt has launched a pilot screening program in October 2007. This program is coordinated by Dr. Dorria Salem, Prof. of Radiology Cairo University and Head of Women's Imaging Unit. The purpose of this program is to screen women from 45 years old for:

1. Breast cancer (digital mammography exam)
2. Diabetes (blood sugar test)
3. Hypertension (blood pressure test)
4. Obesity (weight and height measurement)

The women recruitment process is based on the presence of mobile vans where all of the above exams take place. Few weeks before a van is moved to a district, the population is informed about the importance of screening, thanks to posters and pamphlets distributed in mosques, churches, and streets. Women eligible for screening (i.e., 45 years old or more) are contacted by phone or visited by heath workers of the Red Crescent to encourage them to come to the vans. Only women without breast complains are admitted for breast cancer screening. The complaining patients can go to the women's imaging unit at Al-Kasr Al-Ainy teaching hospital.

The pilot phase of the project has begun in October 2007. By February 2009, 25 different locations in Cairo, Giza, and Alexandria governorates were visited; up to 22,000 women had been screened, 406 were referred for further diagnosis, 75 (18 %) turned out to be false positive. Out of the real positive, 59 (18 %) were operated, 73 (22 %) refused diagnosis or treatment, 35 (11 %) were not reachable, and the remaining were into the diagnosis or treatment process.

One of the main problems encountered is to convince women who have a suspicious mammogram, to go for diagnosis and treatment as some refuse or disappear. Health workers from the NGO "Hope" are dedicated to this task. This kind of problem is frequently observed in developing countries when screening for breast cancer.

A TV media campaign about screening has taken place during the autumn 2008 to raise awareness about breast cancer and facilitate acceptance of screening, as well as a campaign on the local radio station Nogoom FM; a new TV campaign should start soon [12].

The Breast Cancer Cairo Trial

The BC Cairo Trial is a research project designed to evaluate the efficiency of screening by clinical breast examination (CBE) in the context of primary health care (PHC). The project has been designed by Pr. Tony Miller, Epidemiologist at the Public Health Sciences Department of Toronto University (Canada), and is headed in Cairo by Dr. Salwa Boulos, radiologist in charge of the mammography unit at the Italian hospital until recently and now at El-Gallaa Hospital. The project has been financially supported by the Italian embassy in Cairo and the European School of Oncology (Milan).

The study has been launched in other countries of the region (Yemen, Iran, Sudan) but Cairo was the first and is thus the more advanced center of the study. The study was launched in May 2000 and has begun by a pilot phase (phase I) followed by a classical randomized trial (phase II and III).

Phase I (Pilot Study)

The initial target group was women 35–64 living in a geographically defined area (eight blocks) around the Italian Hospital (Abasseya district). In this pilot phase, 4116 women were contacted by social health worker (door to door visit) to attend designated PHC centers for Clinical Breast Exam at pre-determined date and time.

Table 9.4 Preliminary comparison of the stage distribution in the Cairo Trial

	Screened group (%)	Control groups (%)
Stage I	30	8
Stage II	43	18
Stage III	20	44
Stage IV	7	30

Of the women targeted, 60 % ($N=2481$) attended, of those who attended 12 % ($N=291$) were found to have abnormalities, of these 82 % ($N=236$) attended the Italian hospital for diagnosis, and of these 3.4 % (20 women) were diagnosed with BC. This latest number corresponds to a quite high prevalence of BC: 8/1000. Only one BC patient was less than 40.

Phases II and III

The target group was restricted to women 40–64 and divided in two groups based on residential blocks (four blocks each). The group A was offered active screening as in the pilot phase, the group B received only health education. Two additional areas were identified each with 5000 women aged 50–65 who were cluster randomized. The reputation of the trial preceded subject recruitment and there was higher acceptance than in the pilot phase, with 85–91 % of women accepting to go for screening.

Although follow-up of all groups is yet to be completed, preliminary results are encouraging. Stage distribution in both screened and control groups are given in Table 9.4.

This trial is testing an approach to early detection which is promising for Egypt; it would be beneficial to extend this trial to other centers/towns of Egypt. However this requires important resources, especially human resources, i.e., dynamic and dedicated local PIs, not mentioning international specialists.

It has to be mentioned that the idea of screening by clinical breast exam usually receives very little support from the medical community in low- and middle-income countries; CBE is erroneously perceived as inefficient because of its low-tech nature. This is a misconception that could be tackled in Egypt by an increased publicity about the Cairo Trial [13].

Remarks on the Two Screening Experiments Taking Place in Egypt

The populations at risk of BC in Egypt, i.e., the women above 45 years of age, are approximately 8.5 millions. The 22,000 women screened by the MOH mammography program in 1.3 years and the 15,000 women screened by the Cairo Trial screened women in 8 years represent, respectively, 0.26 % and 0.17 % of this target population. Such percentages are a little demoralizing in view of the dedication, effort, and resources which were put in these two screening programs. However these programs are pilot studies and they are not aiming at a rapid national expansion, especially the Cairo Trial which should be viewed as a research project, but their results raise some concerns about the feasibility of a national screening program in a country like Egypt in a foreseeable future [13–15].

Fakkous and Port Said Program

A program in the rural region of Fakous and the urban region of Port Said used local resources to increase awareness of breast cancer and its treatment by organizing home visits from primary care workers and meetings with local women resulted in a substantial reduction in cases of advanced breast cancer. About 20 % of breast cancer cases in Port Said were amenable to conservative breast cancer surgery in 2008, and the number of stage III and IV cases had halved by 2004–2008 compared with 1992–2003 [16]. Conversely, early detection programs without access to treatments would be fruitless and frustrating for both patients and health professionals.

The Breast Cancer Foundation of Egypt

The Breast Cancer Foundation of Egypt (BCFE) was established in 2003 by a small group of health care professionals, survivors and public spirited citizens as a nongovernmental, nonprofit organization under the Ministry of Social Solidarity. At that time, there was no established BC awareness governmental program and no other NGO was working in this area. The public in general was not receptive to information about cancer. The topic was considered taboo in Egypt.

The BCFE philosophy is to advocate for BC awareness and services by serving the public in a manner that generates happy clients and positive recognition. BCFE partners with the National Cancer Institute (NCI) for teaching health care professionals. It is a mutually beneficial arrangement that does not involve the exchange of money.

In the past few years BCFE has done educational presentations and opportunistic screening programs wherever asked for, i.e., private companies and ministries. The BCFE staff designed the screening program, all the tools for implementing it, the training program for doctors and nurses to provide screening services. BCFE surveyed the facilities of hospitals that wanted to establish an early detection clinic and recommended changes to support a good patient flow, privacy, and efficiency. These services were provided free of charge to any facility requesting this assistance. The cost was supported by the sponsored screening program.

BCFE deals directly with many patients. Quick referral mechanisms and the link to treatment services are ensured. Poor patients are referred to free clinics of NCI. If they are covered by insurance they are advised WHERE and WHO to go to. If they do not want to go to NCI and are not covered by insurance, BCFE arranges for treatment for them at a low cost facility, or through a doctor that will charge reasonably [17].

Egyptian Society for Promotion of Women's Health

Egyptian Society for Promotion of Women's Health (ESPWH) is a nonprofit organization, nongovernmental organization under the Ministry of Social Solidarity, established in June 2009; Dr. Karima Elshamy is the founder and executive director. The aim of establishing ESPWH was to improve and promote the health of women, increase women's awareness regarding many diseases, especially cancer awareness, control and prevention, reducing cultural barriers and detecting cancer as early as possible, also for education of people, health care personnel, and research. ESPWH is a member of Alliance of African & Mediterranean French Speaking Leagues Against Cancer.

Liver Cancer Prevention

Many countries, including the USA, are experiencing a decades-long trend of increasing rates of liver cancer. The most common type of liver cancer, hepatocellular carcinoma (HCC), has a high mortality rate and limited therapeutic options, to which most populations have limited access.

The prevention of this type of cancer is especially urgent in developing countries. Among the major contributing factors to the development of HCC are chronic infections with hepatitis B (HBV) or hepatitis C (HCV) virus, and food contaminated with aflatoxins (toxins secreted by molds that infect improperly stored grains and nuts).

Fortunately, these factors are amenable to prevention, including protections against blood-borne viral infections, vaccination against HBV, and improved food safety.

But would such strategies work in a developing country, such as Egypt, and why would Egypt be an appropriate place to test the effectiveness of liver cancer prevention programs?

The research group began studying HCC in Egypt more than 10 years ago, following ground-breaking work on HCV led by Dr. G.T. Strickland of the University of Maryland, Baltimore. Dr. Strickland's studies of HCV in communities in Egypt revealed that the country has the highest rates of HCV in the world, the unintended consequence of a massive public health campaign that used injected drugs to halt the suffering from a type of parasitic infection (Schistosoma species) native to the Nile River valley.

The evidence suggests that improper sterilization techniques applied to the needles in that campaign resulted—over a span of 50 years—in the spread of HCV and other viruses to a large segment of the population. The situation resulted in massive epidemics of chronic liver disease, cirrhosis, and HCC that have not yet reached their peak. The rate of HCC is about four times higher in Egypt than in the USA, and rising at a faster rate. Each year, over 15,000 Egyptians die from liver cancer.

Dr. Karima Elshamy mentioned that the major risk factors for HCC in Egypt, in addition to chronic infections with HCV and HBV, are occupational exposures to chemicals, pesticides, and contamination of the diet with aflatoxins (alcohol abuse is uncommon due to religious customs that forbid drinking).

Each of these factors is preventable; yet beyond HBV vaccination, scant attention is being paid to preventive research or effective interventions, even in the more developed countries. In fact, a recent report by the U.S. Institute of Medicine concluded that the lack of knowledge and awareness of viral hepatitis among members of the public and policy-makers were major barriers to prevention.

Added to the burden of viral hepatitis in Egypt is the unsafe handling of pesticides in agriculture—its predominant industry—and the lack of awareness of safe food handling practices regarding aflatoxins. A program of health education focused on these and other risk factors for HCC could deliver appropriate information at low cost, aimed at empowering households to interrupt the current cycle of viral hepatitis transmission and carcinogenic exposures.

Over the long term, this approach could be used by many countries to reduce the human, economic, and societal costs of this fatal and rising type of cancer.

To fit the specific needs of Egyptians in the context of their society and culture, a community-based health education approach tailored to the population at risk for cancer would offer many advantages. Community-based participatory research involves members of local communities in all aspects of a study-from design to dissemination-to ensure that the proposed intervention reflects the specific needs of the communities, and to strengthen the capacity of the community to implement public health activities.

Moreover, the engagement of peer educators to deliver the health education program, which has been shown by Sarah Dalglish and others to be highly effective in such issues as tobacco prevention and reproductive health interventions, would be highly innovative in the context of HCC, where little or no such work has been previously reported [18].

Egypt's Infection Control Program (ICP) was designed in collaboration with the WHO and is considered the reference for the Eastern Mediterranean region. In 2001, MOHP began by assessing infection control policies, indicating a need for action. For example, only 16 % of HCW were vaccinated against HBV, hand washing rates were extremely low, and needle stick injuries occurred at a rate of 4.9 % per worker per year.

The resulting program includes training of HCW; the establishment of infection control committees at the levels of the governorate, the directorate, and the hospital; and regular monitoring by local and national teams. As of January 2008, the plan has been implemented in 283 hospitals, representing all MOHP hospitals with more than 50 beds in 21 governorates. Further, all HCW in all MOHP facilities, including primary health care units, have been vaccinated against HBV in six governorates (Cairo, Alexandria, Sharkia, Monofiya, Menia, and Qena). In 2009, MOHP will add the remaining 70 hospitals with more than 50 beds, to cover all 27 governorates, and vaccinate all health care workers in these facilities nationwide.

The National Committee on Viral Hepatitis, under MOHP, mandated the development of the Control Strategy 2008–2012 to ensure the strengthening and expansion of the national, multicultural response to viral hepatitis. This plan builds on what has already been achieved and is based on the best epidemiological estimations of viral hepatitis in Egypt and the latest scientific knowledge [18].

Egyptian National Control Strategy for Viral Hepatitis 2008–2012

The National Control Strategy for Viral Hepatitis is the first comprehensive approach to reducing the prevalence, incidence, and burden of disease associated with hepatitis B and C in Egypt. It represents a comprehensive, multisectoral response to the challenge of this major public health issue and is informed by the latest medical and scientific research on viral hepatitis in Egypt. The Strategy seeks to provide guidance to various government ministries and agencies, as well as to nongovernmental partners, in order to ensure coordination and cooperation among them. The plan has been elaborated in concert with the Egyptian National Committee on Viral Hepatitis and in consultation with officials from the Ministry of Health and Population, the Ministry of Higher Education, various UN agencies and the WHO (Geneva and Cairo), as well as researchers at Egyptian universities and other local and international stakeholders involved in the fight against viral hepatitis [5].

Research

One of the most successful elements of the fight against viral hepatitis in Egypt has been the creation of an international research network called the Liver Disease Research Unit. The network brings together Egyptian, French, American, Swedish, and Finnish universities and research institutes. External funding has been provided by USAID, the National Institutes of Health (USA), the European Commission, the French ANRS and Ministry of Foreign Affairs, and the Welcome Trust, among others.

Diagnosis and Treatment of Cancer

Viral hepatitis cannot be treated at the periphery of the health care system (e.g., in primary health care units), since its management requires special training for physicians and special equipment for diagnosis, follow-up, and drug storage. Some 100 hospitals in Egypt are currently equipped to treat patients with advanced liver disease, and there are approximately 400 specialists in advanced liver disease working mostly out of major cities. However, the quality of care and degree of access to drugs may be heterogeneous throughout these facilities.

Recently, ten National Treatment Reference Centers were opened under the supervision of the National Committee on Viral Hepatitis, providing care for patients with HBV and HCV according to standardized guidelines and at subsidized costs. The Egyptian government provides 20,000 LE for the treatment of each HCV patient treated under HIO and or at government expense, categories which include 94.1 % of the 12,089 patients having started treatment as of February 2008. These outlays do not include financial expenditures required for monitoring, testing, facilities, and related costs. The total cost to the government is thus a not insignificant percentage of the annual MOHP budget.

Transplants are currently available at approximately 10 public and private facilities, though donors can be difficult to come by and cadaveric livers are not yet available in Egypt. As of 2008, the cost is high (220,000–400,000 LE), though some government assistance is available [19].

Surveillance and Monitoring

The most recent population-level surveillance study is the 1996/7 Egyptian household and workers national survey. It is impossible to say with any confidence how prevalence rates have changed in the 10 years since the completion of this study; however, an upcoming (2008) DHS survey will provide new figures on the prevalence of HBV and HCV infection.

There is currently no ongoing sentinel surveillance of chronic HBV and HCV, with the exception of monitoring of infection rates in Hemodialysis units as part of the national Infection Control Program. Additionally, the MOHP's Epidemiological Surveillance Unit, established in 1999 with the cooperation of WHO, EMRO, and the CDC, coordinates surveillance of 26 communicable and noncommunicable diseases. Forty-two cases of acute hepatitis A, B, and C are reported monthly from the network of 256 district surveillance units.

However, surveillance figures do not accurately reflect the number of cases for several reasons: underreporting due to time constraints on health care workers (HCW); the lack of a reliable IgM assay for acute HCV, making it more difficult to diagnose than HAV or HBV; and the fact that surveillance only covers MOHP facilities. Participation by private facilities is voluntary, and thus difficult to enforce. The laboratory support for surveillance also needs strengthening, as labs are not always fully equipped [19].

Pain Relief and Palliative Care in Egypt

In most of the world, the majority of the cancer patients present with advanced disease. For them, the only realistic treatment option is pain relief and palliative care. Effective approaches to palliative care are available to improve the quality of life for cancer patients. Lack of access to basic pain relief continues to make living and dying with cancer in Egypt a very different experience from that in developed countries.

The National Cancer Institute (NCI) in Cairo was established in 1969 as a specialized institute, affiliated with Cairo University. In 2004, palliative care was included in the oncology medical training program at the National Cancer Institute at the University of Cairo. In 2006, there were two organizations providing hospice palliative care in Egypt: the Cairo Evangelical Medical Society (which has hospice facilities in Cairo and Alexandria) and the National Cancer Institute (which puts an emphasis on cancer pain relief). In 2010, the NCI, Cairo, has cared for 18 156 new patients which comprised 70–80 % of all cancer patients in Egypt. A total of 70 % of all new cancer patients were diagnosed with an advanced stage of the disease. NCI's first initiative towards the development of palliative care services was in 1981 when the first pain clinic was established as part of the Department of Anesthesiology. This clinic handles 120–150 patients daily, while slow release morphine tablets are the only available pain medicine [20].

At the present, NCI is running a pain care clinic at its outpatient pain department. This clinic operates on a the capacity of a 24 h/7 days basis, and its staff comprises pain management physicians, specialized nurses, clinical social workers, pharmacists, psychiatrists, dietitians and administrative manpower. In addition, a hotline service was established, thus enabling easier access to the experts on the team. In addition to the NCI, Cairo, the El-Kasr El-Aini Cancer Center in Cairo also runs a pain clinic and a palliative care service (started in 2007). The new Children's Cancer Hospital 57357 in Cairo runs pediatric palliative care services including psychological support. The Cairo Evangelical Medical Society provides inpatient and day care hospice services (opened in 2001), while similar services are provided by the Elhadra Elromany hospice in Alexandria [20].

Palliative care in Egypt is in an early stage of development with very few palliative care activities available even in all of the above specialized centers. At this stage, research is crucial to develop suitable palliative care models with respect to the needs, culture, and resources in Egypt.

Opioid consumption figures in Egypt are among the lowest worldwide indicating largely inadequate cancer pain control. Based on the data published in the most recent annual report of the International Narcotics Control Board, the average opioid consumption in Egypt during 2008–2010 was 62 defined daily dosed for statistical purposes (S-DDD) per million inhabitants per day. With this figure Egypt was ranked 115th among 184 countries [21].

Ethical, Religious, and Cultural Issues

All patients probably undergo the stages of acceptance of terminal cancer in the same fashion. The difference between Egyptian and Western cultural practices would likely be in the culturally specific coping strategies. Ultimately, the physician and other health care providers have to assess the patient in his cultural context and find out what would help the patient the most to go through the terminal phase of the disease. The community bond amongst Muslims is very strong, most end-of-life issues are preferably taken care at home amongst family members rather than in hospice facilities.

In dealing with a patient, a physician must take into account the degree of his cultural inclinations as well as that of his family in order to communicate and provide best medical treatment effectively. Invariably, communication and empathy are indispensable in achieving this. In an increasingly westernizing society, a physician should be wary of imposing generalized belief models on patients without first understanding their background and preferences.

Islam is the dominant religion in Egypt, and observant Muslims believe that having an illness represents an opportunity to enhance the Muslim's degree or expiating personal sins. Yet, Islamic teaching encourages Muslims to seek treatment when they fall sick, as it is believed that Allah did not send down a sickness but rather a medication for it [22]. Muslim's beliefs attribute to occurrence of pleasure and suffering to the will of Allah, and that every effort should be made to relieve suffering. Moreover, Islamic teaching considers the relief of suffering to be highly virtuous [23]. According to Islam, adults of both genders are granted the full right to accept or decline medical intervention. In reality, close family members are more often directly involved with the decision-making process. Generally, parents, spouses, and older children, in descending order, have greater decision-making power than the other members of the family [24].

Islamic teaching encourages the community members to visit the sick and the sick to welcome their guests. Patients, therefore, may entertain a larger number of visitors during their hospitalization [22]. The use of drugs that might affect consciousness is strictly prohibited in Islam. However, medically prescribed opioids are generally permissible because of their necessity. Usually, patients and families accept the use of opioids for symptom management, provided the rationale for their use is clearly explained to them. Of great importance is to explain patients and their relatives the possible side effects, as there are great concerns about an imposed drowsiness [25].

Issues that relate to end of life are compounded spiritually and ethically, and are open for interpretations. While discussing the prognosis of the loved one, Muslim families are often skeptical about receiving clear cut massages from the treating physician. The former are for the most part more comfortable receiving less concrete information and quite often would respond with: "This is in Allah's (God's) hands, and we are not to predict the fate of the patient." Such a response is largely due to the Islamic belief that the life expectancy of every person is only up to Allah, who is the one to determine the timing of death. Families, however, are very appreciative being updated as to the patient's condition, in order to enable them to carry out the traditional funeral rites. Taking all of the above into consideration, caregivers in Egypt exercise all the precautions and sensitivity while talking to terminally ill patients and their families [20].

Barriers for implementing Egyptian palliative care include the following:

Health Care Systems and Policies

- The big challenge to Egyptian palliative care professionals is the development of hospice systems along with well-organized home-based services.
- Lack of national health policies in support of palliative care development
- Focus on acute care
- Poor understanding and awareness of the role of palliative care in community
- Lack of legislation and accreditation of this new specialty discipline
- Lack of facilities and resources for palliative care
- Palliative and end-of-life care not prioritized in health care strategies
- Lack of long-term care and community services
- No statistical data about how and where patients die, how many receive PC, and the characteristics of the caring process
- Insufficient supplies and equipment

Health Care Professionals

- Inadequate training for both health care professionals and general public about the necessity and importance of palliative care as integral part of cancer care
- Palliative care as a discipline is being seen as less prestigious
- Lack of interdisciplinary concepts and teams
- Negative attitude towards caring for dying patients
- Fear of opioid use (fear of side effects and/or fear of prosecution)
- Resources focused on curative treatments and acute care
- Perceived sense of failure

Patients and Families

- Fear of addiction to opioids
- Fear of abandoning family members
- Unrealistic hopes of cure
- Families also refuse admission to hospice which is considered as a place of death, isolated and unfriendly
- Diversity in religious interpretation of death and dying

Drugs

- General lack of opioids and unavailability of opioids in remote areas
- Very strict opioid prescription and dispensing policies
- Lack of other essential medications lists
- Poor accessibility of essential palliative care drugs

Education and Training

- Lack of palliative care education programs at all levels
- Lack of funds for setting up education programs or hiring experts

The National Cancer Registry Program of Egypt

The National Cancer Registry Program of Egypt (NCRPE): Population-based cancer registry, it was initiated through a protocol of cooperation between the ministries of Communication and Information Technology, Health, and Higher Education. The Supreme Committee of the Program decided to start by population-based registration of incident cancer cases and to explore the possibility of establishing a national cancer database through eventual inclusion of hospital-based cancer registries in due time. The registry program started in 2008 and covered Aswan Governorate followed by ElMinia, Beheira, and Damietta. Governorate of Gharbiah already has a registry that was established 10 years ago and will be included in the national registry program in a subsequent phase. Egypt will thus be covered by a network of population-based registries geographically spread all over the country. The Metropolitan Cairo is not covered by population-based registration due to logistic difficulties. Nonetheless, comparison of program results with those of the National Cancer Institute in Cairo would give a clue to the profile of cancer in the Metropolitan Cairo Area and complete the picture for Egypt [26].

Government Involvement in the Care for Cancer Patients

The ministry of health and population is responsible for overall health and population policy as well as the provision of public health services, and is responsible for health insurance organization that provides services too, cancer registration, access to public health awareness through working as change agents, increase health awareness and literacy, educating patients on patients' rights, encouraging volunteerism, and public campaigns and community outreach, access to early detection through: leading the Egyptian breast cancer program, increasing accessibility of early detection services, and improving the quality of services across the country. Also, accreditation program through capacity building of health care providers from all sectors, access to quality cancer treatment, and prioritizing quality cancer care.

The Ministry of Higher Education

The ministry of higher education is however responsible for health profession education (medical, nursing, dentistry, and pharmacy) and also runs university teaching hospital, access to research through creating an enabling environment for research and academics, moving toward evidence-based decisions at the national level and pushing boundaries of clinical research, in addition to community services.

Nongovernmental Organization Responsibilities

Nongovernmental organizations focus on the prevention and early detection of cancer. The nongovernmental sector is an important source of technical knowledge, skills, and resources relevant for cancer care and research, this involvement implies either direct provision of the services or acting as funding institutions. Furthermore, nongovernmental organizations provide an important ability to reach out to the professional and public communities, advocate for cancer prevention and control, offer cancer education and screening services in our community, support cancer patients and survivors. They have access to patient support, patients support groups, financial support, transportation, accommodation, food coupons, and the sharing of survivors' stories. Nongovernmental and voluntary organizations can, therefore, play a significant role in assisting the efforts of the government health system in reducing disparities in coverage regarding cancer care services.

Prof. Dr. Karima Elshamy (Head of Gerontological Nursing Department, Faculty of Nursing, Mansoura University, Egypt and AORTIC Vice President of North Africa) reported that it is very important for all organizations to be aware of the complexity of cancer control, and of the role they should play in achieving the goals of the cancer control program or strategy, through a unified effort with other sectors. Improved cancer control will, to a substantial degree, relate to prevention strategies and early detection programs, including information campaigns and population-based screening programs. Success of the early detection programs will rely on effective and optimal use of treatment possibilities.

Cancer Education in Medical, Nursing, and Pharmacy Schools in Egypt

More than 1500 Egyptians have postgraduate qualifications in clinical and medical oncology. The medical and health-related educational system in Egypt has advantages and limitations. Medical education includes a unique system of 3-year community-based public health training, but better planning and collaboration among schools could notably increase new physicians' knowledge of cancer detection and prevention. Nurses and pharmacists exert great influence in the provision of health care. Yet, their training includes neither cancer education nor information about prevention. The medical and health-related educational system in Egypt has many limitations, but it has the structure and inherent ability to achieve cancer education goals [27]. Prof. Dr. Karima Elshamy added that many nursing researches, master and doctoral thesis in faculty of nursing, Mansoura University focus on cancer and palliative care.

Interrelationship Between Cancer Care and Local Culture

Culture refers to a set of shared attitudes, values, goals, and practices that characterize a group. Cancers are known to be a result of both genetics and lifestyle factors. Lifestyles emanate from cultural beliefs, values, and practices. Thus culture affects both the risk factors for cancers and the meaning of the disease by influencing the behavior responding emotionally, cognitively, and socially to this disease. Culture will determine approaches to prevention, early detection, treatment choices, and management of side effects such as pain, appropriate psychosocial support, rehabilitation efforts, survivorship issues, hospice use, and effective end-of-life care.

Cultural values, beliefs, and assumptions influence health care. In every clinical encounter, providers decide what to say and what not to say, who to include in important discussions, how to provide patient teaching, and when to schedule follow-up care. When providers are working with someone from another culture, these decisions may be influenced by assumptions and stereotypes about what people from that culture are like. If the assumptions are wrong, a person's health can be seriously jeopardized.

Cultural Influence in Cancer Screening

There has been much debate regarding cultural influence on cancer screening, especially that regarding culturally sensitive regions of the body such as the breasts, cervix, and colon. Cultural factors have been shown to play a vital role in women's attitudes to breast cancer screening. Cervical cancer screening has been widely implemented and has been subject to much study [28].

Cultural Influence in Cancer Diagnosis and Disclosure

Confucius teaches that in a society, every person has a role and obligations to fulfill. In the context of cancer diagnosis, this phenomenon is particularly acute. To a parent of a young family, a diagnosis of cancer immediately brings the burden of the possibility of being unable to fulfill his or her duties to raise the young and provide for the family. This may produce intense feelings of guilt, shame, and anger. These reactions must be taken into consideration by the health care provider in relating to the patient.

Another factor relates to the phenomenon of reciprocity and filial piety (righteousness). As the parents grow old and the children come to maturity, the role of the provider is gradually passed to the children and in the twilight years, it often comes to pass that the family will make most of the decisions for the elderly ones. It is widely observed in local medical practice that in Egyptian families, the children often wish to conceal the diagnosis of cancer from the patient. At times, the diagnosis is explained to the children who stay behind in the consultation room after the patient leaves. This is entirely opposite to the grain of Western bioethics of medical confidentiality and patient disclosure. Indeed, this practice is not usually seen in clinics in the West where the very opposite occurs: the patient attends the consultation alone and certainly would hold the confidentiality of his medical information dear.

Amongst the Muslims, again the concept of God's will influence the willingness to accept bad news and even mishaps and regard it as fate and thus may be more forgiving to the carers. Research has shown that distribution of BC is within the younger age group of Egyptian patients, the majority of cases occurring between 30 and 60 years of age. The median age at diagnosis is 49 years, one decade younger than the corresponding age in Europe and North America [29].

Reduction in mortality from BC depends to a large extent on interventions aimed at early detection and treatment; including breast self examination, clinical breast examination, and mammography [30]. Lack of early detection programs is the primary reason for the escalation of the mortality rate from BC in developing countries [31].

Not seeking medical advice unless one is ill, followed by the women's beliefs that physical checkups were not worthwhile were the most common personal barriers revealed by the present participants. In their study among women from rural Egypt, Younes et al. stated that many Egyptian women suffered in silence, endured much pain and discomfort before they would admit to being ill, and would mostly only seek treatment when their symptoms became severe [32].

Unsurprisingly, a significant proportion of the women in the present study reported they were afraid of discovering that they had cancer, and embarrassment by the screening was a personal barrier. Generally, there are many personal obstacles for women to access prevention services. The fear of discovering cancer, embarrassment, and fear of the screening procedure were among the most commonly reported personal/cultural barriers to using the screening services [7, 33]. Spirituality and religion have been identified as major determinants of fear and fatalism with regard to BC in previous research [33]. Personal barriers can be overcome by promoting health seeking behavior and educating the public on the importance of early detection of cancer with a message that empowers women to take charge of their own health.

The Impact of Culture and Religion on Truth Telling at the End of Life

In Islamic ethics, family and community are intrinsically linked with each individual's well-being [34]. Similarly, in many Asian cultures, illness is a shared family event rather than an individual occurrence [35]. The family provides a source of strength, hope, and connectedness to others. Accordingly, the principle of autonomy does not bear the same weight as it does in many Western cultures and thus the family is the locus of the decision-making process [36]. A Japanese study [37] found that 46 % of the population felt it was the family's duty to provide "a protective role in shielding the patient from a painful diagnosis" [38]. Equally, in Ethiopia and Saudi Arabia, information regarding a patient's illness belongs to the family, who then use the information in the best interests of the patient [39, 40]. Physicians, consequently, respect the "autonomy of the family as a unit" [36].

Society Reaction Towards Cancer Patients

Cancer is one of the oldest diseases of human beings. Diagnostic and therapeutic aspects have advanced significantly. The life span of a cancer patient of today is increased considerably because of multifarious approach by scientists and medical personnel. However nothing much is done regarding the status of the patient in relation to the society and the mental, behavioral, and physical aspects.

Social reaction towards the cancer patient ranges from total nonnormalcy to almost normalcy. Most of the families believed in "God's Way," the others were showed no significant reaction. Children of the patient were more concerned, affectionate, and sympathetic to their mother than the others. The husbands were either badly affected psychologically or kept up calm to face the situation. This was more so in educated ones. Some families encouraged the patients to gain strength and to face the disease which in turn has helped the patient to lead an almost normal life. The non-acceptance in the society, based on no firm grounds, is leading the patient to despair. However, avoidance of the patient in one pretext or the other is prevailing in significant number of cases.

Anger, irritation, sense of inferiority, insecure feeling, emotional stress, and total lack of hope of survival were the main feelings. Given a proper atmosphere of normalcy and affection, the quality of the life and survival time would be enhanced significantly. Philosophy has come as important source of solace to many affected families [41].

Summary and Recommendations

In Egypt, cancer is already an important health problem and will become increasingly important not only in terms of rank order, as infections are better controlled, but also in terms of incidence and mortality. The commonest sites were liver and breast among men and women, respectively. Based upon the results of National Cancer Registry Program, Egypt is expected to experience the highest increase by 2050; the following recommendations could enhance the effectiveness of cancer care in Egypt.

1. The ministry of health and population should recognize palliative care as a new subspecialty for nurses, and expansion of palliative care services to a larger number of patients and illnesses throughout the country, considering home-based palliative care service is urgently and badly needed.
2. National Committee for Pain Relief and Palliative Care should be developed, and the latter committee should develop a national plan that involves: education, clinical practice including opioids availability, accessibility and disposal, research, public policy, and evaluating and monitoring care plans and activities.
3. Strengthening health care systems; focusing on patient centered care that optimizes outcomes for patients that are patient focused and are based on the patients need as opposed to prognosis, optimal care to optimizes systems and access to services within available resources to provide the best care for the patient that is high quality and safe, also, management, monitoring and evaluation of interventions to ensure they are effective and remain effective. Making real improvements in management will require the proactive efforts of many organizations, and we believe that education as well as discipline should be the cornerstone of efforts to improve cancer care in general and pain relief and palliative care specifically.
4. Education at all levels to be undertaken to all staff members in the oncology units throughout Egypt would gain basic practical training in dealing with cancer patients suffering from pain and other physical, psychological, and spiritual symptoms. In order for such a plan to come about a ministerial-driven program is needed, whereby trained oncologists and oncology specialized clinical nurses be educated and trained in the following topics: communication skills between the clinical caregivers, the patients and their families, basic concepts of pain pathophysiology, pain assessment, choosing of analgesics and their dosing, management of visceral, somatic and neuropathic pain, management of other symptoms such as nausea, vomiting, constipation, and delirium, wound care, management of last hours of life including dyspnea, and how to overcoming cultural barriers. Also, to focus on subspecialties on the psychological, behavioral, physical, and spiritual.
5. Effective cancer prevention programs customized to the community should be fostered, particularly for prevention of hepatitis B and C infection, and breast cancer awareness and early detection, and encourage community share in the program by money donations, hospice places, volunteers, and training.
6. Pain and palliative care education and training should be incorporated in the training curricula of all medical schools, family residents training program and all postgraduate oncology and other chronic disease nursing training program, also palliative-care certified physicians are going to be central in coordinating this kind of care, clinical nurse specialists in palliative care, who provide palliative care at both institutional and community settings throughout the country are also needed.
7. Setting up hospital-based palliative care support teams would be the biggest foreseeable challenge; as currently there are neither nurses nor physicians

trained in palliative care within the public hospitals. These teams working within hospitals will offer an in-house consultant service, and facilitate their transfer to the community. The hospital-based teams will continually liaise with other services within the hospital as well as the home care teams to improve continuity of care, as well as provide education for both hospital and community health care professionals.
8. Many important BC screening barriers have been identified among this group of Egyptian women. Women's perception of these barriers was associated with some sociodemographic characteristics. Identifying barriers to breast screening in the local community will help to remove those obstacles and design more culturally relevant strategies to increase the utilization of breast screening service and to ensure adequate breast care of these women.
9. Changing the current opioid dispensing regulation and ensuring the availability of essential drugs.
10. Training and workforce capacity building are needed to improve research into cost-effective cancer-control interventions and clinical trials.

Acknowledgment The author acknowledges the important and fantastic role played by Prof. Michael Silbermann in increasing health care awareness and establishing palliative care in Middle East Countries, Executive Director, Middle East Cancer Consortium.

Conflict of Interest: The authors declare that there is no conflict of interests regarding the publication.

References

1. Ibrahim AS, Hussein MK, Nabiel NM, Hoda B, Hossam K. Cancer incidence in Egypt: results of the National Population-Based Cancer Registry Program. J Cancer Epidemiol. 2014;2014:18. Article ID 437971.
2. World Health Organization. Towards a strategy for cancer control in the Eastern Mediterranean Region. 2009.
3. EGYPT CIA—The World Factbook. 2011. Accessed 18 Apr 2011.
4. World Health Organization. The Country Cooperation Strategy. 2013.
5. Egyptian National Control Strategy for Viral Hepatitis 2008–2012.
6. The Demographic Profile of Egypt. United Nations, World Population Prospects. 2012. http://esa.un.org/wpp/unpp/panel_indicators.htm
7. Younis N, Khattab H, Zurayk H, ElMoelhy M, Amin M, Farag A. A community study of gynaecological and related morbidities in rural Egypt. Stud Fam Plann. 1993;24(3):175–86.
8. Stefan DC, Elzawawy AM, Khaled HM, Ntaganda MM, Asiimwe A, Wiafe Addai B, Wiafe S, Adewole IF. Developing cancer control plans in Africa: examples from five countries. Lancet Oncol. 2013;14(4):e189–95.
9. WHO. Global Health Observatory data repository. NCD country capacity survey 2010. 2013. http://apps.who.int/gho/data/
10. National cancer control programmes. Policies and managerial guidelines. 2nd ed. 2002.
11. Anwaar A. Breast cancer in Egypt: the challenges include education and detection. The Washington Times (online). 2011. http://communities.washingtontimes.com/neighborhood/egypt-pyramids-and-revolution/2011/oct/11/breastcancer-egypt-challenges-education-treatment/

12. Information provided by Dr Dorria Salem, head of the digital mammography screening project. MOHP Women Health outreach program. www. whop.gov.eg/
13. Information provided by Dr Tony Miller, designer of the trial, and Dr Salwa Boulos, PI of the trail in Cairo. Information retrieved in the following scientific publications.
14. Boulos S, Gadallah M, Neguib S, Essam E, Youssef A, Costa A, Mittra I, Miller AB. Breast screening in the emerging world: high prevalence of BC in Cairo. Breast. 2005;14(5):340–6.
15. Miller AB. Practical applications for clinical breast examination (CBE) and breast self-examination (BSE) in screening and early detection of BC. Breast Care. 2008;3:17–20.
16. Omar S, Elzawawy A, Omar A. Down staging of the breast cancer in a low resource setting, rural (Fakous Cancer Centre) and urban (Port Said)—Egypt. Global summit on international breast health, Chicago, IL, USA, June 9–11, 2010.
17. http://portal.bhgi.org/GlobalPortfolio/globalsummit/Documents/Presentations/OMAR.pdf. Accessed 18 Feb 2013.
18. Information provided by Dr Mohamed Shaalan, Professor of Surgery, BCFE Founding Chairman, Co-Director of prevention and early detection unit, NCI, and Lois Crooks, Volunteer Executive Director, General Secretary (2004–2008) and Founding Member.
19. Prevention & Control of Viral Hepatitis Infection. World Health Organization. 2012.
20. Egypt Health Sector Reform Program. MOHP. 2003.
21. Fahmi R, Mostafa KA. Palliative cancer care in Middle Eastern countries: accomplishments and challenges. Ann Oncol. 2012;23 Suppl 3:iii15–28.
22. International for Narcotics Control Board. Narcotic drugs: estimated world requirements for 2011; statistics 2009. New York: United Nations; 2011.
23. Daher M. Challenges and barriers for pain management in cancer patients. J Pediatr Hematol Oncol. 2010;32:425–8.
24. Tuncer M, Ozgul Gultekin M. National Cancer Control Program 2009–2015. Ankara: Turkish Ministry of Health Publication; 2011. www.kanser.gov.tr. Last accessed 16 Dec 2011.
25. Ozgul N, Koc O, Gultekin M, et al. Opioids for cancer pain: availability, accessibility and regulatory barriers in Turkey and the Pallia-Turk Project. J Pediatr Hematol Oncol. 2011;33: S29–32.
26. Al-Jibaly M. The inevitable journey, Part I—sickness: regulations and exhortations. Arlington: Al-Kitaab & As-Sunnah; 1998. p. 1998.
27. Towards a National Population-based Cancer Registry for Egypt (NPCR): Amal Samy Ibrahim: ppt.
28. Soliman AS, Nasser SS, El-Hattab O, Sobeih T, Chamberlain RM. Cancer education in medical, nursing, and pharmacy schools in Egypt: features applicable to other countries. J Cancer Educ (Impact Factor: 1.05). 2003;18(1):12–4. doi:10.1207/s15430154jce1803s_2.
29. International Agency for Research in Cancer. Lyon, France.
30. Holroyd E, Twinn S, Adab P. Socio-cultural influences on Chinese women's attendance for cervical screening. J Adv Nurs. 2004;46(1):42–52.
31. Shi JF, Qiao YL, Smith JS, Dondog B, Bao YP, Dai M, Clifford GM, Franceschi S. Epidemiology and prevention of human papillomavirus and cervical cancer in China and Mongolia. Vaccine. 2008;26 Suppl 12:M53–9.
32. Solomon D, Breen N, McNeel T. Cervical cancer screening rates in the United States and the potential impact of implementation of screening guidelines. CA Cancer J Clin. 2007;57(2): 105–11.
33. Thompson HS, Littles M, Jacob S, Crystal C. Cancer surveillance and follow-up care experiences of breast cancer survivors of African descent: an exploratory qualitative study. Cancer Nurs. 2006;29:478–87.
34. Flynn P, Betancour H, Tucker J, Garberoglio C, Riggs M. Culture, emotions, and breast self-examinations among culturally diverse women. Presented at the annual conference for the American Psychological Association, San Francisco, CA, August 2007.
35. Beyene Y. Medical disclosure and refugees. Telling bad news to Ethiopian patients. West J Med. 1992;157:328–32.

36. Sachedina A. End-of-life: the Islamic view. Lancet. 2005;366:774–9.
37. Searight HR, Gafford J. Cultural diversity at the end of life: issues and guidelines for family physicians. Am Fam Physician. 2005;71:515–22.
38. Chattopadhyay S, Simon A. East meets west: cross-cultural perspective in end-of-life decision making from Indian and German viewpoints. Med Health Care Philos. 2008;11:165–74.
39. Surbone A. Cultural aspects of communication in cancer care. Support Care Cancer. 2008;16:235–40.
40. Seo M, Tamura K, Shijo H, et al. Telling the diagnosis to cancer patients in Japan: attitude and perception of patients, physicians and nurses. Palliat Med. 2000;14:105–10.
41. Younge D, Moreau P, Ezzat A, et al. Communicating with cancer patients in Saudi Arabia. Ann N Y Acad Sci. 1997;809:309–16.

Chapter 10
Cancer Care in Lebanon, New Trends and Challenges

Michel Daher

General Introduction

Cancer is a global issue; it is the second leading cause of death after heart disease and stroke. Its impact is devastating, but especially so for poor, vulnerable, and socially disadvantaged people who are more often diagnosed with advanced disease and die sooner [1].

The number of new cancer patients worldwide was estimated at over 14 million new cancer cases, 8.2 million cancer deaths and 32.6 million people living with cancer (within 5 years of diagnosis) in 2012 worldwide. Fifty-seven percent (8 million) of new cancer cases, 65 % (5.3 million) of the cancer deaths and 48 % (15.6 million) of the 5-year prevalent cancer cases occurred in the less developed regions [2].

The burden induced by cancer, both on health care practitioners and on the whole system, is considerable and it is rapidly growing. As a matter of fact, the overall number of cancers has grown twofold during the last three decades of the past century, and it is estimated that this number will double between 2000 and 2020, and almost triple by 2030. Some of the determinants of this evolution include the increasing number of elderly, group with highest prevalence of cancer, the decrease of mortality caused by communicable diseases, and the increase of exposure to some risk factors [3].

There's no one single family in the world that is spared by this plague. The social harms caused by cancer are immense, not only in terms of sufferings by the patients themselves, their families and friends, but also in terms of high economic burden [4].

M. Daher, M.D., F.A.C.S., F.E.B.S. (✉)
Saint George Hospital University Medical Center, Achrafieh,
P.O. Box 166378, Beirut 1100 2807, Lebanon
e-mail: mndaher@inco.com.lb

M. Silbermann (ed.), *Cancer Care in Countries and Societies in Transition*,
DOI 10.1007/978-3-319-22912-6_10

Disparities and Inequalities in Cancer Care in ME Countries

Cancer incidence in Middle Eastern countries WHO Eastern Mediterranean Region (EMRO), most categorized as low- and middle-income, reached 555,000 cases, and a mortality of 367,000. It is predicted to double in the next 10 years, greater than in any other part of the world [2, 5].

It is the fourth leading cause of death in this region. It is expected that deaths from cancer in these countries could reach 760,000 per year by the year 2020 [2, 6]. While progress has been made in cancer diagnosis/treatment, much remains to be done to improve palliative care for the majority of patients with cancer who present with advanced disease.

This region includes a wide range of economically diverse countries, from technically advanced countries with high level cancer care to countries with little or no cancer treatment capabilities. There are large differences in population size, wealth, and health expenditure. Although the incidence of cancer is still well below that in developed countries, the ME countries are expected to experience an increase in cancer in the coming two decades, attributed to many factors including population aging and exposure to risk factors, such as smoking, unhealthy diet and physical inactivity and environmental pollution [7, 8].

The availability and quality of treatment is another factor. Cancer is not only often caught sooner but also usually treated more successfully in some countries compared to less developed ones. The relative survival rate can be 50 % or better, but in less developed countries it is only 30 % [7].

At present, resources for cancer control in the ME countries as a whole are not only inadequate but also directed almost exclusively to treatment. The curability of cancer is directly related to its stage at the time of diagnosis, and in the majority of countries of this region, cancer is generally diagnosed when it is at a relatively advanced stage [9–11]. Thus, recommendations are tailored, to the extent possible, to different resource levels, both among countries and in different regions or populations within the same country.

Cancer in Lebanon: Situation Analysis

Lebanon is a small middle-income country on the Eastern Mediterranean shore—with a current population of 4.4 million—, is at the third stage of its demographic transition characterized by a decline in both fertility and mortality rates [12] (Fig. 10.1).

It is estimated that just less than 10 % of the population is above the age of 65 years and 1.5 % above the age of 85—a small proportion compared to Western Europe and the USA, but quite high regionally. The United Nations estimates that the average life expectancy in Lebanon will rise from approximately 74 years for men and 77 years for women (as little as 50 years ago, it was 60 years) to 78.7 years between 2014 and 2050, leading to an increase in the median population age from 28.8 to 41.7 years as well as the percentage of older population aged 60 years and above from 10.3 to 25.8 % [13] (Fig. 10.2).

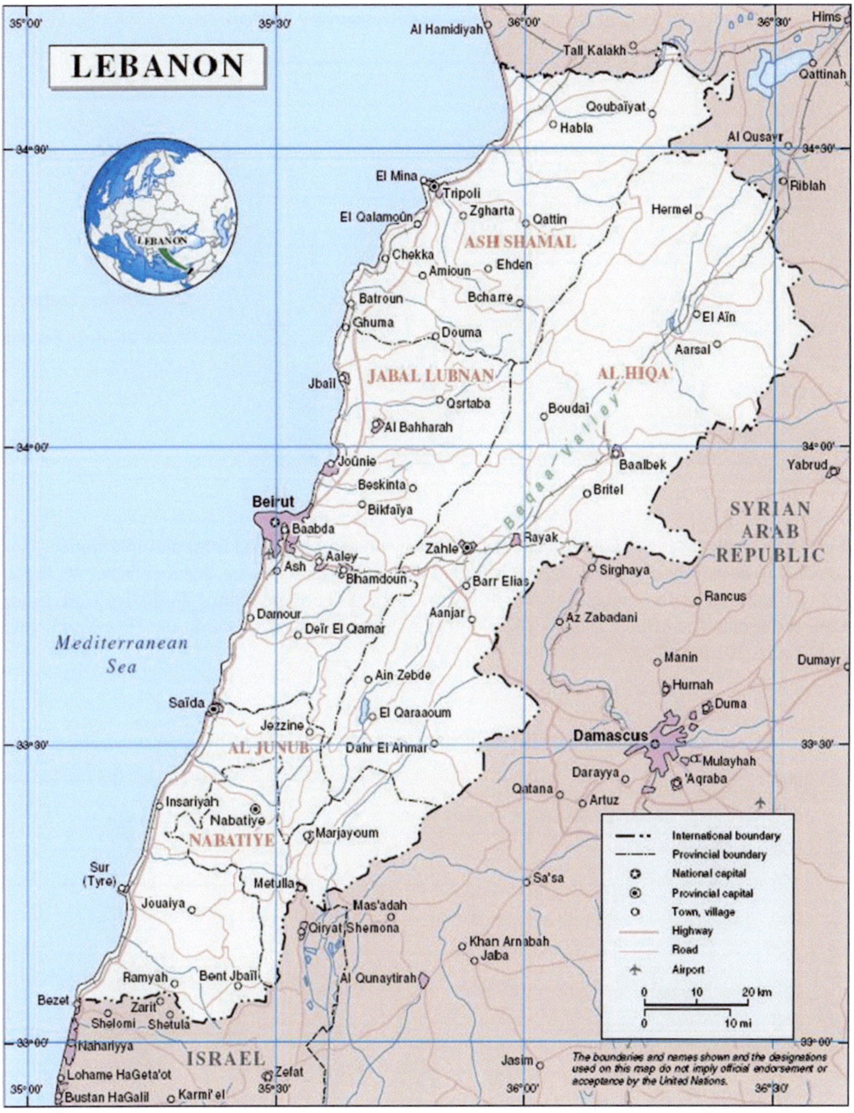

Fig. 10.1 Map of Lebanon

With an aging population, comes chronic, costly, and serious illness, including many types of cancers, of which the Lebanese health care system is ill-prepared to deal with. All-cause cancer incidence peaks at around age 70 [14, 15] (Fig. 10.3).

The number of new cases of cancer in Lebanon has increased steadily over the past decade, according to the National Cancer Registry of the Ministry of Health and the World Health Organization (WHO). In 2004, almost 7200 new cases of cancer were reported in Lebanon, compared to over 8400 in the most recent report [14, 16].

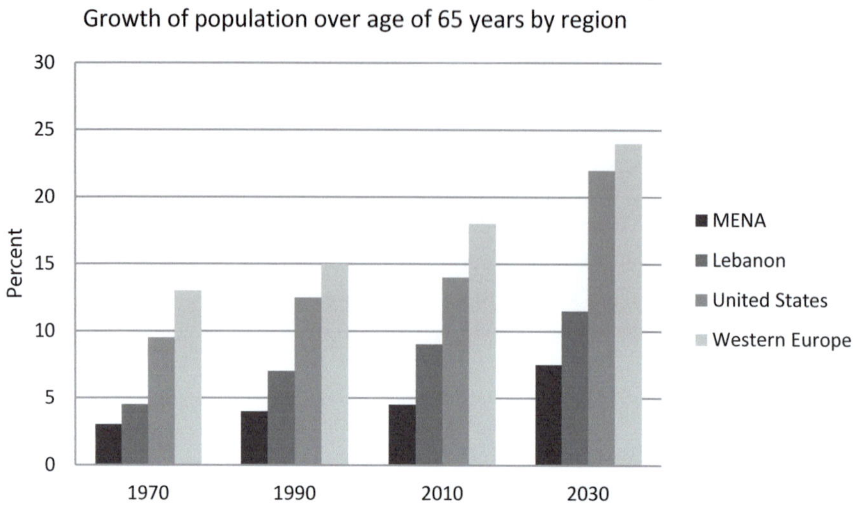

Fig. 10.2 Growth of population over age 65 years by region. Compiled from multiple sources, and rounded to nearest half percent. *MENA* Middle East and Northern Africa. *Source*: Daher M, Hajjar RR. Palliative care for cancer patients in Lebanon. In: Silbermann editor. Palliative Care to the Cancer Patient: The Middle East as a Model for Emerging Countries, 1st edition. New York: Nova Publishers, 2014: 125–40

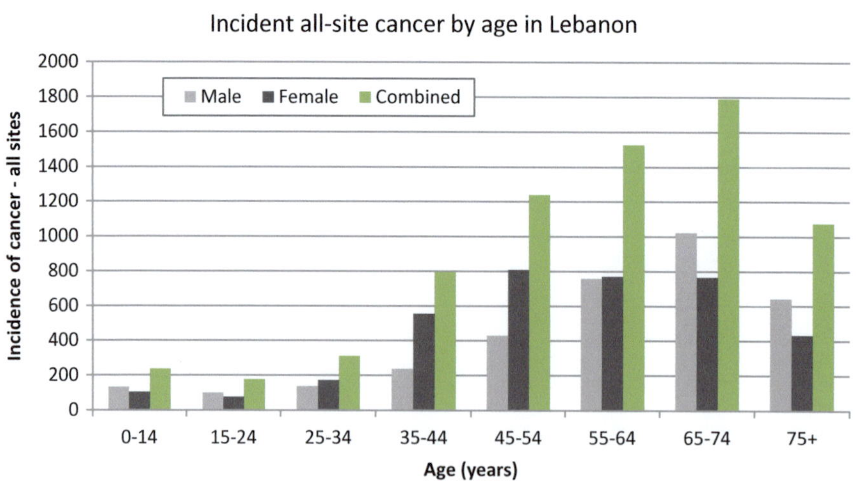

Fig. 10.3 Incident cancer cases in Lebanon by age-2003. All-case cancer excludes non-melanoma skin cancer. *Source*: National Cancer Registry (NCR). Cancer in Lebanon 2004 with an update of 2003, Beirut, Lebanon

This worrisome trend is not entirely due to aging; expanded screening efforts and improved registration methods have likely contributed significantly. It is estimated that by 2030, the number of new cancer cases will approach 12,000 [17].

The situation in Lebanon is as alarming as in ME countries and other countries in transition:

Incidence: The National Cancer Registry (NCR) was implemented within the Ministry of Public Health NCD Programme and was integrated into the Epidemiological Surveillance Programme (ESP) in 2007. Cancer notification has been made mandatory through Ministry of Public Health Decision 1/511 in 2002. The first annual report on national cancer incidence data was published in 2003 (about 7400 cases), noting age-standardized incidence rates of 191.3 and 190.7 per 100,000 for males and females, respectively [16].

Top cancer sites: The highest burden among cancers in both sexes is breast, prostate, lung, bladder, non-Hodgkin lymphoma, and colorectal cancers, all of which form approximately 65 % of cancer cases. The present incidence rates for the five most common cancers in males and females reported that cancers of prostate, bladder, lung, colon, and non-Hodgkin were the most common among males, and cancers of the breast, colon, lung, non-Hodgkin, and ovary were the most common among females. During the period (2003–2008), reported by the NCR, males and females presented with an overall 4.5 % and 5.4 % annual increase, respectively. Significant increases were observed for cancers of the liver and prostate among males, and for cancers of the liver, thyroid, and corpus uteri among females [16, 17] (Figs. 10.4 and 10.5).

Although there are no reliable data on cancer incidence and mortality in Lebanon in recent years, (the last official report was about 8500 new cases in 2008), estimates from the International Agency for Research on Cancer (IARC) indicate 9059 new cancer cases in 2012 (4321 cases among men and 4738 cases in women) per annum. The estimated number of deaths from cancer in 2012 was 4831 (2588 cancer deaths among men and 2243 among women) [GLOBOCAN 2012] (Tables 10.1 and 10.2).

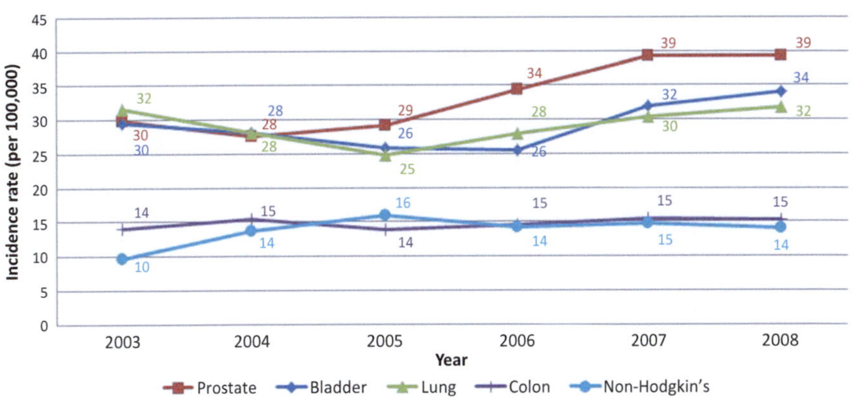

Fig. 10.4 Cancer incidence of the five most common cancers in males (2003–2008)

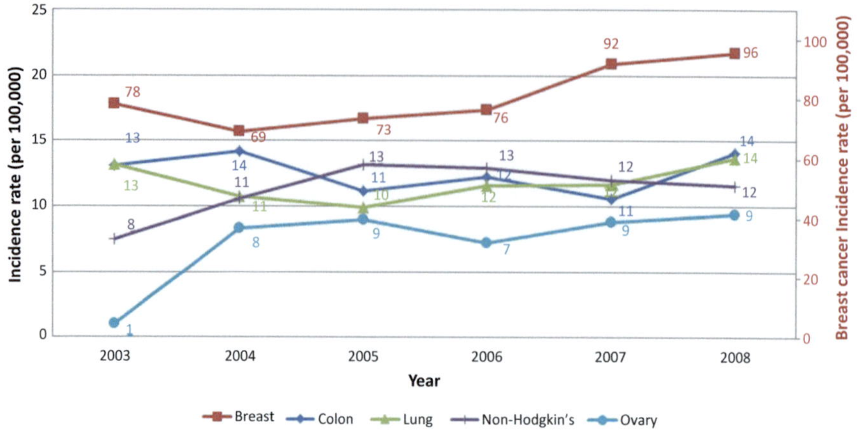

Fig. 10.5 Cancer incidence of the five most common cancers in females (2003–2008)

Table 10.1 Cancer incidence among top five cancer sites (*Source*: GLOBOCAN 2012)

Cancer incidence estimates					Total 9059				
Male					Female				
Cancer site	Number of cases	% of cancers	Crude rate	ASR[a]	Cancer site	Number of cases	% of cancers	Crude rate	ASR[a]
Prostate	807	19	38.5	37.2	Breast	1934	41	88	78.7
Lung	625	14	29.8	30.2	Colorectum	338	7	15.4	13.5
Bladder	618	14	29.5	29.1	Non-Hodgkin lymphoma	282	6	12.8	11.5
Colorectum	407	9	19.4	19.1	Lung	272	6	12.4	11
Non-Hodgkin lymphoma	310	7	14.8	14.7	Corpus uteri	187	4	8.5	7.7
Total**	4321	100	206.3	203.9	Total**	4738	100	215.7	192.8

[a]*ASR* Age Standardized Rate using world population **excluding non-a melanoma skin cancer

Table 10.2 Cancer mortality among top five cancer sites (*Source*: GLOBOCAN 2012)

Cancer mortality estimates					Total 4831				
Male					Female				
Cancer site	Number of deaths	% of cancers	Crude rate	ASR[a]	Cancer site	Number of deaths	% of cancers	Crude rate	ASR[a]
Lung	559	22	26.7	26.9	Breast	599	27	27.3	24
Prostate	411	16	19.6	17.1	Lung	240	11	10.9	9.6
Bladder	243	9	11.6	11	Colorectum	190	8	8.6	7.4
Colorectum	229	9	10.9	10.5	Non-Hodgkin lymphoma	166	7	7.6	6.6
Non-Hodgkin lymphoma	183	7	8.7	8.6	Ovary	116	5	5.3	4.7
Total**	2588	100	123.5	119.5	Total**	2243	100	102.1	89.6

[a]*ASR* Age Standardized Rate using world population **excluding non-a melanoma skin cancer

Particular Cancers in Lebanon

Breast cancer: In Lebanon, the incidence of breast cancer among women in general is increasing (APC=5.4 %) and is projected to continue to cause the highest morbidity burden compared to other cancers (33–44 %). It occurs at a younger age (50 % of all breast cancer patients are below the age of 50), with a median of 50 years, compared to western countries where the median age approaches 63 years [18].

Moreover, these trends can be partly explained by widespread national breast cancer awareness campaigns since the early 2000s, with the wide adoption of mammography screening programs at reduced fees within NGOs and primary health care centers. The recommended age as the starting point for such a screening in Lebanon is 40 years. Awareness campaigns increase women's personal motivation to utilize the diagnostic services and sensitize physicians to suspect and diagnose signs and symptoms of potential breast tumors [18].

Further, significant changes in social behaviors, like higher ages of marriage and less children, are likely to increase the likelihood of breast cancer incidence in the country [19]. Breast cancer is also altered by changes in dietary habits [20, 21]. The nutritional transition, characterized by an alteration in the food choices from the traditional Mediterranean diet to a more Westernized diet is currently underway [22, 23].

Bladder cancer: It was always surprising to observe a high incidence of bladder cancer relative to other cancers among males and females. Although the incidence of bladder cancer has been related to exposure to chlorinated water and its by-products and caffeine consumption [24, 25], smoking remains one of the most direct risk factors [26–28].

Prevention Strategy

Prevention is the most successful approach in public health and economically the most efficient for a long-term control of the disease. As a matter of fact, about 40 % of cancer cases can be avoided by preventing, modifying, or reducing vulnerability of persons exposed to the main risk factors, that is to say smoking, overweight and obesity, inadequate consumption of fruits and vegetables, the lack of physical activity, drinking of alcoholic beverages, infections (HBV, HPV), and air pollution.

Considering Lebanon's cancer burden, it is encouraging that the country's most common cancers (lung, head and neck, and bladder) are eminently preventable, through tobacco and obesity control. Lebanon signed and ratified the WHO Framework Convention on Tobacco Control (FCTC) in 2004 and 2005, respectively, and it entered into force in March 2006.

Although parliament passed a Tobacco Control Law in 2011, it has not been fully implemented and is currently not monitored. The law includes provisions for health education on the harmful aspects of tobacco use, tobacco taxation, advertising, labelling of tobacco products, and a ban on sponsorship and tobacco use in public places.

However, current measures to reduce tobacco consumption through enforcement of the tobacco control law are sporadic, and further activities to promote physical activity and healthy diet are recommended.

Early Detection Strategy

Early detection activities are essential in reducing the burden of certain cancers. In fact, we may reduce about one-third of the cancer burden through early detection and treatment of cases at the onset of the disease, the phase where treatment is most efficient. This can be done by keeping the population aware of the early signs of cancer and by undertaking screening programs for risk persons in order to detect the disease even before the appearance of the first symptoms. Control of lymphomas, breast, prostate, and colorectal cancers rely predominantly on early detection and appropriate treatment.

No population-based, organized breast cancer, colorectal, and prostate cancer screening programs exist in Lebanon, although activities for early detection of these cancers are in place. Breast cancer awareness campaigns are initiated annually during the last 3 months of each year with provision of free mammography at government hospitals. Although no population-based colorectal cancer screening program is in place, the Ministry of Public Health is exploring ways to implement such a program. Although there is no national guideline or recommendation for systematic prostate cancer testing by prostate-specific antigen (PSA) among the asymptomatic population, men are prescribed PSA testing in some private primary care facilities.

Diagnosis and Therapeutic Management Strategy

Cancer is a priority health problem in Lebanon. Cancer diagnosis is performed late in a multitude of cases. Therefore, a large proportion of cases are locally advanced with reduced chances of cure. Infrastructure for diagnosis (staging) and treatment is adequate at the private tertiary-level system. However, there is a challenge regarding integration between primary care network (prevention and early diagnosis), and specialized hospital care network. This situation impedes the continuum of care.

The diagnostic and treatment capacity, particularly in the private sector, is a notable strength. However, the discrepancies in terms of services and technology between the public and private sector is skewed heavily in favor of private practice. There is adequate access to all modalities of cancer treatment (surgery, chemotherapy, radiotherapy) in Lebanon, though a significant portion of the Ministry of Public Health budget is allocated for four chemotherapy drugs.

Capacity in Diagnosis

There are 24 nuclear medicine centers in Lebanon, all of which had single, aging SPECT gamma camera equipment. It is clear that as the private sector is focused on profits these units will not be upgraded as scintigraphy does not generate revenue due to the cost of isotopes. However, metastatic work-up for cancer patients requires bone scintigraphy before surgery. This needs to be developed to match radiology services.

As relates to nuclear medicine services, it is evident that many gamma cameras in operation are old and have a low work load. This is evident as service providers are private hospitals and conventional nuclear medicine has a high cost for generators and kits (which is not highly profitable). Therefore, there is an availability of greater than necessary positron emission tomography-computed tomography (PET-CT) units (though not gamma cameras) as they are part of metastatic work-up.

Currently, Lebanon has seven operational PET/CT units and two more in the pipe line. This is quite satisfactory for current cancer control capacity. Lebanon uses F18, FDG, FLT, Choline, and Ga68 for oncology purposes.

Though it is inexpensive and highly effective in conservative breast surgery, sentinel lymph node procedures are not broadly performed for proper conservative breast cancer surgery.

Radiotherapy Capacity of Lebanon

According to the Ministry of Public Health, there are nine radiation oncology centers (eight in the private sector and one in public). The technology platform is heterogeneous in its geographical distribution, in addition to its qualitative and quantitative characteristics. All centers have basic infrastructure for delivering standard 3-D CRT. Some private centers have an advanced platform to deliver high quality radiation therapy including IMRT and IGRT.

With regards to equipment needs in Lebanon, there were reported 9554 new cancer patients in 2012. Assuming that 60 % will require radiotherapy, the number of new cancer cases requiring radiotherapy is roughly 5700. Considering that roughly 500 patients may be treated on a single radiotherapy unit, it is estimated that 11 radiotherapy treatment units are needed in Lebanon.

The number of specialists in radiation oncology is between 10 and 12, according to the Ministry of Public Health. The European Society for Therapeutic Radiology and Oncology (ESTRO), following a review of all European guidelines, recommends to have a radiation oncologist for every 250 patients treated.

Palliative Care Strategy

Major strides have been made in the last few years to develop the field of PC and make it an integral part of the health care delivery system in Lebanon; but much remains to be done to improve palliative care for the majority of patients with cancer who present with advanced disease.

Top barriers include lack of designated palliative care beds/services, community awareness, staff training, access to hospice services, and personnel/time. The non-existence of functioning home-based and hospice services leaves families/providers unable to honor patient wishes.

Considering that a sizeable portion of cancer patients are diagnosed at advanced stages of disease, palliative care services should be a priority in Lebanon. There is currently no organized, specialized palliative care service in any of the main hospitals providing cancer care. Pain management services are provided in some hospitals in Lebanon and administered mainly by anesthetists who conduct consultations for patients in pain, but none of these have received training in palliative care. Further, only inpatient services are provided as no outpatient PC services exist in Lebanon [29].

The development of palliative care services has been inconsistent in Lebanon and implementation of a national strategy faces many challenges, including:

No postgraduate training fellowships in palliative care or pain management programs; lack of a financial reimbursement system for outpatient palliative care and pain services; no clear strategy regarding the interactions between cancer management and other NCDs in palliative care and pain management (although Ain Wazein Hospital has been providing palliative care for patients with various end-stage diseases, and starting at the AUH); a deficiency of data on patients in different stages of cancer and other NCDs in order to estimate the number of patients in advanced stages who may be in need of palliative care; lack of clarity on Do Not Resuscitate (DNR) policies for Lebanon.

Weak opioids such as codeine and tramadol and strong opioids such as oral and patches of Fentanyl are available. Morphine (IR), oxycodone, and hydromorphone are not available. Only oncologists and pain specialists (palliative care specialists and some other specialists more recently) are allowed to prescribe opioid medications.

Despite these numerous challenges, there have been a series of developments in Lebanon over the past decade that indicate a steady upward trend in the advancement of services in the country.

Timeline of PC Developments: In 2000, a pain relief and palliative care group was established under the auspices of the Lebanese Cancer Society to educate health care providers. Since that time, a number of initiatives have advanced the development of palliative care. On 4 May 2011, the Ministry of Public Health formed the National Committee for Pain Relief and Palliative care with a mission focusing on improving education, field practice and research as well as developing public policy. In October 2012, the first International Conference on Palliative Care was held.

Following this conference, the national committee on pain relief and PC has made a number of recommendations in the domains of education, practice, research, and public policy which can be summarized as follows:

- Training of all health care professionals in basic principles of PC through the inclusion of PC content in undergraduate and graduate curricula.
- Creation of continuing education programs in PC.
- Provision of specialist training in PC for physicians and nurses.
- Development of professional standards and multidisciplinary clinical practice guidelines to guide PC practice.
- Coordination of care and rapid-access to PC services.
- Integration of PC services throughout the health care delivery systems.
- Development of PC research priorities and funding mechanisms for research.
- Revision of legislation governing the delivery of opioid analgesics.
- Development of a model to fund PC services.
- Launching of public awareness campaigns to raise the profile of palliative and end-of-life care in the country.

All the above recommendations will have significant implications for the provision of PC services for children and adults. Additionally, high quality research is still needed in PC. For now, PC research is limited to cancer, is descriptive in nature, and in most cases lacks the quality to contribute to evidence-based care. As a result, more research in this field is warranted [30, 31].

On 28 July 2013, hospital-based palliative care services gained new momentum following the addition of palliative care to the current list of specialties recognized in Lebanon through the ministerial special decree No. 1/1048 [32].

National Plan for Cancer Control

In sum, we can note that Lebanon has many elements in place for successful implementation of a national cancer control program, namely a strong commitment on the part of national authorities to fight cancer, a generally high level of diagnostic and treatment services (primarily in the private sector), facilities and capacity for training in all areas of cancer control (with exception of palliative care) and strong dedication among health professionals working in cancer to carry activities forward.

At present, Lebanon has neither a fully endorsed national cancer control plan nor a national committee representing major stakeholders in cancer control. The National Cancer Registry is currently a pathology-based registry and may serve as a strong basis to develop a population-based cancer registry. Establishment of a national cancer control plan and building the capacity of the current registry are critical activities to set a framework for long-term planning and implementation of a sustainable cancer strategy. These components will be supported by a communication and social mobilization program, along with the strengthening of legislation and regulation.

Final thoughts about three issues that are not yet enough studied and need attention in the future:

1. Lebanon is experiencing a large wave of refugees from the neighboring countries due to the war and lack of security (around two million representing the third of the current population). We don't have until now any data as for the exact number, the health problems, the specific diseases (especially concerning cancer), and their burden. We will need a time before getting some objective conclusions.
2. On the other hand, we don't have any study, or observational report about a difference of incidence or behavior of cancer disease from a community to another (only more bladder cancer is observed in Armenians which can be due to a special diet and tobacco consumption?), or from a geographical area to another.
3. Disparity and inequalities in cancer care are only related to age (elderly people have less adapted treatment for cancer), and geographical reason: the control of cancer is less good in the peripheral areas of the country. I think this is common in many countries in transition too.

Priority Recommendations

In the light of the situation analysis and the commitment on the part of national authorities to fight cancer, the following recommendations can be made:

Cancer Control Program

1. Establish a national cancer control steering committee.
2. Conduct a situation analysis for the top priorities for cancer control (for example, a significant number of cancers can be prevented with tobacco and obesity control).
3. Develop a cancer control plan with specific timelines and budget based on the priorities identified.

Cancer Registration

4. Upgrade the National Cancer Registry to a population-based registry and ensure its sustainability by allocating greater technical and financial support.
5. Improve the accuracy of cancer incidence data (completeness and validity). Increase coverage and quality of the vital statistics system, and improve cause of death reporting; link the mortality database to the cancer registry.

Prevention

6. To facilitate reduction in tobacco consumption, enforce sub-decrees regarding smoke-free environments, place health warning labels and 'shock' photos on tobacco product packages, ban advertisements for tobacco products, prohibit the sale of tobacco products to minors and substantially increase tobacco taxation so that excise taxation on finished tobacco products rises to 67–80 % of retail price.
7. Develop a comprehensive national policy to promote healthy diets and increased physical activity in daily routine activities.

Early Detection

8. Improve population and professional awareness of early symptoms and signs of common cancers among population and professionals, and strengthen referral pathways to ensure prompt diagnosis and treatment.
9. Organize and implement a national breast cancer early detection program according to international standards.
10. Given the increasing burden of colorectal cancer in men and women, implement a pilot study on the feasibility and acceptability of colorectal cancer screening.

Diagnosis and Treatment

11. Within the context of the national cancer control plan, create an inclusive national task force comprised of relevant stakeholders to standardize national protocols for treatment of most common cancers. Place special emphasis on development of the national essential oncology medicines list.
12. Within the context of the national cancer control plan, design a plan for development of facilities for pathology, radiology, radiotherapy, and nuclear medicine services in the public sector to compensate for geographical differences in access to technology.
13. Create a national training program for medical physics and radiotherapy technologists (RTTs).

Palliative Care

14. Establish a training program in palliative care and pain control.
15. Establish national guidelines for palliative care services.
16. Improve legislation with regards to opioid prescriptions.

Conclusion

Whether we consider incidence, mortality, early detection, or treatment rates, it is clear that there exist significant opportunities to save lives and reduce suffering in the ME countries. Unfortunately, the single most important trend in cancer in these countries today (and in developing countries in general) is the growing gap between what we know and what is actually being done to reduce human suffering and to save lives. Given the impact of the late presentation problem, palliative care is of paramount importance in the ME countries [33].

Fighting cancer is a lifelong mission. It implies a long struggle which enhances our humanity and teaches us humility, solidarity, and hope. When the Lebanese Cancer Society was created in 1954, the dedicated group of doctors who founded it was aware of the scale of the challenge, the immensity of the task, and the extent of the commitment required. And then the consecutive Presidents and members of the Board of the Administration of the LCS had an obligation to achieve concrete results, which means we had to act quickly and efficiently to alleviate suffering, shine a light of hope and make sure programs and actions were sustainable.

The health care system in Lebanon will be required to adapt to the growing burden of cancer in our population. As is the case in developed countries, Lebanon needs now a National Plan for Cancer Prevention and Control. This will need an effective partnership between the LCS and other associations, and the Ministry of Health.

The plan, which takes into account Lebanese specificities, is developed in light of existing and potential resources. It advocates new approaches in terms of screening, treatment, and social support, all of which are consistent with our cultural values and based on the active involvement of the entire society. The implementation of this plan will have a significant impact on the fight against cancer.

References

1. World Cancer Day 2014. Myth 2—cancer is a disease of the wealthy, elderly and developed countries.http://www.worldcancerday.org/myth-2-cancer-disease-wealthy-elderlyand-developed-countries. Last accessed 13 May 2014.
2. International Agency for Research on Cancer: GLOBOCAN 2012. Estimated cancer incidence, mortality, and prevalence worldwide in 2012. http://globocan.iarc.fr/Pages/fact_sheets_cancer.aspx. Last accessed 13 May 2014.
3. Center for Disease Control and Prevention. National Vital Statistic System. http://www.cdc.gov/nchs/nvss.htm. Accessed 26 Nov 2013.
4. American Cancer Society. The global economic cost of cancer. http://www.cancer.org/acs/groups/content/@internationalaffairs/documents/document/acspc-026203.pdf. Accessed 30 Jan 2014.
5. Boseley S. Global cancer surge fueled by alcohol, smoking, and obesity predicted by WHO. The Guardian. February 3, 2014. http://www.theguardian.com/society/2014/feb/03/alcoholsugar-smoking-fuel-cancer-surge. Last accessed 13 May 2014.
6. Revised global burden of disease (GBD) 2002 estimates. Geneva: World Health Organization; 2002. http://www.who.int/healthinfo/bodgbd2002revised/en/index.html
7. Rastogi T, et al. Opportunities for cancer epidemiology in developing countries. Nat Rev Cancer. 2004;4:909–17.
8. Pisani P, et al. Estimates of the worldwide prevalence of cancer for twenty five sites in the adult population. Int J Cancer. 2002;97:72–81.
9. Cancer prevention and control. Alexandria, WHO Regional Office for the Eastern Mediterranean, 1997 (EMRO technical paper series 2).
10. Cancer incidence report in Gulf Cooperation Council countries. Gulf Center for Cancer Registration, Executive Board of Health Ministers Council for GCC States. Riyadh: The Research Center, King Faisal Hospital; 2000.
11. Cancer in Lebanon 2003. National Cancer Registry. Ministry of Public Health, Beirut, Lebanon. http://www.cancer.org.lb/public/NationalCancerRegistryReport2003.pdf
12. Sibai AM, Sen K, Beydoun M, Saxena P. Population ageing in Lebanon: current status, future prospects and implications for policy. Bull World Health Organ. 2004;82:219–25.
13. United Nations—Department of Economic and Social Affairs—Population Division: World population prospects: the 2008 revisions, highlights and advances. Working paper no. ESA/P/WP.210. United Nations; 2011.
14. Lebanese Ministry of Public Health, National Cancer Registry (NCR). Beirut, Lebanon: Cancer in Lebanon 2004 with an update of 2003.
15. Hall S, Petkova H, Tsouros AD. Palliative care for older people: better practices. World Health Organ. 2011;3:1–59.

16. Lebanese Ministry of Public Health: National Cancer Registry—cancer surveillance. 2012. http://www.moph.gov.lb/Prevention/Surveillance/Pages/Cancer.aspx. Accessed 1 Aug 2012
17. Shamseddine A, et al. Cancer trends in Lebanon: a review of incidence rates for the period of 2003–2008 and projections until 2018. Popul Health Metrics. 2014;12:4. http://www.pophealthmetrics.com/content/12/1/4
18. El-Saghir N, Khalil M, Eid T, El Kinge AR, Charafeddine M, Geara F, Seoud M, Shamseddine AI. Trends in epidemiology and management of breast cancer in developing Arab countries: a literature and registry analysis. Int J Surg. 2007;5:225–33.
19. Rashad H, Osman M, Roudi-Fahimi F. Marriage in the Arab world. Population Reference Bureau; 2005. http://www.prb.org/pdf05/marriageinarabworld_eng.pdf
20. Yahia N, Achkar A, Abdallah A, Rizk S. Eating habits and obesity among Lebanese University students. Nutr J. 2007;7(32). doi:10.1186/1475-2891-7-32.
21. Sibai AM, Nasreddine L, Mokdad A, Adra N, Tabet M, Hwalla N. Nutrition transition and cardiovascular disease risk factors in the MENA countries: reviewing the evidence. Ann Nutr Metab. 2010;57:193–203.
22. Sibai AM, Hwalla N, Adra N, Rahal B. Prevalence and covariates of obesity in Lebanon: findings from the first epidemiological study. Obes Res. 2003;11(11):1353–61.
23. Nasreddine L, Naja F, Chamieh MC, Adra N, Sibai AM, Hwalla N. Trends in overweight and obesity in Lebanon: evidence from two national cross-sectional surveys (1997 and 2009). BMC Public Health. 2012;12(1):798. doi:10.1186/1471-2458-12-798.
24. King WD, Marrett LD. Case-control study of bladder cancer and chlorination by-products in treated water. Cancer Causes Control. 1996;7(6):596–604.
25. Pelicchi C, La Vecchia C. Alcohol, coffee and bladder cancer risk: a review of epidemiological studies. Eur J Cancer Prev. 2009;18(1):62–8.
26. Freedman ND, Silverman DT, Hollenbeck AR, Schatzkin A, Abnet CC. Association between smoking and risk of bladder cancer among men and women. JAMA. 2011;306(7):737–45.
27. International Agency for Research on Cancer. World cancer report. Lyon: IARC Press; 2008. 9789283204237.
28. Lee R, Droller M. The natural history of bladder cancer: implications for therapy. Urol Clin N Am. 2000;27(1):1–13.
29. Abu-Saad Huijer H, Abboud S, Doumit M. Symptom prevalence and management of cancer patients in Lebanon. J Pain Symptom Manage. 2012;42(1):147–54.
30. Daher M, Hajjar RR. Palliative care for cancer patients in Lebanon. In: Silbermann M, editor. Palliative care to the cancer patient: The Middle East as a model for emerging countries. 1st ed. New York: Nova; 2014. p. 125–40.
31. Daher M. Implementation of palliative care in Lebanon. J Pediatr Hematol Oncol. 2010; 32(1):44.
32. Daher M, Doumit M, Hajjar R, Hamra R, Naifeh Khoury M, Tohme A. Integrating palliative care into health education in Lebanon. J Med Liban. 2013;61(4):191–8. http://www.lebanese-medicaljournal.org/articles/61-4/review1.pdf
33. Daher M. Palliative care in Arab countries: challenges and achievements. ACCESS Health J. 2013;(2):89–94.

Chapter 11
Cancer Care in an Economically Torn Country: Cyprus

Haris Charalambous

Introduction

Cyprus is situated in the eastern part of the Mediterranean Sea, between Greece, Turkey, Syria, Lebanon, Israel, and Egypt. Cyprus gained its independence from the UK in 1960. There are two main ethnic communities in Cyprus; the Greek Cypriot constituted the majority of the population (close to 80 %) and the Turkish Cypriots the minority (around 18 %). In 1974 following a military group d'état by Greek Cypriot nationalists, Turkey invaded Cyprus, resulting in the island being divided; in the south, the area under the effective control of the Republic of Cyprus, comprising about two-thirds of the island's area, and the Turkish-controlled area in the north. The northern part is recognized as an independent state only by Turkey. This separation has dominated Cypriot life over the last 40 years and despite numerous attempts there has been no political solution as yet in the Cyprus problem, resulting in communities moving further away from each other. This separation has also a significant impact on provision of health services in the two communities [1]. For the purposes of this chapter, we are going to discuss Cancer Care in relation to the Republic of Cyprus, excluding discussion about the Turkish-controlled area.

In 2004 the Republic of Cyprus joined the European Union and in 2008 it joined the Euro. According to the 2011 latest census, the population is 838.897 inhabitants with 659.350 Cypriot citizens and 176.547 foreign citizens; with 112.424 coming from the European Union [2]. Since its independence Cyprus has developed as a centre in the Eastern Mediterranean for offshore businesses, financial services, shipping and tourism [2], and is considered to be among the world developed countries with very high Human Development Index, ranking in the 32nd position in 2013 among 187 countries [3]. In fact, until recently and before the economic and

H. Charalambous, B.M., M.R.C.P. (UK), F.R.C.R. (UK) (✉)
Bank of Cyprus Oncology Centre, Nicosia, Cyprus
e-mail: haris.charalambous@bococ.org.cy

M. Silbermann (ed.), *Cancer Care in Countries and Societies in Transition*,
DOI 10.1007/978-3-319-22912-6_11

financial crisis in Cyprus, the GDP (gross domestic product) per capita adjusted for purchasing power at 28,961 USD (2010) was around the average of the European Union (EU27). Since the crisis in 2012–2013, brought on by a large fiscal deficit and problems in the banking sector, as a result of exposure to Greek National Bonds and poor lending, this has been reduced considerably with an estimate of US$ 24,181 for 2014 [4]. There have been in fact now three successive years with a large decrease in GDP; in 2012 this was −2.4 %, in 2013 −6.0 %, and the estimate for 2014 was −3.0 %.

As a result of this major economic and financial crisis, Cyprus has received financial bailout from the European Union, the European Central Bank, and the International Monetary Fund, known collectively as the Troika. This has been in addition to the bail-in of bank deposits, applied worldwide for the first time in Cyprus. Under this financial assistance programme, the European Stability Mechanism (ESM) will provide up to nine billion euros, and the International Monetary Fund (IMF) is expected to contribute around one billion euro. The financial assistance came with the enforcement of an economic adjustment (austerity) programme for Cyprus to cover the period 2013–2016.

The Health Care System in Cyprus in Brief

Health Care in Cyprus is provided within two parallel delivery systems, a public Health Care System (HCS) and a separate private HCS. The public HCS is highly centralized and almost everything regarding planning, organization, and administration is regulated by the Ministry of Health (MoH) [5]. It is financed by the state budget, with services provided through a network of hospitals and health centers. More specifically, health services in the public sector are provided by six hospitals (five district hospitals; one in each district of Nicosia, Limassol, Larnaca, Paphos, and Ammochostos and one hospital dedicated to Paediatrics and Gynaecology; Makarios Hospital in Nicosia), four specialist centers (the Bank of Cyprus Oncology Centre BOCOC, the Institute of Neurology and Genetics, the Thalassaemia Centre, and the Arodafnousa Hospice/Palliative Care Centre), three small rural hospitals, 38 health centres (Kentra Ygeias Gk) similar to facilities for General Practitioners in the UK, as well as many subcenters for primary services [5]. The public HCS however does not secure universal coverage for all in Cyprus, as only around 83 % of the population has right to access to the public health system free of charge [5]. The rest of the population to use the public HCS have to pay according to the fee schedule set by the MoH or alternatively could pay privately to use the private health care sector [5]. The private HCS largely consists of independent providers and facilities (including private hospitals) which are often physician-owned, or private companies in which doctors are usually shareholders [5]. The majority of private physicians however work out of their own premises/offices conducting mainly outpatient type of consultations, and carrying out less complicated procedures/investigations, e.g., echocardiograms and endoscopies.

The majority of doctors, dentists, and pharmacists work in the private sector while the majority of nurses are employed in the public sector. Over the last decade most of the newly qualified physicians have pursued careers in non-primary care specialties. As a result there has been a decrease of 20 % on the number of GPs between 1995 and 2005 [5]. Since patients have direct access to specialist care, GPs mainly treat minor illnesses, provide prescriptions, and order laboratory tests.

Total Health expenditure in Cyprus in 2010 accounted for 6 % of GDP, with 41.5 % of health care expenditures being government (public health care sector) funded and 58.5 % privately funded [5]. In fact the Health expenditure share of total Government expenditure at 5.3 % is the lowest of all EU countries. Private Health Care expenses are partly covered by private medical insurance (about 20 % of the population have voluntary health insurance through workers' unions or semi-state organizations), although a significant part is covered by Out Of Pocket (OOP) payments [2, 5]. OOP payments are the dominant private source of health care expenditures, whilst Cyprus has one of Europe's highest proportions of health care spending by household [5].

A major limitation of the current Cyprus HCS is the absence of an organized Primary Care level/sector, with only a few trained General Practitioners operating in Cyprus predominantly in the private sector, essentially resulting in patients' care provided by the secondary and tertiary level providers [2, 5]. Physicians employed at the public health care centres (Kentra Ygeias) have predominantly internal medicine background and no consistent training in other specialties, e.g., Gynaecology and Paediatrics, as is the training for General Practitioners in the UK.

Deficiencies of the Current HCS in Cyprus

1. Incomplete coverage and high Out Of Pocket spending
2. Lack of an organized primary care sector
3. Inefficient use of resources through lack of management in the public sector and overcapacity and duplication in the private sector
4. Poor communication among health care providers resulting in poor continuity of care
5. Unenforced quality standards

Another major weakness of the current HCS is the fragmentation of the services with little coordination among health care providers within and between the private and public sectors [5]. This results in inefficiencies in both sectors, in the public sector as a result of lack of proper structures and management and in the private sector as a result of duplication and underutilization of services [5]. For instance, as a result of this duplication of services, Cyprus has a very high number of CT and MRI scanners compared with the OECDO average, with most of them being concentrated in the private sector [5].

Furthermore there are no established referral/treatment pathways for patients, linked with poor communication between doctors and other health care providers, resulting in poor continuity of care, when patients need to transition from different specialties or from hospital to home the community and vice versa. Finally despite talk to the contrary, there is little evidence of guidelines being used and audits being undertaken to ensure high standards of the quality of care either in the public or private sectors.

Despite these shortcomings the overall health status of the population is good. There is complete eradication of communicable diseases (such as Malaria, Tuberculosis, and Echinococcus), low infant mortality, low prevalence of HIV infection, high levels of immunization coverage [5], and a good sanitation system. As a result life expectancy in Cyprus for 2010–2011 was 79 years for males and 82.9 years for females according to the MOH's report on deaths and causes of deaths (2004–2011) [6].

Since 2013 and following the crisis, legislation was enacted to introduce fees for doctor appointments, blood results, and drugs, even for those previously entitled to free health care. User charges however are low. Public sector workers are also required to contribute for their access to "free" public health care. These measures have also affected cancer patients, which were also previously exempt from any charges.

The Proposed New National General Health Care System

In recognition of these problems, especially the lack of universal coverage for health care of all people living in Cyprus, the Parliament approved legislation in *2001* to set up a national General Health Care System (GHCS) to provide universal health care cover for all citizens in Cyprus through a General Health Insurance System (GHIS) [5]. Despite a number of studies on expected costs of the GHIS, there has been a major delay in its implementation, mainly due to concerns over costs, which have been exacerbated by the economic crisis [5]. Amendments to the legislation regarding the GHIS have just been proposed (December 2014) and are currently under public consultation, prior to the implementation of such a system in 2015.

The original proposal specified that the new GHCS provides universal coverage under a single payer system financed by contributions from employers and employees (including self-employed and pensioners), the government budget and OOP spending; however, the Government more recently is considering to involve the private health insurance industry and convert the system to a multi payer one. A study to this effect is currently under way. Other key features of the new GHCS include:

- Fostering competition between public and private providers by offering patients free choice of providers
- Providing public hospitals and health centres with financial and managerial autonomy
- Requiring all patients to register with a family doctor who will function as the gatekeeper of the system and may also help coordinate care. Reimburse family doctors based on a capitation payment with performance incentives
- Specialists to be paid on a fee-for-service basis under a global budget, while hospital care to be reimbursed based on a Diagnosis-Related-Group system (DRG)

- Introduction of bulk purchasing of goods and services
- The creation of a pharmaceutical Health Technology Assessment (HTA) committee
- Reform of the MoH into a planning and regulatory body

In fact implementation of the new GHCS is part of the agreement with the International Lenders, and according to the Memorandum of Understanding the new GHCS System must be implemented in three phases as below:

- Phase I (01/07/2015)—Primary Health Care Services (includes visits to the family doctors and pediatricians).
- Phase II (01/01/2016)—covers additional outpatient services, including all services of specialists and outpatient drugs.
- Phase III (7/1/2016)—Full implementation of the GHCS, which will also include all the secondary and tertiary health care, laboratory and clinical tests, inpatient hospitalization.

Given that there is still public consultation about the final legislation regarding the GHCS, it is likely that there is going to be further delay in the above timetable for implementation.

Cancer Epidemiology in Cyprus

Cancer is the second commonest cause of death in Cyprus after cardiovascular disease causing 22.1 % of all deaths in Cyprus compared to 39.2 % of deaths due to cardiovascular disease according to the 2004–2011 MoH report [6, 7]. On average about 1100 people in Cyprus die from cancer each year, compared to 2035 by cardiovascular disease [6]. Of note that there is a much higher increase in cancer deaths compared to deaths due to cardiovascular disease; in the period of 2004–2011 this was 19 % for cancer and only 5.3 % for cardiovascular disease [6, 7]. The crude rate of cancer mortality in 2011 was 162.29 for males and 116.02 for females per 100,000 [7]. Finally, according to Eurostat and European Community Health Indicators, cancer death rates in Cyprus are the lowest in the European region [7].

In 2010, which is the last year for which there are published records from the Cyprus Cancer Registry, there were 3035 new patients diagnosed with cancer in Cyprus (crude cancer incidence), with an Age Standardized Rate (ASR) for men of 249.3 and 225.3 for women per 100,000 population [8]. The European Network of Cancer Registries (EUCAN) website operated by the International Agency for Research in Cancer (IARC) has *estimates* of the different European countries' Age Standardized Cancer Incidence Rates (ASR), Mortality and Prevalence for 2008 and 2012. For 2008 the actual ASR in Cyprus for men was 249.9 and 225.7 for women per 100,000 population [9]; this can be compared to a European Union (27 countries) rate for 2008 for both gender of 372.2 as estimated by EUCAN [10]. For 2012 the ASR for both gender, is estimated by EUCAN for Cyprus to be 290.4 per 100,000 population, which is again considerably less than the corresponding European Union average (27 countries) at 382.0 per 100,000 population [10].

Table 11.1 Cancer incidence in Cyprus (2010)

Men			Women		
Cancer type	Crude incidence/%	ASR per 100,000	Cancer type	Crude incidence/%	ASR per 100,000
Prostate	418/26.4	71.4	Breast	496/34.0	87.0
Colon/rectum	206/13.1	35.7	Colon	161/11.0	24.2
Lung	204/13.0	35.6	Thyroid	158/10.8	32.0
Bladder	112/7.1	19.8	Uterus	94/6.4	15.4
NHL	61/3.9	11.4	NHL	70/4.8	12.0

Adapted from the latest Cyprus Cancer Registry Report covering Incidence Data for the period of 1999–2010 [8]

Table 11.2 Comparison of ASRs between Cyprus and EU (27): EUCAN 2012 estimates

	Thyroid cancer	Breast cancer	Prostate cancer	Lung cancer
Cyprus	10.1	104.3	85.9	23.6
EU (27)	6.5	108.8	110.8	44.1

From the EUCAN website at: http://eu-cancer.iarc.fr/EUCAN/Default.aspx. Accessed 29 Dec 2014

According to the latest Cyprus Cancer Registry Report [8] for 2010 prostate cancer is the commonest cancer in men followed by Colon, Lung, Bladder cancer, and Non-Hodgkin's lymphoma, whilst the commonest cancer in women is Breast cancer followed by Colon, Thyroid, Uterus, and Non-Hodgkin's Lymphoma (see Table 11.1).

Comparison of Cyprus incidence rates for 2012 with the EU (27) as estimated by EUCAN reveals significant deviations; for instance for thyroid cancer the ASR is higher at 10.1 in Cyprus compared to 6.5 in the EU (27), whilst for both the usually screening-detected prostate and breast cancers the rates are close, whilst for Lung Cancer there is a much lower incidence in Cyprus almost half of the EU (27) average (see Table 11.2). These observations are currently under further investigation.

Cancer Services in Cyprus

Regarding cancer prevention, educational activities are organized by the MoH in collaboration often with patients' organizations and advocacy groups. A smoking cessation clinic operates in Nicosia General Hospital with plans to set up similar clinics in all general hospitals.

Regarding screening activities, a comprehensive national breast cancer screening programme has been in place since 2007, which is free for all women between the ages of 50 and 69 years [7]. There is no formal comprehensive screening for cervical, colorectal, and prostate cancer in Cyprus, instead individuals present themselves to their physicians either for other reasons (opportunistic screening) or specifically to request screening. The high prostate cancer incidence in Cyprus (see Table 11.2) suggests that the practice of PSA testing is widespread. A pilot programme for colorectal cancer screening has been recently initiated. Finally in terms of cervical screening, health surveys from 2003 to 2008 suggest that there is a reduction in the percentage of women undergoing pap tests; 80.9 % of women surveyed in 2003 had a pap test compared to 73 % in 2008 [7, 11, 12].

Genetic testing is available for hereditary predisposition and familial cancer syndromes especially in relation to Breast and Colon cancer in the Cyprus Institute of Neurology and Genetics [13].

Treatment of all patients with cancer is provided in the two public/government oncology units, located in the Nicosia and Limassol General hospitals and also in the Bank of Cyprus Oncology Centre (BOCOC). The BOCOC is a not-for-profit organization, co-founded and co-funded by the Bank of Cyprus and the Cyprus Government, and is the only purpose built Oncology tertiary referral centre in Cyprus [14]. The BOCOC essentially operates as a public oncology centre, accepting all patients eligible for health care in Cyprus without charging patients any additional fees (over and above those charged in the public hospitals). The BOCOC provides comprehensive specialized nonsurgical oncology services, including both Chemotherapy and Radiotherapy, whilst the public hospitals oncology units provide only chemotherapy. In terms of radiotherapy facilities the BOCOC is equipped with three linear accelerators, with Image Guided and Intensity Modulated Radiotherapy as well as Stereotactic Radiotherapy capabilities, a superficial orthovoltage treatment unit and a High Dose Rate (HDR) Brachytherapy system. In terms of chemotherapy facilities, there is a day care unit for outpatient chemotherapy administration (19 beds), with a separate room for infusions with four couches and four chairs (for iv zoledronic acid and Trastuzumab). This is supported by an aseptic suite for the reconstitution of cytotoxic drugs, a pharmacy and dispensary. There is also a day care unit for supportive care (13 beds/couches) and two wards for hospitalization of patients with difficult-to-control symptoms and inpatient treatment with chemotherapy and radiotherapy (38 beds).

There is a limited number of private oncologists, based in private hospitals, which see and treat a small percentage of cancer patients, although often act as a source of second opinion for patients treated at the BOCOC or at the public hospitals oncology units. Of note that three medical schools have been set up in the last 4 years in Cyprus offering undergraduate medical courses (St George's, University of London in association with the University of Nicosia, the University of Cyprus, and the European University). Although all are affiliated with local hospitals in Cyprus, none of the Medical Schools is involved in providing oncology services or has dedicated oncology facilities.

From the 2013 Annual report for the BOCOC it is stated that 2108 new patients were seen in 2013; and in total in excess of 26,000 patients were seen since its foundation in 1999 [15]. Furthermore in 2013 there were 34,449 outpatient clinic visits, 10,175 outpatient chemotherapy administrations with a further 2796 targeted therapies including zoledronic acid administrations, and 1540 inpatient chemotherapy administrations. From the Nicosia General Hospital (NGH) annual report for 2013, it is stated that there were 6084 outpatient visits at the NGH Oncology clinic compared to 7070 in 2012, with 2201 outpatient chemotherapy treatments provided [16]. At the Limassol General Hospital (LGH) Oncology unit in 2013, there were 593 new patients seen, 9396 outpatient clinic visits, and 3721 chemotherapy and other intravenous treatments [17].

In terms of radiotherapy activity, 32.251 fractions of external beam Linear Accelerator radiotherapy were delivered at the BOCOC in 2013, in addition to 192 brachytherapy treatments (predominantly for gynaecological cancers) and 1.271 fractions of superficial orthovoltage radiotherapy for skin malignancies [15]. There are currently no waiting lists for Radiotherapy treatment in Cyprus, as a result of the efficient use of the three Linear Accelerators, delivering each close to 11,000 fractions of external beam radiotherapy per year, whilst using the new advanced Radiotherapy techniques, including the use of Image Guided and Intensity Modulated Radiotherapy. This compares very favourably with recommendations from the UK, which suggest that for the UK the average number of fractions per linear accelerator should increase to 8700 fractions per linear accelerator per year by 2016 [18].

From the Cyprus Cancer Registry 2011 progress report covering 2006–2008 data [9], the number of patients registered at the different Oncology providers, i.e., the BOCOC/the General Hospitals and private hospitals, can be seen in Table 11.3.

In terms of geographical citing of oncology services, Nicosia is in the middle of the island, where both radiotherapy and chemotherapy services are available whilst Limassol is in the south and west of the island, with only chemotherapy services available. In terms of distances that patients have to travel to Nicosia, the furthest east town of Paralimni is 75–85 km away, in the south the town of Larnaca and Limassol are less than 70 km away, whilst the furthest away district by far is in the west of the island, Paphos, is around 120 km away (see Fig. 11.1, Map of Cyprus). Between all main towns in Cyprus (Nicosia, Larnaca, Limassol, Paphos, and Paralimni) there are new, modern, dual carriage motorways, allowing for both safe and fast travel between the main towns [2].

Table 11.3 Cyprus cancer registry: cancer cases abstracted from various sources, 2006–2008

Facility	Count	%
Bank of Cyprus Oncology Centre	4686	54.2
Nicosia General Hospital	1141	13.2
Lemesos General Hospital	792	9.2
Larnaca General Hospital	225	2.6
Limassol Private Hospital 1	172	2.0
Paphos General Hospital	153	1.8
Makario Nosokomio Lefkosia	109	1.3
Paphos Private Clinic 2	73	0.8
Nicosia Private Hospital 4	65	0.8

From the Cyprus Cancer Registry 2011 Report covering data for 2006–2008 [9]

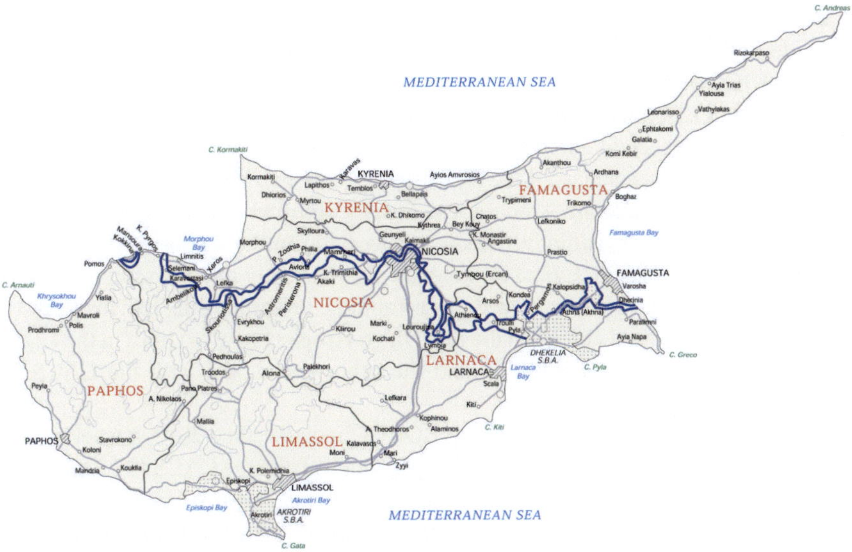

Fig. 11.1 Map of Cyprus. *_Blue line_: border since 1974. North of Nicosia is the occupied part of Cyprus controlled by Turkey

Palliative Care Services in Cyprus

Palliative Care (PC) services in Cyprus are mainly provided by NGOs (Non-government Organizations), whilst there are currently no organized public PC services [1, 2, 19]. Furthermore these services provide almost exclusively to adult cancer patients, given that there are no organized paediatric PC services. Patients with other life-threatening but non-cancer related conditions, are rarely referred to these PC services [1, 2]. The main NGOs in the Republic of Cyprus are the Cyprus Anti-cancer Society (CACS) [20] and the Cyprus Association of Cancer Patients and Friends (PASYKAF) [21], which were founded in 1971 and 1986, respectively [2]. Both NGOs provide a home-based/specialist nurse delivered community-type PC service. The Cyprus Anti-cancer Society (CACS) also operates the main hospice in Cyprus, called Arodafnousa.

Both organizations have shared a major commitment for continuous training and education, and have encouraged their staff beyond attending training courses, also to work and attain higher degrees in PC [1, 2]. Through consistent training and education of PC staff, alongside their dedication to cancer patients in Cyprus, PC staff have been able to provide high quality service to cancer patients in Cyprus, both in the Arodafnousa hospice and in the community [2].

Beyond the CACS and PASYKAF, there are smaller NGOs, e.g., ELAZO which is the association for the patients of the Nicosia General Hospital, the "Friends of Life" Limassol, and "Friends of the Hospice" Paphos (run by expatriates from the UK) fundraising and helping with PC especially in the districts of Limassol and

Paphos [2]. Supportive and PC, sometimes extending to end of life care, is also provided by the two Public Hospital Oncology Units in Nicosia and Limassol and by the BOCOC.

The main PC services provided across the Republic of Cyprus-controlled part of the island can be seen in Table 11.4.

In terms of PC specialists, there are currently only two physicians trained in PC in Cyprus; both work at the Arodafnousa hospice. Furthermore there is an oncologist with a diploma in Palliative Medicine, working in the Oncology Unit of the Limassol General Hospital. Finally there are also currently three physicians undergoing specialist PC training in a 3 year training program with the Institute of Palliative Care (formerly based in the San Diego Hospice, now in Ohio) in the USA; two of them work at the BOCOC and the other one works with the CACS in Limassol [2].

Other initiatives regarding PC in the BOCOC include since 2010, a weekly outpatient PC clinic being run by the two PC physicians from the CACS [2]. This helps both to improve patients' difficult-to-control symptoms, but also encourages earlier introduction of PC in patients with advanced/metastatic cancer and facilitates referral of patients to the Arodafnousa hospice [2]. Furthermore, since 2012 with two physicians in the BOCOC receiving specialist training in PC, there has been the ability to form a hospital PC team and run daily a supportive/PC unit/drop in centre, to address urgent symptom control problems for cancer patients attending the BOCOC [2].

Regarding the availability of opioids in Cyprus, all four opioids on the WHO list are available, i.e., codeine, oral morphine immediate and controlled release forms and injectable morphine, whilst from the International Association for Hospice and Palliative Care (IAHPC) list there is also availability of fentanyl transdermal patches, methadone, and oxycodone long release preparations, whilst oxycodone immediate release is available, but patients in Cyprus have to pay for this [2, 22]. There is however no availability of buprenorphine and hydromorphone in Cyprus [2].

Examining the current legal framework in Cyprus for prescription of opiates compared to the guidelines for assessment of national opioid regulations of the World Health Organization [23], there is no significant overregulation for opioids in Cyprus; however, there is no legal framework to facilitate emergency prescribing and dispensing [2, 22].

In terms of opioid consumption for cancer patients in Cyprus, three studies examining physicians' prescribing habits for cancer pain both within and outside the BOCOC undertaken in 2010 showed that only 56.0, 48.1, and 57.7 % of patients with pain were prescribed analgesia, with the majority of patients being prescribed paracetamol and nonsteroidal anti-inflammatory drugs, and, respectively, only 8.6, 11.5, and 0 % of patients being prescribed strong opioids [22]. In the last two studies, following their oncology appointment the prescription of analgesia to patients with pain increased to 80.8 % and 73.1 %, respectively, whilst the prescription of strong opioids to 28.8 and 34.6 %, reflecting oncologists' practice within the BOCOC, hence providing evidence of an improvement in adequate pain management

Table 11.4 Palliative care provision in Cyprus, 2013

Organization delivering service	Hospice/PC unit	Hospital unit	Hospital support team	Psycho/social service	Home care team	Day care	Supportive-PC unit/ drop in centre	Grand total
PASYKAF				1	1	1		3
CACS	1			1	1	1	2	6
Public Hospital oncology units								
• Nicosia General Hospital Oncology Unit							1	1
• Limassol General Hospital Oncology Unit							1	1
Not-for-profit NGO								
• Bank of Cyprus Oncology Centre			1	1			1	3
Total	1		1	3	2	2	5	14

Produced with permission from Charalambous H, Pitsillide B, Nestoros S. Palliative Care in Cyprus: Current Status (chapter 1. pp. 1–21) in: Palliative Care to the Cancer Patient. The Middle East as a Model for Emerging Countries. First edition, 2014

Table 11.5 Cyprus opioid consumption in Morphine Equivalence (ME) mg/person

	2003	2005	2007	2009	2011	2012
ME mg/person	7.4	10.7	12.6	17.7	35.0	52.9

Data derived from the Pain and Policy Studies Group of the University of Wisconsin website relating to Cyprus [24]

by oncologists within the BOCOC compared to pain management by general physicians in the community [22].

Of interest is the substantial increase (sevenfold) in the annual opioid consumption over the last 10 years in Cyprus, as can be seen in Table 11.5, expressed as total Morphine Equivalence (ME) in mg per person [24]. The last available data from 2012 from the Pain and Policy Studies Group of the University of Wisconsin is close to the global average of 61.7 mg/person.

Systematic high quality training courses in PC for Oncology and PC staff in Cyprus were initiated by the Middle East Cancer Consortium (MECC) [2]. MECC is an intergovernmental organisation, which was set up in 1996 by the governments of Cyprus, Egypt, Israel, Jordan, the Palestinian Authority, and the USA, through the National Cancer Institute of the United States of America [25]. The goal of MECC is to "raise cancer awareness in the Middle East and, ultimately, to reduce the burden of cancer in the region" [2]. MECC has been organising PC courses on an annual basis for health care professionals from its constituent members working in the Oncology or PC field with the first one taking place in 2004, in Larnaca, Cyprus, to which key members of staff from both NGOs, the BOCOC, and the General Hospitals' Oncology Units over the years have participated. It is likely that this sevenfold increase in opioid consumption seen in the last 10 years (2003–2012), as well as general improvement in PC in Cyprus, at least partly reflects the impact of the work of MECC in promoting PC activities and providing training for health care professionals in Cyprus.

In terms of the four stages of development of PC (first stage is when no Services are identified, the second stage is that of Capacity Building, the third stage of Localized provision, and the final/fourth stage is that of Approaching Integration) it is currently accepted that Cyprus in terms of PC services is approaching integration [2, 26]. However further work needs to be done especially in providing organized PC within the main public hospitals, which is currently the main problem with PC in Cyprus [1, 2]. This results in patients in all the public hospitals having no input from specialist PC teams, and this applies both for cancer patients and for patients with other life-threatening illnesses, e.g. End stage Heart or Respiratory Failure [2]. Another main problem of PC services in Cyprus is that there is little cooperation between the two NGOs, resulting in a fragmented service, where currently each home care service only covers the patients at home between 8 am and 6 pm [1, 2, 19]. There are currently however efforts to unite the services of both CACS and PASYKAF, whilst a pilot program is currently being tried by PASYKAF to offer a true 24-h service in Limassol and subsequently in Nicosia, which is being facilitated by a European grant [27].

Impact of the Financial Crisis on Palliative Care Services

The financial crisis exposed the fundamental problem of the NGOs that their budgets and financial sustainability depends to a very large degree on donations and charitable contributions. The financial crisis by increasing unemployment and by negatively affecting peoples' incomes resulted in reduced incomes for both the main NGOs, and as a result to a significant financial budget deficit for both of them. The contribution of the Government to both NGOs also decreased by a small amount. For the PASYKAF the 220,000 euros annual grant from the government was reduced by approximately 10 % to 195,000 euros, whilst for CACS the reduction was slightly less from 600,000 euros to 585,000 euros (in recognition of the costs to support the running of the Arodafnousa hospice).

To respond to decreased fundraising and the resultant budget deficit PASYKAF went ahead with a 16 % pay cuts for all its staff members in 2013 and 2014, but managed as a result to keep all services running. A similar proposal for pay cuts was however rejected by staff at CACS, hence as a result the Board of CACS, among other measures to decrease expenditure, had to lay off a small number of members of staff, with the resultant closure of three hospice beds in Arodafnousa and abolishing the home physiotherapy service, in 2013 [2]. However, with renewed enthusiasm new sources of funding were identified in 2014, and as a result new qualified nurses were recruited, hence currently the hospice operates its full capacity of 15 inpatient beds.

Also as a result of the current financial crisis in Cyprus, the two small hospice units in Limassol, at Chrysovalantou Clinic paid by the Friends of Life (Limassol) NGO, and in Paphos at the Evangelismos Hospital, funded by the Friends' of the Paphos Hospice NGO, ceased to operate in 2013 [2]. Instead Friends for Life Limassol NGO is making a financial contribution to the CACS towards the running of the Arodafnousa Hospice, whilst Friends for Hospice in Paphos has managed to reopen a limited number (3) hospice inpatient beds in Paphos at the St Georges private clinic in 2014.

Finally, a new purpose built hospice, including facilities for children with cancer, Archangel Michael Hospice in Mesa Chorio village in Paphos is ready to start operating, awaiting final local authority approval [28]. Archangel Michael Hospice was planned to start operating in 2013; however, again due to the financial crisis there was a delay until sufficient funds were in place to ensure the smooth running of this facility in the future [2, 28].

Hence as a result of the financial crisis, there were only 12 inpatient hospice beds available in Cyprus in 2013, compared to 24 beds in 2011. Through hard work from all PC NGOs, and the set up of the completely purpose built hospice in Mesa Chorio, the capacity in 2015 is going to be 26 hospice beds (including two paediatric hospice beds in Archangel Michael hospice), which is clearly much better than in 2013 in the aftermath of the financial crisis and a little better than 2011, prior to the financial crisis (see Table 11.6). This is however still inadequate to cover the needs of a population close to one million, when compared with the European guidelines from the

Table 11.6 Inpatient hospice beds for Cyprus 2011 compared to 2013 and 2015

Name	District	Beds 2011	Beds 2013	Beds 2015	Population [2] (approximately)
Arodafnousa Hospice	Nicosia/Larnaca/ Ammochostos	15	12	15	515,000
Chrysovalantou Clinic	Limassol	4	Closed	Closed	235,000
Evangelismos Hospital	Paphos	5	Closed	Closed	90,000
St George's Hospital		–	–	3	
Mesa Chorio Hospice		–	–	8	
Total	Cyprus	24	12	26	840,000

Modified from Charalambous H, Pitsillide B, Nestoros S. Palliative Care in Cyprus: Current Status (chapter 1. pp. 1–21) in: Palliative Care to the Cancer Patient. The Middle East as a Model for Emerging Countries. First edition, 2014

European Association of Palliative Care (EAPC) White Paper [29], where the original need for 50 PC care beds needed per million population has been upgraded to 80–100 beds per million population in view of the needs of non-cancer patients and the prevalence of chronic diseases due to the aging of the population [2].

As a result of the scarcity of inpatient hospice beds, patients with palliative care needs, including end of life care, who are unable to remain at home with home PC support, are often accommodated at the Oncology centres (BOCOC and the Oncology Units in Nicosia and Limassol General Hospitals), where they originally received their oncology treatment [2].

Impact of Financial Crisis and Austerity Measures on Cancer Services

Until 2013 all services to cancer patients were free. In August 2013 legislation was enacted to introduce conditions for patients to be entitled access to cancer care and also to introduce nominal fees for patients whilst accessing this care. Under this legislation patients to be allowed access to cancer care have to fulfill the following two conditions: firstly to have paid for at least 3 years social security contributions and secondly to have filled in their tax return form at the time/year of seeking medical treatment. Furthermore a cap of 150,000 euros of family income was set to allow access to "free" cancer care, whilst patients with family income over this amount would have to pay for the full cost of their care. Furthermore, since 2013 cancer patients have now to pay a nominal fee of 6 euro to see an oncologist per outpatient visit (no fees for inpatient stays), and they also have to pay half a euro per drug/ blood test prescribed. Charges for blood tests are waived when they undergo chemotherapy. Equally chemotherapy drugs remain free, even when patients opt to have treatment privately; the same applies for radiotherapy treatment [2].

Furthermore the financial crisis has resulted in reduced ability of patients to pay for private health care (e.g., due to some patients becoming unemployed or patients suffering from large pay cuts), and hence shifting more activity to the public sector, resulting in a further unused capacity in the private sector. At the same time the Public Health care expenditure has been reduced from a peak of 605 million euros in 2011 [30] to 530 million euros, and private sector expenditure from 704 to 580 million euros [30]. This is in the background of a country already dedicating less proportionally of its GDP to health care compared to other European Countries even prior to the financial crisis; in 2011 Cyprus spent 7.3 % of its GDP towards health care, which is lower than the 8.9 % average of the European Union [30].

As a result of the austerity budget of the MoH for both 2014 and 2015, significant cutbacks were made to Cancer Services expenditure across the board, beyond the new charges introduced for cancer patients. For the BOCOC, funding from the government went down from 15.8 million in 2012 prior to the crisis to 14.7 million in 2015, despite a significant increase of activity levels over this period. Equally financial support of the BOCOC suffered as a result of the financial difficulties of the Bank of Cyprus (BOC), resulting in a cap of donation from the BOC to 2.5 million, whilst the commitment for future equipment replacement is going to be reviewed on a year-by-year basis. In terms of public sector Oncology services, previous plans for two new radiotherapy centres are currently under review.

The total Drugs Budget was also reduced by 10 %. As a result the Cyprus Pharmaceutical Services (responsible for the overall Drugs Budget in Cyprus) have been involved in a major effort to identify potential cost savings. Savings were made possible by a conscious effort on behalf of the Pharmaceutical Services to introduce generic drugs, with the expiry of patents for a number of important anticancer agents in the last couple of years (Imatinib, Temozolomide, Capecitabine, and Zoledronic acid), and to negotiate discounts from Pharmaceutical Drug Companies for cancer drugs currently in the formulary, when new orders for stock are placed. As an example of these policies on behalf of the Pharmaceutical Services, despite a significant year on year increase in patient activity and chemotherapy use in the BOCOC, the Cancer Drugs Budget at the BOCOC went down from 12.6 million in 2012 prior to the crisis to a projected 9.2 million for 2015.

However despite these savings, and due to the 10 % reduction in the Pharmaceutical Services Drugs Budget, there was a need to introduce more intense rationing for access to oncology drugs, and as a result no new chemotherapy/targeted drugs have been approved in the last 2 years 2013–2014. This has resulted in significant gaps in the available treatment options, for a number of different cancer types. As an example for patients with metastatic melanoma there are currently no targeted agents approved, despite the major breakthroughs made in the last couple of years with the use of both checkpoint inhibitors and B-Raf inhibitors in this disease (see Table 11.7).

How HCS cope with the funding of expensive drugs in oncology and in other disciplines however is not a problem unique to Cyprus. It can be argued that under the current financial circumstances, new expensive oncology drugs should not be

Table 11.7 Approval of anticancer targeted therapies in Cyprus

Cancer type	New Targeted Drugs approved in Cyprus	Drugs NOT approved in Cyprus
Breast	Trastuzumab* for HER2 + ve Everolimus* for ER/PR + ve post AI failure	Pertuzumab
Colon	Bevacizumab and Cetuximab* only one agent allowed per patient	Regorafenib
NSCLC	Pemetrexed first line treatment	Crizotinib
	Gefitinib* with EGFR mutations	Nintedanib
	Erlotinib* as 2nd/3rd line treatment	Pemetrexed maintenance
SCCHN	Cetuximab* with platinum and 5FU first line metastatic setting	
Kidney cancer	Sunitinib, Everolimus	Axitinib
	Sorafenib* only for patients not able to tolerate sunitinib or sorafenib	
Prostate cancer	Abiraterone	Alpharadin
		Cabazitaxel
HCC	Sorafenib	
Melanoma	None	Ipilimumab
		Vemurafenib
Gastric	None	Ramucirumab
Thyroid	None	Sorafenib
		Vandetanib
Bone metastases	Zoledronic acid	Denosumab

approved in Cyprus. However it is also important that these decisions are made based on cost-effectiveness criteria, as opposed to whether a drug gets EMA (European Medicines Agency) approval before the financial crisis and hence is available for use, whilst drugs gaining EMA approval after the financial crisis in 2013, are just simply not approved in Cyprus. In the past and until now, no consistent rules for approving oncology drugs existed. Clearly this would need to be addressed, and setting a threshold over above no drug is going to be deemed cost effective, i.e., agreeing on what the Incremental Cost Effectiveness Ratio (ICER) for the Cyprus HCS is absolutely essential. The current crisis however with the involvement of the Troika has meant that a long overdue mechanism to carry out Health Technology Assessments (HTAs) has been finally set up, so that appropriate decisions in relation to approving cost-effective therapies are going to be made in the future.

The introduction of nominal fees for outpatient appointment (6 euros) and 0.5 euros per drug/blood test probably did not impact significantly for the majority of cancer patients, although for some patients this may have been a problem. The measure dictating 3 years of social security contributions has however impacted disproportionately for Turkish Cypriot patients, who unless they are currently staying/working in the Republic of Cyprus or worked in Cyprus prior to 1974, would not be

Table 11.8 New Turkish-Cypriot cancer patients' registrations at the BOCOC

Year	First semester	Second semester	Year total
2004	66	49	115
2005	36	26	62
2006	32	29	61
2007	42	43	85
2008	59	49	108
2009	76	60	136
2010	56	39	95
2011	27	26	53
2012	40	44	84
2013	25	14	39
2014	11	4	15

Source: BOCOC Patients' Registration Office

able to meet this condition for access to the HCS in Cyprus. This is evident from a large decrease in registration of new cancer Turkish Cypriot patients at the BOCOC in Nicosia (Table 11.8) dating back to the second semester of 2013 (legislation was enacted in August 2013).

The austerity measures, resulting in very significant salary cuts for all public workers, staff in all hospitals and BOCOC (close to 20 % of their salary) alongside the introduction of other taxes/contributions, may have also impacted negatively on retention of oncologists in Cyprus, especially in the Public Hospitals Oncology Units. Three (3) Greek Oncologists in 2013–2014 resigned from their posts in Nicosia General Hospital (NGH) Oncology units, with two of them moving back to work in Greece and one going to the UK. In their place it was made possible to employ two oncologists, one who completed training in Germany and another one from Greece. Equally another oncologist resigned in 2014 from the BOCOC to work in the UK, with his replacement being an oncologist from the private sector in Cyprus.

Impact of the New GHCS on Cancer Services

The setting up of the new national GHCS is also a source of concern, as it is currently unclear how this is going to affect funding of cancer services, whilst its long term financial viability is uncertain. At the same time, this is going to bring with it, the setting up of primary care, which is going to be especially helpful for both patients and also for oncologists/cancer services, given that in the absence of an organized primary care sector, often oncologists ended up fulfilling the role of the general practitioner/family doctor, with cancer patients making use of cancer services for problems unrelated to their disease. Equally the GHCS, with centralized funding, has the potential to enforce standards, e.g. by selecting high quality/high volume centres-services that are going to be funded, whilst not funding service providers with low quality standards. Finally the new GHCS is going to fund Palliative Care (PC) services; therefore, the PC NGOs are no longer going to be dependent on charity contributions for running their services. This direct funding of PC services has the potential to allow expansion of PC services by all PC providers.

Critical Clinical Issues: Organization of Cancer Services in Cyprus

Currently Cancer Care in Cyprus suffers from a fragmentation of services in terms of both surgical and nonsurgical oncology, lack of collaboration between the three main Oncology providers (BOCOC, NGH Oncology Clinic, and LGH Oncology Clinic) and lack of agreed treatment pathways for cancer patients in Cyprus. An important issue that needs to be taken into consideration in planning Cancer Services in Cyprus is the combination of a small population (under one million) associated with a low cancer incidence compared to the EU average (as analysed in the Cancer Epidemiology section), that give rise to only a small number of patients treated per year by each of the three Oncology Providers when looking at individual cancer types. To illustrate the low number of cancer patients in Cyprus, in Table 11.9 there is a list of the top 20 cancers in Cyprus, including both men and women, with the exclusion of Hematological cancers.

By excluding the top six cancers in Cyprus, i.e., Breast, Prostate, Colorectal, Lung, Thyroid, and Bladder; each of them accounting for at least 4–5 % of all cancer patients in Cyprus, it can be seen that from the 7th to the 20th commonest cancer in Cyprus there are from 15 to 94 cancer patients per cancer type diagnosed per year in Cyprus. Taking into account, that in these numbers diagnosed per year, include patients who are not fit to receive treatment, and patients who have early disease,

Table 11.9 Crude cancer incidence in Cyprus (2010): cumulative for both gender (excluding hematological cancers)

Rank	Cancer type	Crude incidence/% of total cases	Rank	Cancer type	Crude incidence/% of total cases
1st	Breast	501/16.5	11th	Melanoma	56/1.9
2nd	Prostate	418/13.8	12th	Brain	50/1.6
3rd	Colorectal	367/12.1	13th	Ovary	46/1.5
4th	Lung	261/8.6	14th	Liver	34/1.1
5th	Thyroid	197/6.5	15th	Cervix	34/1.1
6th	Bladder	133/4.4	16th	Larynx	29/1.0
7th	Uterus	94/3.1	17th	Sarcoma	24/0.8
8th	Stomach	79/2.6	18th	Testis	21/0.7
9th	Pancreas	66/2.2	19th	Gallbladder	20/0.7
10th	Kidney	58/1.9	20th	Bone	15/0.5

Adapted from the Cyprus Cancer Registry Report covering 1999–2010 [8]

where surgery is curative and no additional chemotherapy or radiotherapy treatment is required, it can be concluded that there are small number of patients being treated with chemotherapy/radiotherapy per individual cancer type per year in Cyprus. Furthermore, for chemotherapy services, this small number of patients, e.g., patients with testicular cancer, ovarian cancer, sarcoma, hepatocellular cancer, and renal cancer, are further divided into having treatment in three different Oncology centres/units, hence restricting the number of patients treated per year per oncology provider even further.

Similar issues apply to surgical oncology. For instance data from the BOCOC show that 72 individual surgeons operated on 381 women with breast cancer in 2013. Among those 72 surgeons, 5 surgeons operated on 170 patients (i.e., 45 % of total), whilst the other 67 surgeons operated on the other 211 women, with 45 surgeons operating on only one or two patients in 2013! Equally in thyroid cancer, 43 different surgeons performed thyroid surgery on the 198 patients seen at the BOCOC in 2013, and only five surgeons operated on ≥5 % of patients each. Similar data exist for Colo-Rectal Cancer. More concerning is that even for more complex surgery, e.g., for pancreatic cancer, there may be a number of different surgeons/teams operating on these patients per year. Of course the current mixed private–public HCS does not help in setting up treatment pathways, i.e. providing guidance or putting rules in place regarding where complex oncological surgery should be taking place; however, this is an important issue that needs to be resolved hopefully with the set up of the new national GHCS and the reorganization of cancer services.

The relatively small number of patients treated per year per cancer type in Cyprus as illustrated above, in combination with a significant fragmentation of cancer services, hence resulting in even smaller number of patients treated per Oncology Centre/Unit in Cyprus, can potentially have a detrimental effect on quality of care, as a result of a lack of a critical mass of patients to maintain expertise in treatment of rarer cancers and difficulty to maintain Multi-Disciplinary Teams (MDTs) for each of the three centres [31]. Furthermore it can result in an increase in the cost of care, as a result of lower activity levels and decreased cost-effectiveness for each one of the Oncology providers, with a resulting low value for money in unit cost terms [31, 32]. Worldwide there is remarkably consistent evidence, on the impact of centralization on oncological outcomes, showing that the more experience doctors/hospitals or HCSs have with a procedure, the better the results are [32–35]. In fact it was calculated that out of 128 published studies, 123 showed some evidence of a "volume-quality" relationship [32, 33].

Finally in the last few years there has been an ongoing debate in Cyprus about commissioning new radiotherapy facilities. In fact the current National Cancer Control Plan for Cyprus [36] specified the setting up of two new Radiotherapy centres in both Nicosia and Limassol General Hospitals. It has however been argued that the commissioning of two new radiotherapy centres, by further fragmentation of services may have adverse impact on quality of care, as well as an increase in the cost of Radiotherapy services, as a result of the relatively small population in Cyprus and the low cancer incidence compared to the European average. In this debate, attention was given to guidelines from the UK about "Commissioning Arrangements for Radiotherapy" suggesting that centralization of Radiotherapy Services is in fact needed to maintain quality of care and optimal outcomes in view of Radiotherapy being the most complex treatment modality provided in any hospital and that this is especially relevant for less common cancers, as well as for more highly specialist Radiotherapy modalities such as stereotactic Radiotherapy, paediatric Radiotherapy, and brachytherapy, where there is even a higher need for centralization of services due to the critical mass of patients required to maintain clinical expertise and the highly specialized multidisciplinary teams to undertake all the above [31]. The same guidelines suggest that given "the high-cost of buildings and capital equipment, Radiotherapy service can only become affordable for a high volume service, hence centres with a large catchment population, with high activity levels and clinical effectiveness would deliver remarkably high value for money in unit cost terms" [31]. For these reasons, the Calman Hine Report [37] set as the minimum population to be served by a radiotherapy centre in the UK to be one million (catchment population), whilst this model of centralization has also been followed in the Netherlands [38] and other European countries especially in Northern Europe. A significant consideration however for commissioning of Radiotherapy facilities is patients' access (distance/travel time) to Radiotherapy centres. Taking into account distance for patients to travel from the periphery (see map in Fig. 11.1), and specifically in view of the travelling distance from the Paphos district, exceeding 1½ hour, it has been proposed to commission a second Radiotherapy centre/or a Satellite Radiotherapy unit in Limassol to improve access to patients from Paphos and Limassol districts by decreasing travel time to less than 1 hour.

Following the financial crisis in 2013, and at a time of limited resources, this has served as an opportunity to rethink the strategy set in the current Cancer Control Plan of commissioning two new Radiotherapy centres in Nicosia and Limassol, and question whether this indeed is going to improve services or by further fragmentation of service, the quality of care is going to suffer. Hence a decision has been made to commission a study to be undertaken by a team of Australian specialists headed by Dr. Liz Keany, to make recommendations as to commissioning and citing of new Radiotherapy Centres/Satellite Units in Cyprus.

In conclusion the low cancer incidence and small population in Cyprus resulting in a small number of cancer patients per cancer type (for most cancer types) needs to be taken into consideration, when planning the reorganization of cancer services in Cyprus. Key principles of centralization of services for both surgical and nonsurgical oncology would need to apply especially for less common cancers and treatment pathways would need to be determined for all different cancer types. The Cancer centre / unit approach adopted in the UK in 1995 by Calman Hine (37), with a clear distinction between services offered at the centre and units should also be considered. For instance it can be proposed that patients with common cancers, e.g., breast, lung, colon, and prostate cancer, can be treated with chemotherapy/hormonal treatment/targeted therapy in all three Oncology centres/units or even in peripheral clinics in all districts, whilst patients with rare cancers, e.g., patients with melanoma, sarcoma, kidney cancer, and germ cell tumours, are treated in one centre to allow the development of expertise and the setting up of specialized Multi-

Disciplinary Teams. Greater degree of centralization is likely to be needed for Radiotherapy services.

Finally such a reorganization of services is going to address the deficiencies in the existing set up/organization of Cancer services that does not allow for cooperation between the BOCOC and the oncology clinics in the NGH and LGH, apart from referrals for radiotherapy to the BOCOC, and result in more efficient use of manpower resources. Furthermore it would deal with the difficulty in site specialization of the oncologists working in the two oncology units in the NGH and LGH, due to the small number of oncologists (3–4 in each one), who have to treat many different cancer types, compared to site specialization of oncologists at the BOCOC, where each oncologist treats only 2–3 cancer types (sometimes even one, e.g., only Breast Cancer).

Interrelationship Between Cancer Care and Local Culture

As in other countries in Southern Europe and the Middle East, within the local culture in Cyprus is embedded a tradition of having very strong family ties and close relationships between family members. This can be a very valuable asset in the care of cancer patients, as invariably families see it as their obligation to look after their sick relatives at home, quite often well into the end of life [19].

The close family members feel it as their duty beyond the caring role, also to assume a protective role towards the patient, especially regarding disclosure of information by health care professionals. Truthful disclosure of information about the diagnosis of cancer can sometimes be considered a threat by families in Cyprus. As a result, not uncommonly there is a request of collusion by family members towards oncologists in Cyprus; i.e., a request by close family members to withhold either information about the cancer diagnosis or potential treatment options to the patient [39]. Often relatives request, prior to the oncologist seeing the patient, that the patient is not told the diagnosis, or that they should control the information or treatment options given to the patient. Normally families or relatives mention psychological reasons or the patient's inability to cope with the truth or the proposed treatment, or that the patient is going to become depressed and distressed if he/she ever found out, as the main reasons for asking for collusion. Collusion occurs when the medical professional agrees to the requests of third parties to give either false or misleading information/different treatment to the patient.

In a European survey of Oncologists regarding information disclosure to cancer patients there was a North versus South and a West versus East divide, with more oncologist agreeing to collusion and withholding information from patients in South and East Europe compared to North and West Europe [40]. It is the author's understanding that collusion was also commonly practiced in the past in Cyprus in the field of Cancer care. Two studies were enacted in 2011 to look into this issue in more detail and to elicit Cypriot patients' preferences for disclosure of information, information needs as well as families' preferences for disclosure of information to the patient and the practice of collusion. The Cassileth questionnaire, enriched with questions relating to the control of information and collusion, was given to 100 consecutive *new patients* attending the BOCOC. Of interest that prior to seeing an oncologist, 75 % said that they knew their diagnosis, 17 % did not, whilst 8 % did not complete the questionnaire. In terms of their general preference for information, 79 % said that they want as much information as possible, with 7 % wanting additional information only if it is good news, and 6 % did not want to know any details. In Table 11.10 are the answers to six additional questions asking about information needs relating to their illness.

Regarding control of information and the practice of collusion, 62 % of patients wanted to know everything and for them to decide how much their family would know, whilst 19 % wanted their family to know everything and the family to decide how much the patient would know; of note that 16 % did not complete this question [39].

In the second study, the views of the relative(s) accompanying the same 100 consecutive new patients attending the BOCOC, enrolled in the first study, were sought. The results showed that 68 % of relatives agreed that the patients should have all the information regarding their disease whilst 14 % disagreed, with 14 % of patients attending alone, hence the questionnaire could not be filled out and 4 % of relatives refusing to fill in. Only 6 % thought that the true diagnosis should be kept from the patient, whilst 76 % did not agree that it was right to withhold the diagnosis. Regarding collusion, 36 % of relatives felt that the family should decide on what the patient should know, whilst 46 % did not think that this was appropriate [41].

Table 11.10 New cancer patients' preferences for information in Cyprus

	Absolutely need this (%)	Would like this info (%)	No views (%)	Would not like this info (%)	Do not want this info (%)	Not completed (%)
Exact name of disease	76	13	1	1	1	8
Whether it is cancer?	75	10	1	2	4	8
Weekly progress	71	15	2	2	2	8
Cure possibilities	78	13	1	0	0	8
Prognosis	72	12	2	2	4	8
Possible treatments	77	13	1	0	1	8
Side effects of treatment	78	10	2	1	1	8

From Charalambous H, Koukides A., Avgousti V, Gavrielidou D. Cancer patients preferences for information in Cyprus. Support Care Cancer (2012) 20 (Suppl 1): abstract 1008. S 241

Hence these two studies show that the majority of cancer patients in Cyprus would like to have information about their illness, treatment, and prognosis, whilst a little over a third of relatives still feel that the family should filter what information the patient is going to receive (with the rest believing that the cancer patients should be informed about their disease). Health professionals in Cyprus need to take these findings into consideration in their consultations with cancer patients and relatives.

The local culture has also been in the not too recent past associated with an element of mistrust for Oncologists in Cyprus, with patients and families seeking often second opinions, especially from oncologists in Israel, Greece, Germany, and the UK (although seeking multiple opinions is commonly seen in all aspects of Health Care in Cyprus, stemming from prejudices that treatments abroad are better than in Cyprus). This has however improved considerably over the last few years, and is now the exception as opposed to being the rule, possibly as a result of better information provided to patients, the presence of a Specialized Oncology Centre in Cyprus at the BOCOC, as well as the return to Cyprus of a number of Cypriot oncologists, who had previously trained and worked for many years in the UK, Germany, the USA, and Greece.

Another aspect of the local culture, which is very relevant to cancer treatment, is the lack of acceptance of death, similar to other Western societies. This can often complicate end of life care, and usually results in overtly aggressive care towards the end of life [19]. With increased PC input, and earlier discussions by oncologists, it is the author's understanding that this is being reversed. No studies have been however conducted about patients' preferences for information or treatment (e.g., aggressive anticancer treatment versus PC) for patients entering the end of life, or studies looking at symptom control/quality of life near the end of life for patients in Cyprus.

Society Reaction Towards Cancer Patients

Until the last 10–15 years there was a fear and a stigma associated with cancer, and people were frightened and embarrassed to talk openly about it. People in Cyprus would often try to avoid using the word Cancer, instead they would refer to cancer as "that disease" or they would use the phrase "η επάρατη νόσος"(Gk), which means the disease which is cursed or incurable (είναι καταραμένη και/ή ανίατη: Gk). Essentially cancer was a taboo subject, especially for the older generations and for the less well educated. More recently however, and as a result of the work that all cancer patients advocacy groups do, especially Europadonna Cyprus (the Breast Cancer Advocacy Group), and the PC NGOs PASYKAF and CACS, there is less fear about cancer, there is more understanding about the disease and an openness to discuss issues relating to cancer diagnosis and treatment. This has been achieved through tv and radio programs, discussing cancer issues, education and charity events as well as promotion and advertising in the media, carried out regularly by the advocacy groups (with their proceeds being used to fund services for cancer patients), highlighting the fact that cancer can be a curable and treatable disease. Furthermore, these events are often attended by both local celebrities and politicians, helping further to get rid of the stigma of having a cancer diagnosis. Furthermore a number of politicians have come forward publicly making it known that they suffer from Breast Cancer, also again raising awareness, and helping to make cancer now less of a taboo topic in Cyprus, as compared to the past. Finally there was a recent event, where in public Cypriot women have shared their experience about living with advanced Breast Cancer [42].

Individualized (Personalized) Oncology in Focus

Individualized oncology treatment/personalized medicine, especially in relation to targeted therapy, is a very important goal of cancer care today. However individualized treatment should not be restricted just to the search for a druggable genetic abnormality in the patient's tumour biopsy, that can be targeted with a new tyrosine kinase inhibitor or a new monoclonal antibody, but instead should cover all aspects of a cancer patient's care. For instance, in terms of disease directed therapy, treatment should be provided by "experienced specialist multidisciplinary teams" to ensure that "all patients have the benefit of the range of expert advice needed for high quality care" [37, 43]. Multi-Disciplinary Team (MDT) Meetings were set up at the BOCOC in 2006 for the first time in Lung Cancer, and subsequently MDT meetings were set up for Breast, Gastro-intestinal, Head and Neck, CNS, and Gynaecological Cancers, to allow discussion of patients' proposed treatment, and ensure that the more appropriate decisions are made [2], whilst such meetings are also now taking place at the NGH.

The American Society of Clinical Oncology (ASCO) in a statement with the title "Individualized Care for Patients With Advanced Cancer" gives guidance and recognizes deficiencies in the standard oncology care today in terms of providing true individualized care. The ASCO statement recommends that beyond disease-directed therapy, there should be "attention to symptom management and attention to quality of life" [44]. This raises a very important issue of personalized cancer care: to provide each cancer patient with good symptom control, addressing not only physical, but also psychological, social, and spiritual consequences of disease and its treatment. Unfortunately a number of studies show that oncologists often fail to manage adequately even the simplest of the physical symptoms, that of pain [45, 46], never mind to address psychological, social and spiritual consequences of cancer and also toxicity of cancer treatment. Studies of pain management in Cyprus corroborate this finding [22]. It is vital therefore that oncologists receive more palliative care training to improve their symptom control skills and be able to provide basic PC [47], and that care for patients especially with advanced cancer includes input from multidisciplinary teams including PC physicians and nurses, psychologists, social workers, etc. that can help to address these problems, as is also recommended by ASCO in another provisional clinical opinion [48]. This in a way is the message from studies of early PC, that early introduction of PC can improve patients symptoms, quality of life, and possibly even improve survival [48, 49].

In Cyprus there have been a number of initiatives to provide personalized cancer care according to this definition, including high quality supportive and palliative care. An Advanced Palliative Care Course was organized in Cyprus between the 5th and 9th of December 2011 with Dr. Frank Ferris, Director of the Institute of Palliative Medicine from the USA, providing training to fifty (50) health care professionals working in cancer care in the General Hospitals, the BOCOC, CACS, and PASYKAF. Also joint training through lectures for both oncology and palliative care staff has been organized at the BOCOC helping to foster collaboration between the two specialties. Other initiatives within the BOCOC to facilitate referral of patients to specialized PC services include the weekly PC clinic set up at the BOCOC and being run by the PC physicians from CACS, and a weekly PC MDT meeting, where patients with PC needs are discussed, and appropriate referrals are being made to the different members of the Multidisciplinary team and to staff from PASYKAF and CACS [2].

Furthermore the ASCO statement on Individualized Cancer Care recommends that "care for patients with advanced disease, should include an individualized assessment of the patient's needs, goals, and preferences throughout their illness," and they further highlight that "realistic conversations about prognosis, the potential benefits and limitations of disease-directed therapy, and the potential role of palliative care, occur late in the course of illness or not at all" [44]. This highlights another important aspect of personalized cancer care relating to patient communication and involvement in decision-making. Important ground work has been done with the information disclosure studies in Cyprus, which show that the majority of new patients would like to be informed about their disease, and would also like to be involved in the decision-making. It is therefore important that Cypriot oncologists do not assume what patients would or would not like to know about their disease or prognosis, as in a significant proportion of cases, the assumption is going to be wrong, and patients are either going to be denied information they wished to know, or they are going to be given information they did not wish to have [50]. The challenge therefore for oncologists in Cyprus is to be able to deal with collusion and to be able to discuss these issues ensuring that not only patients but also caregivers and family are happy with the disclosure of information. Training in communication skills is particularly useful to tactfully elicit preferences regarding the disclosure of information from each patient and often from a number of different family members and to negotiate solutions to the various dilemmas and conflicts that may arise in relation to the patient and his/her family [50]. In Cyprus steps in the right direction have been made with an Advanced Communication Skills training course taking place in March 2011 in Cyprus for Oncologists, Nurses, and Psychologists, from both the BOCOC, NGH, and LGH Oncology units and the NGOs: CACS and PASYKAF provided by Professor Fallowfield's team from the UK [51].

It is unknown however whether patients with more advanced disease in Cyprus, who have had already treatment, and are now less likely to respond to further anti-cancer treatment, have the same preferences for information disclosure, as compared to their initial appointment to the oncology centre. It is also unknown to what degree truthful End of Life discussions take place in Cyprus, and to what extent the alternative option of no further anticancer treatment but instead PC treatment, is offered to patients, and this should be an area for further research.

Local Achievements and Innovations for the Future

A major achievement for Cancer care in Cyprus has been the set up of the BOCOC in 1999. The BOCOC has broadly fulfilled its main mission to provide high quality Cancer treatment in Cyprus and to collaborate with public hospitals, clinics, and patient organizations [14]. This has been achieved through hard work and dedication from the staff, the generous contribution from the BOC to allow the centre to expand and upgrade its diagnostic and therapeutic facilities, and of course through the major contribution from the MoH covering the running expenses of the centre for the last 15 years. Testament to this achievement is the number of patients treated over the last 15 years at the BOCOC (over 28,000 new patients) and its broad recognition within both the medical community and the public in Cyprus. Further evidence of its accomplishments come from its quality accreditation from the largest accreditation organisation for hospitals in Europe in 2007, whilst in 2010 the Centre was reevaluated by the accreditation body and the results were excellent [15]. It is also important to reflect on the other areas in its mission statement, whereby the BOCOC failed to perform so well [14]. There are many reasons for those, including difficulty to work closely with the MoH, and as a result failure to influence government policy in terms of prevention/screening and organization of Cancer services in Cyprus. In terms of research, there has been significant progress in relation to entry of patients to clinical trials, but the lack of resources including clinicians time/and support with more staff, did not facilitate more original research to be carried out, and hence failed to gain more of a regional/international reputation. These areas remain challenges that would need to be addressed in the very near future.

Initiatives bringing closer the BOCOC as an Oncology provider and the two main PC organizations, PASYKAF and CACS, have been particularly successful, with joint training courses/lectures, the set up of PC clinics and joint PC MDT meetings within the BOCOC, and have resulted in overall better quality of care for patients with difficult symptom control problems as well as facilitating respite and end of life care. In the future there should be consideration in applying in conjunction with the PC providers for recognition as an ESMO (European Society of Medical Oncology) Designated Centre of Integrated Oncology and Palliative Care [52].

Special recognition is also due to the hard work by both CACS and PASYKAF over the years to provide PC services for cancer patients in Cyprus and to have developed PC services so that it is currently accepted that Cyprus has now reached the top level of PC development, that of approaching integration [2, 26]. Furthermore praise should be given to PASYKAF for securing European funding to start a pilot project to provide true 24 h—Home PC service. The project benefits from a grant from Iceland, Liechtenstein, and Norway through the EEA Grants. The aim is that by offering a continuous 24 h service there is going to be better symptom control for patients at home, and that this is going to facilitate the ability of patients to stay at home towards the end of life. Beyond helping to fulfill patients'/families' preferences, this is also likely to have a positive impact by releasing beds at the BOCOC, the NGH, and LGH Oncology Units. As a result this is likely to have a positive financial impact, as care in the community is considerably cheaper than within hospitals or the hospice. The project started in the district of Limassol in October 2014, and will extend to the district of Nicosia in February 2015. At the completion of the project, the plan would be to set up this 24-h home care service across the whole of Cyprus [27].

Summary and Recommendations/Challenges for the Future

Major progress has been made in the last 15 years in the provision of Cancer Services in Cyprus, especially following the set up of the purpose built BOCOC, whilst steady progress has also been made by the NGH and LGH Oncology Units. The financial crisis in 2013, with a significant decrease in the GDP, increase of unemployment close to 20 % and the bail in and austerity program, has resulted in a significant reduction of the Health Care Budget necessitating the introduction of fees for cancer patients as well as the reduction in funds allocated to Cancer Services. Reduction in the Cancer Drugs budget has resulted in a significant limitation in the use of new targeted therapies in Cyprus, with no new targeted agents approved in 2013 and 2014. The financial crisis however presents a major challenge to achieve more at a time of limited resources, to consider carefully and strategically the direction of Cancer Services and to allocate resources using cost-effectiveness criteria. As a result a plan to build two new radiotherapy centres in Nicosia and Limassol is under review, as more careful considerations in terms of the impact of the fragmentation of the service are being made, whilst an external review of Radiotherapy Services and the needs for Radiotherapy for the future is currently being undertaken by Australian Oncologists. Similarly progress with the implementation of Comparative Effectiveness Research (CER) at the level of the MoH and the new national GHCS with the setting up for the first time of a body to undertake regularly Health Technology Assessments in Cyprus represents an opportunity to consider what are the most cost-effective and beneficial interventions for Cancer Care in Cyprus and to allocate resources accordingly. Equally the crisis has drawn attention to the fact that investing in PC services can provide gains for patients' quality of life and symptom control, whilst being very cost effective, as a result of decreased expenditure of looking after patients with advanced disease in the community instead of admitting patients for end of life care in hospitals.

The financial crisis as well as the setting up of the New National HCS is also an opportunity to improve on organization of cancer care in Cyprus. Reorganization of

Cancer Services with better collaboration between all three oncology providers, centralization of services for rare cancers, with clear treatment pathways, i.e., where patients get treated, with compulsory discussion of all patients in Multi-Disciplinary Team meetings and treatment offered by experienced MDT as evidenced by workload and regular monitoring of outcomes is urgently needed. The centralization of services beyond the improvement in quality of care is likely to result also in more cost-effective care.

Finally areas that need to be addressed in more depth, as part of a comprehensive Cancer Control Plan for Cyprus, include initiatives for Cancer Prevention (with the need to invest more in public campaigns for smoking cessation and to tackle alcohol abuse and obesity), Screening (with the need to fund fully cervical and colorectal screening), and Survivor care (with the need to establish follow up guidelines to be endorsed by all oncology providers in Cyprus).

Acknowledgments For valuable comments to the manuscript I would like to acknowledge the input of Mr. Alecos Stamatis, CEO of the BOCOC, and Dr. Chrystala Charalambous, Ph.D. Candidate, Open University and Ministry of Health, Cyprus.

References

1. http://www.lancaster.ac.uk/shm/research/ioelc/international/pdf/cyprus_country_report.pdf.
2. Charalambous H, Pitsillide B, Nestoros S. Palliative care in Cyprus: current status. In: Silbermann M, editor. Palliative care to the cancer patient. The Middle East as a model for emerging countries. 1st ed. New York: Nova; 2014. p. 1–21. (Chapter 1) ISBN: 978-1-63117-709-5.
3. http://hdr.undp.org/en/content/table-2-human-development-index-trends-1980-2013. Accessed 12 Dec 2014.
4. http://www.gfmag.com/global-data/country-data/cyprus-gdp-country-report#axzz1sYmGJiRR. Accessed 13 Dec 2014.
5. Theodorou M, Charalambous C, Petrou C, Cylus J. Cyprus: health system review. Health Syst Transit. 2012;14(6):1–128.
6. Report for deaths and causes of death for 2004–2011. Available December 2012. Health Monitoring Unit, Ministry of Health, Republic of Cyprus.
7. Farazi PA. Cancer trends and risk factors in Cyprus. Ecancermedicalscience. 2014;8:389. doi:10.3332/ecancer.2014.389. eCollection 2014.
8. Cyprus Cancer Registry Report: Covering 1998–2010: http://www.moh.gov.cy/MOH/MOH.nsf/All/9245B3902339397CC22579C60026560F/$file/Cyprus%20Cancer%20Registry%20-%20Summary%20Results%201998-2010.pdf. Accessed 29 Dec 2014.
9. Cyprus Cancer Registry 2011 Progress report (covering data 2006–2008). http://www.moh.gov.cy/MOH/MOH.nsf/0/A0B4FEC0AC7BB073C22579C7002A9683/$file/%CE%88%CE%BA%CE%B8%CE%B5%CF%83%CE%B7%20%CE%A0%CF%81%CE%BF%CF%8C%CE%B4%CE%BF%CF%85%20%CE%B3%CE%B9%CE%B1%20%CF%84%CE%BF%20%CE%AD%CF%84%CE%BF%CF%82%202011%20(%CE%A3%CF%84%CE%BF%CE%B9%CF%87%CE%B5%CE%AF%CE%B1%202006-2008).pdf. Accessed 13 Dec 2014.
10. http://eu-cancer.iarc.fr/EUCAN/Cancer.aspx?Cancer=0. Accessed 13 Dec 2014.
11. Republic of Cyprus Statistical Service. Health survey 2003. Nicosia: Printing Office of the Republic of Cyprus; 2005.
12. Republic of Cyprus Statistical Service. European health survey 2008. Nicosia: Printing Office of the Republic of Cyprus; 2010.

13. Cyprus Institute of Neurology and Genetics (CING): genetic counseling service. http://www.cing.ac.cy/easyconsole.cfm/id/313. Accessed 14 Dec 2014.
14. Bank of Cyprus Oncology Centre website. http://www.bococ.org.cy. Accessed 13 Dec 2014.
15. Bank of Cyprus Oncology Centre Annual report 2013. http://www.bococ.org.cy/cache/1145a30ff80745b56fb0cecf65305017.pdf. Accessed 13 Dec 2014.
16. Nicosia General Hospital Oncology Unit 2013 Report. http://www.moh.gov.cy/MOH/ngh/ngh.nsf/All/850670F92D9777F2C2257DB3002CD467/$file/Ετήσια%20Έκθεση%202013.pdf. Accessed 13 Dec 2014.
17. Limassol General Hospital Oncology Unit. Workload data: Personal communication Dr Simon Malas, Head of Limassol Oncology Unit; 2013.
18. Radiotherapy: developing a world class service for England. Report to the Ministers from the National Radiotherapy Advisory Group; 2007.
19. Silbermann M, Arnaout M, Daher M, et al. Palliative cancer care in Middle Eastern countries: accomplishments and challenges. Ann Oncol. 2012;23 Suppl 3:15–28.
20. Cyprus Anticancer Society website. http://www.anticancersociety.org.cy/anticancer1/page.php?pageID=1&langID=0. Accessed 19 Dec 2014.
21. Cyprus Association of Cancer Patients and Friends (PASYKAF) website. http://www.pasykaf.org/en. Accessed 19 Dec 2014.
22. Charalambous H, Protopapa E, Gavrielidou D, Avgousti V. Physicians' prescribing habits for cancer pain in Cyprus. Ann Oncol. 2012;23 Suppl 3:79–83.
23. World Health Organization. Achieving balance in national opioids control policy: guidelines for assessment. Geneva: World Health Organization; 2000.
24. Annual opioid consumption in Cyprus in morphine equivalence. http://www.painpolicy.wisc.edu/sites/www.painpolicy.wisc.edu/files/country_files/morphine_equivalence/cyprus_me.pdf. Accessed 29 Dec 2014.
25. The Middle East Cancer Consortium (MECC). http://www.cancer.gov/aboutnci/organization/global-health/research-programs-initiatives/mecc. Accessed 29 Dec 2014.
26. Bingley A, Clark D. A comparative review of palliative care development in six countries represented by the Middle East Cancer Consortium (MECC). J Pain Symptom Manage. 2009;37(3):287–96.
27. Personal communication Mr Nicolas Philippou, General Director/Chief Executive Officer PASYKAF.
28. Archangel Michael Hospice website. http://archangel-michael-hospice.com/. Accessed 29 Dec 2014.
29. Standards and norms for hospice and palliative care in Europe—The EAPC White Paper. Lukas Radbruch, Sheila Payne and the Board of Directors of the European Association for Palliative Care (EAPC). http://ukz.katolik.cz/texty%20sokrates/eapc.pdf. Accessed 29 Dec 2014.
30. The MERCER report: actuarial study of the Cyprus National Health Expenditure and National Health System. http://www.hio.org.cy/docs/mercer_report_october2013.pdf. Accessed 29 Dec 2014.
31. Commissioning arrangements for radiotherapy a response from the Royal College of Radiologists (RCR) the Society and College of Radiographers (SCOR) and the Institute of Physics and Engineering in Medicine (IPEEM).
32. Charalambous H, Marcou Y, Katodritis N, Kountourakis P, Andreopoulos D. Radiotherapy capacity in Europe. Lancet Oncol. 2013;14(6):e196.
33. Smith TJ, Hillner BE, Bear HD. Taking action on the volume-quality relationship: how long can we hide our heads in the colostomy bag? J Nat Cancer Inst. 2003;95:695–7.
34. Birkmeyer JD, Siewers AE, Finlayson EV, et al. Hospital volume and surgical mortality in the United States. N Engl J Med. 2002;346(15):1128–37.
35. Wuthrick EJ, Zhang Q, Machtay M, et al. Institutional clinical trial accrual volume and survival of patients with head and neck cancer. J Clin Oncol. 2015;33:156–64. pii: JCO.2014.56.5218.
36. Cyprus National Cancer Plan—in Greek Εθνική Επιτροπή για τον Καρκίνο; 2012.
37. Calman K, Hine D. A policy frame world for commissioning cancer services a report by the expert advisory group on cancer to the chief medical offices of England and Wales quittance from purchasers and providers of care. London: Department of Health; 1995.

38. Slotman B, Vos PH. Planning of radiotherapy capacity and productivity. Radiother Oncol. 2013;106:266–70. pii: S0167-8140(13)00058-3. doi:10.1016/j.radonc.2013.02.006.
39. Charalambous H, Koukides A, Avgousti V, Gavrielidou D. Cancer patients preferences for information in Cyprus. Support Care Cancer. 2012;20 Suppl 1:S241. abstract 1008.
40. Cherny NI, Catane R, Chasen MR, et al. Factors influencing the attitudes and behaviors of oncologists regarding the truthful disclosure of information to patients with advanced and incurable cancer. Psychooncology. 2011;20(12):1269–84.
41. Charalambous H, Avgousti V, Gavrielidou D, Koukides A. Relatives preferences for disclosure of information to cancer patients in Cyprus. Support Care Cancer. 2012;20 Suppl 1:S245. abstract 1025.
42. Talking about the experience of living with advanced Breast Cancer in Cyprus. http://cyprus-mail.com/2014/11/02/projecting-the-invisible-woman/. Accessed 13 Dec 2014.
43. The UK NHS Cancer Plan. http://www.thh.nhs.uk/documents/_Departments/Cancer/NHSCancerPlan.pdf.
44. Peppercorn JM, Smith TJ, Helft PR, et al. American society of clinical oncology statement: toward individualized care for patients with advanced cancer. J Clin Oncol. 2011;29(6):755–60.
45. Fisch MJ, Lee J-W, Weiss M, et al. Prospective, observational study of pain and analgesic prescribing in medical oncology outpatients with breast, colorectal, lung, or prostate cancer. J Clin Oncol. 2012;30:1980–8.
46. Breuer B, Fleishman SB, Cruciani RA, et al. Medical oncologists' attitudes and practice in cancer pain management: a national survey. J Clin Oncol. 2011;29:4769–75.
47. Charalambous H, Silbermann M. Clinically based palliative care training is needed urgently for all oncologists. J Clin Oncol. 2012;30(32):4042–3.
48. Smith TJ, Temin S, Alesi ER, et al. American Society of Clinical Oncology provisional clinical opinion: the integration of palliative care into standard oncology care. J Clin Oncol. 2012; 30(8):880–7.
49. Temel JS, Greer JA, Muzikansky A, et al. Early palliative care for patients with metastatic non-small-cell lung cancer. N Engl J Med. 2010;363:733–42.
50. Silbermann M, Epner DE, Charalambous H, et al. Promoting new approaches for cancer care in the Middle East. Ann Oncol. 2013;24 Suppl 7:vii5–10.
51. Training in Communication skills by professor Leslie Fallowfield in Cyprus. http://www.bococ.org.cy/index.php?s_id=38&a_id=1469. Accessed 13 Dec 2014.
52. ESMO designated centre for Oncology and Palliative Care. http://www.esmo.org/Patients/Designated-Centres-of-Integrated-Oncology-and-Palliative-Care. Accessed 13 Dec 2014.

Chapter 12
Cancer Care in a Country Undergoing Transition: Turkey, Current Challenges and Trends for the Future

Rejin Kebudi and Fatma Betul Cakir

Introduction

Cancer and cancer care are increasingly recognized as a major worldwide challenge given their global, financial, social, and health implications. The prevalence of cancer, primarily a disease of aging, is increasing with the increasing life-span and the adaptation of Western lifestyle in both high and low income countries. Of the 14 million people diagnosed with cancer worldwide in 2012, more than 60 % live in low and middle income countries (LIC/MIC). 70 % of the cancer deaths worldwide occur in LIC/MIC as well. Global cancer incidence is predicted to reach 25 million by 2030, 70 % of which is expected to be reported in developing countries [1]. Turkey, according to the World Bank's classification for income is considered as an upper middle income country. Turkey is located on two continents Europe and Asia, located at the crossroads of East and West; it also has parts in the Mediterranean and the Middle East. At the beginning of the millennium, the performance of Turkey's health system in terms of public health, insurance of the patients, and the patient satisfaction was at the bottom of the Organisation for Economic Co-operation and Development (OECD) countries and in the European Region of World Health Organization (WHO) [2]. Turkey has undertaken the Health Transformation Program (HTP) from 2002 on, including major reforms to transfer and improve the health system and its outcomes and the situation has improved in the following decade.

R. Kebudi (✉)
Istanbul University Cerrahpasa Medical Faculty, Istanbul, Turkey

Istanbul University Oncology Institute, Istanbul, Turkey
e-mail: rejinkebudi@yahoo.com

F.B. Cakir
Bezmialem Vakif University Medical Faculty, Istanbul, Turkey

M. Silbermann (ed.), *Cancer Care in Countries and Societies in Transition*,
DOI 10.1007/978-3-319-22912-6_12

Current Status of Cancer Care in Turkey

The population in Turkey is about 76 million. The population annual growth rate is 11.2‰ for 2013. The average life expectancy is 75 years (F 77, M 72). One fourth of the population is 14 years of age and younger [3–9]. The gross national income (GNI) was reported as 10,830 US dollars per capita in 2012. The incidence of cancer is 227 per 100,000 which means about 175,000 new patients each year [10]. Cancer is the second cause of death with a rate of 20 % after cardiovascular diseases (39.9 %) in adults in Turkey [3, 10–12]. The most frequent cancers in adult females are breast (28 %) and thyroid (10.3 %); and in adult males are lung (31.2 %) and prostate (13.7 %) [3, 10–12]. The most significant difference of Turkey from developed countries has been the higher number of cancers caused by tobacco. Turkey had one of the highest smoking rates in the OECD in 2007 [13]. It was reported that cancer incidence had increased annually by 6 % due to the tobacco problem. For men, the cancer incidence rate of 165.8/100,000 for years 1993–1998 had increased to 216.3/100,000 by year 2003. For women, the cancer incidence rate had increased from 97.3 to 152.2/100,000 in the same decade [11, 12]. In Turkey, the incidence of lung cancer is 63 %, and incidence of the cancer of the larynx is 10 %, whereas the same incidences in the European Union are 55 % and 8 %, respectively [11, 12]. Many patients have delays in diagnosis and are diagnosed at advanced stages [3, 4, 10–12].

Turkey became a smoke-free country on July 19, 2009—the use of tobacco in all areas except open air areas was banned by law. This has led to a significant decrease in the use of tobacco in Turkey. The success of the law is reflected in the most recent data which show that exposure to secondhand tobacco smoke has decreased substantially since 2008 [13]. In 2010, Turkey was awarded for this achievement by WHO Director General's Special Recognition Award [13]. It is expected that cancers induced by tobacco such as lung cancer will decrease in the future. For pediatric cancer, survival rates are around 80 % in the USA. Approximately 250,000 children worldwide develop cancer each year, of whom 200,000 live in MIC and LIC. Every year in Europe 15,000 children aged 0–14 years and 20,000 teenagers and young adults aged 15–24 years are diagnosed with cancer [14]. In Europe, overall survival at 5 years continuously improved from 76.1 % in 1999–2001 to 79.1 % in 2005–2007 [14]. However, 6000 young people in Europe still die of cancer each year despite best available treatments. Across Europe there are still major disparities in 5-year survival, for example, Eastern Europe reports 10–20 % lower survival rates [15]. Cancer remains the commonest disease causing death beyond the age of 1 year in Europe. The types of cancer occurring in this age group in Europe are similar to those observed in the rest of the world [16]. Middle East includes countries from North Africa to central Asia. This region includes a wide spectrum of economically diverse countries, from technically advanced countries with high level cancer care to countries with little or no cancer treatment capabilities. There are large discrepancies in population size, wealth and health expenditure, and availability of quality of treatment. The relative overall cancer survival rate can be around 60 % in some; however, it is only 30 % in most [17].

The International Union Against Cancer (UICC) initiated a world cancer campaign in 2005 to increase awareness, improve care, and coordinate the training professionals using the support offered by the NCI (USA), International Society of Pediatric Oncology (SIOP), and the International Confederation of Childhood Parent Organizations (ICCCPO) and Sanofi–Aventis [18, 19]. This project promotes twinning programs to transfer information, technology, and other supports required to improve cancer care for those children with inadequate access to curative and palliative care. The current president of UICC, T Kutluk, is a Turkish pediatric oncologist.

According to childhood mortality, cancer is the fourth cause of death (7.2 %) in Turkey, after infections, cardiac deaths, and accidents [3, 20]. Each year in Turkey, 2500–3000 new childhood cancer cases are expected [20–22]. According to the Turkish Pediatric Oncology Group (TPOG) and Turkish Pediatric Hematology Society (TPHD) Registry, that was initiated in 2002, about 2000 new pediatric cancer cases are reported each year [20]. The distribution of major cancers in children are leukemia (32 %), lymphoma (17 %), and central nervous system neoplasms (13 %). Five-year survival rate in children with cancer in Turkey is reported as 65 % [20–22]. Higher survival rates are reported in specific cancer centers. Among 2413 patients, mostly solid tumors, diagnosed and treated between 1990 and 2012 in the Istanbul University, Institute of Oncology, Division of Pediatric Hematology–Oncology, the 5-year survival rate is reported as 74 % [22].

Both adult and pediatric oncology national groups are established in Turkey. The Turkish Society of Medical Oncology (TSMO) was established in 1996. Palliative Care Society was established in 2006 and cooperates with European Society of Medical Oncology (ESMO) Palliative Group. The Turkish Radiation Oncology Group (TROG) was established in 1993. TPOG and TPHD were established in 1997 and 1999, respectively. The first group has the main role of management of children with cancer and improvement of pediatric oncology in Turkey via meetings and courses. The second group chiefly focuses on nonmalignant hematology, also leukemias and transplantation [3]. Aforementioned three oncology groups (TSMO, TROG, TPOG) together organize the national cancer meetings with parallel sessions for medical doctors and nurses. In cooperation with the Ministry of Health, TPOG has been organizing regional pediatric oncology postgraduate courses in different regions of Turkey for general practitioners, physicians, and nurses to increase awareness of pediatric cancer throughout the country. To date, education has been provided to 850 professionals in 12 different cities. European Society Medical Oncology (ESMO), European Society for Radiotherapy and Oncology (ESTRO), Middle East Cancer Consortium (MECC), Asian Pacific Organization for Cancer Prevention (APOCP), and SIOP congresses and postgraduate courses have been organized in Turkey. Furthermore, these societies and other non-governmental organizations (NGOs) come together at the National Cancer Week Symposium held by Ministry of Health, annually. Turkey is a member of the MECC that aims to promote cancer registry, epidemiology, and mortality and also supports palliative cancer care and encourages cancer education and research through meetings held in various Middle East countries, including Turkey [3].

The Ministry of Health cooperates with numerous national and international institutions and agencies in the fight against cancer. The Ministry has put the National Cancer Control Program in cooperation with the following international organizations: WHO, International Agency for Research on Cancer (IARC), International Association for Cancer Registry (IACR), UICC, National Cancer Institute (NCI), APOCP, MECC, National Health Service (NHS) [3–5, 20]. The program includes five main headings: Registry, Prevention, Screening and Early Diagnosis, Treatment and Palliative Care.

According to our regulations, after completing 6 years of education in the medical faculty, the title of "medical doctor" (MD) is obtained [3]. An MD has to complete a 4-year training resident program in internal medicine or pediatrics to be a "specialist in internal medicine or pediatrics." Afterwards, a further 3-year fellowship program in medical oncology/pediatric hematology–oncology has to be completed to become a specialist in medical oncology (medical oncologist) or pediatric hematology and oncology (pediatric hemato-oncologist) [3]. The specialty and subspecialty training is given in university hospitals or government tertiary training and research hospitals authorized to provide training by the High Education Council and the Ministry of Health. The specialty and subspecialty certificates are awarded by the Ministry of Health. The nurses in Turkey are either graduated from high school for nursing or from universities for nursing. Clinical nursing education is carried out by faculty members of nursing schools after completion of or in conjunction with theoretical courses. Since April 2007, men have been accepted into nursing programs in Turkey [23].

In general, there are no certified PC/hospice care specialist nurses. PC in general has not been incorporated yet into the curriculum of nursing at both undergraduate and postgraduate level. There are prominent psychologists and psychiatrists only in a few oncology centers, in most others a psychology/psychiatry consultation is requested from the related department as needed. There are scarce social workers and almost no art therapists employed in most oncology centers. There are no specifically trained spiritual counselors both for adults and children. The doctors and nurses try to cover the role of the psychologist, social care worker in many centers. Recently, Ministry and Ankara University collaborative training program has been started for spiritual counselors [3].

Interrelationship Between Cancer Care and Local Culture in a Transforming Society

Turkey is a country where the cultural aspects of the society are blended both by the Eastern and Western societies. A myth about cancer treatment is common among Turkish community. Patients having mass in their viscera are often reluctant to undergo surgery because they believe "if there is a cut through a cancerous mass, it will spread all over the body" [24]. This misbelief has changed in recent years with the success of advances in medicine and increased awareness of the society.

Screening for some types of cancer has led to early diagnosis, thus increased survival, although it yet needs much improvement. Gynecological or breast cancers may present with symptoms that women are reluctant or shy to visit a doctor, and they might be less willing to undergo necessary examinations to investigate the cause of such symptoms, and this may cause delay in diagnosis [25, 26].

In Turkey, most patients diagnosed with cancer receive the standard oncological treatment which is completely funded by the government. In addition, most use some herbal medicines as well. The study of traditional uses of plants in the world in general and in the Mediterranean region in particular has been progressively increasing during the past few decades [27, 28]. According to WHO, the international market of herbal products is estimated to be US$ 62 billion which is poised to grow to US$ 5 trillion by the year 2050 [29]. Turkey is one of the richest countries in terms of plant diversity. Approximately 10,500 plant species have been identified and 30 % of this is endemic [30]. There are around 347 medicinal plants used in Turkey, 139 of which are exported [31]. A study performed at a university hospital in the Mediterranean region of Turkey, established that 50 % of the patients used mainly medicinal herbs, and the most frequently used (87 %) plant was stinging nettle (*Urtica dioica*) [32]. However, the majority used more than one item. The study also showed that the other remedies were honey, pollens, "pekmez" (a traditional syrup obtained mainly from boiled grape juice or other fruits), garlic, olive oil, rosehips, parsley, spice mixtures, avocado, bango tea, chestnut honey, carrots, hemp, mushroom tea, oregano, turnip seed, black grape seed, red berries, extracts of *Salvia officinalis*, *Semen nigellae*, and oleander [32]. Interestingly, the most popular complementary methods, such as prayer, meditation, massage, relaxation, and special diets reported from western countries, were not the remedies of Turkish people. Other plants used frequently in various parts of Turkey may be listed as:

Sonchus asper, *Urtica dioica*, *Viscum album*, *Asphodelus aestivus*, *Cynarascolymus*, *Ficus carica*r, *Hypericum perforatum*, *Lagenaria siceraria*, *Matricaria chamomilla*, *Neriumoleander*, *Picnomon acarna*, *Pinus brutia*, *Plantago major*, *Portulacaoleracea*, *Rosa canina*, *Urtica pilulifera*, *Calendula arvensis*, *Cichoriumintybus*, *Dracunculus vulgaris*, *Pistacia terebinthus*, *Anthemis tinctoria*, *Zea mays*, *Anthemis tinctoria*, *Heracleumtrachyloma*, *Astragalus brachycalyx*, *Thymus kotschyanus* [33–37].

In many Middle East countries, many individuals believe in their own spirituality and faith when coping with illness. In addition to standard cancer treatment, this might contribute positively to the outcome of the cancer. Positive way of thinking might influence serotonin pathways in the brain that regulate mood and possibly pain [24, 38]. In a survey, it was stated that many patients believed that "everything comes from God and one should never give up hope of God's mercy." This belief could be a reason for high levels of hope [39, 40]. Advances in technology, cancer treatment and supportive care, adequate family support, and the presence of governmental health insurance were reported as other factors for high levels of hope. Financial problems were reported to negatively affect the psychological distress and thus adversely affect the level of hope in this study [39]. The future subscale and total hope scores of patients were found to increase with their information level about the disease. Similarly, in the study of Durusoy et al. [41], more than half of the patients (63 %) stated that they would like to know all the details about their disease.

Future of Individualized Oncology in Focus

In the USA and other developed countries, most children <15 years are treated in clinical trials and the high survival rates achieved is suggested to be due to building up protocols according to statistically significant data resulting from trials. In adults, the number of cancer patients treated in clinical trials is less than in pediatrics, even in developed countries, but most are treated according to guidelines or accepted protocols.

Adolescents are sometimes treated by pediatric oncologists, sometimes by medical oncologists in most countries. They usually are not put into trials due to physicians' or patients' choice. In some developed countries, adolescents and young adult (AYA) clinics have been developed that address the physical and psychological needs of this age group. Recently, in the USA, many COG studies recruit adolescent and young adults in pediatric treatment trials, since there are reports that the survival rates in some cancer types have increased when pediatric protocols were used. According to recent regulations in Turkey, all cancer patients up to 18 years of age are treated by pediatric oncologists.

Most centers in Turkey treat their patients according to worldwide accepted US- or European-oriented protocols. Medical oncologists in some oncology centers in Turkey, mainly in universities in big cities, participate in phase II and mostly phase III international clinical trials that are designed mostly by the USA or European centers [42, 43]. In Turkey, children with cancer are treated either by national protocols/trials developed by TPOG or by international clinical trials/protocols developed mostly in the USA or Europe such as protocols by SIOP and Children's Oncology Group (COG). Some of the pediatric oncologists have also participated in phase III international trials such as the SIOPEL liver tumor randomized treatment trials or brain tumor trials [44, 45]. Also, pediatric oncologists in Turkey, as the first author of this chapter (RK), has participated in some international guidelines such as febrile neutropenia for pediatric cancer [46] and some treatment strategies for developing countries [47]. Among TPOG protocol studies, Wilms tumor [48] and neuroblastoma studies [49] can be mentioned. A nationwide pediatric cancer registry is also active under TPOG governance since 2002 and is currently conducted by both TPOG and TPHD [6, 20].

Personalized medicine is the tailoring of therapies to the patients based on the stage of the disease, the response to therapy or risk of adverse events. The goal in cancer treatment should be to use the most effective and the least toxic therapy. Currently, risk-adapted treatment approaches are used both in adult and pediatric cancer. Risk-based treatment leads to decreased toxicity and late effects by decreasing treatment intensity in low risk patients. Chemotherapy intensity may be alleviated or diminished according to the treatment responses. The number of chemotherapy courses has decreased to 2–4 courses in early stage Hodgkin's disease. Radiotherapy (cranial prophylactic radiotherapy) has been successfully omitted from most acute lymphoblastic leukemia protocols in children except in high risk patients and some special conditions.

Targeted treatment has also proved to be successful in some cancers. In patients having t(9;22) acute lymphoblastic or chronic myeloid leukemia, targeted therapies like imatinib has led to revolutionary results. Furthermore, monoclonal antibodies such as brentixumab, in relapsed/refractory non-Hodgkin's lymphomas or Hodgkin's disease, have led to successful responses.

In Turkey, standard cancer treatment and care has been funded by the government for all citizens. Targeted therapies are also funded by the government [50]. In an international survey, patients in Turkey, were the least likely to pay for medical expenses out of pocket, compared with the US or other emerging markets (<1 %) [51].

In Turkey, although oncologists advise and apply standard treatment protocols, they also respect patients' and their families' wishes. Mostly, it is the families rather than the patients who participate in the decision. In pediatric cancer, the families are informed of the malignancy and the prognosis of the disease in detail, the child is informed of the malignancy in words that they may understand according to their age. Most parents do not want the doctor to tell the child that they have "cancer," and the doctor tries to convince the parents to at least use the term "tumor" in the first session. In adults, especially in the elderly, most families do not want the patient to know that he/she has cancer. Changing the orientation towards a more patient-centered approach as is in the USA and Europe needs time [50].

Current Challenges Facing Critical Clinical Issues in Cancer

Cancer is the second most common cause of death after cardiovascular diseases in Turkey; therefore, it is an important public health issue. There are cancer centers within the universities and public teaching and education hospitals [3]. There are also three oncology Institutes in Turkey; one in Istanbul (Istanbul University Oncology Institute), one in Ankara (Hacettepe Oncology Institute) and one in Izmir (Dokuz Eylul University Oncology Institute). In Turkey, all medication and hospital services for patients with cancer are provided by the government in university or government training hospitals free of charge [2]. Almost all standard and new chemotherapeutics, including many targeted agents, are available in the market [50]. Taking into account the large number of patients, especially in big cities where the majority of patients are located, hospital beds are always full, the number of patients per doctor is high and the number of nurses experienced in oncology is low [2, 3]. In general, the number of beds in long-term care hospitals (not only for cancer) has increased from 6841 in 2000 to 8469 in 2010 [2, 52]. The number of physicians per 100,000 people (167 in 2010) has grown moderately, but is still lower than that of Greece, Italy, Spain, and Portugal, as well as of the average for the European Union

(EU) [5, 52]. Similarly, the number of nurses per 100,000 people (156 in 2010) is the lowest among the countries mentioned. Palliative experts are indeed scarce [2, 3]. Recently, private university hospitals have also taken part in care of this population. The Ministry of Health has planned to build big city hospitals including cancer centers in big cities. There is a serious lack of psychological (psychologist and psychiatrist) support services specific for cancer patients; no social worker, no art therapist in most centers [3]. Due to high number of patients, limited time is dedicated to cancer research. The current health system in Turkey has been designed primarily for the daily care of the patients both at inpatient and outpatient clinics. Despite the heavy clinical burden, academic staff in the university try to do research. Mostly, scientists other than clinical physicians are able to do full time research. Research conducted according to priorities in the society such as the genetic differences in cancer in a particular setting or environmental effect may have relevant results. For this issue, specific tumor tissue banking was planned. A pilot study was performed at Dokuz Eylül University Breast Tumor DNA Bank (DEUBTB) to facilitate sharing of tumor DNA/RNA [53]. At interim phase, the authors suggested that biobanks need to be controlled by the government or regulatory authorities for the necessary funding and quality standards of ethical, legal, and social regulations.

Insights on Palliative Care

The Pallia-Turk project, in the Turkish national cancer control program, focuses on implementation of a palliative care (PC) model with family physicians, nurses, and home-care teams so that patients with chronic diseases can receive basic PC services [3, 54–56]. This project also integrates NGOs and local municipals to cover the psychosocial, economic, and religious needs of the patients. The project secondarily aims new legislations for morphine prescription to increase morphine availability and to train the medical staff against "opiophobia."

The Pallia-Turk project has three levels of organization: Primary, Secondary, and Tertiary Palliative Care Centers. Tertiary centers take care of complex patients who cannot be managed at the primary or secondary levels. These centers also will plan research and training activities of doctors, nurses, and social workers and interact with NGOs within time [3, 54, 55]. Home-care units, 290 in number, related to the government hospitals have been planned in 71 cities, although chronic patients such as those with diabetes and neurological disorders have used these services, cancer patients using these services constituted only 4 % of the patients. This may be due to the physicians and nurses feeling inadequate for cancer supportive care management, and the patient and family desiring to be treated by the doctor, nurse, or center that they have been treated by for their cancer. Currently, Turkey has ten PC units, five in governmental hospitals, and five in university hospitals. Additionally; there is a private unit for pediatric cases and some pain units across the country [3, 5, 54, 55]. However, most of the oncology staff provide some form of PC in their inpatient or outpatient clinics by way of consultations with the related disciplines [3]. Formal comprehensive PC curriculum is not yet present both for physicians and nurses [3, 23, 54, 55]. Hospice care and home care for palliative care in cancer is highly needed in Turkey.

Regarding medication for pain relief in cancer, there are regulations for prescriptions and distribution of opioids in Turkey. These are controlled by the Ministry of Health. Thus, illegal use of opioids is avoided. Opioids can be prescribed by all physicians including family physicians [3, 54–60]. The Ministry of Health has also planned to decrease the unnecessary legislation according to European Union guidelines by 2015 and e-prescriptions, like the prescriptions of other drugs, are also planned for opioids [3].

Local Innovations

Each country has its own needs, and the focus of research and clinical care activities should be defined according to these realities. An agenda is needed to set priorities for cancer research, to identify strategies for overcoming barriers, and to develop a workforce and international collaboration.

The NCCN–Middle East and North Africa (MENA) project was established to address the need for guidelines according to evidence-based medicine involving social, cultural, and economic realities of this region [61]. This project is a very good example of regional collaboration based on local experience but also on standard global evidence.

The WHO 58th World Health Assembly approved a program to develop partnership between low and middle income countries and the high income countries on cancer prevention and control in 2005 [18]. IUCC, in 2006, reported World Cancer Declaration to increase awareness, improve care, and coordinate training of professionals, by the support of National Cancer Institute (USA), SIOP, ICCCPO, and to reduce cancer burden in the world by 2020 [62, 63]. The ASCO International Affairs Committee, having the role of supporting the improvement of oncology in less-developed countries, developed a series of programs [64]. "The International Development and Education Award Grant (IDEA/G)" supports these oncologists by giving them opportunity to visit the USA or Canada and make a strong relationship with a mentor. The second author (FBC) of this chapter by the support of the first author (RK) as the national mentor received IDEA on palliative care in 2014 and had the opportunity to join the annual ASCO meeting and also visited the pediatric advanced care team at Dana-Farber Cancer Institute in Boston. Each program serves to facilitate relationships for knowledge exchange between ASCO mentors from high-resource countries and new ASCO members from the developing world [64].

There are many health websites that serve the global health community. "Cure4Kids" is the pediatric cancer website of St. Jude Children's Research Hospital that introduces a platform to provide real time access to protocols, education, and professional development opportunities [65]. The first author (RK) of this chapter is one of the international editorial board members of Oncopedia, in Cure4Kids.

Cancer prevention and early detection continue to represent areas where effective strategies have the potential to yield the greatest impact on overall reduction of morbidity and mortality from cancer. The Ministry of Health National Cancer Control Program in Turkey has organized programs for prevention and screening and early diagnosis of breast, cervical, and also colorectal cancers since 2009 [4, 12].

Government Involvement in the Care for Cancer Patient

Turkey's health care system has undergone radical changes since 2003 both in the provision and financing of health care services. The most important of these was the removal of different accessibility rules between social security schemes and applying the same rules to all of them. Under the General Health Insurance Scheme, all citizens are covered by the Social Security Institution. Health services are predominantly government-based managed through a social security scheme by the Ministry of Health [5]. When the patient has a chronic disease such as diabetes, hypertension, or cancer, the patient receives full reimbursement [5]. Total expenditure on health as a proportion of gross domestic product (GDP) has risen from 2.4 % in 1980 to 6.1 % in 2008.

The National Cancer Department, in coordination with NGOs and universities has carried out breast, cervical, and colorectal cancer screening throughout the country since 2009 [15, 16]. Epidemiological studies are being performed regarding cancers caused by environmental factors. Turkey has a "National Mesothelioma Control Program." It's a rare lung and peritoneal cancer globally, but is 4000 times more prevalent in Tuzköy town in Nevsehir city, compared to the rest of the world. This has led to the decision to relocate the town for the solution of the problem. A mineral fiber called "erionite" is suspected in the development of mesothelioma [15].

In the Black Sea Region, a study has been carried out to investigate the effects of radiation after the accident at Chernobyl Nuclear Plant in 1986. According to the results, cancer incidence rate is similar (1.85 %) both in the Black Sea Region and in the control group in Isparta Eğirdir. No radiation-specific evidence had been found in terms of cytogenetic methods in the cancer patients. The development of thyroid cancers which is related with radiation also did not indicate a difference between the Black Sea Region and the control regions [15].

Epidemiological studies showed that cancer have become the leading cause of death in Kocaeli Dilovası area, where dust and smoke from many factories pollute the air. Daily measurement of SO2 and smoke values in the air have been initiated at six different locations [15].

The studies on the impact of the power plant to the environment are planning in Afsin-Elbistan and Muğla Yatağan region, where Fossil Fuel Power Plants have commenced energy generation [15].

There is not sufficient data concerning the HPV level and types in Turkish women. HPV DNA obtained from 1500 patients with invasive cervical cancer and from 3500 cervical smear samples of healthy women has been studied to determine the HPV frequency and genotype variety [15].

For the establishment of the National Cancer Institute, studies have been carried out by TEPAV (Economic Policy Research Foundation of Turkey) and almost completed [15].

Cancer Early Diagnosis and Screening Centers (KETEM) have been established in order to implement screening programs for cancers [15]. By the end of the year 2008, the Ministry has established 84 centers in 81 provinces. The duties of KETEMs are to organize the training and to inform the health personnel and the public on the issue of cancer and to raise awareness, to provide diagnosis in early stages through population-based screening programs (on breast, cervical (cervix uteri), colorectal cancers, etc.) on identified risk groups, to refer the patients diagnosed with cancer to treatment centers, to carry out patient follow-up evaluations, and to provide possible social, psychological, and medical support. Screening services are provided free of charge [15].

Cancer Care to Foreigners in Turkey

Multidisciplinary cancer treatment in Turkey is quite advanced in comparison to most countries in the region. Some cancer patients from some Middle East countries, Balkan countries, and Turkic origin or Turkic-speaking countries in the northeast of Turkey such as Azerbaijan, Kazakhstan, come to Turkey for an accurate diagnosis and/or treatment, they also come for transplantation. Some of these patients come to private hospitals that have cancer centers and/or transplantation units. There are also refugees coming to Turkey from neighboring areas of conflict. Since the onset of the civil war of Syria in March 2011, over one million Syrians (around one million 350,000) have come to Turkey according to Government estimates. Authorities at all levels of the government have shown great sensitivity and taken pioneering role to attract the attention of the United Nations (UN) and the EU [66]. Since the beginning of the crisis in 2011, Disaster and Emergency Management Residency (AFAD), an organization activated for crisis circumstances promoted ordinary daily life, regular education facilities, and health services. In April 2013, Turkey put its first asylum law, the "Law on Foreigners and International Protection" regulating all proceedings for refugees living in Turkey [66]. According to AFAD survey, about 10 % of refugees report problems with noncommunicable diseases, including hypertension, diabetes, cancer, asthma, and renal failure [67].

Over the last 4 years, the financial requirements for United Nations High Commissioner for Refugees (UNHCR)'s operation in Turkey have increased dramatically.

Refugees with cancer can be treated at tertiary government and university hospitals free of charge. The patients usually have very advanced stage diseases at diagnosis, so that they have poor outcome.

Turkey also has seen an important increase in the number of non-Syrian asylum applications over 2 years mainly from Iraq, Iran, and Afghanistan. It is estimated that there are over 100,000 refugees in Turkey in 2014, not including Syrians [66].

Institutional Involvement

Most cancer treatment in Turkey is provided free of charge, within the cancer center/units in the government university hospitals or public training and education hospitals. The number of private hospitals in Turkey has increased in recent years, however, most provide outpatient care [5].

Most of the patients treated at private hospitals have voluntary health insurance (VHI). This kind of insurance provides a very small share of health expenditure as 3.7 % of total health expenditure in 2000 [5]. Only 15 % adult cancer patients and 1–2 % pediatric ones get treatment at private setting. Bone marrow and stem cell transplantation facilities have been governed by the university hospitals; however, the capacity was limited. Currently, particularly in Istanbul, transplantation is done in private centers, most of which are fully reimbursed by the government.

Society Reaction Towards Cancer Patients in a Modernizing Society

At the traditional Turkish family style, there is close relations within the family; physical, social, and psychological needs of a sick member is supported by the rest of the family members at their own home. Home is still the most common place for death in rural areas [6]. However, through 2000s, particularly in the western part of Turkey, the place of death inclined towards hospitals as women are working outside and are not available to care for their sick relatives at home.

Turkish patients suffering from cancer clearly express their desire of being told about cancer diagnosis and prognosis [26, 27]. However, families believe that cancer is "that is not to be named" since nothing can be done to treat it and it is always fatal [6, 22, 27]. While this is dishonesty, it is also an expression of the individual's desire to protect a loved one from cancer—the bad news. However, the family members also deprive the patient of the right to make decisions about his or her life [6]. Physicians tend to respect the patients' right to know the truth but are limited from the family pressure [27, 28].

The right of dying patients has just been established by law in Turkey, and do-not-resuscitate (DNR) orders for patients are now legal. End-of-life care is given mostly in the inpatient setting. Although most of the patients or family members in rural areas prefer to stay at home at their end-of-life period, most patients in urban areas and most families of children prefer to stay in the hospital in the terminal stage, in contrary to many countries in the Middle East [3]. The patient should be offered an integrated model of palliative care that continues throughout the course of the illness, regardless of the outcome. Sometimes, families resist PC consultations because this may symbolize evidence of the patient's deterioration, which may be difficult to face. All cancer care must be provided respecting patients' or families' spiritual, cultural background. So health care professionals should be sensitive and tolerable of various beliefs in order to meet the spiritual needs of patients and families and ensure a "good death" and healthy bereavement.

Summary and Recommendations

Turkey, according to the World Bank's classification for income is considered as an upper middle income country. Turkey is located on two continents, Europe and Asia, located at the crossroads of East and West; it also has parts in the Mediterranean and the Middle East. Turkey has undertaken the Health Transformation Program from 2002 on, including major reforms to transfer and improve the health system and its outcomes and the situation has improved in the following decade.

Each year, about 175,000 new cancer patients is expected. The most frequent cancers in adult females are breast (28 %) and thyroid (10.3 %); and in adult males are lung (31.2 %) and prostate (13.7 %). The number of cancer caused by tobacco was very high in Turkey. Turkey had one of the highest smoking rates in the OECD in 2007. Turkey became a smoke-free country in 2009 when smoking was banned in all indoor areas. This has led to a significant decrease in the use of tobacco in Turkey. Thus, it is expected that cancer induced by tobacco such as lung cancer will decrease in the future.

Cancer is the second cause of death after cardiovascular diseases in adults; cancer is the fourth cause of death in children. In children, 2500–3000 new cancer cases are expected in Turkey. The survival rate in pediatric cancer is 65 % in Turkey.

Cancer care in Turkey is quite advanced in comparison to many countries in the region. All cancer treatment is reimbursed by the government in cancer center/units in the government university hospitals or public training and education hospitals. Some cancer patients from neighboring countries come for diagnosis and treatment to Turkey. Most cancer treatment is provided free of charge to refugees coming from areas of conflict to Turkey. The government provides free health. The residency and fellowships program in medical oncology, in radiation oncology, in pediatric hematology–oncology, and in surgical oncology is very well organized for years and most physicians in oncology are well qualified. However, the number of doctors and the number of nurses for oncology patients are not adequate, nor is the number of beds for oncology patients. Palliative care needs improvement. Government, non-governmental organizations and health care professionals should collaborate to improve palliative care in Turkey.

References

1. Lyerly HK, Abernethy AP, Stockler MR, Koczwara B, Aziz Z, Nair R, Seymour L. Need for global partnership in cancer care: perceptions of cancer care researchers attending the 2010 Australia and Asia pacific clinical oncology research development workshop. J Oncol Pract. 2011;7(5):324–9.
2. Tatar M, Mollahaliloğlu S, Şahin B, Aydın S, Maresso A, Hernández-Quevedo C. Turkey: health system review. Health Syst Transit. 2011;13(6):1–186.
3. Kebudi R, Cakir FB, Gultekin M. Palliative care to the cancer patient in Turkey. In: Silbermann M, editor. Palliative care to the cancer patient: the Middle East as a model for emerging countries. New York: Nova; 2014.

4. Tuncer M. (ed.). National cancer program, 2009–2015, Ankara: Ministry of Health (Turkey), Department of Cancer Control; 2009. Ministry of Health publication no. 760. [Turkish].
5. Ozgul N, Gultekin M, Koc O, Goksel F, Bayraktar G, Ekinci H, et al. Turkish community-based palliative care model: a unique design. Ann Oncol. 2012;23 Suppl 3:76–8.
6. Kutluk T. The epidemiology of childhood cancer. In: Tuncer M, editor. Cancer control in Turkey. Ankara: The Turkish Republic Ministry of Health, Department of Cancer Control; 2008. p. 159–67.
7. http://data.worldbank.org/country/tr.
8. http://sbu.saglik.gov.tr. 2011.
9. Silbermann M, Arnaout M, Abdel Rahman Sayed H, Sedky M, El-Shami M, Ben-Arush M, et al. Pediatric palliative care in the Middle East. In: Knapp C, Madden V, Fowler-Kerry S, editors. Pediatric palliative care: global perspectives. Amsterdam: Springer; 2012. p. 127–59.
10. Turkish Ministry of Health, Cancer Statistics, 2008. http://www.kanser.gov.tr/daire-faaliyetleri/kanser-istatistikleri.html.
11. Turkish National Statistics Institute, 2012. http://tuikapp.tuik.gov.tr/demografiapp/olum.zul.
12. http://portal.org/sites/default/files/plans/Turkey NATIONAL CANCER PROGRAM 2-1.pdf.
13. http://www.euro.who.int/en/health-topics/Health-systems/health-systems-governance/publications/2012/turkey-health-system-performance-assessment-2011.
14. Vassal G, Fitzgerald E, Schrappe M, Arnold F, Kowalczyk J, et al. Challenges for children and adolescents with cancer in Europe: the SIOP-Europe agenda. Pediatr Blood Cancer. 2014;61(9):1551–7.
15. Gatta G, Botta L, Rossi S, Aareleid T, Bielska-Lasota M, Clavel J, et al. Childhood cancer survival in Europe 1999–2007: results of EUROCARE-5-a population-based study. Lancet Oncol. 2014;15:35–47.
16. Pritchard-Jones K, Kaatsch P, Steliarova-Foucher E, Stiller CA, Coebergh JW. Cancer in children and adolescents in Europe: developments over 20 years and future challenges. Eur J Cancer. 2006;42:2183–90.
17. Silbermann M, Epner DE, Charalambous H, Baider L, Puchalski CM, Balducci L, Gultekin M, Abdalla RF, Daher M, Al-Tarawneh MR, Smith TJ. Promoting new approaches for cancer care in the Middle East. Ann Oncol. 2013;23 Suppl 7:5–10.
18. UICC 2005. World cancer campaign: the time to act is now. Geneva: International Union against Cancer (UICC); 2005.
19. Burton A. My child matters initiative awards: combating cancer in children in the developing world. Lancet Oncol. 2006;7:13–4.
20. Kutluk T, Yeşilipek A. Turkish National Pediatric Cancer Registry 2002–2008 (Turkish Pediatric Oncology Group and Turkish Pediatric Hematology Society). J Clin Oncol. 2013;31(Suppl); abstr. 10067.
21. Kebudi R, Turkish Pediatric Oncology Group. Pediatric oncology in Turkey. J Pediatr Hematol Oncol. 2012;34 Suppl 1:S12–4.
22. Kebudi R, Uludag D. for the Istanbul University. Demographic, clinical and survival features of childhood cancers in Istanbul University, Oncology Institute (1990–2012). 46th SIOP Congress, Pediatr Blood Cancer. 2014;61:S2,S291. Toronto, Canada, 22–25 October, 2014.
23. Can G. Nursing education in Turkey. Nurse Educ. 2010;35(4):146–7.
24. Daher M. Cultural beliefs and values in cancer patients. Ann Oncol. 2012;23 Suppl 3:66–9.
25. Lagnado L. In Some Cultures, Cancer Stirs Shame. The Wall Street Journal, 2008; p. A1. http://online.wsj.com/article/SB122304682088802359.html.
26. Ashing-Giwa KT, Padilla G, Tejero J, et al. Understanding the breast cancer experience of women: a qualitative study of African American, Asian American, Latina and Caucasian cancer survivors. Psychooncology. 2004;13:408–28.
27. De Natale A, Pollio A. Plants species in the folk medicine of Montecorvino Rovella (inland Campania, Italy). J Ethnopharmacol. 2007;109:295–303.
28. Polat R, Satıl F. An ethnobotanical survey of medicinal plants in Edremit Gulf (Balıkesir-Turkey). J Ethnopharmacol. 2012;139:626–41.
29. WHO. WHO Traditional Medicine Strategy 2002–2005. Geneva: World Health Organization; 2002.

30. Guner A, Ozhatay N, Ekim T, Başer KHC. Flora of Turkey and the East Aegean Islands, vol. 11. Edinburgh: Edinburgh University Press; 2000.
31. Yeşilada E, Sezik E. A survey on the traditional medicine in Turkey: semi quantitative evaluation of the results. In: Singh VK, Govil JN, Singh G, editors. Recent progress in medicinal plants VII: ethnomedicine and pharmacognosy. Houston: SCI Tech; 2002. p. 389–412.
32. Samur M, Bozcuk HS, Kara A, Savas B. Factors associated with utilization of nonproven cancer therapies in Turkey: a study of 135 patients from a single center. Support Care Cancer. 2001;9:452–8.
33. Sargın SA, Akçicek E, Selvi S. An ethnobotanical study of medicinal plants used by the local people of Alaşehir (Manisa) in Turkey. J Ethnopharmacol. 2013;150:860–74.
34. Tetik F, Civelek S, Cakilcioglu U. Traditional uses of some medicinal plants in Malatya (Turkey). J Ethnopharmacol. 2013;146:331–46.
35. Cakilcioglu U, Khatun S, Turkoglu I, Hayta S. Ethnopharmacological survey of medicinal plants in Maden (Elazig-Turkey). J Ethnopharmacol. 2011;137:469–86.
36. Kaval I, Behçet L, Cakilcioglu U. Ethnobotanical study on medicinal plants in Geçitli and its surrounding (Hakkari-Turkey). J Ethnopharmacol. 2014;155:171–84.
37. Polat R, Cakilcioglu U, Tetik F. Traditional uses of medicinal plants in Solhan (Bingöl-Turkey). J Ethnopharmacol. 2013;148:951–63.
38. Koenig HG. Religion, spirituality and medicine: application to clinical practice. J Am Med Assoc. 2000;284:1708.
39. Kavradim ST, Ozer ZC, Bozcuk H. Hope in people with cancer: a multivariate analysis from Turkey. J Adv Nurs. 2013;69(5):1183–96.
40. Bozcuk H, Erdoğan V, Eken C, Çıplak E, Samur M, Özdoğan M, Sava B. Does awareness of diagnosis make any difference to quality of life? Determinants of emotional functioning in a group of cancer patients in Turkey. Support Care Cancer. 2002;10:51–7.
41. Durusoy R, Karaca B, Junushova B, Uslu R. Cancer patients' satisfaction with doctors and preferences about death in a university hospital in Turkey. Patient Educ Couns. 2011;85(3):285–90.
42. Baum M, Budzar AU, Cuzick J, Forbes J, Houghton JH, Klijn JG, Sahmoud T, ATAC Trialists' Group. Anastrozole alone or in combination with tamoxifen versus tamoxifen alone for adjuvant treatment of postmenopausal women with early breast cancer: first results of the ATAC randomised trial. Lancet. 2002;359(9324):2131–9.
43. Smith IE, Pierga JY, Biganzoli L, Cortés-Funes H, Thomssen C, Pivot X, ATHENA Study Group, et al. First-line bevacizumab plus taxane-based chemotherapy for locally recurrent or metastatic breast cancer: safety and efficacy in an open-label study in 2,251 patients. Ann Oncol. 2011;22(3):595–602.
44. Kebudi R, Emiroglu HH, Gorgun O, Akıcı F, Tugcu D, Ayan I. Pediatric malignant liver tumors: results of a single center. Int J Hematol Oncol (UHOD). 2012;22(1):1–8.
45. Wolff J, Wrede B, Peters O, Kebudi R, Pietsch T, Finlay F. Choroid plexus tumors in CPT-SIOP 2000: update March 2006. Pediatr Blood Cancer. 2006;47:382 (abstract O.100).
46. Lehrnbecher T, Phillips R, Alexander S, Alvaro F, Carlesse F, Fisher B, International Pediatric Fever and Neutropenia Guideline Panel, et al. Guideline for the management of fever and neutropenia in children with cancer and/or undergoing hematopoietic stem-cell transplantation. J Clin Oncol. 2012;30(35):4427–38.
47. Magrath I, Steliarova-Foucher E, Epelman S, Ribeiro RC, Harif M, Li C, Kebudi R, et al. Pediatric cancer in low-income and middle-income countries. Lancet Oncol. 2013;14(3):e104–16.
48. Akyüz C, Yalçin B, Yildiz I, Hazar V, Yörük A, Tokuç G, et al. Treatment of Wilms tumor: a report from the Turkish Pediatric Oncology Group (TPOG). Pediatr Hematol Oncol. 2010;27(3):161–78.
49. Aksoylar S, Varan A, Vergin C, Hazar V, Akici F, Dagdeviren A, et al. High-dose chemotherapy and autologous stem cell transplantation in patients with high-risk neuroblastoma: results of Turkish pediatric oncology group—Neuroblastoma 2003 (TPOG-NBL 2003) protocol. Blood. 2013;122(21):3411.

50. Kockaya G, Polat M, Vural IM, Akbulat A, Dedeoglu BD, Akar H, Karman S. Off-label and unlicensed oncology medicine use in Turkey: a retrospective analysis of computer records of the Turkish Ministry of Health. JPHSR. 2011;2:53–7.
51. Lammers P, Criscitiello C, Curigliano G, Jacobs I. Barriers to the use of trastuzumab for HER2+ breast cancer and the potential impact of biosimilars: a physician survey in the United States and emerging markets. Pharmaceuticals (Basel). 2014;7(9):943–53.
52. Akdağ R. The progress so far. Turkey: Health Transformation Program. Ankara, Sağlık Bakanlığı Hıfzıssıhha Mektebi Müdürlüğü; 2007. http://ekutuphane.tusak.gov.tr/kitaplar/the_progress_so_far_health_transformation_program_in_turkey_november_2002_june_2007.pdf. Accessed 20 July 2011.
53. Cavuşoğlu AC, Saydam S, Alakavuklar M, Canda T, Sevinç A, Kiliç Y, et al. A pilot study for human tumor/DNA banking: returned more questions than answers. Med Oncol. 2008;25(4):471–3.
54. Ozcelik H, Fadiloglu C, Karabulut B, Uyar M. Palliative care activity in the field of oncology in Turkey. J Palliat Care. 2010;26(4):305–10.
55. Komurcu S. Current status of palliative care in Turkey. J Pediatr Hematol Oncol. 2011;33 Suppl 1:S78–80.
56. Silbermann M, Fink RM, Min SJ, Mancuso MP, Brant J, Hajjar R, Al-Alfi N, Baider L, Turker I, ElShamy K, Ghrayeb I, Al-Jadiry M, Khader K, Kav S, Charalambous H, Uslu R, Kebudi R, et al. Evaluating palliative care needs in middle eastern countries. J Palliat Med. 2015;18(1):18–25.
57. Silbermann M, Al-Hadad S, Ashraf S, Hessissen L, Madani A, Noun P, et al. MECC regional initiative in pediatric palliative care: middle eastern course on pain management. J Pediatr Hematol Oncol. 2012;34 Suppl 1:S1–11.
58. Elcigil A, Maltepe H, Esrefgil G, Mutafoglu K. Nurses' perceived barriers to assessment and management of pain in a University Hospital. J Pediatr Hematol Oncol. 2011;33:S33–8.
59. Ozgul N, Koc O, Gultekin M, Goksel F, Kerman S, Tanyeri P, et al. Opioids for cancer pain: availability, accessibility, and regulatory barriers in Turkey and Pallia-Turk Project. J Pediatr Hematol Oncol. 2011;33 Suppl 1:S29–32.
60. Mutafoglu K. Challenges and obstacles facing the oncologist in pain management. J Pediatr Hematol Oncol. 2010;32:424–5.
61. Içli F, Akbulut H, Bazarbashi S, Kuzu MA, Mallath MK, Rasul KI, et al. Modification and implementation of NCCN guidelines on colon cancer in the Middle East and North Africa region. J Natl Compr Canc Netw. 2010;8 Suppl 3:S22–5.
62. United Nations: Resolution adopted by the General Assembly: 64/265. Prevention and control of non-communicable diseases. http://www.who.int/nmh/events/2011/UN_resolution_prevention_control_ ncds.pdf.
63. International Union Against Cancer: The World Cancer Declaration. http://www.uicc.org/declaration/world-cancer-declaration.
64. Patel JD, Galsky MD, Chagpar AB, Pyle D, Loehrer Sr PJ. Role of American Society of Clinical Oncology in low and middle-income countries. J Clin Oncol. 2011;29(22):3097–102.
65. Kellie SJ, Howard SC. Global child health priorities: what role for pediatric oncologists? Eur J Cancer. 2008;44(16):2388–96.
66. https://data.unhcr.org/syrianrefugees/download.php?id=3780. 2014 Syria Regional Response Plan of Turkey.
67. https://data.unhcr.org/syrianrefugees/download.php?id=4085. Syrian Refugees in Turkey, 2013. Republic of Turkey Prime Ministry Disaster and Emergency Management Presidency (AFAD) Field Survey Results.

Chapter 13
Cancer Care in Sudan: Current Situation and Challenges

Nahla Gafer, Esther Walker, Mohja Khair Allah, and Ali Elbaghir

Abbreviations

APCA	African Palliative Care Association
CCST	Comboni College of Science and Technology
HAU	Hospice Africa Uganda
IAHPC	International Association for Hospices and Palliative Care
IASP	International Association for the Study of Pain

Country

Sudan, in northeast Africa, after a long civil war and separation of the South of Sudan in 2011, is still one of the largest countries in Africa (a million km^2). Sudan's total population is 35 million; 67 % of the population live in rural areas. More than five million people live in Khartoum, the capital city. The main language is Arabic with many local dialects (e.g. Nobian, Fur), and the main religion is Islam with a small Christian minority. The Nile runs through Sudan and has influenced the lives of Sudanese people throughout the course of its history until today. Cities and towns form all along the Nile and its main tributaries: the Blue Nile and the White Nile. Inland from the Nile, much of Sudan is desert, home to nomadic tribes.

Armed conflict, poor transport, and infrastructure, in addition to administrative problems, have impeded the provision of humanitarian assistance to populations

N. Gafer, M.D. (✉) • M.K. Allah, M.B.B.S. • A. Elbaghir, M.D.
Radiation and Isotope Center, Khartoum, Sudan
e-mail: nahla.gafer@yahoo.com

E. Walker, M.B.E., B.S.C.
St. Catherine Hospice, Crawley, West Sussex, UK

M. Silbermann (ed.), *Cancer Care in Countries and Societies in Transition*,
DOI 10.1007/978-3-319-22912-6_13

affected by war—currently in the west, south, and a small area in the east. Poor services in remote areas make people feel marginalized, and their voices unheard.

Cancer has been one of the major ten killer diseases for many years in Sudan, and the number of people developing and dying from cancer is predicted to continue to increase steadily both in Sudan and worldwide. Sudan is witnessing double epidemic: high incidence of communicable diseases and an increasing incidence of noncommunicable diseases.

An increasing number of cancer patients every year are faced by poor and slow improvement in cancer services, care delivery, and treatment capacity across the country. In fact, low awareness and negative beliefs among Sudanese community about cancer are likely to contribute to the delayed presentation of cancer, leading to worst prognosis. Furthermore, there is too much unwarranted variation in the quality of care across and treatment protocols leaving the cancer patient affected by cost of treatment and inaccessible services.

Administratively, the Republic of Sudan is governed by a federal system, comprising 18 states. The Federal Ministry of Health is committed through a national cancer policy and strategy to give a high priority to cancer care as part of the overall health system.

Huge efforts were intended to strengthen the war effort against cancer by diverse governmental and nongovernmental bodies, but unfortunately are delivered through fragmented services and poor referral scheme.

Non-communicable diseases (NCDs) are emerging as one of the major health problems in Sudan [1–3]. Being an African country, Sudan has its share of cancer burden. However, population-based data in cancer incidence, prevalence, and mortality in Sudan were not available, and most published cancer cases were based on estimates from hospital-based information sources. Most of these sources are maintained by individual health institutions and are mostly paper based.

Culture

Sudan, like other developing countries, has many challenges regarding cultural status. There is a low public awareness due to lack of efficient health education at schooling; there is weak healthcare services and inequity of distribution; there is stigma and reliance on traditional healers and herbal medicines and a population living mainly in rural communities resulting in relatively costly and long-duration travel to and from Khartoum.

Although Islam and Holy Quran frequently refer to life and death [4], including how to prepare ourselves for after death, many Sudanese health professionals, patients, and their families avoid talking about death and dying. Consequently, many seek futile treatment outside Sudan resulting in patients dying away from their home and family.

Cancer has a strong stigma. Some families will not mention if a member is diagnosed with cancer for fear that nobody would marry the girls of the family. Lack of insight is common. Family members, particularly male members are told of the diagnosis, and they may not reveal this information to the patient themselves, especially if female.

Families and patients sometimes do not go to the oncology services after referral, instead, they deny the diagnosis, especially if the patient has few symptoms, and later when the disease burden has increased, they rush with the patient to the oncology center with advanced disease or with a dying patient.

Socioeconomic Status

Sudan is an extremely poor country that has experienced protracted social conflict, civil war, and, in July 2011, the loss of three-quarters of its oil production due to the secession of South Sudan. For nearly a decade, the economy boomed on the back of rising oil production, high oil prices, and significant inflows of foreign direct investment. Since the economic shock of South Sudan's secession, Sudan has struggled to stabilize its economy and make up for the loss of foreign exchange earnings. Sudan is also subject to comprehensive US sanctions. Sudan is attempting to develop non-oil sources of revenues, such as gold mining, while carrying out an austerity program to reduce expenditures. The world's largest exporter of gum Arabic, Sudan produces 75–80 % of the world's total output. Agriculture continues to employ 80 % of the work force. Sudan introduced a new currency, still called the Sudanese pound, following South Sudan's secession, but the value of the currency has fallen since its introduction. Sudan also faces rising inflation, which reached 47 % on an annual basis in November 2012, but subsided to 25 % in 2013.

Ongoing conflicts in Southern Kordofan, Darfur, and the Blue Nile states, lack of basic infrastructure in large areas, and reliance by much of the population on subsistence agriculture keep close to half of the population at or below the poverty line.

Despite the economic hardships suffered, the Sudanese are very social and kind people, have genuine hospitality and a very strong sense of family responsibility which encompasses caring of their sick relatives and support them physically, morally, and financially.

Cancer Services

Historically, the first national cancer registry had been functioning in 1966–1980s in the National Health Laboratory (NHL) under the sponsorship of the International Union against Cancer (IUCC). The data was collected from only two pathology laboratories, hence affecting the registry with bias reports since cancer was based on a laboratory diagnosis only. This initiative concluded in the 1980s due to the lack of sustaining funds. Another cancer data source is the hospital-based case series at the only two oncological centers of the country, both located in the densely populated Central Sudan, i.e., the Radiation and Isotope Center in Khartoum (RICK), which is the oldest and biggest center for managing cancer patients, witnessing more than two folds increase in the number of patients between the year 2000 and the year 2014, and the National Cancer Institute of the University of Gezira (NCI-UG) in Wad Medani, Gezira State.

During the year 2000, cancer was the third of the identified leading causes of death in Sudanese hospitals, after malaria and pneumonia, accounting for 5 % of all deaths [5]. It must be underlined that this figure, which appears quite low, most likely reflects severe shortcomings in cancer diagnosis and data collection [6].

The National Cancer Registry (NCR) was established in 2009 under the auspices of Sudanese Ministry of Federal Health and is located in the capital Khartoum. A recent report from NCR showed that among all registered cancer cases with available information, breast cancer was the most common cancer, followed by leukemia, lymphoma, prostate cancer, colorectal cancer, oral cancer, cancer of esophagus, liver cancer, stomach cancer, and cancer of cervix. These cancers together made up 68.9 % of all reported primary cancer sites. A positive association between incidence rate of the top five most common cancer sites and age was observed in both adult women and men [7].

Health system in Sudan is composed of Federal states (18 states) and local governments. Health care is delivered through primary health care, secondary hospitals, and tertiary hospitals. At the primary level, there are no significant ongoing activities in cancer control. Some of the secondary and tertiary hospitals are doing some cancer care activities, with a weak referral system and links. There are two national bodies working subsidiary with the cancer control program.

The National Cancer Council (2008) of 28 different professionals, the other body is the Cancer Advisory Committee, belongs to the directorate of curative medicine. The main tasks of the program include development of strategies, plans, guidelines, and protocols, and building the capacity of workers in the field of cancer control at different levels. Another main objective is building partnership with all related sectors and raising the awareness among public care providers. Efforts are underway to formulate national management guidelines for all types of cancer. In fact, guidelines on prevention and early detection of the most common cancers: breast, cervix, and oral cancers were developed and printed. There are two standard management guidelines protocols already published for breast and prostate cancers [8].

The Radioisotope Center Khartoum (RICK) started functioning at 1967 as a center for the treatment of cancer under the auspices of the IAEA, and the Sudan Government. A vertical national cancer control program has been established at RICK since 1982.

Till April 1999, the Radiation & Isotopes Centre (RICK) in Khartoum was the only specialized center for cancer patient management in Sudan. In April 1999, the Gezira Centre (NCI) (initially named INMO—Institute of Nuclear Medicine, Molecular Biology & Oncology) was opened. RICK and NCI are both located in central Sudan with only 200 km distance between them. This obviously limits access for patients who live far from them. This number of centers is definitely below the recommendation by IAEA which suggested one center for each 2–5 millions of population [9].

Shendi Cancer Center (University of Shendi) in River Nile State was established in 2010, started by a medical oncology unit, providing only chemotherapy, hormonal therapy, and nuclear medicine for diagnosis. The center was equipped recently with radiotherapy machines. There are other three proposed centers, Khartoum (Soba), AlFasher (MoH), and Merowe (MoH). Two other proposed centers at Alobied and AlGadarif are planned but challenges are fund shortages.

The number of working radiotherapy units is greatly below the need of the country and the international standards. Only four cobalt machines and one linear accelerator exist for a population of over 30 million. In Sudan, with the current number of cancer patients, the real need of radiotherapy machines is 16, according to the standard of 1 machine/500 cancer patients [10]. With this limited number of radiotherapy machines, and the machines being out of order large parts of the year (no maintenance contract) leads to very long waiting lists of patients.

The chemotherapy drugs are free of charge for all cases; targeted therapy, immunotherapy, and other supportive treatments are not included. The problems related to chemotherapy, hormonal therapy, and new agents as targeted therapy include: estimation of real needs, availability and sustainability, rising cost, rising number of patients, inadequate budget to support poor patients, inadequate number of well-trained staff: pharmacists, chemo-nurses, and inadequate facilities to administer chemotherapy agents.

Regarding prevention, in Sudan, tobacco use, obesity, and infections are prevalent. As yet unpublished NCR study in all the States highlighted poor lifestyles with high risk for cancer [11]. More than a third of respondents smoked cigarettes; one in four used tumbak (snuff); one in five used shisha; and nearly one in seven mentioned drinking alcohol. Half of these were long-term users more than 15 years. The public awareness regarding cancer prevention and control is poor. There are limited cancer preventive activities.

There is a shortage in histopathology services; there is one national health laboratory (NHL) at Khartoum state. Very few states have this service, largely due to lack of retention of skilled staff. This lack of accessible high quality diagnostic services undoubtedly contributes to the late treatment of cases with the resulting poor outcomes. There is anecdotal evidence of missed diagnosis and erroneous diagnosis.

Records and pathology reports are individually designed by labs, and this contributes to lack of accurate information for patient management and for cancer registry records.

Main Cancers in Sudan

New cancer cases are in the increase. There is no proper community-based cancer registry. Apart from NCI, there are no population-based cancer statistics. People feel a great increase in incidences, but if no exact population figures are available, the size of increase cannot be judged. For sure improvement in education, diagnosis and transport also leads to increased cases presenting to oncology centers.

Breast cancer is the most common cancer in Sudanese women living in Khartoum. The incidence rate is higher than that reported of black women in Harare and Kampala, and also higher compared to North Africa, e.g., Benghazi, Tunisia, or

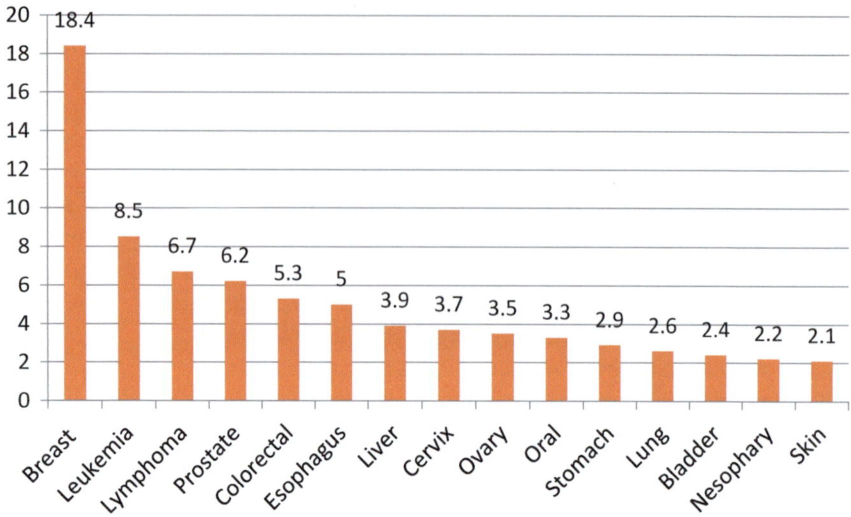

Fig. 13.1 The most common types of cancer among Sudanese patients, 2009–2010. National cancer strategy, Sudan 2012–2016

Garbiah, Egypt. This relatively high risk is quite surprising and might be due to urbanization, increased infertility, and overweight (which till recently was a sign of beauty and wealth in this community).

Although cervical cancer used to be the most common cancer among women in sub-Saharan and East African countries, the incidence rate of cervical cancer in Khartoum is low. It might be due to under-reporting as Sudanese women under 55 years of age, are usually not open about their gynecological problems with family (husband or sons are the ones financially responsible for treatment). Lack of screening tests and awareness and low prevalence of human papilloma virus and human immunodeficiency virus infection in the general population may contribute to this low level of cervical cancer cases [7].

There are certain cancers with an observed high incidence in certain areas of the country. Women from the east have higher incidence of squamous cell esophageal cancer. It is unknown whether it is due to peculiar drinking coffee habits, chronic anemia, or something genetic. There are more young patients with cancer of the breast and cancer of the rectum, as in other African countries. Hepatocellular carcinoma and cervical cancer are more prevalent in the west of the country (Fig. 13.1).

Early Detection in Sudan

There are some efforts to train primary healthcare workers in cancer awareness and suspicion, but these have not been scaled up or systematized. Early detection guidelines have been developed for breast, oral, and cervical cancer [12]. There are no organized screening programs other than sporadic efforts in the private and NGO sectors. Some states as Gezira and River Nile practiced a small scale or pilot screening for breast cancer. At North Kordofan there was a demonstration project for use of Visual Inspection with Acetic acid (VIA) test in cervical cancer. The shortcomings in cancer diagnosis and early detection, and health education are demonstrated by the late presentation of cancer.

In addition to centralization of the health services, the majority of cancer services based in Khartoum and neighboring states (Medani-Gezira state & Shendi—River Nile state). Tobacco control measures need urgent attention for high incidences of oral and lung cancer.

While much is being done for the treatment of cancer, less attention has been paid to important components: prevention and early detection. At the time of RICK's inception in 1967, an estimated 85–90 % of cancer cases presented late. This trend has not changed noticeably in the 45 years since its opening. The National Health Insurance offers access to mammography and blood exams at basic centers, sometimes of poor quality. The MoH is educating newly appointed medical officers on cancer early detection, signs and symptoms, screening and referral, but lack of facilities at primary health centers impedes the work. Several civil society associations are highly involved in education and screening about breast and oral cancers. More work is still needed to be done.

Treatment

A challenge facing proper diagnosis is the lack of reagents (or availability of reagents of poor quality) in the pathology laboratories which result in ineffective diagnosis and later improper treatment of cancer. There is scarcity of pathologists. Proper pathological diagnosis is possible in only two cities: Khartoum and Madani. The MoH is availing the chemotherapy drugs for free benefiting even foreigners residing or passing by the country. Lack of planning and proper management of resources (e.g., opting for brand names) leads to some shortages in basic chemotherapeutic agents for periods that might reach 2 months. Apart from drug availability, a lot needs to be done in organization, training, and provision of service in order to improve patients' care.

There is a local training for clinical oncologists that started in the late 1990s. It helped a lot in providing trained staff committed to work in the country. Before that training cancer centers witnessed huge loss of staff qualified abroad.

The are two main oncology centers in Sudan (RICK and NCI) have: histopathology labs, radiotherapy (external beam, and high dose brachytherapy) nuclear medicine, and chemotherapy facilities. Surgical oncology services at these centers are still to develop. There is an increase in a number of private centers offering care for certain diseases (e.g., Khartoum Breast Care center) or offering a certain modality of management, mainly chemotherapy administration at private rooms; certain hospitals are specialized in surgical management of some cancers, esp. Soba University Hospital (SUH) and Ibn Sna Hospital for GIT tumors and liver surgeries, respectively.

Palliative Care

Palliative care is a relatively new concept in Sudan. Three centers are offering dedicated palliative care units/beds: RICK (started 2010), SUH (2011) and NCI (2015). With international collaboration (especially in terms of training), palliative care services were introduced in the country, mainly the IAHPC, HAU, APCA, MPCU, Cairdeas International, and the IASP. The latter recently sponsored a multidisciplinary Health Professionals Training in Pain Management covering 22 hospitals in the State of Khartoum. That training in collaboration with CCST (the only and first approved course in the country) had the objective to avail oral opioids, which are used in these three centers only, by improving health professionals' knowledge, dispersing unrealistic fears of morphine. Further efforts are needed to help provide palliative care services in different hospitals, especially in the states.

The current palliative care services at all three centers are still facing a lot of challenges especially in remuneration to the staff, and incomplete staffing of the palliative care teams, especially there is the absence of psychologists, social workers, and religious advisors. Palliative care does not enter as an item in these centers' budgets. Services include out-patient clinic, consultation to in-patients, and a limited home care (limited due to lack of dedicated vehicles and hospital commitment).

The Future

Progress is going on at all levels, in spite of the limited financial resources. The WHO has made cancer in developing countries a priority. Through a national cancer control program relevant to Sudanese settings, these can lead to an impact on cancer even on the least developed countries [13].

References

1. Federal Ministry of Health, Sudan—Annual Health Statistical report; 2009.
2. Sudanese Federal Ministry of Health and WHO. STEPS risk factor indicator survey (Khartoum); 2006.
3. Federal Ministry of Health. Sudan Household Health Survey; 2010.
4. Zafir al-Shahri M, al-Khenaizan A. Palliative care for Muslim patients. J Support Oncol. 2005;3(6):432–6.
5. Hamad HM. Cancer initiatives in Sudan. Ann Oncol. 2006;17(8):viii 32–6.
6. Dafaallah K, Mariani-Costantini R, Eldin N. Science of the total environment cancer in the Sudan: an overview of the current status of knowledge on tumor patterns and risk factors. Sci Total Environ. 2012;423:214–28.
7. Saeed IE, Weng H-Y, Mohamed KH, Mohammed SI. Cancer incidence in Khartoum, Sudan: first results from the Cancer Registry, 2009–2010. Cancer Med. 2014;3:1075–84.
8. Federal Ministry of Health. Standard care management protocols for breast and prostate cancer; 2010.

9. IAEA. Setting up a radiotherapy programme: clinical, medical physics, radiation protection and safety aspects. Vienna: IAEA; 2008.
10. Levin V et al. Improving cancer care: Increased need for radiotherapy in developing countries. IAEA BULLETIN, 43/2/2001.
11. National Cancer Registry. Risk factor survey in States. Unpublished; 2011.
12. Federal Ministry of Health. Early detection guideline for breast, oral and cervical cancer; 2011.
13. Reeler AV, Mellstedt H. Cancer in developing countries: challenges and solutions. Ann Oncol. 2006;17:viii7–8.

Chapter 14
Cancer Care in Countries in Transition in Africa: The Case of Uganda

Amos Deogratius Mwaka, Henry Wabinga, and Christopher Orach Garimoi

Introduction

The concept of transition may apply to demographic and/or epidemiologic transition. The latter includes the multitude of usually sequential and complex changes in disease and health patterns in specific human populations and countries, usually over a long period of time. Such changes are intricately related with and manifest as social, economic, and demographic transformations within societies. The transition might take the form of a health system dominated by communicable diseases and poverty-related conditions including poor sanitation, lack of clean potable water, inadequate or unhealthy diet and nutrients intake, poor housing, and low education attainment to a health system predominated by chronic non-communicable diseases (NCDs) including cancers and degenerative illnesses [1]. Uganda is clearly undergoing an epidemiologic transition as the incidence of communicable diseases including tuberculosis and HIV are matched by an increasing incidence of noncommunicable diseases such as diabetes, hypertension, heart diseases, and cancers associated with infections and western lifestyles [2–11].

A.D. Mwaka, M.B.Ch.B., M.Med. (✉)
Department of Medicine, School of Medicine, College of Health Sciences, Makerere University, P.O. Box 7072, Kampala, Uganda
e-mail: mwakaad@yahoo.com

H. Wabinga, M.B.Ch.B., M.Med., M.D.
Department of Pathology, Kampala Cancer Registry, School of Biomedical Sciences, College of Health Sciences, Makerere University, Kampala, Uganda
e-mail: hwabinga@chs.mak.ac.ug

C.O. Garimoi, M.B.Ch.B., M.P.H., Ph.D.
Department of Community Health and Behavioural Sciences, School of Public Health, College of Health Sciences, Makerere University, P.O. Box 7072, Kampala, Uganda
e-mail: cgorach@hotmail.com

M. Silbermann (ed.), *Cancer Care in Countries and Societies in Transition*,
DOI 10.1007/978-3-319-22912-6_14

The countries in transition do not only face the double jeopardy of communicable diseases and noncommunicable diseases including infections-related cancers and cardiovascular diseases but also the fact that the cancers affect the younger productive age groups thus crippling the economic productivity, further leading to entrenchment of poverty in these communities [12–14]. What is needed to control the dual burden of communicable and noncommunicable diseases is an integrated primary care approach based on lessons learnt from long-term experiences with communicable diseases while taking advantage of the favorable global health policy environment [15]. The infrastructures and organizational arrangements used to combat communicable diseases need to be transformed into a more dynamic system to deal with the rocketing burden of noncommunicable diseases.

Uganda Country Profile: Location and Population

Uganda is located in East Africa between 1° 12′ South and 4° 12′ North Latitude, and 29° 34′ East and 35° 0′ East Longitude. It has an area of 241,038 km^2 of which the land area covers 197,323 km^2 [16]. Uganda population is projected to between 40.6 and 43.4 million people by 2017. The annual population growth rate is currently about 3.5 % per annum [16].

Uganda has a high total fertility rate (TFR) of 6.7 [17]. The life expectancy at birth is expected to increase from 50.5 for females and 45.7 for males in 1991 to 54 and 53, respectively, in 2017. The population of the older persons in Uganda (those aged >60 years) is projected to increase from an estimated 1.29 million in 2007 to approximately 1.83 million in 2017 [16]. More cancer diagnoses are therefore expected in Uganda in the near future because the older populations are at greater risk of developing cancers. Worldwide, about 45 % of all the new cancer diagnoses in 2002 were among people aged >65 years [18].

Current Status of Cancer Care in Uganda

This section will include a brief review of the incidence and burden of cancer and the resources and facilities available for cancer care in Uganda.

Incidence and Burden of Cancer

The incidences of cancers have steadily increased worldwide. There is disproportionately marked increases in the low- and middle-income countries (LMICs). In 2002, the number of new cancer diagnoses was estimated at 12.4 million worldwide. About 5.1 million of the new cases of cancer were in developed countries and

5.8 million new cases in developing countries. An estimated 530,000 of the new cases of cancer occurred in sub-Saharan Africa [19]. In 2008, about 12.7 million new cancer cases occurred worldwide; 56 % were in the less developed regions of the world [20]. The rising trend in cancer incidence is expected to continue with the least developed countries being disproportionately affected [21]. In the recent 20 years, data from the Kampala Cancer Registry (KCR) in Uganda show an overall increase in the risk of cancers in both women and men. Greatest increases in risk were noted for prostate (5.2 % annually) and breast (3.7 % annually) cancers [9].

Facilities for Cancer Research and Care

Until the last decade, there was only one established center of excellence for cancer care, training, and research—the Uganda Cancer Institute (UCI) built in 1967 as a center for research and treatment for Burkitt's lymphoma. The UCI provides chemotherapy for cancer patients referred from all over the country [22]. However, with the increasing cancer incidence and burden on the population, two missionary not-for-profit private hospitals, St. Mary's Hospital Lacor and St. Francis Hospital, Nsambya, started to increase their scope of cancer care. In 2010, St. Francis hospital, Nsambya, started providing cancer care services majorly for gynecological malignancies including choriocarcinoma, cervical cancer, and breast cancer. Nsambya Hospital has worked with an Italian nongovernmental organization AISPO and in support with a local catholic bank, Centenary Rural Development Bank, to finance and construct a state-of-the-art center for cancer care. The rotary club of Kampala has contributed in raising funds for the construction of this cancer center through cancer runs campaigns. Both UCI and Nsambya hospitals are located in the capital city, Kampala. Located in the north of the country, St. Mary's Hospital Lacor has collaborated with the International Network for Cancer Treatment and Research (INCTR) to improve its status in the management of Burkitt's lymphoma. It is expected that the cancer treatment center will now grow to provide sustainable quality cancer care for the population of northern Uganda. The center is expected to enhance its surgical oncology services in addition to chemotherapy for childhood Burkitt's lymphoma.

There are two national and 15 regional referral hospitals in Uganda. Most of these referral hospitals have resident general surgeons and gynecologists who do some aspects of cancer care including biopsy for diagnosis and operative management of surgical and gynecologic malignancies including colorectal, ovarian, cervical, and breast cancers. These services are provided by general surgeons. There are hardly any specialist oncology surgeons, e.g., breast surgeons in Uganda.

There is currently only one functional radiotherapy machine (Cobalt-60) in Uganda located in Mulago National Referral Hospital in Kampala [23]. This center is often overcrowded with advanced stage cancer patients, and the machine frequently breaks down leading to long waiting time for patients to complete their radiotherapy sessions. Lacor Hospital had ever provided radiotherapy services for cancers, but this stopped during the mid-1990s as the civil conflict that engulfed northern Uganda for more 26 years since 1987 escalated.

In terms of cancer intelligence and registration, there is only one active population-based cancer registry, the Kampala Cancer Registry (KCR) that documents incidences and monitor trends in cancer rates and mortality [24]. The KCR provides relevant cancer statistics used for projection of cancer incidences and cancer planning in Uganda. It is one of the oldest cancer registries in sub-Saharan Africa, and it has been accredited by the International Agency for Research in Cancer (IARC) for providing quality data [24]. Recently, a new population-based cancer registry has been set up in St. Mary's hospital, Lacor in collaboration with the INCTR. This registry is expected to serve a population of about 664,000 from Aswa, Kilak, Omoro, and Nwoya counties in northern Uganda.

Hospice Africa Uganda (HAU) has been active in management of pain among cancer and HIV/AIDS patients since 1993. The head office for hospice is in Kampala but has branches in Mbarara and Hoima. The principles of operations of hospice include use of community volunteers, hospital-based care, and community outreaches [25]. Home-based care predominates hospice approaches because local researches among terminally ill patients in Uganda revealed that patients and their families prefer to be cared for and die at their homes in the company of their loved ones [26]. In order to increase availability of quality hospice care in the country, Hospice developed training programs for nurses, medical clinical officers, and medical officers in pain management principles and use of oral morphine for the management of cancer pain. Hospice provides scheduled short-term and long-term courses for various cadres of health workers. Since 1998, hospice has worked with the various health training institutions to incorporate hospice care and principles of pain assessment and management into many curricula in Uganda [25]. Hospice has contributed to the realization of pain control and palliative care for terminally ill patients in Uganda. To achieve its broader and long-term goals, hospice has fostered collaboration with the Uganda Ministry of Health to legalize the prescription of oral morphine by lower cadres of healthcare professionals including nurses and clinical officers who have received additional training from hospice. In addition, palliative care has also been included among the essential clinical services in the Uganda national health policy and the health sector strategic and investment plan [27].

Human Resources for Cancer Care

Currently, there are about seven oncology physicians and one oncology pediatrician directly involved in clinical care for cancer patients in Uganda. There are a handful of experienced gynecologic and surgical oncologists based in Mulago National Referral Hospital in Kampala. A limited number of other general surgeons and gynecologists in the regional referral hospitals have keen interest in and often contribute to surgical management of common malignancies including colorectal, breast, and cervical cancers. The radiotherapy unit in Mulago Hospital is run by four radiation oncologists.

In addition to these available human resources engaged in clinical oncology, there are visiting oncologists from collaborating institutions in the developed countries including Fred Hutchinson Cancer Research Center (FHCRC) in the US and Regina-Helena hospital, Italy. Clearly, this limited number of specialists is inadequate to meet the demand for timely diagnosis and prompt treatment for the common cancers in Uganda. Uganda and many other LMICs need to invest more in capacity development including in-service training and retaining oncology specialists in order to improve cancer care and reduce morbidity and mortality from cancers.

International Collaborations in Cancer Care

Decades of collaborations geared towards planning for cancer control, strengthening researches, improving quality of clinical care, building capacity of local physicians, and improving institutional capacity to deliver holistic high quality cancer care have existed between international institutions and cancer centers in Uganda. These collaborations started way back in the 1960s when the National Cancer Institute, USA, together with Mulago Hospital and Makerere University mutually agreed to build a cancer treatment, research, and training center known as Uganda Cancer Institute [22, 28]. This early collaboration was aimed at the development of treatment and research on a common childhood tumor, Burkitt's lymphoma, and later research into liver and esophageal cancers. Recent collaborations include the Fred Hutchinson Cancer Research Center and University of Washington in the USA with the Uganda Cancer Institute, the Case Western Reserve University and the UCI, Italian AISPO with St. Francis Hospital Nsambya, and International Network for Cancer Treatment and Research with St. Mary's Hospital Lacor [29, 30]. These collaborations have emphasized different aspects of cancer control as follows:

1. The FHCRC/University of Washington and UCI has been involved in training of oncology specialists in their center of excellence in the USA in both clinical oncology and research, and carrying out multitude of formative and clinical researches in the fields of infections-related cancers especially herpes virus- and HIV-related malignancies [29].
2. AISPO/Nsambya Hospital collaborations set up one of the first facility-based cervical and breast cancer-screening centers in Uganda as well as providing outreaches for cervical screening. This collaboration has also led to the establishment of chemotherapy center in Nsambya Hospital specializing in cervical, breast, and choriocarcinoma treatment/management.
3. INCTR/Lacor Hospital collaboration has concentrated on research and treatment of childhood Burkitt's lymphoma mainly in northern Uganda. In addition, Lacor has been involved in the Epidemiology of Burkitt's Lymphoma in East African Children and Minors (EMBLEM) research collaborations between the US NCI and Uganda, Kenya, and Tanzania geared towards improving the management of children with Burkitt's lymphoma [29].
4. INCTR and the African Cancer Registry Network (AFCRN) in collaboration with Lacor Hospital and the Kampala Cancer Registry have established a new

population-based cancer registry in Gulu, northern Uganda. The objective is to generate quality data from two population-based registries on exposures associated with specific cancers, incidence, mortality, stage distribution, treatment patterns, and outcome to inform planning and guide government and policy interventions relevant for cancer control [31].

Diagnostic Capacity and Accuracy

The histopathology laboratory at the department of pathology, Makerere University College of Health Sciences (medical school) has provided morphological diagnoses of cancers since the 1930s [28]. More recent histopathology laboratories have been established including in the pathology department of Mbarara University of Science and Technology, St. Francis Hospital Nsambya, Rubaga Hospital, Mengo Hospital, and St. Mary's Hospital Lacor. In addition, several private histopathology laboratories have emerged in the capital city, Kampala, over the last decade and have contributed to prompt tumor histology diagnoses. However, only a limited number of these histopathology laboratories provide immunohistochemistry studies to further characterize tumors and improve morphologic descriptions.

Recent studies have shown that morphologic descriptions are not adequate to accurately characterize tumors. In addition, morphological diagnoses require invasive approaches to obtain bigger chunks of tissues while in flow cytometry, small tissues samples suffice [32]. To minimize the rates of false positivity and negativity findings, it is important to do additional tests to determine cell surface receptors and characteristics with adjuvant tests including DNA-image-cytometry (DNA-ICM), immunocytochemistry, and Polymerase Chain Reaction (PCR) [33–35].

These adjuvant tests can be used in combination or solely to accurately diagnose cancers. In a recent review to assess accuracy and quality of pathological diagnoses in Uganda, review of tissue samples were done in external laboratories that used these adjuvant tests to augment their diagnostic capabilities. In one such case, an external international laboratory review of histopathology blocks locally diagnosed as Burkitt's lymphoma in the histopathology laboratory in Lacor Hospital showed that there were inconsistent applications of laboratory procedures and suboptimal tissue fixation and staining. The agreement between the local laboratory and external laboratory for tissues that were adequately fixed was about 82 % [36]. Similarly, an international histopathology laboratory in the Netherlands reviewed tissue blocks diagnosed as Non-Hodgkin's lymphoma (NHL) by the Makerere University histopathology department. The agreement between the two laboratories was 36 % (95 % CI 28–46; kappa 0.11; $P=0.046$) [37]. In both the Lacor and Makerere University histopathology laboratories studies, there were a substantial minority of patients assigned lymphoma diagnoses when they actually did not have lymphoma nor have any cancers at all [36, 37]. This illustrates the limitations of using only haematoxylin & Eosin (H&E) for morphologic diagnosis of various cancer types [38, 39]. Ancillary diagnostic tests including immunohistochemistry tests are therefore urgently needed to improve the quality of cancer diagnoses in Uganda.

Cancer Stage at Diagnoses

In Uganda, the majority of cancer patients are diagnosed with advanced stage cancers and experience poor survival [40–42]. Patients in advanced stage III/IV have higher risk of death than those in early stage of cancers [40, 43]. Even for potentially curable cancers such as Burkitt's lymphoma, diagnoses are often made after substantial delays. Most of the delays reported by caretakers of patients with BL in Uganda were attributed to the patient interval [44]. Kaposi sarcoma diagnoses were also made when the cancers were in advanced stage despite the fact that most of the patients included in that study were under regular care by clinicians providing HIV/AIDS care in Kampala [45]. Factors that lead to advanced stage of cancer at diagnoses include long patients and diagnostic intervals [46, 47]. And factors that influence these intervals vary depending on the sociocultural and/or geopolitical circumstances affecting people's beliefs and barriers to medical health seeking. In northern Uganda, women with cervical cancer inappropriately attributed their symptoms to other illnesses including sexually transmitted diseases and engaged in home-based management of these illnesses. While the majority of the women with cervical cancer did not perceive personal risk for cancer, they reported that they would have sought care early if they knew their symptoms were due to cancer [48].

Members of community influence the health seeking pattern of cancer patients. Lay consultations for cervical cancer symptoms often lead to enforcing advice for prompt health seeking. Community members in northern Uganda believed that use of traditional medicines are important remedies for cancers. The reasons for use of the traditional medicines stemmed from sociocultural beliefs about intrinsic effectiveness, low costs, payment methods for traditional medicines including credits but also the multitude of barriers to medical healthcare seeking [49]. Community perceived barriers to cancer care were similar to healthcare professionals' perceived barriers which included long distances to and unavailability of medicines at health facilities, disrespectful and discouraging behaviors of healthcare professionals, patients' inability to pay for health services and transport to health facilities, and inadequate knowledge about services [50].

Interrelationships of Cancer Care and Local Culture

Only limited studies have examined the relationship between cancer care and local cultural beliefs and care practices in Uganda and most of LMICs. This is in spite of the fact that culture is a strong determinant of a person's life. Culture can explain how illness, disease, and their causes are perceived; the behavior of patients in seeking healthcare; and the views and values of those delivering healthcare [51]. The culture of any given group helps determine what it means to be healthy; it influences acceptable methods for attaining, maintaining, and regaining health, and also influences how health and illness are described [52] and what sources of care are available for the different diseases. Thus, culture has important positive and/or negative influences on access to healthcare.

Different communities have local cultures with special description of every kind of illnesses or categories of illnesses. These cultural representations carry lots of meaning to that society and contain ideas and recommendations about the appropriate sources of treatments or action for the illnesses or illness categories. Choice of source of help-seeking also depends on what the particular community considers the probable causes of the illness. If a community believes that a certain illness, e.g., cervical cancer is caused by witchcraft activities directed to some person, the culture may prescribe help-seeking directed to some traditional practices [53]. These cultural beliefs and illness representations drive and explain the basis of choices of source of care and are thus very important in control of chronic diseases including cancers. Care that is not culturally competent can result in missed and/or delayed diagnoses of cancer and inadequate treatment for patients with cancer.

Illnesses have social significance and are socially shaped. How we perceive, experience, and cope with disease is based on our explanations of sickness [54] which in turn influences our expectations and perceptions of symptoms [55], and the way we label particular diseases and respond to them [56]. In northern Uganda, cervical cancer is perceived by some lay people as caused by use of family planning pills and injections, repeated use of condoms, and/or not washing a woman's genital immediately after sexual intercourse. Some members of the studied community in northern Uganda believed that poor diet and/or unhealthy foods distributed to them while in internment camps could account for an observed increase in number of cervical cancer cases among the women [57]. Consequently, in addition to some perceived barriers to medical health seeking, this community believed that cervical cancer could be best treated with traditional medicines rather than modern medicines [49]. Notably, there is increase in use of traditional medicines for the treatment of cancers in most parts of the world, and this may be explained by cultural beliefs about the causes of cancers and the perceived outcome of treatment with different treatment modalities [58–61].

Insights on Palliative Care

Until about 1993, many countries in Africa had never incorporated palliative care into their healthcare structure and budgets. Consequently, cancer patients that presented with advanced stage disease suffered avoidable pain [62]. In Uganda, palliative care has been successfully implemented through home- and community-based care approaches. Community volunteers and resource persons identify patients in need of chronic care and pain control and liaise with hospice staff members that then carry home visits to assess and enroll the patients into care. While this approach has been cost-effective and successful in delivering hospice care to the community, it faces a number of challenges related to inadequate number of volunteers, lack of transport means for the volunteers and staff, limited number of clinical staff to supervise volunteers, and lack of money to support needy patients [63].

Summary and Recommendations

Uganda currently has an estimated population of 35 million inhabitants, with high growth rates of 3.5 %, low life expectancy of 50.5 years for females and 45.5 years for males, respectively. However, the number of elderly persons who are at higher risks of cancers is rising and is currently estimated at 2.7 million.

Uganda is undergoing an epidemiologic transition. It currently faces a double burden of rising incidence of both communicable, e.g., tuberculosis and HIV/AIDs and non-communicable diseases including hypertension, diabetes, heart diseases, and cancers.

Although the incidence of cancer is rising worldwide, there is a marked increase in low- and middle-income countries. In Uganda, data from the Kampala cancer registry show an increase in the risks of prostate cancer (5.2 %), and (3.7 %) for cancer of the breast annually.

Uganda has few health facilities for cancer care. These include the Uganda Cancer Institute and a few private not-for-profit hospitals. The country has one of the oldest cancer registries that was opened in the 1960s. Uganda is currently collaborating with several organizations in cancer research and management.

The capacity for cancer management in Uganda is limited. Capacity is low in the areas of human resources for clinical management of cancers, as well as capacity of laboratory services to undertake various histopathological diagnostics tests for cancers.

Available evidence shows that societal reactions to cancer diagnoses and causes vary in different parts of the country. In central and northern Uganda, it has been found that cultural beliefs related to the causes of cancer influences choice of care for cancer [57, 64]. Fear of conventional chemotherapy and radiotherapy compromise use/uptake of these modalities of treatment. Treatment such as total mastectomy has cultural implications and is often rejected. Survival from cancer is thus hampered by late reporting and diagnosis in advanced stages at which time benefit of treatment is minimal [40, 41, 65].

There are important lessons that we do learn from developed countries. These include development of capacity—so as to have adequate number and equitable distribution of skilled human resources for management of cancers, better and advanced diagnostic equipments and technology, and increasing cancer awareness in the communities. We do recommend appropriate knowledge, skills, and technology transfer to developing countries so as to improve cancer care/management. This will contribute to improving the management of cancers and survival and quality of lives of cancer patients in low-income settings.

References

1. Frenk J, Bobadilla JL, Sepuulveda J, Cervantes ML. Health transition in middle-income countries: new challenges for health care. Health Policy Planning. 1989;4(1):29–39.
2. Kiwanuka N, Ssetaala A, Nalutaaya A, Mpendo J, Wambuzi M, Nanvubya A, et al. High incidence of HIV-1 infection in a general population of fishing communities around Lake Victoria, Uganda. PLoS One. 2014;9(5):e94932.

3. Nantongo JM, Wobudeya E, Mupere E, Joloba M, Ssengooba W, Kisembo HN, et al. High incidence of pulmonary tuberculosis in children admitted with severe pneumonia in Uganda. BMC Pediatr. 2013;13(1):16.
4. Seeley J, Nakiyingi-Miiro J, Kamali A, Mpendo J, Asiki G, Abaasa A, et al. High HIV incidence and socio-behavioral risk patterns in fishing communities on the shores of Lake Victoria, Uganda. Sexually Transm Dis. 2012;39(6):433–9.
5. Okiro EA, Bitira D, Mbabazi G, Mpimbaza A, Alegana VA, Talisuna AO, et al. Increasing malaria hospital admissions in Uganda between 1999 and 2009. BMC Med. 2011;9(1):37.
6. Jagannathan P, Muhindo MK, Kakuru A, Arinaitwe E, Greenhouse B, Tappero J, et al. Increasing incidence of malaria in children despite insecticide-treated bed nets and prompt anti-malarial therapy in Tororo, Uganda. Malaria J. 2012;11:435.
7. Mayega RW, Makumbi F, Rutebemberwa E, Peterson S, Östenson C-G, Tomson G, et al. Modifiable socio-behavioural factors associated with overweight and hypertension among persons aged 35 to 60 years in eastern Uganda. PLoS One. 2012;7(10):e47632.
8. Mayega RW, Guwatudde D, Makumbi F, Nakwagala FN, Peterson S, Tomson G, et al. Diabetes and pre-diabetes among persons aged 35 to 60 years in eastern Uganda: prevalence and associated factors. PLoS One. 2013;8(8):e72554.
9. Wabinga HR, Nambooze S, Amulen PM, Okello C, Mbus L, Parkin DM. Trends in the incidence of cancer in Kampala, Uganda 1991–2010. Int J Cancer. 2014;135(2):432–9. Epub 2014/03/13.
10. Musinguzi G, Nuwaha F. Prevalence, awareness and control of hypertension in Uganda. PLoS One. 2013;8(4):e62236.
11. Maher D, Waswa L, Baisley K, Karabarinde A, Unwin N. Epidemiology of hypertension in low-income countries: a cross-sectional population-based survey in rural Uganda. J Hypertens. 2011;29(6):1061–8.
12. Parkin DM. The global health burden of infection-associated cancers in the year 2002. Int J Cancer. 2006;118(12):3030–44. Epub 2006/01/13.
13. Parkin D, Bray F. The burden of HPV-related cancers. Vaccine. 2006;24 Suppl 3:S3/11–25.
14. Kostelecky B, Trimble EL, Bhatia K. Learning lessons from cancer centers in low-and middle-income countries. Infect Agent Cancer. 2013;8(1):44.
15. Maher D, Smeeth L, Sekajugo J. Health transition in Africa: practical policy proposals for primary care. Bull World Health Organ. 2010;88(12):943–8.
16. Uganda Bureau of Statistics UBOS. Projections of Demographic Trends in Uganda 2007–2017. UBOS UBoS, editor: Government of Uganda; 2007.
17. Ministry of Health (MOH). Uganda Demographic and Health Survey (UDHS). Kampala: Government of Uganda; 2006.
18. Thun MJ, DeLancey JO, Center MM, Jemal A, Ward EM. The global burden of cancer: priorities for prevention. Carcinogenesis. 2010;31(1):100–10.
19. Ferlay J, Bray F, Pisani P, Parkin DM. GLOBOCAN 2002: cancer incidence, mortality, and prevalence worldwide. Lyon: International Agency for Research on Cancer; 2003.
20. Ferlay J, Shin HR, Bray F, Forman D, Mathers C, Parkin DM. GLOBOCAN 2008: cancer incidence and mortality worldwide. Lyon: International Agency for Research on Cancer; 2010.
21. Bray F, Moller B. Predicting the future burden of cancer. Nat Rev. 2006;6(1):63–74.
22. Savage L. Former African cancer research powerhouse makes plans for a return to greatness. J Natl Cancer Inst. 2007;99(15):1144–5. Epub 2007/07/27.
23. Abdel-Wahab M, Bourque JM, Pynda Y, Izewska J, Van der Merwe D, Zubizarreta E, et al. Status of radiotherapy resources in Africa: an International Atomic Energy Agency analysis. Lancet Oncol. 2013;14(4):e168–75. Epub 2013/04/09.
24. Davies JNP, Knowelden J, Wilson BA. Incidence rates of cancer in Kyadondo County, Uganda, 1954–1960. J Natl Cancer Inst. 1965;35(5):789–821.
25. Merriman A. Going the extra mile with the bare essentials: home care in Uganda. Progr Palliative Care. 2010;18(1):18–22.
26. Kikule E. A good death in Uganda: survey of needs for palliative care for terminally ill people in urban areas. BMJ (Clinical Research ed). 2003;327(7408):192–4.

27. Jagwe J, Merriman A. Uganda: delivering analgesia in rural Africa: opioid availability and nurse prescribing. J Pain Symptom Manage. 2007;33(5):547–51.
28. Olweny CLM. The Uganda Cancer Institute. Oncology. 1980;37(5):367–70.
29. Adewole I, Martin DN, Williams MJ, Adebamowo C, Bhatia K, Berling C, et al. Building capacity for sustainable research programmes for cancer in Africa. Nat Rev Clin Oncol. 2014;11(5):251–9.
30. Orem J, Wabinga H. The roles of national cancer research institutions in evolving a comprehensive cancer control program in a developing country: experience from Uganda. Oncology. 2009;77(5):272–80.
31. Parkin D. The role of cancer registries in cancer control. Int J Clin Oncol. 2008;13(2):102–11.
32. Paul T, Gautam U, Rajwanshi A, Das A, Trehan A, Malhotra P, et al. Flow cytometric immunophenotyping and cell block immunocytochemistry in the diagnosis of primary Non-Hodgkin's Lymphoma by fine-needle aspiration: experience from a tertiary care center. J Cytol. 2014;31(3):123.
33. Böcking A, Stockhausen J, Meyer-Ebrecht D. Towards a single cell cancer diagnosis. Multimodal and monocellular measurements of markers and morphology (5M). Analyt Cell Pathol. 2004;26(1):73–9.
34. Onofre ASC, Pomjanski N, Buckstegge B, Böcking A. Immunocytochemical diagnosis of hepatocellular carcinoma and identification of carcinomas of unknown primary metastatic to the liver on fine-needle aspiration cytologies. Cancer Cytopathol. 2007;111(4):259–68.
35. Böcking A, Nguyen VQH. Diagnostic and prognostic use of DNA image cytometry in cervical squamous intraepithelial lesions and invasive carcinoma. Cancer Cytopathol. 2004;102(1):41–54.
36. Ogwang MD, Zhao W, Ayers LW, Mbulaiteye SM. Accuracy of Burkitt lymphoma diagnosis in constrained pathology settings: importance to epidemiology. Archiv Pathol Lab Med. 2011;135(4):445–50.
37. Orem J, Sandin S, Weibull CE, Odida M, Wabinga H, Mbidde E, et al. Agreement between diagnoses of childhood lymphoma assigned in Uganda and by an international reference laboratory. Clin Epidemiol. 2012;4:339.
38. Wittekind D. Traditional staining for routine diagnostic pathology including the role of tannic acid. 1. Value and limitations of the hematoxylin-eosin stain. Biotech Histochem. 2003;78(5):261–70.
39. Simpson PT, Reis-Filho JS, Lakhani SR. Breast pathology: beyond morphology. Semin Diagn Pathol. 2010;27(1):91–6.
40. Wabinga H, Ramanakumar AV, Banura C, Luwaga A, Nambooze S, Parkin DM. Survival of cervix cancer patients in Kampala, Uganda: 1995–1997. Br J Cancer. 2003;89(1):65–9.
41. Gondos A, Brenner H, Wabinga H, Parkin DM. Cancer survival in Kampala, Uganda. Br J Cancer. 2005;92(9):1808–12.
42. Coghill A, Mutyaba I, Okuku F, Phipps W, Harlan JM, Orem J, et al. Treatment recommendations for patients with NHL at the Uganda Cancer Institute. Blood. 2013;122(21):2960.
43. Mike M, Ronald W, Fabian N. Survival factors of Burkitt's lymphoma patients at discharge: the case of St. Mary's Hospital Lacor in Northern Uganda. Am J Health Res. 2014;2(1):9.
44. Buckle GC, Collins JP, Sumba PO, Nakalema B, Omenah D, Stiffler K, et al. Factors influencing time to diagnosis and initiation of treatment of endemic Burkitt Lymphoma among children in Uganda and Western Kenya: a cross-sectional survey. Infect Agent Cancer. 2013;8(1):36.
45. De Boer C, Niyonzima N, Orem J, Bartlett J, Zafar SY. Prognosis and delay of diagnosis among Kaposi's sarcoma patients in Uganda: a cross-sectional study. Infect Agent Cancer. 2014;9(1):17.
46. Gyenwali D, Khanal G, Paudel R, Amatya A, Pariyar J, Onta SR. Estimates of delays in diagnosis of cervical cancer in Nepal. BMC Womens Health. 2014;14(1):29.
47. Gyenwali D, Pariyar J, Onta SR. Factors associated with late diagnosis of cervical cancer in Nepal. Asian Pac J Cancer Prev. 2013;14(7):4373–7.

48. Mwaka AD, Okello ES, Wabinga H, et al. Symptomatic presentation with cervical cancer in Uganda: a qualitative study assessing the pathways to diagnosis in a low-income country. BMC Women's Health. 2015;15(1).
49. Mwaka AD, Okello ES, Orach CG. Barriers to biomedical care and use of traditional medicines for treatment of cervical cancer: an exploratory qualitative study in northern Uganda. Eur J Cancer Care. 2015;24:503–13.
50. Mwaka AD, Wabinga HR, Mayanja-Kizza H. Mind the gaps: a qualitative study of perceptions of healthcare professionals on challenges and proposed remedies for cervical cancer help-seeking in post conflict northern Uganda. BMC Fam Pract. 2013;14:193. Epub 2013/12/18.
51. Szczepura A. Access to health care for ethnic minority populations. Postgraduate Med J. 2005;81(953):141–7.
52. Kagawa-Singer M, Kassim-Lakha S. A strategy to reduce cross-cultural miscommunication and increase the likelihood of improving health outcomes. Acad Med. 2003;78(6):577–87.
53. Igun UA. Stages in health-seeking: a descriptive model. Social Sci Med. 1979;13A(4):445–56.
54. Kleinman A, Eisenberg L, Good B. Culture, illness, and care: clinical lessons from anthropologic and cross-cultural research. Ann Intern Med. 1978;88(2):251–8.
55. Mechanic D. Social psychologic factors affecting the presentation of bodily complaints. N Engl J Med. 1972;286(21):1132–9.
56. Waxler NE. Culture and mental illness. A social labeling perspective. J Nerv Ment Dis. 1974;159(6):379–95.
57. Mwaka AD, Okello ES, Kiguli J, Rutebemberwa E. Understanding cervical cancer: an exploration of lay perceptions, beliefs and knowledge about cervical cancer among the Acholi in northern Uganda. BMC Womens Health. 2014;14(84):1472–6874.
58. Pud D, Kaner E, Morag A, Ben-Ami S, Yaffe A. Use of complementary and alternative medicine among cancer patients in Israel. Eur J Oncol. 2005;9(2):124–30. Epub 2005/06/10.
59. Ku CF, Koo M. Association of distress symptoms and use of complementary medicine among patients with cancer. J Clin Nurs. 2012;21(5–6):736–44. Epub 2011/11/10.
60. Oh B, Butow P, Mullan B, Beale P, Pavlakis N, Rosenthal D, et al. The use and perceived benefits resulting from the use of complementary and alternative medicine by cancer patients in Australia. Asia-Pacific J Clin Oncol. 2010;6(4):342–9. Epub 2010/12/01.
61. Ezeome ER, Anarado AN. Use of complementary and alternative medicine by cancer patients at the University of Nigeria Teaching Hospital, Enugu, Nigeria. BMC Complement Alternat Med. 2007;7:28.
62. Minja BM. Cancer pain control in Africa (state of the art). J Palliative Care. 1989;5(2):31–4.
63. Harding R, Higginson IJ. Palliative care in sub-Saharan Africa. Lancet. 2005;365(9475):1971–7.
64. Koon KP, Lehman CD, Gralow JR. The importance of survivors and partners in improving breast cancer outcomes in Uganda. Breast. 2013;22(2):138–41.
65. Gondos A, Chokunonga E, Brenner H, Parkin DM, Sankila R, Borok MZ, et al. Cancer survival in a southern African urban population. Int J Cancer. 2004;112(5):860–4. Epub 2004/09/24.

Chapter 15
Cancer Care in Pakistan

Muhammad Shamvil Ashraf and Ahsan Jamil

Introduction

Pakistan is the sixth most populous country with 184.35 million people and an area of 796,095 km^2. It is a low to middle income developing country with per capita income of US$ 1368. The literacy rate is 58 %, and average life expectancy from birth is 65.7 years. Almost 21 % people live below poverty line. The human development index in 2013 was 0.515 making Pakistan 145 out of 187 in the world rankings [1].

The gross domestic product (GDP) in 2013 was US$ 236.62 billion [2]. As far as the GDP allocation on health is concerned, it is not only suboptimal but is far below the international standards. The Government of Pakistan since last 10–15 years is spending 0.6–1.19 % of its GDP and 5.1–11 % of its development expenditure on health. Over the last 5 years, this budgetary allocation has further dropped, and the recent figures 2012–2013 in term of percentage are 0.35 % of GDP [3].

Mortality trends in Pakistan give an idea of the state of maternal and child health in Pakistan. We are far below in achieving our goals to comply with MDGs targets [4]. Pakistan demographic health survey (PDHS) preliminary report for 2012–2013 although shows a declining trend (Table 15.1), but when we analyze the data in detail, it becomes pretty obvious that one in every 14 children born in Pakistan die before reaching his or her first birthday [5].

It would be logical and prudent to have an idea of the health system of Pakistan, before discussing the state of cancer care in our country. Federal government has a "stewardship" role as far as health system is concerned. This means articulating the vision and translating them into meaningful actions. Provincial government's role basically revolves round health system delivery. Based on this role functioning, all

M.S. Ashraf, M.B.B.S., D.C.H., M.C.P.S., M.R.C.P., F.C.P.S. (✉)
A. Jamil, M.B.B.S., M.Sc.
Department of Pediatric Oncology, The Indus Hospital, Karachi, Pakistan
e-mail: shamvil.ashraf@tih.org.pk

M. Silbermann (ed.), *Cancer Care in Countries and Societies in Transition*,
DOI 10.1007/978-3-319-22912-6_15

Table 15.1 Mortality Trends in Pakistan

Indicator	Between 1960–1970	Between 1990–2000	Current	2015
Under 5 mortality	227	128	89	52
Infant mortality	145	105	74	40
Maternal mortality	600	340	300–340	104

policy directions are given by the Federal government, and all activities are executed at the provincial level thorough multifunctional modes of delivery that ranges from Basic Health Units and Rural Health Units to district hospital and dispensaries. On top of this, there are many vertical programs interspersed within the health system with focused and targeted aims and objectives like, e.g., TB DOTS, and POLIO. Then, there are few primary health care programs, targeting the general population of our country and trying to achieve the goal of health for all. There are obvious gaps in the "Stewardship role" of successive governments in Pakistan and on a detailed analysis this is disconnect of health policy with evidence.

At the same time, there is a burgeoning private sector where an integrated system of health is being practiced localized predominantly in urban areas. There is significant philanthropic support in healthcare. In Pakistan, many hospitals are run totally on charity some of them providing tertiary care free of cost. The health insurance has started but limited to major cities.

With this backdrop, we have to see and evaluate the state of cancer care in Pakistan. This means we have to analyze a difficult situation, i.e., cancer care in the most vulnerable and high risk population of Pakistan in a health care system, where the service delivery is not standardized.

Current Status of Cancer Care

As there is no national cancer-based population registry in Pakistan and whatever data of cancer received is through the International Agency for Research on Cancer Registry (IARC), therefore the estimates on the burden of disease related to cancer are not exact. According to Globocan 2012, in Pakistan 148,000 people are diagnosed with cancer every year. Age-standardized rate, i.e., incidence per 100,000 people/year is 111.8. Risk of getting cancer before age 75 is 11.8 %. 101,000 people die from cancer every year [6]. As far as cancer in the pediatric population is concerned, the first population-based data came from IARC registry in Karachi [7]. Based on this data and current population, it is estimated that about 8000 children (<18 years) get cancer every year in Pakistan [8]. When we assess the burden of cancer in Pakistan, we must not forget Afghanistan where cancer treatment facility is minimal and substantial numbers of patients travel to Pakistan for treatment. The most common cancer seen in male and female is shown in Tables 15.2 and 15.3 [9]. The most common cancer seen in children at Children Cancer Hospital is shown in Table 15.4 [7].

Cancer treatment has gradually evolved from an individual to standard multidisciplinary treatment over last three decades in Pakistan. Before 1980s, cancer was treated

Table 15.2 Top 10 cancers in males

Site	Percentage
Lung	10.5
Lip, oral cavity	10.5
Stomach	7
Other pharynx	5.6
Oesophagus	5.4
Leukemia	5.2
Colorectum	4.7
Bladder	4.6
Larynx	4.3
Other and unspecified	42.1

Table 15.3 Top 10 cancers in females

Site	Percentage
Breast	26
Cervix uteri	15.7
Lip, oral cavity	6.6
Ovary	4.8
Oesophagus	4.2
Stomach	3.4
Leukemia	3.3
Colorectum	3.3
Non-Hodgkin's lymphoma	2.4
Other and unspecified	30.3

Table 15.4 Common pediatric cancers

Type of cancer	Children Cancer Hospital Karachi 1997–2011 (%)	IARC data of Karachi region 1995–1999 (%)
Leukemia	38	26
Lymphoma	18	22
Sarcoma	7	5
Bone tumor	7	10
Brain tumor	7	13
Retinoblastoma	6	4
Wilms tumor	4	4
Germ cell tumor	4	2
Neuroblastoma	4	2
Others	5	11

Note: IARC indicates International Agency for Research on Cancer

mainly by the surgeons and radiotherapists often without standard multimodality treatment. Now, there are centers providing standard multimodality treatment; however, the numbers are far too little considering the burden. Majority patients still do not have access to standard of care multimodality treatment.

With the exception of hematological malignancies, most patients present to surgeons and are initially treated by the surgeons. Most of these surgeons have no surgical oncology training hence oncological surgical principles are not followed, and many patients do not get standard treatment. College of Physicians and Surgeons Pakistan (CPSP) has recently recognized fellowship in surgical oncology, but this training is currently available only in one center.

Radiotherapy units have been the first and major cancer treatment facilities in Pakistan. Radiotherapy units have been working in few government hospitals since 1960s. At the same time, Pakistan Atomic Energy Commission (PAEC) established cancer centers that initially focused primarily on the provision of radiation treatment. Gradually, they have come to deliver chemotherapy in addition to radiation treatment, but do not have surgery or palliative care services. Currently, there are 17 PAEC centers all over the country. The new patients registered in all the PAEC cancer hospitals was 46,000 in 2010 covering almost one third of cancer burden in Pakistan. In addition to these radiotherapy centers, radiation facility also exists in private hospitals. According to a nationwide survey done in 2010, there were 41 mega-voltage teletherapy machines, 632 patients per physicist, and 549 patients per radiation oncologist [10]. While there was an increase in the number of radiation therapy centers, equipment and human resources, this was insufficient to comply with international guidelines and meet the demands.

The specialty of medical oncology has slowly developed since 1980s. The slow growth has been largely due to the absence, until the mid-1990s, of a formal national training program and continuous brain drain. There are currently less than 30 fully trained medical oncologists practicing in the country, and most cancer patients will never see a medical oncologist throughout the course of their treatment [11].

Like medical oncologists formally trained pediatric oncologist first returned to Pakistan in 1980s. However, major development has occurred only in the last two decades both in terms of manpower and facilities. There are 13 centers in Pakistan, where pediatric cancer care is provided. All these centers are limited to four cities in Pakistan [7]. Till to date two provinces, i.e., NWFP/Baluchistan, are devoid of a pediatric cancer facility. There are limited numbers of trained pediatric oncologists in Pakistan, and postgraduate training programs accredited by College of Physicians and Surgeons (CPSP) have been recognized recently and are limited to four centers of the country. With the existing dearth of pediatric cancer facilities in Pakistan, it becomes very obvious that substantial number of children with cancer remain undiagnosed and the remaining who are diagnosed are reported late, which further complicates the situation.

Interrelationships Between Cancer Care and Local Culture

Cancers are known to be a result of both genetics and lifestyle factors. Lifestyles emanate from cultural beliefs, values, and practices. Thus, culture affects both the risk factors for cancers and the meaning of the disease by influencing the behavior responding emotionally, cognitively, and socially to this disease. Culture will determine approaches to prevention, early detection, treatment choices, and management of side effects such as pain, appropriate psychosocial support, rehabilitation efforts, survivorship issues, hospice use, and effective end-of-life care [12].

Reflecting this on Pakistan, it is to be noted that although the nation articulates its vision through Islamic value system, but there is a strong local cultural bonding that has its roots in the Indus valley civilization. Pakistan is a multilingual nation which at the same time has strong ethnic background embedded with strong regional cultural values.

From a pure socioeconomic perspective, it is a fact that almost 65–70 % of the population of Pakistan has a rural background and agriculture being the main source of income. This rural environment has its inequities, and a system of unjust distribution of wealth exists afflicting our rural population. This feudal stricken environment does not take into account the basic human needs, and most of our rural population is deprived of basic human needs, like clean water and sanitation. This case mix makes our population vulnerable to disease and with time the growing incidence of cancer in Pakistan is quite explainable keeping the sociocultural and economic context in mind. The urbanized society is ill organized and unplanned. Health system is neither structured nor integrated, so a double burden of disease phenomenon presently exists in Pakistan, and we see a surge of communicable and noncommunicable diseases in our urban settings. Cancer is the most prominent disease that has emerged as a challenge.

While it is true that modesty along with a fatalistic bent of mind is a prominent attribute of our general population, but with the growing awareness and media influence urbanized population's demand for healthcare in an integrated fashion is growing day by day. Recent media coverage on a high infant mortality rate in Sind province has raised questions in the overall health delivery system. We are in a transitional phase at the moment where there is a prevalence of a certain concept of fatalism, "God's will or destiny" along with a conscious awareness for health for all. On most occasions, people believe that cancer is "inevitable and thus taking preventive measures may be moot." This may influence the active participation in screening and preventive measures, but contrary to this belief especially in urbanized dwellings there is a growing awareness of cancer and screening programs, for example, for breast cancer are becoming popular. Our social fabrics have its constraints by virtue of which the bread winner, i.e., elderly male is given preference as far as provision for healthcare is concerned. Pediatric population especially males within a household is the second preference and women are the worst neglected. Late diagnosis of cancers is the outcome of this preferential social system. Slowly and gradually, things are changing because of the growing awareness of the fact the cancer has a "hope," the sooner it is diagnosed the better is the outcome. Still what is being diagnosed is to be considered as the tip of the iceberg.

In spite of all disparities, inequities, and odds, Pakistani society has a strong "family system," and the interrelationships between the family members have an important role to play, especially in times of stress. It is a common finding that whenever a case of cancer is diagnosed whatever the settings may be the entire family comes together and emerges as a unit. Social safety nets in the form of family support are extremely heartwarming and a friend in need is a friend indeed becomes the order of the day. This enables the affected family to sustain the stressful situation and natural coping mechanisms come at the forefront. All these protective mechanism helps in the disclosure of unfavorable news to the physicians. Moreover, the head of the family does not face any intense feeling of guilt, anger, frustration, and shame of not being able to fulfill the responsibilities. At the same time, all critical decisions that are related to management, treatment, end-of-life care, palliation, and financial matters are family decisions and in most of the cases everyone owns them. Above all the concept of God's influence, the willingness to accept bad news and even mishaps is astonishing and in most of the cases is a strong psychological support to the patient as well as to the family.

In short while dealing with a patient and family with cancer, a physician must take into account the degree of their cultural inclinations, belief system, and the overall social fabric in order to communicate and provide best medical treatment effectively in the best possible circumstances. Invariably, compassion and empathy are indispensable in achieving this. For societies in transition like ours, a physician should be wary of imposing generalized belief models on patients without first understanding their background and preferences.

Individualized Oncology in Focus (The Perception of Personalized Oncology in the Individual Countries)

To address this issue, we have to see and evaluate the functioning of our health care system. Secondly, we have to acknowledge our societal norms and general behavior of our public towards cancer. On moral and ethical grounds and as articulated in our Constitution, health and well-being of the people of Pakistan is State's responsibility, but somehow the State is unable to exert its influence on the executive, as a result of which our health system's performance is suboptimal. General public's out of pocket expenses for procuring health services is considerable, but the dilemma that we face at the moment is that despite this personal contribution in procuring health services, the services available lack standards and even with massive expenditure the services received has many limitation. Prevailing situation is encountered with all cross sections of our society and is across the board, i.e., in rural as well as in urban areas.

This situation clearly mandates that for cancer a practice for provision of individualized care is out of question. Neither we have the trained manpower nor the infrastructure base to provide these services. Home health is being practiced in some urbanized dwellings, but very limited services are being provided through home health.

At the facility level, although cases are individualized on merit but the cancer protocols being practiced are "generic" although validated, time tested, and comply with the best practiced clinical guidelines. Service provision at the door step level is yet to be initiated. Patient with cancer is a "high demanding" patient and only facility-based individualized options can be thought of.

Critical Clinical Issues that Is Being Faced by the Health Care System

There are many critical clinical issues faced in the delivery of comprehensive cancer care in Pakistan. The important problems highlighting the inadequacies of our health care system are:

Manpower/Training-Related Issues

There is a severe dearth of trained manpower in oncology. This includes physicians as well as nursing. Nationally, in 2012 there were approximately 125 oncologists of all descriptions with some sort of postgraduate qualification practicing medical and radiation oncology [13]. There are approximately 20 pediatric oncologists for estimated 7–8 thousands annual new cases of childhood cancer in Pakistan. This state of affair is not only due to limited training centers but also due to continuous brain drain as a result of prevailing socioeconomic stagnation and law and order situation in Pakistan.

Undergraduate training in oncology is minimal [14] and contributes to lack of awareness among physicians as to how to screen, diagnose, and refer cancer. Communication skills and training in breaking bad news, both so important in cancer management, are other areas which receive scant attention in the undergraduate curriculum [15]. Postgraduate training is more structured, with 1–2-year diploma program, or more formal fellowships of the CPSP in medical oncology, radiation oncology, pediatric oncology, and now also in surgical oncology. There are currently only six sites nationally which are approved for training leading to the Fellowship of the College of Physicians and Surgeons (FCPS) in medical oncology and only four centers are recognized for fellowship in pediatric oncology. Radiation oncology is a stand-alone specialty, with its own exit examination and FCPS diploma.

As far as middle-tier oncology professionals such as physicists, technicians, and specialist nurses are concerned, the available resource are far from satisfactory and that there is a dire need for further training and for improving the quality of care provided [16]. With growing awareness and need assessment, in some centers designated diploma courses in oncology nursing have been initiated, duly accredited by Pakistan Nursing Counsel (PNC).

A gap analysis of one of the most prominent centers of pediatric oncology in Pakistan was conducted, taking 2014 AAP (American Academy of Pediatrics) guidelines for pediatric oncology as reference, showed that out of 16 international standards related to human resource; only 31 % met the international requirements, rest of the standards were partially met.

Infrastructure Facilities

Although there are specialized cancer hospitals and pediatric oncology centers in Pakistan, their numbers are far less than needed and in most of these centers level of infrastructure needed for providing comprehensive cancer care under one roof does not meet international criteria. A gap analysis of one of the most prominent centers of pediatric oncology in Pakistan was conducted from facility management perspective, taking 2014 AAP (American Academy of Pediatrics) guidelines for pediatric oncology as reference, showed that out of six international standards, the standards that were met were five, i.e., 83 %, but most of them, i.e., 60 % were outsourced.

Support Services

As far as capabilities in support services are concerned, most centers are lacking in this aspect. Out of the 20 international standards as per American Academy of Pediatrics (AAP), standards that were met were only 8, rest of the standards were either partially met or unmet. These were the findings of a self audit conducted in a notable cancer facility, based on AAP guidelines. Paucity of these services is a major cause of high morbidity and mortality in cancer patients resulting in poor survival and quality of life. There is a dire need for the development of adequate support services in facilities treating cancer across the country.

Abandonment

This is one of the toughest challenges in dealing the patients with cancer. The abandonment in pediatric oncology units in Karachi is as high as 20–25 %. This challenge has many dimensions and is multi-faceted. In most of the cases, the abandonment after a diagnosis is related to patient, family, and community psyche. Cancer is still synonymous with death in the illiterate and poor strata of society. Patient and family start fearing death as a direct and immediate consequence of cancer and refusestreatment upfront. Treatment of cancer is fraught with many complications, hazards, and risks particularly related to chemotherapy. Sometimes, the fear of side effects of chemotherapy is the only reason for abandonment and patient seeks treatment with alternative medicine. Long distance from the treatment center is another contributing factor. In a resource constrained situation with poor socioeconomic background, even if treatment is provided free of cost, managing residence and food away from home becomes impossible and family often discontinue curative treatment. All this mandates an "integrated approach"—an approach that takes into loop some financial assistance for poor and neglected patient, residence during treatment, counseling, and education in easy and comprehendible language.

High Infective Mortality and Morbidity

Infection-related mortality and morbidity among cancer patients is alarmingly high in Pakistan. Several factors like malnutrition, poor hygiene practices, unsafe water and food, lack of immunization, overcrowding, delay in seeking medical advice, and other comorbidity contribute to this. In one study, 24 % children died during treatment of Acute Lymphoblastic Leukemia due to toxicity and 85 % of those were related to infection [17]. In resource-poor country like Pakistan, giving intensive chemotherapy regimens alone is not likely to improve overall outcome, unless simultaneous major reforms are made in the supportive care facilities and infection control measures.

Lack of Uniformity of Care

One of the major factors leading to improve cancer survival in developed countries is employment of clinical trial methodology and following standard guideline for treatment. There is marked disparity and inadequacy of treatment offered in different treatment centers due to lack of following uniform guideline. The culture of working together and following a uniform treatment protocol has not developed yet in Pakistan. Pakistan Society of Pediatric Oncology (PSPO) is taking initiative to start a common protocol for the treatment of Acute Lymphoblastic Leukemia in children.

Lack of Awareness of Cancer

Majority of patients tend to present at a late stage in their disease [8]. The delay occurs at all stages from first consultation to referral to oncologist and diagnosis to treatment. The reasons for these delays are multifactorial including poor awareness among general public and physicians, inability to afford investigation, and distance from treatment center.

Insights on Palliative Care: Preferred Formats for Cancer Palliative Care

Given the large cancer burden, advanced stage at presentation and low cure rate the need of palliative care in Pakistan cannot be overemphasized. Development of palliative care services with prioritization of pain control were main objectives of WHO National Cancer Control Plan initiated in Pakistan in 2002 [18]. Unfortunately, implementation of the plan has been poor, particularly with regard to the development of services for early detection, palliative care, and morphine availability. As a result, most patients still present with advanced disease in need of palliation from the start, face abandonment when terminally ill and usually die of poorly controlled pain [19].

Palliative care in Pakistan is still at its developmental stage. With the exception of foreign qualified one palliative care physicians, there are no formally trained palliative care doctors in a country with an enormous cancer burden. Palliative care remains unrecognized at all level of medical education in Pakistan. There is no module of palliative care in any undergraduate and postgraduate medical curriculum except in oncology. There is no formal training, course or diploma offered by any medical and nursing institutions. In most places, palliative care is led by oncologist working in the organizations.

Palliative care nursing is also in the undeveloped phase. Very few institutions have trained nurses in their palliative care team with no formal qualification. Most of them are trained on job by physicians or have attended short courses or workshops. Pakistan Nursing Council the licensure body of nursing in Pakistan does not offer any certification or diploma in palliative care nursing [20].

The "registered" narcotics theoretically available for use are oral and parenteral formulations of morphine sulfate, parenteral pethidine and fentanyl, oral codeine phosphate, oral and parenteral buprenorphine, and fentanyl patches. The newly formed Drug Regulatory Authority of Pakistan (DRAP) has formulated new rules wherein any narcotics not already registered in Pakistan cannot be imported. The rules state that only companies approved by the DRAP can import narcotics [11]. Opioid availability is a major problem. Procurement of morphine in any institution is a complex, complicated, and cumbersome task. It has to go through four authorities: Federal and provincial health ministries, narcotic board and excise department. The whole process takes long team and often by the time it is procured the expiry is limited to 1.5 years. Morphine supply was sporadic but now with an increase in usage it is available most of the time [19].

Palliative care services are offered only in few hospitals and hospices in Pakistan. There are no community-primary health center services for palliation. Home-based service is only offered at a private hospital in Karachi.

There are fewer than five hospices limited to three major cities with no systemic approach to palliative care. These centers are mainly used for terminal care. At some of these centers, chemotherapy is also provided and they function more like a cancer hospital. They are looked after by oncologists and nurses. Psychosocial support is nonexistent or minimal. Most of them are run by NGOs with philanthropic support. Many of them have morphine available, but there is no multidisciplinary and pain management team.

A full multidisciplinary palliative care team exists only in two or three institutions in Pakistan. Other hospitals have some form of pain and symptom control. Other aspects like psychological, social, and spiritual support are mostly unmet.

Pediatric palliative care also remains in the early stages of development. Only one or two pediatric units have multidisciplinary palliative care team with physicians, nurses, psychologist, social worker, and spiritual counselor. Lack of trained personnel, insufficient supply of morphine, and the absence of outreach continue to remain major problems [8].

As far as format of palliative care in cancer patients is concerned, the awareness of new format of palliative support from the beginning of diagnosis is limited to professionals working in some oncology units while most of the places are still following old model, where patients are referred to palliative care team once curative option is exhausted.

Local Innovations

Oncologists and caregivers of oncology in a developing country like Pakistan have advantage to adopt evidence-based guidelines and protocol not only in treatment but also in the diagnosis and risk stratification of different types of cancer. With the availability of internet and web-based knowledge, there are huge learning and training resources for all interested health professionals. The most important thing that needs to be learned by the oncologists in our part of the world from developed countries is the culture of working together to ensure uniformity of treatment protocol. One has to document, analyze, and learn from the failures. It is also important to note that the contextuality of patient demographics, available resources, and availability of treatment modality sometimes does demand local modification and innovation. While on the one hand there is lot to be learned from developed countries, oncology in developing countries provide an opportunity for develop countries to learn about epidemiology and biology of different types of cancers due to large number of cases.

Role of Government, Private Sector, and Nonprofit Organizations in Cancer Care

As mentioned earlier, in Pakistan all health care policy directions are given by the Federal government and activities are executed at the provincial level. As far as cancer care is concerned, Pakistan Atomic Energy Commission (PEAC), a federal government institution, plays a major role looking after 25–30 % burden in 17 centers across the country. These are primarily radiotherapy centers, but most of them also deliver chemotherapy. They do not have surgery or palliative care services. The treatment is subsidized but not free.

At provincial level, there are facilities for radiotherapy and oncology units in few government hospitals of major cities. There is disparity among provinces; some have better facilities and care than the others. Most of the government hospitals however have no facility for diagnosis and treatment of cancer. The level of care given in these hospitals is also far from satisfactory. With few exceptions most of the time patients have to do out-of-pocket expense for cancer treatment even in government hospitals.

In the absence of free cancer care for all from government and very limited health insurance, a good number of patients seek treatment in private hospitals. There are oncology units providing standard of care multimodality treatment in both teaching and non-teaching hospitals. These are obviously limited to major cities; treatment is expensive and beyond reach of common person. Lot of patients start treatment in private hospitals but due to financial constraints abandon the treatment. These oncology units however are playing an important role in teaching, training, and setting the standard of oncology care. There are regular tumor boards and other CME activities related to oncology.

There is substantial contribution of philanthropy in delivery of cancer care in Pakistan both as a public–private partnership and stand-alone cancer center. The oncology unit at Sindh Institute of urology and transplant and National Institute of Child Health Karachi are evident examples of public–private partnership and Shaukat Khanum Cancer Hospital Lahore and Indus Hospital Children Cancer Centre Karachi are good examples of philanthropic culture prevailing in Pakistan.

There is no national statistics on access to pediatric cancer care in Pakistan. An exercise done by the author estimated that out of approximately 7000 children under 15 diagnosed with new cancer annually, almost one third have no access to any pediatric treatment center; 40 % are treated by pediatric oncologists, remaining are treated by pediatricians and adult oncologists.

Society Reactions Towards Cancer Patients

Pakistani society follows a collectivistic paradigm, where the social structure is firmly entrenched in social mores and values and traditions. The social fabric of society is glued together on the basis of relationships, traditions, and boundaries that have been set by our ancestors. Pakistani families will stick together through thick and thin and relatives will be supportive and compassionate and will help with time and money. We have seen relatives register shock and then the outpouring of sympathy and support begins, which is one of the most beneficial offerings of our society. It is not unusual to see siblings and uncles and aunts or grandparents and cousins staying at the hospital to look after the patient, opening up their homes and hearts to the afflicted family.

However as treatment is prolonged, the resources are drained especially when the reserve is scarce; the relatives and family start to lose their initial motivation; there is helplessness, frustration, and hopelessness. This pushes the family to the brink of emotional and financial bankruptcy. The support and sympathy from friends and extended family will thin out, except a few resilient ones.

On the other hand, we have strata of society where cancer is viewed as a dangerous malaise brought upon by the vengeance of God as a result of evil deeds of parents or kith and kin. Parents are asked to beg for forgiveness for their sins. People whose family has a cancer patient may become social pariahs and will be shunned by relatives and friends alike. In support groups run for the provision of further psychological assistance to the parents of children suffering from cancer, it was found that paternal side of the family often distance themselves from the person suffering from cancer and their family. There have been cases where the husband and wife have fallen out due to the stressors.

Families often become more closely knit, cancer will bring the family together even further as they turn towards spiritual healing to help in their emotional healing, thus hoping to ease the suffering of the patient. It has been seen that families who turn more towards spiritual support will feel more calm and peace and the distress levels of the patient and their families have been markedly less than in those who turn away from spiritual healing. That is not to say that one is wrong and the other is right but that which one of these philosophies aids in lowering distress levels and subsequently aiding families in adjusting to the challenges that are thrown in their path. This further helps in dealing with society's responses be they supportive or nonsupportive. And a society which is taught to be compassionate will be able to provide the kind of support and empathy required for patients suffering from cancer and their families.

Pakistan as a nation is a "giving nation" and our per capita donations for projects related to social welfare and health are phenomenal in spite of all our short comings at the state level, along with a misaligned health system. In the field of cancer, Shaukat Khanum Cancer Hospital and Children Cancer Hospital are evident examples of philanthropic culture prevailing in Pakistan. Society is willing for all help and support especially for cancer patients. At the facility level, optimal utilization of these philanthropic grants has to be ensured and if a facility has this kind of confidence in Pakistan, then it is seen quite vividly that sustainability of funds are ensured.

Summary and Recommendations

In summary, cancer care in Pakistan is in developmental phase facing many challenges. These are multi-faceted from huge cancer burden, dearth of trained manpower, paucity of training opportunities, lack of infrastructure, poor awareness, advanced stage presentation to poor spending by government on cancer prevention and treatment.

At the State level, the per capita expenses on health have to match the international standards. Cancer care will not improve unless the State takes the ownership. This provision in health budget has to be translated into an integrated system of health, with primary, secondary, and tertiary care facilities. Within the ambit of tertiary care, cancer care should be envisioned in a holistic fashion, designated cancer care centers meeting international standards. All this has to be complemented with a sound training environment for physicians, nurses, and technicians. Provision and procurement of medicines have to be easy and cheap, which means local manufacturing has to be thought of. Social Welfare at the state level has to be ensured. At the services level in order to avoid patient overcrowding and congestion, controlled home health, extended patient triaging are likely service innovation that can reduce the incoming patient load but are cost-effective infection control strategies.

An enhanced partnership is needed between the public, private, and philanthropic organizations for comprehensive cancer control program. The culture of working together needs to be inculcated among different centers not only for uniformity of care but also for training and research.

Acknowledgement The author would like to thank Erum Khan Ghazi for help in writing section of society reactions towards cancer patients.

References

1. http://www.pk.undp.org/…/pakistan/…/human-development. Accessed 11 Dec 2014.
2. http://www.tradingeconomics.com/pakistan/gdp. Accessed 11 Dec 2014.
3. http://www.heartfile.org/gateway1. Accessed 8 Dec 2014.
4. www.undp.org/…/pakistan/docs/MDGs/MDG2013Report/UNDP-Report13. Accessed 8 Dec 2014.
5. www.nips.org.pk/abstract_files/Priliminar Report. Accessed 8 Dec 2014.
6. http://www.cancerindex.org/Pakistan#sthash.3pTH7gnr.dpuf. Accessed 11 Dec 2014.
7. Bhurgri Y, Bhurguri A, Hassan SH, et al. Cancer incidence in Karachi, Pakistan. Int J Cancer. 2000;85:325–9.
8. Ashraf S. Pediatric oncology in Pakistan. J Paed Hematol Oncol. 2012;34:S23–5.
9. http://globocan.iarc.fr/factsheets/populations/factsheet.asp?uno=586. Accessed 10 Dec 2014.
10. Begum N, Nasreen S, Shah AS. Quantification of trends in radiation oncology infrastructure in Pakistan, 2004–2009. Asia Pac J Clin Oncol. 2012;8:88–94.
11. Yusuf A. Cancer care in Pakistan. Jpn J Clin Oncol. 2013;43(8):771–5.
12. Cheng C. Relationships between cancer characteristics and culture in Singapore. www.senkyo.co.jp/…/apcc0017.
13. Noronha V, Tsomo U, Jamshed A, et al. A fresh look at oncology facts in south central Asia and SAARC countries. South Asian J Cancer. 2012;1:1–4.
14. Jeeva I, et al. Oncology curriculum in developing countries and the lessons to be learned. J Clin Oncol. 2007;25:e12–15.
15. Jameel A, Noor SM, Ayub S. Survey on perceptions and skills amongst postgraduate residents regarding breaking bad news at teaching hospitals in Peshawar, Pakistan. J Pak Med Assoc. 2012;62:585–9.
16. Javed AA. Progress of oncology in Pakistan. Indian J Med Paediatr Oncol. 2006;27:54.

17. Asim M, Alia Z, Ghaffor T, et al. Death analysis of childhood Acute Lymphoblastic Leukaemia; experience at Shaukat Khanum Memorial Cancer Hospital and Research Centre, Pakistan. J Pak Med Assoc. 2011;61(7):666–70.
18. Nishtar S. National action plan for the prevention and control of non-communicable diseases and health promotion in Pakistan-prelude and finale. J Pak Med Assoc. 2004;54:S1–8.
19. Shad A, Ashraf S, Hafeez H. Development of palliative-care in a developing country, Pakistan. J Pediatr Hematol/Oncol. 2011;33 Suppl 1:S62–3.
20. Rehana P, Ashraf MS. Palliative care in Pakistan. In: Silbermann M, editor. Palliative care to the cancer patient: the Middle East as a model for emerging countries. New York: Nova Science; 2014. p. 165–70.

Chapter 16
Cancer Care in India

Suresh Kumar

Introduction

The republic of India with a population of 1.2 billion is located in Southern Asia, and covers an area of around 3,288,000 km^2. According to the United Nations human development index (HDI) India is ranked 127/177 countries worldwide (value 0.602). This places India in the group of countries with medium human development.

Cancer is a major health problem in India. Mention of various disease conditions with signs and symptoms similar to cancer dates back to Sushrutha Samhita, the classical Sanskrit text of Medicine dating back to sixth century BC [1]. But pooling together these conditions under the common diagnosis of cancer happened only with the entry of western medicine in India.

As per available data, the rate of incidence of cancer in the country is only one-fourth of the rate in Western Europe. But the high number of deaths from cancer, particularly of patients at a younger age group than in the West, and the projected doubling of the incidence in the next 20 years make it a priority in health care. Absolute number of deaths due to cancer is expected to rise from the present 700,000 per year to 1.2 million by 2035 [2]. Cancer burden of the country is further complicated by socioeconomic inequalities creating problem with access to and affordability of treatment [3, 4]. These factors complemented by inadequate screening and early detection facilities have caused the low incidence but high mortality paradox in cancer in India.

In the absence of proper facilities for treatment and the necessary social support system to support, for the majority of patients, a diagnosis of cancer in India mean catastrophic personal health expenditure and more or less sure death for the average citizen [5, 6].

S. Kumar, M.B.B.S., D.A., M.A., Dip. Pall. Med. (✉)
Institute of Palliative Medicine, Calicut, Kerala, India
e-mail: drsuresh.kumar@gmail.com

M. Silbermann (ed.), *Cancer Care in Countries and Societies in Transition*,
DOI 10.1007/978-3-319-22912-6_16

Current Status of Cancer Care in India

Disease Burden and Outcome

Actual data on the incidence and prevalence of cancer in India are not available. Under-registration is a major factor resulting in inaccuracies in incidence and prevalence data. Estimates based on data from National Cancer Registry Program by Indian Council of Medical Research are the main source of GLOBOCAN data on India. ICMR projections based on available NCRP data show a current incidence of 1 to 1.1 million cancer patients in the country [7]. The age-adjusted incidence of cancer in India of 98 per 100,000 by GLOBOCAN is only almost half of the global average of 182 per 100,000 populations.

The main cancers in men are oral, lung, stomach, colorectal, pharyngeal, and oesophageal cancers. Main cancers in women are breast, cervical, and colorectal cancers. All other cancers have an incidence of less than 5 per 100,000 population and will come under the definition of orphan diseases according to the USA and European Union definitions [8]. Breast cancer is the most frequently diagnosed cancer in women, followed by cancer of the uterine cervix. Mortality from cancer in women also follows the same pattern. Oral and lung cancers are the most frequent in men. Lung and stomach cancers lead cancer mortality in men.

Oral cancers account for over 30 % of all cancers reported in India. Estimated age-adjusted rates of oral cancer in the country are 20 per 100,000 population as against 10 per 100,000 in the USA, and less than 2 per 100,000 in the Middle East. This is particularly important from the treatment point of view because early detection of oral cancer offers good treatment outcomes and long term survival in theory. Oral cavity is accessible for visual examination and diagnosis is not difficult as oral cancers and premalignant lesions have well-defined clinical diagnostic features. But the majority of patients with oral cancer in India end up with poor treatment outcome due to delays in diagnosis and lack of access to proper treatment facilities [9]. Tobacco consumption habits including chewing betel quid or khaini and smoking bidis and cigarettes have been identified as the common cause of oral cancer [10]. Available evidence also points to an association between alcohol consumption and oral cancer. A significant dose response relationship between intake frequencies, duration, and risk with an increased hazard ratio of 49 % among current drinkers and 90 % among past drinkers has been observed [11].

Though the incidence is less, cancer survival in India is poor when compared to the High-Income Countries. Available data indicates that fewer than 30 % of Indian patients with cancer survive 5 years or longer after diagnosis as against the 5 year survival of 60 % in High-Income Countries. International Agency for Research on Cancer estimated indirectly that about 635,000 people died from cancer in India in 2008, about 6 % of all deaths in India. This number is also about 8 % of all estimated global cancer deaths [2]. India is a culturally diverse country, with huge regional and rural-to-urban variation in lifestyles and in age-specific adult death rates [12]. The number and rates of cancer deaths in India is anyhow projected to increase because of population growth, increasing life expectancy, increases in the age-specific cancer risks of tobacco smoking [13].

A recent nationally representative survey on cancer mortality in India showed that cancer deaths accounted for 8.0 % of the 2.5 million total male deaths and 12.3 % of the 1.6 million total female deaths at age 30–69 years. In 2010, at all ages, the rates of cancer deaths were about 59 per 100,000 for men and about 52 per 100,000 for women. But the rates of cancer deaths per 100,000 individuals rose sharply with age and at age 30–69 years, these were about 98 for men and 95 for women. The survey also revealed that 71 % cancer deaths occurred in people aged 30–69 years. The three most common fatal cancers in this group were oral (including lip and pharynx), stomach, and lung (including trachea and larynx) in men, and cervical, stomach, and breast in women. Tobacco-related cancers represented 42.0 % of male and 18.3 % of female cancer deaths. Age-standardized cancer mortality rates per 100,000 were similar in rural (men 95.6 per 100,000 deaths and women 96.6 per 100,000 deaths) and urban areas (men 102.4 and women 91.2). Mortality rates varied greatly depending on the states and educational status of the patients. Men aged 30 in northeastern India had the greatest risk (11.2 %) of dying from cancer before the age of 70, where as the death risk for men was less than 3 % in the adjacent states of Odisha, Bihar, and Jharkhand. Women in the northeastern states of India also had the greatest risk (6.0 %) of dying from cancer before the age of 70. Mortality rates were two times higher in the least educated than in the most educated adults [14].

Cancer Care

Getting treated properly for cancer is not easy for an average patient in India. India's public expenditure on health is one of the lowest in the world. Naturally, public health spending in cancer care is grossly inadequate to deliver a basic set of care for all cancer patients in the country [15]. For example, the ratio of radiotherapy machines available per population in India is 1 per 2–5 million, 10–20 times less than the ratio in High-Income Countries [16]. Health care remains highly privatized and commercialized for majority of patients in India and those with cancer are not an exception. Payment is mostly out-of-pocket despite the introduction of government-funded schemes in many states. It is estimated that more than 80 % of outpatient care and 40 % of inpatient care in cancer is provided by the private sector. Health insurance coverage is poor. Only around 15 % of the country's population has some degree of health insurance coverage [17].

Lack of trained professionals is also a major issue in the area of cancer care, particularly in rural India. This has created the problem of limitations of patients to access competent professionals. A study of resource poor regions in India has shown that a huge majority (more than 90 %) of patients from rural households with cancer first report to private practitioners, majority of whom (79 %) are not qualified in modern medicine [18].

Cancer is expensive to treat. Households affected by cancer spent the equivalent of 36–44 % of the annual expenditures of control households on inpatient expenses alone [19]. When they have access to treatment facilities in public sector, most of the patients reporting to these cancer centers in public sector find that waiting times are unjustifiably long. Such prolonged waiting times, in addition to delaying treatment, causes substantial expenditure due to related issues like lost income, cost of accommodation near the treatment center, and expenses for food [20].

The issue of oral cancer, with potentially good treatment outcomes, typically demonstrates the complexities of cancer care in India. The greatest threat of the oral cancer burden exists among people belonging to lower socioeconomic strata in the country. This segment of the population is the most vulnerable because of higher exposure to tobacco. They are also the segment of the population with most limited access to education, early detection and primary prevention of the disease and treatment with the result that treatment is delayed or not accessible/affordable and treatment outcomes becomes poor [21].

Individualized Oncology in Focus

Early Detection of Cancers

Most individuals in India lack access to facilities for early detection of cancer. Not many centers or programs for cancer screening are available in the country. For example, screening facilities for cervical cancer is available only in some district-level government hospitals (each hospital catering to a population of more than 30 million people) as a free test and in some of the private hospitals on a payment basis. Visual inspection with acetic acid is available in a few Tertiary Cancer Centers. Human papilloma virus based molecular tests are mainly available only through corporate private hospitals [22]. Clinical examination is recommended as the method to screen breast cancer, though many private hospitals offer mammography in line with the approach in high-income countries. The main approach to detection of oral cancers is through clinical visual examination.

Treatment of Cancers

Since most patients present with advanced disease, surgery and radiotherapy remain two of the most important areas of intervention. A recent study on economic burden of cancer treatment estimated the average economic cost of treatment of a typical cancer patient in a government facility in India to be about US$ 600 [23].

Cost of cancer drugs are a major issue. Most of the newer molecularly targeted drugs from the multinational pharmaceutical companies are beyond the purchasing capacity of average citizen in India [24]. The question of interests of the patient vs.

profit by drug companies in the light of the recent World Trade Organization directed new patent regulations has already surfaced by a couple of court cases. Pharmaceutical companies are fighting against decisions by the Patent Controller to issue compulsory licenses to local companies. These compulsory licenses will make the otherwise expensive drug available in Indian market at reduced prices. Novartis fighting a case for its leukemia drug, imatinib mesylate and Bayer on the cancer drug sorafenib. Bayer has even been arguing that "challenges faced by the Indian health care system have little or nothing to do with patents on pharmaceutical products"! [25].

Critical Clinical Issues

India is facing a low incidence–high mortality paradox in cancer [2]. The most important issue is that a large percentage of these deaths are preventable. 60 % cancer deaths in India are associated with tobacco or infectious diseases. Tobacco-related cancers represent 42.0 % of male and 18.3 % of female cancer deaths and there were twice as many deaths from oral cancers as lung cancers. The age-standardized death rate of 41.4 per 100,000 in men from tobacco-related cancers corresponds to a cumulative risk of 1.9 % of dying at age 30–69 years in the absence of other diseases. In women, the age-standardized death rate from tobacco-related cancers of 17.6 per 100,000 corresponds to a cumulative risk of 0.8 % of dying at age 30–69 years in the absence of other diseases. Cervical cancer is the leading cause of cancer death in India. The cervical cancer death rate of 16 per 100,000 suggests that a 30-year-old Indian woman has about 0.7 % risk of dying from cervical cancer before 70 years of age in the absence of other diseases [14].

Rates of cancer deaths in India are about 40 % lower in adult men and 30 % lower in women than in men and women in the USA or UK. But these mortality data should be seen in the background of incidence data. In age-adjusted terms the recorded incidence of cancer for India is only 94 per 100,000 people, which is only slightly more than half of the world average of 182 per 100,000, and about a third of the 268 per 100,000 recorded in the more developed countries [2].

Major factors making interventions cancer care less effective have been discussed. The main concerns from the point of view of oncologists that emerged in a study included practical constraints in access and treatment, cultural issues in communication, stigma associated with the disease, and inequalities related to place, gender, and class [26].

Palliative Care

Palliative care services can quickly and dramatically improve the quality of life for cancer suffers, other patients dying of chronic diseases, the elderly terminally ill and AIDS. Palliative care in fact relieves suffering and improves the quality of life of the living and dying. Majority of patients with cancer in India are in need of palliative care.

But with the rapid aging of the Indian population occurring, the highest number of patients needing palliative care will in the future come from the elderly terminally ill. India has a death rate of 7.4/1000 and a population of more than 1.2 billion which gives just under nine million deaths a year. The total number needing palliative care in India can be estimated to be 60 % of all deaths, or 5.4 million people a year.

Palliative care in India is about three decades old. But there is huge regional variation in the availability of services in the country. The south Indian state of Kerala with 3 % of the national population has more than 1000 home based palliative care services, with a quarter of them offering additional outpatient or inpatient services. Beyond Kerala, there are around 200 organizations providing hospice and palliative care services in 16 states or union territories. These services are usually concentrated in large cities and regional cancer centers, with the exception of Kerala, where services are more widespread. There is practically no palliative care service in most regions in the country, where health care professionals are not even aware of the concept of palliative care. There is no known palliative care provision in 19 states or union territories. There are places were excellent palliative care is offered to a lucky few in India, but overall less than 2 % of those needing pain relief and palliative care are getting it. If one takes out patients in Kerala (with more than 50 % coverage) out of this, the national coverage will be less than 1 % [27].

Outside Kerala, cancer palliative care services are not generally available below the level of Tertiary Cancer Centers (TCC) in the country. Some palliative care services are available in most of the TCCs. Most TCCs offer some outpatient clinics, a few inpatient beds, and patchy home care services but it has been observed that palliative care has not been a priority area for the TCCs in the country. Within the cancer centers offering palliative care services, such services are available only to 1–20 % of the patients though the majority of patients reporting to the institutions have advanced disease. A major reason for this can be the lack of the level of awareness about palliative care among doctors and nurses in cancer centers. Availability of basic medicines needed for palliative care is not ensured. Oral morphine is available in all the TCCs, but there are problems with regular use for the needy and uninterrupted supply. There are only a few health care professionals with adequate training (4–6 weeks) in palliative care in TCCs. This is true even of TCCs running palliative care services. There are only less than 30 doctors with a training of more than 1 week in all the TCCs together. The number of nurses with adequate training is still less [28].

Local Innovations

Despite poor progress in the development of proper cancer care services for the majority of the needy (or probably because of this), there have been a few significant local innovations in cancer care in India at the two ends of the management spectrum, namely early detection and palliative care. Both innovations involve the use of grassroots level workers to strengthen/facilitate mainstream health care services.

It has been proven that oral cancer screening by trained health workers can lower mortality of the disease, especially in individuals with a history of tobacco use through a large randomized, controlled trial of almost 192,000 people over an 8-year period. The study could demonstrate a significant reduction in mortality in the intervention arm (29.9 cases per 100,000) as against the control arm (45.4 cases per 100,000), due to detection at an early stage [29]. This project has important implications in early detection of oral cancers in many low- and middle-income countries.

More important probably would be the contribution of India to the concept and practice of community based palliative care services. The South Indian state of Kerala has managed to develop an integrated health service delivery model with community participation in palliative care which can be relevant in other regions of the world and also other areas of cancer care like primary prevention and early detection with community participation [27]. The emerging palliative care system in Kerala tries to address the problems of the incurably ill, bedridden and dying patients, both cancer and noncancer. It is also expanding to areas of community psychiatry and social rehabilitation of the chronically ill. The primary health care system in Kerala plays a major role in these activities.

The main components of Kerala's program are:

1. Community mobilization and ownership by the local community
2. Involvement of the local self-government institutions (LSGIs)
3. Incorporation of palliative care in the primary health care system

The major players in development of this public health model in palliative care in Kerala have been layperson volunteers in the community and Local Self-government Institutions in the state.

The main strategy in palliative care in Kerala has been to encourage local people to address the social needs of patients and families, train community volunteers to offer emotional support, facilitate the development of locally sustainable home care programs and to establish a network of nurses and doctors with expertise in palliative care to support these initiatives. The program has been very popular with the community.

Community volunteers in palliative care have been responsible for setting up most of the existing palliative care units in civil society sector in Kerala. The trained volunteers:

1. Help in identifying need and in initiating and running palliative care units in their locality
2. Visit patients at home (both with the home care unit and on their own)
3. Help at the outpatient clinic (keeping the patients comfortable, talking to them, helping with clerking, and so on)
4. Do administrative work (including clerical work and account keeping)
5. Raise funds for the unit
6. Mobilize support for the patients from the various governmental and nongovernmental agencies

In 2008, the Government of Kerala declared a pain and palliative care policy highlighting the concept of community based care and giving guidelines for the development of services with community participation for the incurably ill and bedridden patients. NRHM Palliative Care Project was initiated by National Rural Health Mission (Kerala) in 2008 with the aim of facilitation of development of a public health model in palliative care in Kerala in line with the Palliative Care policy of government of Kerala. The project has been trying to establish the primary, secondary and tertiary care facilities for all the bedridden, incurably ill and dying patients in Kerala with community participation.

As per the government policy, the Department of Local Self-government got palliative care included in the decentralized system and helped taking it to the whole of the state with the support of NRHM project. All the Local Self-government Institutions in Kerala now have home care programs in palliative care in their regions. The combination of economic, social, psychological, and medical approaches has ensured all-round care of the patients and support to their families, thereby increasing the quality of life and also the quality of death. The efficiency is increased by volunteerism and community involvement. This has facilitated home-based care, which otherwise would have been costly. The clear care and treatment protocols and the rational hierarchy of service provision have contributed to both efficiency and effectiveness. Capacity building with focus on attitudinal changes has further improved the project performance. The high local political priority of the program and its social acceptability and feasibility has helped to pool in other resources—human and financial—to contribute to efficiency.

Government Involvement

Government expenditure on health in India is miniscule. The country is among the lowest ten in the world in terms of public health spending per person. Cancer care is a priority area for the Government and the overall public expenditure is growing slowly, but not at the pace needed to deliver a basic set of cancer care for all cancer patients across the country [15]. Several basic health insurance schemes have recently been initiated by the central and individual state governments. Most of them are nowhere near adequate to cover the huge out of pocket expenditure incurred when getting cancer treated [30]. In the Federal Government system in India, health is a subject of the state governments and there is considerable variability in government expenditure in the area of health care [31]. Insurance schemes launched by South Indian states Karnataka, Andhra Pradesh, and Tamil Nadu are worth mentioning in this context. All the three cover cancer treatment and have reasonably high ceiling for coverage. Government of Kerala has also recently announced a scheme for supporting cancer care for patients in major cancer treatment facilities in the state, but the program is yet to take off in the real sense [32].

Inadequate investment by the Government in cancer care is only one of the problems. Absence of any regulations on private institutions including corporate hospitals providing cancer treatment has also resulted in absence of transparency regarding costs and outcomes. Non-standardized profit oriented inappropriate investigations and treatment are also not uncommon [33].

Government funds for cancer care are spent through complex administrative machinery with some of the components having overlapping roles. Ministry of Health and Family Welfare at the center charged with overall health policy is also responsible for cancer care. Four departments of the Ministry are involved in this process: Directorate General of Health Services, Department of Health, Department of Family Welfare, and Department of Indian Systems of Medicine and Homeopathy. The Directorate General of Health Systems provides technical support for the various health programs. Department of Health deals with health care, awareness campaigns, and all the national health programs. The Department of Family Welfare is responsible cooperation with nongovernmental organizations and international aid groups, and rural health services. The Department of Indian Systems of Medicines and Homoeopathy aims to strengthen research, promote the cultivation of medicinal plants used, and work on pharmacopoeia standards. More or less the same administrative structure responsible for cancer expenditures and planning exists at the state level also [34].

A National Cancer Control Program aimed at reducing cancer related morbidity and mortality was launched by Government of India in 1975 [35]. This program later got integrated with a national program for other noncommunicable diseases. The National Cancer Control program has the four components of prevention, early detection, treatment, and palliative care but the main focus has been on treatment only. India does not have any organized national cancer screening programs or national palliative care program. What is available varies with different states but all are basically opportunistic screening projects mostly through research projects.

Research

Almost all the cancer research in the country is concentrated in Tertiary Cancer Centres and certain central institutions of biomedical science. Progress in this area has been slow. During 1990–2010, the proportion of publications of research papers related to cancer from India in indexed journals increased from 1 % of the world's about 2 % [36]. Government provides the bulk of funding for research. The only other major funder is the US National Institute of Health. Involvement of pharmaceutical companies in research activities in the area of cancer in India is practically nil [36].

A national Cancer Grid has been formed recently by Government of India. This is envisaged to be a network of all the major cancer centers in the country with the mandate of creating uniform standards of patient care across country, making high quality cancer care available to the patients, augmenting human resource capabilities in cancer management and promoting collaborative research in cancer [37].

Involvement of Other Institutions

80 % of total health expenditure in India, from all sources (roughly 4.25 % of GDP) is in private sector business [38]. Almost all of the major cancer care centers in the private sector are non-academic private hospitals. Cost of treatment offered is not affordable to average Indian patients. On the other hand, many of these institutions also cater to patients from more affluent countries or the affluent strata of low-income countries through Medical Tourism. With globalization, increasing numbers of patients are leaving their home communities to seek treatment in countries like India. "Medical tourists" include patients from High-Income Countries trying to avoid treatment delays, people unable to afford health care in their home settings and also rich patients form Low-Income Countries in search of better facilities [39].

Society Reactions Towards Cancer Patients

Stigma occurs when society labels someone as tainted, less desirable, or handicapped. A disease like cancer is likely to generate this type of response from many quarters. Screening camps very often show lower proportion of the marginalized/socially disadvantaged population using the services offered [40]. It has been observed that one of the factors contributing to poor compliance in screening and treatment of cancer is social stigma attached to the disease [41]. A diagnosis of cancer is often perceived as death sentence. Family of the patient very often does not want the patient to know the diagnosis. Family often influences consultation by meeting with the doctor beforehand with a request to withhold information from the patient [42].

References

1. Bhishagratha KL, editor. Sushruta samhita. Varanasi: Choukhamba Orientalia; 1991.
2. Ferlay J, Soerjomataram I, Ervik M, et al. GLOBOCAN 2012 v1.0. Cancer incidence and mortality worldwide: IARC Cancer Base No. 11. Lyon: International Agency for Research on Cancer; 2013. http://globocan.iarc.fr. Accessed 30 Mar 2015.
3. Kawachi I, Subramanian SV, Almeida-Filho N. A glossary for health inequalities. J Epidemiol Community Health. 2002;56:647–52.
4. Balarajan Y, Selvaraj S, Subramanian SV. Health care and equity in India. Lancet. 2011; 377:505–15.
5. Engelgau MM, Karan A, Mahal A. The economic impact of non-communicable diseases on households in India. Global Health. 2012;8:9.
6. Pramesh CS, Badwe RA, Borthakur B, et al. Delivery of affordable and equitable cancer care in India. Lancet Oncol. 2014;15:e223–33. Published online April 11. http://dx.doi.org/10.1016/S1470-2045(14)70117-2.
7. ICMR. Time trends in cancer incidence rates 1982–2005; ICMR Bulletin, vol. 40 No. 2, Feb 2010.

8. Mallath MK, et al. The growing burden of cancer in India: epidemiology and social context. Lancet Oncol. 2014;15:e205–12. Published Online April 11, 2014. http://dx.doi.org/10.1016/S1470-2045(14)70115-9.
9. Kumar S, Heller RF, Pandey U, Tewari V, Bala N, Oanh KTH. Delay in presentation of oral cancer: a multifactor analytical study. Natl Med J India. 2001;14(1):13–7.
10. Khandekar PS, Bagdey PS, Tiwari RR. Oral cancer and some epidemiological factors: a hospital based study. Indian J Community Med. 2006;31(3):157–9.
11. Cancela MDC, Ramadas K, Fayette JM, et al. Alcohol intake and oral cavity cancer risk among men in a prospective study in Kerala, India. Community Dentistry Oral Epidemiol. 2009;37(4):342–9.
12. Registrar General of India and Centre for Global Health Research. Causes of death in India, 2001–2003: Sample Registration System. New Delhi: Government of India; 2009.
13. Jha P. Avoidable global cancer deaths and total deaths from smoking. Nat Rev Cancer. 2009;9:655–64.
14. Dikshit R, Gupta PC, Ramasundarahettige C, et al. Cancer mortality in India: a nationally representative survey. Lancet. 2012;379:1807–16.
15. Prachitha J, Shanmugam KR. Efficiency of raising health outcomes in Indian states. Working paper 70/2012. Chennai: Madras School of Economics; 2012.
16. Samiei M. Challenges of making radiotherapy accessible in developing countries. Cancer Control 2013. http://globalhealthdynamics.co.uk/cc2013/wp-content/uploads/2013/04/83-96-Samiei-varian-tpage-incld-T-page_2012.pdf. Accessed 28 Mar 2015.
17. Thakur J, Prinja S, Garg CC, Mendis S, Menabde N. Social and economic implications of noncommunicable diseases in India. Indian J Community Med. 2011;36 suppl 1:S13–22.
18. Dror D, Putten-Rademaker V, Koren R. Cost of illness: evidence from a study in five resource-poor locations in India. Indian J Med Res. 2008;20:347–61.
19. Datta A. Study finds that half of Indian households affected by cancer have to sell assets to fund care. BMJ. 2013;347:f5147.
20. Nandi A, Ashok A, Laxminarayan R. The socioeconomic and institutional determinants of participation in India's health insurance scheme for the poor. PLoS One. 2013;8:e66296.
21. Coelho KR. Challenges of the oral cancer burden in India. J Cancer Epidemiol 2012 (2012). http://dx.doi.org/10.1155/2012/701932.
22. Saxena U, Sauvaget C, Sankaranarayanan R. Evidence-based screening, early diagnosis and treatment strategy of cervical cancer for national policy in low-resource countries: example of India. Asian Pac J Cancer Prev. 2012;13:1699–703.
23. Mahal A, Karan A, Fan VY, Engelgau M. The economic burden of cancers on Indian households. PLoS One. 2013;8:e71853.
24. Experts in Chronic Myeloid Leukemia. The price of drugs for chronic myeloid leukemia (CML) is a reflection of the unsustainable prices of cancer drugs: from the perspective of a large group of CML experts. Blood. 2013;121:4439–42.
25. Arie S. Bayer challenges India's first compulsory licence for generic version of cancer drug. BMJ. 2012;345:e6015.
26. Broom A, Doron A. The rise of cancer in urban India: cultural understandings, structural inequalities and the emergence of the clinic. Health (London). 2012;16:250–66. doi:10.1177/1363459311403949.
27. Kumar S. Models of delivering palliative and end-of-life care in India. Support Palliat Care. 2013;7(2):216–22.
28. World Health Organisation (India). Review of palliative care in tertiary cancer centres and strengthening of existing palliative care services (APW 2010/144887). Unpublished Report, October 2011.
29. Sankaranarayanan R, Ramadas K, Thomas G, et al. Effect of screening on oral cancer mortality in Kerala, India: a cluster-randomised controlled trial. Lancet. 2005;365(9475):1927–33.
30. Public Health Foundation of India. A critical assessment of the health insurance models in India; 2011. http://planningcommission.nic.in/reports/sereport/ser/ser_heal1305.pdf. Accessed 28 Mar 2015.

31. Rao MG, Choudhury M. Health care financing reforms in India. Working paper No. 2012-100. National Institute of Public Finance and Policy; 2012.
32. Free Press Journal. Kerala becomes first state to provide free cancer treatment. 11 October 2014. http://www.freepressjournal.in/kerala-becomes-first-state-to-provide-free-cancer-treatment/. Accessed 31 Mar 2015.
33. Flores G, Krishnakumar J, O'Donnell O, van Doorslaer E. Coping with health-care costs: implications for the measurement of catastrophic expenditures and poverty. Health Econ. 2008;17:1393–412.
34. Rao MG, Singh N. Political economy of federalism in India. New Delhi: Oxford University Press; 2005.
35. WHO. 2008–2013 Action plan for the global strategy for the prevention and control of noncommunicable diseases. Geneva: World Health Organization; 2008.
36. Lewison G, Roe P. The evaluation of Indian cancer research, 1990–2010. Scientometrics. 2012;93:167–81.
37. Bhaumik S. Network of high quality cancer hospitals is planned for India. BMJ. 2013;346:f2858.
38. World Bank. World development indicators. Nov 21, 2013. http://data.worldbank.org/indicator/SH.XPD.PUBL. Accessed 4 April 2015.
39. Turner L. 'First World Health Care at Third World Prices': globalization, bioethics and medical tourism. BioSocieties. 2007;2:303–25. doi:10.1017/S1745855207005765.
40. Nene B, et al. Determinants of women's participation in cervical cancer screening trial, Maharashtra, India. Bull World Health Organ. 2007;85(4): 264–72. http://dx.doi.org/10.1590/S0042-96862007000400011.
41. Pradeep PV, Aggarwal V, Yip CH, Cheung PS. Spectrum of breast cancer in Asian women. World J Surg. 2007;31:1031–40.
42. Laxmi S, Khan JA. Does the cancer patient want to know? Results from a study in an Indian tertiary cancer center. South Asian J Cancer. 2013;2(2):57–61. doi:10.4103/2278-330X.110487.

Chapter 17
Cancer Care in Afghanistan

Mohammad Shafiq Faqeerzai, Abdul Tawab Saljuqi, and Massoud Samiei

Introduction

Geography and History

Afghanistan is a landlocked country in south central Asia bordered in west with Iran, in east and south with Pakistan and in north with Turkmenistan, Uzbekistan, and Tajikistan. With its strategic geopolitical situation in the cross road of trade routes political powers in Asia, the country has had a rich history of conflict and war during the past four decades. Since 1978 with the occupation of Afghanistan by the Red Army, the turmoil and civil war has never stopped. People had to immigrate to neighboring countries and millions of lives were lost during the fights between two rival factions. The infrastructures were demolished, social texture weakened, and human resources were heavily affected. This trend continued and even worsened over time.

Fortunately, in 2002 after the fall of Taliban, situation changed. International community invested billions of dollars in rebuilding the state and revitalizing the service provisions. Since then, a gradual improvement is seen in terms of government capacity, private sector involvement, and common people's life. During 2002–2005,

M.S. Faqeerzai, P.G.D., M.D. (✉)
Cancer Control, Afghan Society Against Cancer, 5200 Khushal Khan Mena, District 5, Kabul 1010, Afghanistan
e-mail: Faqeerzai@gmail.com

A.T. Saljuqi, M.D., M.P.H., Ph.D.
University of Arizona, USA

Public Health, Afghanistan National Public Health Association, Taimani, Kabul, Afghanistan
e-mail: Tawabsaljuqi@gmail.com

M. Samiei, M.B.A., M.Sc., D.I.C., Ph.D.
Senior Consultant Nuclear Energy/Cancer Control, International Atomic Energy Agency, Wagramerstrasse 5, Vienna 1400, Austria
e-mail: massoud.samiei@gmail.com

M. Silbermann (ed.), *Cancer Care in Countries and Societies in Transition*,
DOI 10.1007/978-3-319-22912-6_17

Afghanistan saw a tremendous progress in all walks of life including security. But after 2005, the insurgent activities augmented and security has started to deteriorate because Taliban regained their strength and regrouped against Afghan government supported by NATO and International Security Autonomous Forces (ISAF). The development pace slowed down after this but was never stopped. The peak of insecurity and instability was during 2013 and 2014. In 2015, NATO forces will leave Afghanistan, and the situation is expected to became worse. The long and unresolved election of 2014 has become another reason for destabilization and dismay in the country.

Population and Sociocultural System

The total population of Afghanistan according to Central Statistics Office (CSO) is 27.5 million [1] out of which 19.7 million is rural and 6.3 is urban. Around 1.5 million is nomad population. The most salient feature of Afghanistan population is its young generation that 46.1 % of it are people under 15 years of age.

Afghanistan is a diverse cultural society. If it is economically a poor nation, socially it has a rich culture. Religion is the upmost cultural drive for all personal beliefs, family behavior, and social norms. Islam is the main religion of the country with minorities of Hindus, Sikhs, and Christians. Tribal culture and style of living influence the social contracts and interactions; even it affects the political processes and decision-makings. Understanding the ethnic diversification of the country will help in understanding the programs that should be designed and implemented. People with different backgrounds have different approaches to disease and its treatment. Thus, good understanding of these nuances would help to provide a clearer account of the cancer care in Afghanistan (Tables 17.1 and 17.2).

Table 17.1 Economic indicators

Indicator	Year	Statistics
GDP: Gross domestic product (million current US$)	2009	12,853
GDP: Growth rate at constant 1990 prices (annual %)		
GDP per capita		456.6
Exchange rates (national currency per US$)	2012	51.5
Energy production, primary (000 mt oil equivalent)	2009	78
Exports (million US$)	2009	403.4
Imports (million US$)	2009	3336.4
Major trading partners (% of exports)	2009	Pakistan (47.4), India (18.8), Iran (10.2)
Major trading partners (% of imports)	2009	Uzbekistan (26.3), China (10.8), Japan (10.1)

Table 17.2 Social indicators

Indicator	Year	Statistics
Population growth rate (average annual %)	2010–2015	3.2
Urban population growth rate (average annual %)	2010–2015	4.7
Rural population growth rate (average annual %)	2010–2015	2.8
Urban population (%)	2010	22.6
Population aged 0–14 years (%)	2010	45.9
Population aged 60+ years (females and males, % of total)	2010	4.0/3.6
Sex ratio (males per 100 females)	2010	107.4
Life expectancy at birth (females and males, years)	2010–2015	45.5/45.5
Infant mortality rate (per 1000 live births)	2010–2015	146.9
Contraceptive prevalence (ages 15–49, %)	2006–2009	18.6 % Age group 10–49 years

Economy

Afghanistan's economy is hugely dependent on the international humanitarian aid with small contribution from general domestic revenue. The national domestic revenue is largely reliant on agricultural products. Dry fruit, carpet, and handicraft are among the key export products.

Health System

The war and conflict has always affected the health system and health service provision. Before war, Afghanistan had a relatively effective system of health provision. The public sector was responsible for both curative and preventive services at all levels of health service provision. The private sector was restricted to private clinics of doctors. During the soviet occupation of Afghanistan (1978–1988), the services inside the communist regime territory continued to rely heavily on government support focused mostly on urban hospitals and clinics. At the same period, the health services were provide to rural Afghanistan by Mujahedeen health services supported financially by international NGOs such as MSH, MSF, Swedish Committee for Afghanistan, and so forth. These services were mostly preventive and emergency. Health system during the rule of Mujahedeen (1992–1995) and Taliban (1995–2001) weakened to the state of collapse. The role of female health workers reduced and even during the Taliban government reduced to zero. It was at this period that slowly the private sector started to emerge, and it was later institutionalized and strengthened after the fall of Taliban government (2002) [2].

Current health system led by the Ministry of Public Health (MoPH) has a better coverage than before (60 % coverage in comparison to 9 % in 2002) [3]. The focus of the current health system is on provision of the basic health needs of the people through implementing Basic Package of Health Services (BPHS) and Essential Package of Health Services (EPHS). Both of these packages funded by the main donors (USAID, EU, and the World Bank) are contracted out to the non-governmental organizations, but the management and oversight is with the Ministry of Public Health [2].

The private sector has seen a tremendous surge in the past decade in the country. Ministry of Public Health developed a private sector policy and thereafter established the Private Sector Support Directorate in the framework of the ministry. Afghanistan National Development Strategy (ANDS) supports the free economy system and thus supporting the private sector in all aspects of life has been one of the government's priorities [4]. The health sector has benefited the most from it, and thus private hospitals, diagnostic centers, and medicinal stores have seen a huge development. The issue of a transparent and good oversight over the private sector though remains an area to be improved [5].

In response to the above developmental challenges facing the country, a very positive development has been the preparation of a 5-year Afghanistan National Development Strategy (ANDS) for 2008–2013 [4]. It provides a road map for transition towards stability, self-sustaining growth, and human development. It is a Millennium Development Goals (MDGs)-based plan that serves as Afghanistan's Poverty Reduction Strategy Paper (PRSP). As an integral component of this strategic plan, the MoPH has formulated the Health and Nutrition Sector Strategy (HNSS) 2008–2013 (updated in September 2009) as Health and Nutrition Strategy 2010–2013—NPNPS [6] that provides strategic directions for reducing morbidity and mortality and for institutional development. Furthermore, based on the identified need for an overall organizing framework for the MoPH, and building on the achievements of the past decade and lessons learned, the Ministry has developed the Strategic Health Plan (2011–2015) [4] with support from international donors. It is designed to enable further health gain for the Afghan people(s) and to strengthen the MoPH itself as an organization, over the next 5 years. This Plan is underpinned by a *Population Health Promotion Model* developed in 1970s and successfully implemented by the Public Health Agency of Canada and now universally adopted [7].

The Strategic Health Plan identifies ten *Strategic Directions*:

1. Improve the nutritional status of the Afghan population
2. Strengthen human resource management and development
3. Increase equitable access to quality health services
4. Strengthen the stewardship role of MoPH and governance in the health sector
5. Improve health financing
6. Enhance evidence-based decision making by establishing a culture that uses data for improvement
7. Support regulation and standardization of the private sector to provide quality health services
8. Support health promotion and community empowerment
9. Advocate for and promote healthy environments
10. Create an enabling environment for the production and availability of quality pharmaceuticals

Strategic objectives and priority interventions are identified for each of the above Strategic Direction for the next 5 years. Some of the key priorities identified are:

- Health system strengthening based on the values and principles of primary health care (main focus: human resource development, stewardship, and governance; health information system and health care financing).
- Social and environmental determinants of health.
- Control of communicable and *non-communicable diseases* (main focus: communicable diseases and mental health).
- Reproductive and child health (main focus: reproductive health and child health).
- Emergency preparedness and response (main focus: emergency preparedness and International Health Regulations (2005)).

In implementing this Plan, the government has recognized that a number of causes of death, illness, and disability in Afghanistan are preventable. International data show that preventing ill health and promoting positive health saves the health care system a lot of money. This also reduces unnecessary suffering and enables people to be more productive and to live longer, happier, and more fulfilling lives.

The formulation of these strategic documents has gone a long way in ensuring that all the stakeholders in the health sector align their priorities and programs with those of the government. The well-defined goals, priorities, and monitoring framework of the ANDS (2008–2013), the Health and Nutrition Strategy (2008–2013), the Strategic Health Plan (2011–2015), and the National Health and Nutrition Policy (2012–2020) ensure that international assistance is in alignment with and contributes to these goals and strategic directions. This is particularly important for the development of any new project to strengthen the national health care system to prevent and control the emerging chronic diseases such as cancer, which is clearly mentioned under the health service delivery of National Health and Nutrition Policy of 2012–2020 (prevent cancer through avoiding or reducing exposure to risk factors, screening of high-risk groups, early detection, diagnosis and treatment of cancer, and improving quality of life of those affected by cancer through public and professional education programs and improvement of services; and encourage and support private sector to invest in the establishment of specialized facilities for this purpose).

For the above reasons, and in line with the World Health Assembly (WHA) resolutions, the MoPH in Afghanistan has established a non-communicable disease (NCD) unit in order to develop the relevant policies and strategies to combat NCDs and cancer. A draft NCD strategy was developed in 2012 and is approved by the MOPH as the national strategy currently under review by the World Health Organization (WHO). Moreover, in line with the provisions of Afghanistan's *Strategic Health Plan 2011–2015*, the MoPH has initiated an action plan to develop a national cancer strategy within the scope of the NCD strategy.

State of Chronic Non-communicable Diseases

Chronic NCDs and mental health remain an important problem in the country. It is estimated that over two million Afghans suffer from mental health problems such as depression, anxiety, schizophrenia, and bipolar disorder. Due to the long period of civil war and conflict, it is estimated that most Afghans suffer from some levels of stress disorder. Mental diseases have not been addressed over the last decades in Afghanistan and little is known about the disease pattern in Afghan society. A study in 2000 compared the mental health status of women living in Taliban controlled versus non-Taliban controlled areas. Major depression among women living in Taliban-controlled areas was recorded at 78 % as against 28 % among women living in non-Taliban controlled areas. Suicidal ideation was alarmingly high—65 % in Taliban-controlled area versus 18 % in the control area and actual suicidal attempts 16 % in the Taliban-controlled area versus 9 % in the non-Taliban controlled area. There has been no demonstrable improvement in the mental health status of the population in the post-Taliban years. A nationwide survey conducted in the first year after the US-led invasion found high levels of depression symptoms (male 59.1 %, female 73.4 %), anxiety symptoms (male 59.3 %, female 83.5 %) and post-traumatic stress disorder (male 32.1 %, female 48.3 %) and confirmed by others. There is a clear correlation between the number of traumatic events and the likelihood of developing psychopathology.

Anecdotal evidence indicates that cardiovascular diseases, and cancer are being diagnosed with increasing frequency, but reliable estimates are not available about their incidence and of the prevalence of related risk factors in the general population (except for cancer data estimated by the International Agency for Research on Cancer as mentioned below).

Among the chronic NCDs, cancer is rapidly becoming a serious burden for the populations and health authorities in all low- and middle-income countries (LMICs). There is no country in the world where cancer does not occur [8], and Afghanistan is no exception. According to the latest WHO statistics, cancer causes around 7.9 million deaths worldwide each year. Of these deaths, around 70 %, that means 5.5 million, are now occurring in LMICs. If no action is taken, deaths from cancer in the developing world are forecast to grow to 6.7 million in 2015 and 8.9 million in 2030. Throughout LMICs, most health systems are designed to cope with episodes of infectious disease. Most LMICs do not have the financial resources, facilities, equipment, technology, infrastructure, staff, or training to cope with chronic care for cancers.

The matter has been given even a higher urgency following the 2012 World Health Assembly's decision to set a global target of 25 % reduction of premature mortality from NCDs by 2025 as a key target, among other targets, for the implementation of the above UN resolution [9].

Current Status of Cancer Care

The situation concerning cancer in Afghanistan is not different from the global cancer scene. Afghanistan a low-income country of nearly 30 million people is typical of many areas of the developing world. Modest increases in life expectancy have led to a subsequent rise in the number of cancer cases. At the same time, changes in lifestyle and eating habits, due to growing urbanization, are causing a surge in cancer and other NCDs. Cancer is already becoming a serious public health issue.

According to International Agency for Research on Cancer (IARC) GLOBOCAN 2008 [9], the cancer incidence in Afghanistan was around 14,355 per year in 2008, of which 11,539 died giving an incidence to mortality rate of over 80 %. Based on the same GLOBOCAN estimates, in 2012 there were around 16,300 new cases of cancer in the country. As there is no proper cancer registry in Afghanistan, the real numbers are not known, although based on experience elsewhere these estimates are close enough for planning purposes. In terms of incidence and mortality, the six most frequent cancers for men are stomach, oesophagus, lung, bladder, colorectal, and leukemia, and for women are breast, stomach, oesophagus, colorectum, cervix uteri, and leukemia. The *top six cancers* for both genders are: Breast, stomach, oesophagus, lung, colorectum, and cervix uteri.

Among the chronic NCDs, cancer is rapidly becoming a serious burden for the populations and health authorities in all low- and middle-income countries (LMICs). There is no country in the world where cancer does not occur [10], and Afghanistan is no exception. According to the latest WHO statistics, cancer causes around 7.9 million deaths worldwide each year. Of these deaths, around 70 %, that means 5.5 million, are now occurring in LMICs. If no action is taken, deaths from cancer in the developing world are forecast to grow to 6.7 million in 2015 and 8.9 million in 2030. Throughout LMICs, most health systems are designed to cope with episodes of infectious disease. Most LMICs do not have the financial resources, facilities, equipment, technology, infrastructure, staff, or training to cope with chronic care for cancers.

Cancer is however not a death sentence; there are proven ways to prevent and cure cancer. The good news is that medicine, health technologies, skills, and experience already exist to treat and cure cancer. Over 40 % of cancers can be prevented, and a third can be successfully cured. In health technologies, radiation medicine knowledge and techniques are indispensable for cancer diagnosis, cure, and care, where radiation and radioactivity play fundamental roles. Worldwide, radiotherapy is a major part of investments in the fight against cancer. Depending on the stage and type of cancer, on average some 50–65 % of all cancer patients require radiotherapy during the course of their disease, either on its own or in combination with surgery, chemotherapy, hormonal therapy, or immunotherapy. Providing equitable and affordable access to cancer care for all who need it and making the essential medicine, health technologies, and specialists available in their own countries are therefore increasingly high priority for most governments in LMICs.

This has also been a priority for many UN agencies beyond WHO, particularly the International Atomic Energy Agency (IAEA), and other active international organizations such as the UICC[1] and INCTR,[2] but has been given a new emphasis following the comprehensive resolution approved by all UN Member States in September 2011 on the prevention and control of NCDs, among which cancer is a leading cause of death.[3] The matter has been given even a higher urgency following the 2012 World Health Assembly's decision to set a global target of 25 % reduction of premature mortality from NCDs by 2025 as a key target, among other targets, for the implementation of the above UN resolution [10].

Afghanistan has had its first tumor registry system before 1968 which has been located at the Pathology department of Kabul Medical Faculty, in Kabul [6]. During a two and half project of registering tumors, 895 benign and malignant neoplasms were identified and diagnosed. The chapter published based on this research in 1969 is comprehensive and could be a baseline for comparing the progress of cancer and its treatment in this country.

A recent ASCO report has confirmed that there is no existing cancer registry or treatment facility in the country. Patients travel to neighboring states for treatment. Cancer assistance camps are one of the unique ways to offer some medical as well as social and educational support to the patients and their families. In 2008, the Indian National Cancer Society, an NGO, organized two such camps at Kabul. Media advertisement was used to invite cancer patients and relatives. Overall, about 350 patients were examined and data from these patients were analyzed. In the series, the commonest malignancy was found to be oesophageal cancer and gastro-oesophageal junction tumors. The second commonest problem was lung cancer. Cases of head and neck cancer were not as common in this study. Among females, breast cancer was in the highest level. The study concludes that the incidence of upper gastrointestinal (GI) cancer is unexpectedly high in Afghanistan. Several cancer risk factors are identified in Afghan society like cigarette smoking (active and passive smokers), air pollution, chronic disease like chronic peptic disease, Helicobacter pylori infection, spoiled food, hot meal, fatty food, obesity, chronic bowel disease, and longstanding use of proton pump inhibitor drugs (due to continuous hypo acidity of the stomach). There is however a definite need to study causative mechanisms or risk factors.

The situation for women with breast, cervix, and other cancers is even more dramatic and complicated with higher mortality to incidence rates due to inequities in health care and ignorance about cancer, among other issues. According to a WHO/ICO report [9], Afghanistan has a population of 6.26 million women ages 15 years and older who are at risk of developing cervical cancer. Current estimates indicate that every year 468 women are diagnosed with cervical cancer and 319 of them die from the disease. Cervical cancer ranks as the 4th most frequent cancer

---

[1] The Union for International Cancer Control, http://wwww.uicc.org

[2] See reference [2] above.

[3] The World Health Organization (WHO), http://www.who.int/nmh/events/un_ncd_summit2011/en/

among women in Afghanistan, and the third most frequent cancer among women between 15 and 44 years of age.

Unfortunately, specific research-based data on morbidity and mortality of breast cancer in Afghanistan is not available. According to a report issued by WHO in 2014, breast cancer annual crude incidence rate per 100,000 is 19.3 % [11].

Diagnostic facilities are very limited and treatment facilities are not available in the country. Since the cancer registry system is not available researchers and the decision makers are facing difficulties. Due to the lack of awareness most of the breast cancer patients go to a doctor at the very late stages. There is no recorded data on the mean age of women while diagnosed with breast cancer because we lack the diagnostic centers and a sound information system to collect this data. Total number of household is estimated to be around 3.6 million. Urban households are slightly larger than rural households. According to the NRVA 2011/2012, the household size in Afghanistan is 7.4. The average number of children under 15 is 3.4 which constitute 48 % of the household. Marriage is universal in Afghanistan, 25 % of women marry at age 15 or and at least 80 % at age 20. Of every six Urban households, one accommodates at least an elderly person while in rural households it is one in four. The households are all headed by male members only a minor percentage of families are headed by female. The NRVA 2011–2012 data indicate that 7.6 % of married women (over 260 thousand) are in union with a husband who has more than one wife. Around two-thirds of these have one co-wife. From the male perspective, 3.1 of all Afghan husbands have more than one wife. A large spousal age difference is the cause of high level female widowhood that is 57 % of women aged 65 and older are widowed [11].

This extremely unfortunate situation of high cancer in Afghanistan mortality is mainly due to late presentations by patients and lack of any reasonable cancer care facilities in the country, in addition to lack of an operational comprehensive cancer control program. The growing cancer epidemic in Afghanistan presents a major challenge to national health system. If present trends continue, the incidence is expected to double by 2030, and if no countrywide concrete actions are taken more and more people will die prematurely and needlessly from cancer in Afghanistan. This serious problem has already been recognized as a new health challenge within Afghanistan's latest *Strategic Health Plan 2011–2015* as highlighted before.

As the population of Afghanistan especially of the Kabul region has considerably increased in the past two decades, the number of cancer patients due to risk factors that already existed (age, family history, diet, smoking, and viruses) has expanded, and there is high demand for cancer treatment, particularly radiotherapy services in the country. However, at present, there are no cancer hospitals, nor any radiotherapy services in Afghanistan. Some surgery exists in ATH, a few private clinics offer limited chemotherapy, and the Indira Gandhi Children Hospital provides some treatment for pediatric leukemia, over 95 % of patients do not get any attention due to the lack of resources. There is a lack of capacity for prevention, public education, screening and early detection, diagnosis and treatment, whether involving surgery, radiotherapy, or chemotherapy, and palliative care. Due to lack of services, a very small percentage of the population who can afford it travel overseas for treatment, but many more die having never been properly diagnosed. Some patients are sent abroad by the government. The cost of treating cancer patients abroad is at least US$ 30,000 per patient and obviously cannot be sustained over a longer period or made available just to a few.

Regulatory Framework and Radiation Safety Infrastructure

As mentioned above, radiotherapy is a major part of investments in the fight against cancer. Depending on the type of cancer, on average some 50–60 % of all cancer patients require radiotherapy during the course of their disease, either on its own or in combination with surgery, chemotherapy, hormonal therapy, or immunotherapy. Over the past 40 years, the IAEA has developed strong technical expertise and acquired unrivalled experience in working with LMICs to build capacity in diagnostic radiology, nuclear medicine, and radiotherapy services at national level. It has mechanisms in place to provide assistance in all relevant aspects, such as needs assessment, planning, training, econometric analysis, implementation, and development of radiation protection, safety, and security infrastructure.

Currently, Afghanistan lacks any radiotherapy services and is therefore planning together with the IAEA to develop a minimum capacity in the country.

However, before initiating construction of a radiotherapy facility, approval has to be obtained from the national regulatory authority. The International Basic Safety Standards for Protection against Ionizing Radiation and for the Safety of Radiation Sources (BSS) produced through the joint work of IAEA, WHO, ICRP, ILO, and several other organizations [11] cover the application of ionizing radiation for all practices and interventions. The BSS can only be implemented through an effective radiation safety infrastructure that includes adequate laws and regulations, an efficient regulatory system, supporting experts and services, and a "safety culture" shared by all those with responsibilities for protection, including both management and workers. Extensive guidance and training on the practical implementation of the standards of safety in medical exposure as established by the BSS is provided by the IAEA [11]. Afghanistan has also received extensive assistance from the IAEA in this area through several technical cooperation projects.

Till 2008, all regulatory activities were carried out through the Radiation Protection Department of the MoPH. As of 21 March 2008, by means of a Presidential Decree, the Afghan Atomic Energy High Commission (AAEHC) was established and assigned the major task of "drafting and processing of the Nuclear Law through the Ministry of the Justice." The regulatory responsibility since then is within a department of the AAECH. The existing capacity in the MoPH will however be maintained to perform dosimetry and quality control services, where radiation is of concern in medical or industrial applications across the country.

The Nuclear Law, written in collaboration with the IAEA, was approved by the Ministry of Justice after certain improvements and passed on to the Council of

Ministers who endorsed it in December 2012 and submitted it to the Parliament for promulgation. In parallel, the regulatory staff is engaged with support from the IAEA in drafting of the following five regulatory documents to be processed after the Law has been promulgated:

1. Radiation protection
2. Control of radiation sources and ionizing radiation machineries
3. Safe transport of radioactive materials
4. Mining practices
5. Licensing

Afghanistan will also be adhering to the IAEA's *Code of Conduct on the Safety and Security of Radioactive Sources.*

Furthermore, since the Radiation Oncology Department of the KMU will be responsible for the operation of the ACCC, and it must apply for construction permit to AAEHC, an IAEA expert mission in January 2013 advised KMU on all safety issues to be evaluated when the application for construction is submitted. These issues included: the international standards and equivalent national regulations, responsibilities of the government, the regulatory body and the licensees, safety features of the radiotherapy equipment, facility layout and shielding, occupational and public protection, medical exposure protection as well as lessons learned from accidental exposures and measures for prevention. As a result of this mission, and in order to ensure the authorization process is fully in line with applicable safety standards and practices, AAEHC, KMU, and the IAEA have agreed on a 2-year work plan, which involves the training of two regulators on licensing and inspection of medical facilities, more specifically on radiotherapy (Annex D).

The IAEA will maintain its close cooperation with the AAEHC, KMU, and the MoPH and will provide the necessary advice and assistance on the licensing process and during construction and future operation of the ACCC.

Interrelationships Between Cancer Care and Local Culture

Islam is the predominant factor in Afghanistan culture. The Islamic beliefs are key to determine how people react towards cancer as a disease and towards cancer patients as the most needy people. Islamic teaching suggests that every Muslim should not put himself/herself in to Tahluka (a condition where death is imminent). This is very important lesson to avoid any risky behavior which may eventually cause any diseases particularly cancer. There are several citations in Quran that proposes that human beings should have mercy on each other and particularly on the ill and sick people. The prophet Mohammad behavior and sayings compiled as Hadith in big volumes emphasizes on the visiting the patients when they are in sickness and they are bed-bound. These teachings that are inseparable part of the Afghan local culture leads the community in an unconscious manner to have a cancer-free society and pay attention to the cancer patients whether they are in recovering phase or at the end-of-life stages.

This type of behavior and social norms can help the future cancer care programs and can be used for national cancer care communication programs.

In a study conducted about Afghan culture and family structure in Iran, almost all participants' responses regarding the Afghan family structure and gender roles were indicative of the conservative Afghan patriarchal tribal practices. One woman explained how male family members, particularly husbands, had a substantial influence on the women's screening decisions: "I don't know how to drive and can't read anything in English, so I need to have someone take me places and my husband is the one that usually does" [source needed].

Forty eight (90 %) of the participants indicated that they were dependent on family members' support, particularly their husbands or male relatives, in scheduling appointments, providing transportation, and interpreting and providing general care during health service.

Most women expressed that men's gatekeeping roles regarding interaction outside of the home, together with the traditional understanding and expectation of men as the head of the household and caretaker of the family had a profound effect on their decision-making power regarding their health care needs.

> In most Afghan family the man makes the important decisions about all things and how to deal with problems, even health problems.

"Husbands wouldn't tell their wives to go to the doctor and get examined." Screening were difficulty in understanding and navigating the health care system, transportation difficulties (including lack of transportation). Forty (75 %) of the participants reported language difficulties, lack of interpreter services, and problems in scheduling appointments as major barrier to health care access. They also commented on the lack of translated material in Farsi/Dari and Farsi/Dari-speaking interpreters at medical centers and clinics and questioned why more Farsi/Dari resources were not available [12].

Individualized Oncology in Focus

Afghanistan does not have reached to the stage to provide individualized oncology at this time. As noted in the previous sections, work on basic health care services for cancer patients is not available, but the individualized oncology is yet a far reached goal for us.

Critical Clinical Issues

According to the WHO, maternal and child health issues and communicable diseases are the critical clinical areas at the moment for Afghanistan. With one of the highest maternal mortality ratios (MMR) in the region (327/100,000 live births) and high burden of communicable such as bacterial diarrhea, cholera, meningitis, pertussis hepatitis A, and typhoid fever; vector-borne disease like malaria and leishmaniasis and animal contact disease as rabies; Afghanistan health system needs to focus on these two areas the most. Some of the communicable diseases are endemic to the country like TB and malaria. These infectious diseases exert a huge burden on health services, but fortunately these can be prevented or treated using low-cost and simple strategies. In spite of lack of reliable data, there is a consensus that HIV/AIDS is emerging as a serious health concern, given the increasing number of drug users. The anthropometric data point to high levels of both acute and chronic malnutrition. So malnutrition cases are high among children [12].

Insights on Palliative Care

Reviewing the current policies of the government and the ministry of public health, it was evident that palliative care in Afghanistan is not part of any policy or strategy. There is no concrete data on this topic. End-of-life patients are taken care by the close family members and are mostly at the risk of being ignored. Religion and traditions has some deep positive values that encourage the families to respect the very ill and elderly. This cultural practice provides some safety net for end-of-life palliative care but institutionally and programmatically there are no services available in Afghanistan. Even there are no educational programs to motivate general public in understanding the importance of palliative care except for Islamic teachings given sporadically through the religious leaders.

Local Innovations

Using mobile technology to improve the health system has started with few public private initiatives. Ministry of Public Health (MOPH) in an attempt to improve the coverage of maternal health services in few districts of Afghanistan has joined Care for Afghan Family (CAF) NGO and Paiwast, a local Information Technology company. The result of this joint work was measured through improvement in health care service utilization as recorded by Health Management Information System (HMIS). Similar technologies and joint efforts can be supported for cancer care both by government and civil society/private sectors.

Government Involvement

Currently, there are no cancer treatment services available in Afghanistan for any patients. Over 40 years ago, Afghanistan had some limited treatment services at the Aliabad Teaching Hospital in Kabul. But in 1992 due to civil war, the health infrastructure including Cobalt Therapy Centre in Afghanistan was destroyed, and the radioactive sources were removed out of the country. The Aliabad Cobalt Therapy Centre was inaugurated in 1967 by Paul Luzinci, the president of Hungary and Dr. Estrofski, the director of Commission of Energy. The project was supported by the International Atomic Energy Agency (IAEA), which provided the radioactive source (5000 Ci). In 1991, a set of radium sources for the treatment of gynecologic cancers was brought from Mumbai, India (Bhabha Atomic Research Centre).

Lacking any cancer care facilities or services, the question of providing affordable means of treating the growing number of cancer patients, particularly in terms of medicine and health technology such as diagnostic imaging and radiotherapy as an integral part of the health care system, has become increasingly of concern in the minds of policy-makers and health authorities, in addition to concerns about the most feasible strategies for cancer prevention and control in Afghanistan. Providing equitable and affordable access to health care for all who need it and making the essential medicine, health technologies, and specialists available in Afghanistan are increasingly high priority for the government as highlighted in the 2011–2015 Strategic Health Plan of the Ministry of Public Health.

In view of the above, the Ministry of Higher Education, which is responsible for the complex containing the Kabul Medical University, Aliabad Teaching Hospital, and a number of other health care facilities, has initiated in coordination with the Ministry of Public Health, the planning of a well-staffed and equipped cancer management center in line with the provisions of the current government strategies, particularly the 5-year Afghanistan National Development Strategy (ANDS) for 2008–2013 and the Strategic Health Plan (2011–2015). The proposed project can be implemented in three phases over a period of 7 years utilizing the existing buildings that formerly accommodated the Cobalt Therapy Centre and can be supported by other clinical services available at the Aliabad Teaching Hospital complex. The equipment, availability of diagnostic imaging and radiotherapy, and the development of full capacity in radiation oncology are essential for the success of the proposed project. However, considering the security issues within the country at present, cobalt radiotherapy may not be an option. Linear accelerators are recommended instead of treatment of common types of cancer in Afghanistan. High dose rate brachytherapy is also required for treatment of the carcinoma of the cervix, oesophagus, and bronchus, which are among the top cancers in the country. Diagnosis of cancer is currently challenging in Afghanistan due to the lack of dedicated imaging and diagnostic equipment. Proper diagnosis and treatment planning of cancer patients requires a well-equipped diagnostic unit in parallel with the radiotherapy center.

Institutional Involvement

Recently after the establishment of the new elected government, the first lady of the country Mrs. Ghani has emerged as the most active advocate of cancer care in Afghanistan. In October 2014, she inaugurated the Breast Cancer Day observation, and on 4th of February 2015 she gave a speech on the World Cancer Day celebration in Kabul. This coincides with the involvement of high profile women from parliament led by one of cancer survivors, Ms. Shinkai Karokhail. She not only started a movement called Cancer Support Group, but she has become a lead advocate in spreading the message about the breast cancer through media and around the country. Afghanistan National Public Health Association (ANPHA) has dedicated its 2014 issue of Afghanistan Journal of Public Health (AFJPH) to non-communicable diseases particularly to tobacco which is one of the key predisposing factors for lung cancer in men. ANPHA has established a collaboration with Afghan Society Against Cancer (ASAC) to conduct a short assessment about cancer care in Afghanistan and the results of which is used for developing this chapter of the book. Based on a survey we conducted among the health workers in Afghanistan, we found out that the top five priorities regarding the cancer care are:

1. Scarcity of preventive measures to change the life style of people in order to avoid cancer diseases at all.
2. Absence of data and information regarding cancer care is a top issue.
3. Absence of comprehensive diagnostic centers in Afghanistan is a key issue in pushing the patients to seek health care services outside the country.
4. Treatment of cancer patients is another priority for Afghanistan. Seldom people are treated in Afghanistan because of lack of diagnosis or lack of expertise. Both radiotherapy and chemotherapy centers are needed for Afghanistan.
5. Absence of expert health workers to provide prevention, early detection, treatment, and palliative care is a key challenge and priority [13].

Other institutions that can play a role in the cancer care program in Afghanistan are Afghanistan Medical Association, Afghanistan Surgeons Association, and Afghanistan Imaging Association.

Society Reactions Towards Cancer Patients

Successful cancer control efforts in most countries rely on civil society action and work at community level by the so-called cancer societies or leagues which act as non-governmental organizations (NGOs). Currently in Afghanistan, there is an active NGO called the Afghan Society Against Cancer (ASAC). ASAC is the leading organization dedicated to increase cancer awareness and advocacy among medical professionals and society at large to help reduce the incidence of cancer and ensure the best cancer care for everyone in Afghanistan. ASAC was established in 2009, as an NGO and as a member of the Union for International Cancer Control (UICC) and registered with the Ministry of Justice with license number 1684.

ASAC's Mission:

To reduce cancer incidence in Afghanistan and improve public awareness level regarding cancer.

ASAC's Vision:

A cancer-free Afghanistan.

Objectives

- Enhancing the society's level of knowledge about cancer and determination of risk factors for cancer in Afghanistan
- Launching of cancer awareness campaigns
- Improving health care providers' level of knowledge about cancer by conducting workshops, seminars, and training programs on cancer
- Initiating the development of a cancer control program in Afghanistan
- Developing a palliative care roadmap and working closely with the health authorities to establish palliative care capacity in Afghanistan
- Encouraging the establishing surveillance system in the country which could provide statistics and data about cancer in Afghanistan
- Encouraging the establishment of early diagnosis facilities utilizing modern technology and standardized approaches as recommended by the World Health Organization
- Encouraging the establishment of cancer treatment and research centers

Since its establishment, ASAC has been the leading voice for cancer patients in Afghanistan through advocacy and outreach on all key cancer issues particularly on cancer prevention, early detection, and treatment. It has developed and submitted to the MoPH two proposals on cancer control planning and capacity building in palliative care in the country. ASAC has also produced informative pamphlets on cancer and has organized a number of national events on World Cancer Day and Breast Cancer Day to increase public awareness and encourage government action. This has been achieved through its main office located in Kabul and support from professionals across Afghanistan. ASAC intends to establish four regional offices throughout the country in the near future, all of which will be involved in providing cancer support programs to the public.

ASAC is well placed to play a pivotal role in the development and implementation of all supportive actions required at society level for the launching of a cancer control strategy and the successful implementation of ACCC.

Summary and Recommendations

In summary, the infrastructure for cancer care in Afghanistan is very weak. The socioeconomical context has made it difficult to prioritize cancer care development in the past decade. Lack of data, lack of trained human resources and most importantly the absence of policies and strategies in this regard is clear. Recently, some efforts have been made by the Ministry of Higher Education and Ministry of Public Health to address the cancer care in a systematic manner. These efforts though uncoordinated are at the policy and programmatic level and needs years to establish a comprehensive system. Community awareness about cancer care is low and few civil society organizations have had the plan and vision to improve it. The main priorities of the cancer care in Afghanistan have been cited above. Here, we present the recommendations briefly; these recommendations are extracted from an online survey that was conducted by the authors.

1. *Prevention*: The policy-makers need to launch the "cancer control program" that would have four elements of prevention, early detection, treatment, and palliative care. Health promotion is the corner stone of the cancer control program where controlling smoking, improving nutrition, and promoting exercise are key steps towards a healthy lifestyle for prevention of cancer. Furthermore, launching a public awareness campaigns is a priority for Afghanistan through which all types of cancer sign and symptoms are explained. These campaigns should call for action which enables the population to detect some type of cancer by themselves and seek medical attention. It is proposed that general awareness should focus on women.
2. *Generating data and compiling information*: The first step towards this goal could be creating a cancer registry in Afghanistan. Establishing a cancer registration in all health care facilities all over Afghanistan could be an ideal vision to know the all incidence and prevalence of cancer in the country. However, we can start with few hospitals in Kabul, and then expand it to the provinces. Targeted surveys and researches can continue to enrich the data house for cancer care, but if these research efforts are strategic and led by one organization then the effect will be several folded.
3. *Establishment of diagnostic center capacity*: Founding a cancer center in Kabul with support of doctors, those who have already gained training in the fields of cancer care could be the first step. Providing state-of-the-art diagnostic and curative services will be the ultimate goal.
4. *Establishment of a radiotherapy center*: The previously cobalt center at Aliabad Hospital can be reestablished and discussion about providing radiotherapy facility inside Afghanistan should be started at the policy level. There is already some efforts and commitment by the IAEA.
5. *Establishment of a chemotherapy center*: The first step could be including cancer chemotherapy medication in essential drug list that makes these medications legal and popular in Afghanistan.
6. *Capacity building of health workers*: Training qualified doctors and personnel for prevention, diagnosis, treatment, and palliative care is important (Saljuqi and Faqeerzai 2014).

References

1. CSO. Central Statistics Organization [Internet]. http://cso.gov.af/Content/files/Population(3).pdf. [cited 25 Sep 2014].
2. Ministry of Public Health. Basic Package of Health Services for Afghanistan, 2005.
3. Afghan Public Health Institute, Ministry of Public Health, Central Statistics Organization (CSO) [Afghanistan], ICF Macro, Indian Institute of Health Management Research (IIHMR) [India], World Health Organization Regional Office for the Eastern Mediterranean(WHO/EMRO) [Egypt]. Afghanistan Mortality Survey 2010. Calverton; 2011.

4. Islamic Republic of Afghanistan. Afghanistan National development Strategy (2008–2013) [Internet]. 2008. http://www.undp.org.af/publications/KeyDocuments/ANDS_Full_Eng.pdf.
5. Amare H, Boccanera R, Intili A, Kissam E, Khuram MD, Williams S. Afghanistan Private Health Sector Survey, 2009.
6. MoPH. National Public Nutrition Policy & Strategy 2010–2013 [Internet]. 2009. http://www.basics.org/documents/National-Public-Nutrition-Policy-and-Strategy_Afghanistan.pdf.
7. Hamilton N, Bhatti T. Population health promotion: an integrated model of population health and health promotion. Health Promotion Development Division, 1996.
8. WHO. National cancer control programmes: policies and managerial guidelines. 2nd ed. Geneva: WHO; 2002.
9. World Health Organization. WHO|65th World Health Assembly closes with new global health measures [Internet]. http://www.who.int/mediacentre/news/releases/2012/wha65_closes_20120526/en/.
10. World Health Organization. Globocan 2012—Home [Internet]. International Agency for Research on Cancer (IARC). 2013. http://globocan.iarc.fr. [cited 25 Sep 2014].
11. IAEA. Radiation Protection and Safety of Radiation Sources: International Basic Safety Standards [Internet]. Vienna: 2011. http://www-pub.iaea.org/MTCD/publications/PDF/p1531interim_web.pdf.
12. Shirazi M, Shirazi A, Bloom J. Developing a culturally competent faith-based framework to promote breast cancer screening among Afghan immigrant women. J Religion Health [Internet]. 2015;54(1):153–9. http://dx.doi.org/10.1007/s10943-013-9793-z.
13. Bruni L, Barrionuevo-Rosas L, Albero G, Aldea M, Serrano B, Valencia B, et al. Human papilloma virus and related diseases in Afghanistan. Summary Report, 2014.

Chapter 18
Kazakhstan

Dilyara Kaidarova

Introduction

Global data shows that morbidity and mortality caused by malignant neoplasms grow all over the world, and according to the estimates of World Health Organization (hereinafter—WHO) by 2020 number of deaths from oncology diseases will get to ten million people. Seven million of those will be contributed by developing countries, including Kazakhstan.

Kazakhstan, officially the Republic of Kazakhstan, is a contiguous transcontinental country in Central Asia, with its smaller part in Europe (Fig. 18.1). Kazakhstan is the ninth largest country in the world by its territory with an estimated population of 17 million people as per 2013. It has borders with Russia, China, Kyrgyzstan, Uzbekistan, and Turkmenistan, and adjoins a large part of the Caspian Sea. The terrain of Kazakhstan includes flatlands, steppe, taiga, rock canyons, hills, deltas, snow-capped mountains, and deserts. The capital is Astana, where it moved from Almaty in 1997.

Kazakhstan was the last of the Soviet republics to declare independence following the dissolution of the Soviet Union in 1991; the current President, Nursultan Nazarbayev, has been leader of the country since then. Kazakhstan pursues a balanced foreign policy and works to develop its economy, especially its dominant hydrocarbon industry.

Kazakhstan has the second largest uranium, chromium, lead, and zinc reserves, the third largest manganese reserves, the fifth largest copper reserves, and ranks in the top ten for coal, iron, and gold. Perhaps most significant for economic development, Kazakhstan also currently has the 11th largest proven reserves of both petroleum and natural gas.

D. Kaidarova, M.D., Ph.D. (✉)
Almaty Oncology Centre, Almaty, Republic of Kazakhstan
e-mail: Dilyara.kaidarova@gmail.com

M. Silbermann (ed.), *Cancer Care in Countries and Societies in Transition*,
DOI 10.1007/978-3-319-22912-6_18

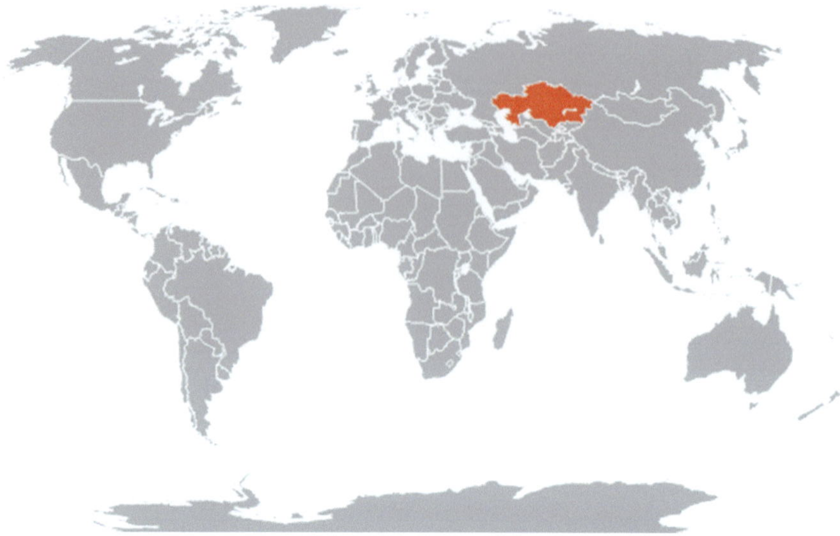

Fig. 18.1 Kazakhstan on the world map

Kazakhstan is populated by 131 ethnicities, including Kazakh (who make up 63 % of the population), Russian, Uzbek, Ukrainian, German, Tatar, and Uyghur. Islam is the religion of about 70 % of the population, with Christianity practiced by 26 %; Kazakhstan allows freedom of religion. The Kazakh language is the state language, while Russian has equal official status for all levels of administrative and institutional purposes.

Health care in Kazakhstan is provided by a network of primary, secondary, and tertiary care facilities. Health care facilities are largely owned and operated by the public sector represented by the Ministry of Health. Health insurance is now primarily provided by the government in the public sector.

Current Status of Cancer Care

In Kazakhstan, oncology mortality takes second place in the structure of mortality causes (Fig. 18.2). Every year over 17,000 people die from cancer in our country, more than 40 % of them are working-age individuals. Over the past 5 years, there is an upward tendency in the absolute number of cases of malignant tumors; annual increase of such patients is 5 %. In 2009, there were 28.3 thousand of oncology affected; by the end of 2013 this number exceeded 32,000.

Mortality rate for the same period decreased by 14.1 % from 113.7 per 100,000 of population in 2006 to 99.6 per 100,000 of population in 2013 (in ppm).

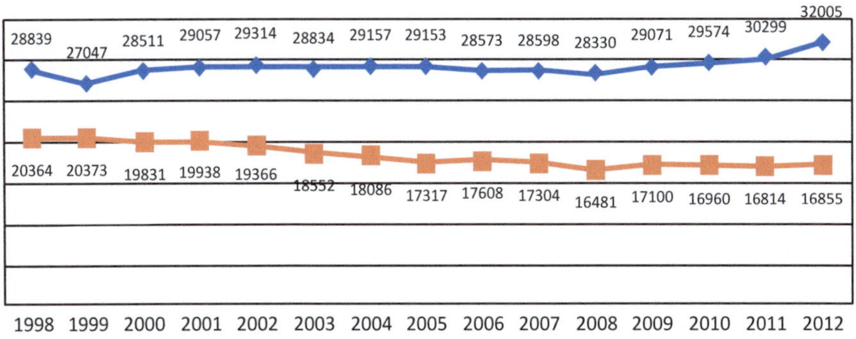

Fig. 18.2 Dynamics of morbidity and mortality in Kazakhstan for 15 years. *Source*: Kazakh Scientific Institute of Oncology and Radiology (2013). *Indicators of Oncology Services in Kazakhstan.* Almaty

Decrease of mortality rate is primarily due to the improvement of early diagnosis of malignant neoplasms and implementation of a national screening system, as well as the development of integrated treatment methods. At the same time, the rate is still below the rates of developed countries because mortality at later stages of cancer is hardly avoidable and very high.

The most common malignant tumors in 2013 in the country were breast cancer (12.1 %), lung cancer (11.7 %), skin cancer and melanoma (11.5 %), and colorectal cancer (9.2 %).

Key indicators describing current situation in Kazakhstan in terms of cancer are revealed in Tables 18.1, 18.2, 18.3, 18.4, 18.5, and 18.6 (*Source*: Kazakh Scientific Institute of Oncology and Radiology (2013). *Indicators of Oncology Services in Kazakhstan.* Almaty).

First place in the prevalence of cancer in the female population belongs to tumors of the breast which is more than 20 %. Then, it is followed by tumors of the skin, cervix, uterus, and stomach cancer. Another problem is that malignant neoplasms are affecting more and more young people. The mean age of women diagnosed with breast cancer is 60 (Tables 18.3 and 18.4).

Within the structure of morbidity among men, leading places are shared by lung cancer, stomach cancer, and skin tumors.

Geographically, leading positions in cancer morbidity and mortality for the last several years held by north and west regions of the country. Figure 18.3 demonstrates dissemination of cancer types among country regions.

History of the Oncology Service of Kazakhstan

History of the oncology service refers to the document "Improving cancer care to the population of Kazakhstan" 1945. Then, first oncology department for 25 beds was established in 1945. Afterwards, on this basis, Republican Oncology Center

Table 18.1 Cancer incidence rates in 2013

Lung cancer (17.6 %)	1
Stomach cancer (12.6 %)	2
Breast cancer (8.1 %)	3
Esophageal cancer (5.9 %)	4
Colon cancer (4.9 %)	5
Pancreatic cancer (4.9 %)	6

Table 18.2 Mortality rates in 2013

Female	Male
Breast 23.8 %	Lung 21.4 %
Skin (+mel.) 11.6 %	Stomach 12.9 %
Cervical 9.6 %	Skin (+mel.) 9.3

Table 18.3 Morbidity by cancer types, women, %

Rank	2012	2013
1. Breast	22.3	21.5
2. Skin	11.1	12.1
3. Cervical	9.2	9.1
4. Uterus	5.6	6.1
5. Stomach	5.7	5.7

Table 18.4 Annual morbidity among women (4000 breast cases)

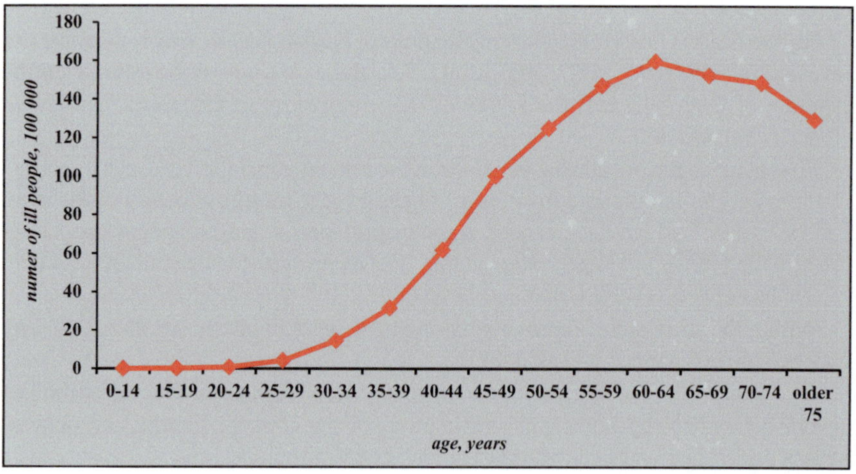

Table 18.5 Morbidity by cancer types, men, %

Rank	2012	2013
1. Lung	20.6	19.9
2. Stomach	12	11.8
3. Skin	9.6	10.1
4. Colorectal cancer	4.6	4.7

Table 18.6 National cancer care development program for 2012–2016

Improvement of life expectancy and quality of life of Kazakhstan citizens by lowering cancer mortality statistics	Objective
Advancement of cancer prevention through the development of screening programs. Increasing the access to high-technology methods of diagnostics and treatment that with proved efficiency. Creation of a modern system of rehabilitation and palliative care for cancer patients	Aims
2012–2016	Term of implementation
Decrease of cancer mortality to 97. 2 per 100 K by 2014, to 95.5 per 100 K by 2016; increase of percentage of I–II Stage cancers to 51.5 % by 2014, to 53.5 % by 2016; increase of 5-year survival rate among cancer patients to 52.0 % by 2014, to 52.5 % by 2016	Target indicators
State and local budgets Overall costs: 178.6 billion Tenge. (*$1.2 bln)	Sources and volumes of financing

Source: Program for Oncology Services Development in Kazakhstan for 2012–2016, Decree of the Government of Kazakhstan, 29 March 2012 #366

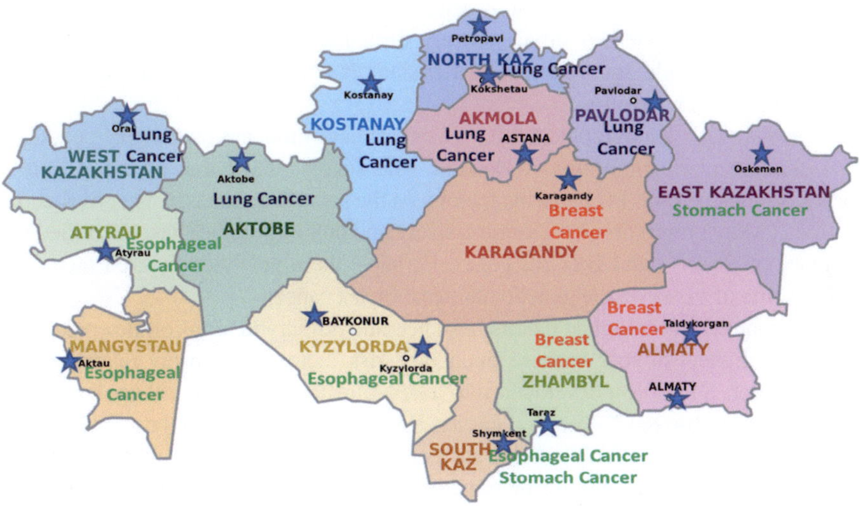

Fig. 18.3 Map of cancer morbidity by types and regions. *Oncological map of Kazakhstan:* Distribution of leading cancers in the various regions of Kazakhstan

was organized in 1947. Later, the oncology care system continued its rapid development. So, in 1947–1949 14 regional oncology centers, 1 city oncology center, 2 oncology departments, and 22 oncology offices were launched. As a consequence of scientific needs, the Kazakh National Scientific Research Institute of Oncology was established in 1960.

Kazakhstan Cancer Care Service

Today, cancer care service comprises 1 National Research Institute, 19 regional centers, and 263 consulting rooms in local outpatient clinics. Hospital and outpatient treatment provide free professional care and medication.

Each year around 350–400 children under age of 15 fall ill with oncological disease. By the end of 2013, there were 1310 children registered with a diagnosis of malignant neoplasm.

Provision of medicines for cancer patients for the last 10 years increased by 17 times from 3.6 mln.euro (2002) to 61 mln.euro (2012). Amount of medical treatment has increased by more than 2.5 times.

Interrelationship Between Cancer Care and Local Culture

Different forms of cancer closely refer to national traditions. Some cases of widely spread cancer are assignable, some—remain a mystery. For instance, the age profile of Kazakhs (both male and female) is very similar to a world one and dominated by young people, while age structure of Russians is closer to Europeans with a predominance of older groups.

There are also demographical differences that have influence on national peculiarities, though most commonly overlooked. The surveys show that breast cancer of Slavic women pertains to endocrine factors. At the same time, breast cancer of Kazakh women (Altay group) progresses aggressively and ongoing studies have identified the absence of BRCA1 and BRCA2 genes. Perhaps, these newly discovered facts will cause shifts of views on the genetic nature of breast cancer.

In recent years, ecological factors have become primary in terms of the epidemiology of malignant tumors because oncogenic risk factors are closely related to the environment; it has been developed into a new direction—"ecological epidemiology of oncological diseases." As stated earlier, Kazakhstan is second in the world by uranium resources. Main uranium fields are located in the North of the country, where an open and underground mining of uranium ore has been conducted intensively for more than 40 years. A big share of radioactive wastes has been accumulated to the present moment. Active and suspended wells and storing facilities—sources of radioactive contamination—pose a big danger to health of local population for those who work on a production and live nearby.

There are following noteworthy environmentally unsafe areas in Kazakhstan.

The *Semipalatinsk Nuclear Test Site* is located in East region. Here, for 40 years, since 1949 the vast majority of Soviet nuclear tests, including nuclear fusion and neutron bombs were conducted. Even though it has been more than 25 years since nuclear tests are over, its bad influence is still affecting not only the inhabitants of the Semipalatinsk region, but also the residents of neighboring regions. These north regions hold stable leading place in morbidity rank, with lung cancer prevalence.

It is still unknown how and to what extent people in regions close to *Baikonur spaceport* are affected. Here, we should note two factors that are harmful to their health and lead to cancer pathology development. First, heptyl that is used as a fuel in heavy liquid-propellant missiles contains many carcinogens, even in products of combustion. While not being fully burned out in disconnected rocket stages, it brings even greater damage to health and nature. Moreover, in case of a crash during the first phase of a rocket launching, liquid heptyl transforms into a droplet suspension, which then can cover significant territory inhabited with people and used for livestock and crop. Less attention is paid to the fact that every launched satellite leads to a hole in the ozone layer of our planet. This process, in its turn, reduces protective features of the atmosphere and increases the ultraviolet impact of the Sun that inevitably leads to an increase in skin cancer incidence on the territory of Kazakhstan around the spaceport.

The tragedy of the *Aral Sea*, which lasts for 30 recent years, has led to real ecological disaster. Desertification, salt marshes covered with sea salt, climate change due to the fact that the water surface has shrunk by its half—all this caused decline in life expectancy in the Aral lowlands, not talking about the growth of cancer pathology in the region.

There is a significant environmental degradation in *Almaty*, former capital and the biggest city of the country. From the south and southeast, it is surrounded by mountains reaching an altitude of over 6000 m above sea level. During the Soviet era, the city was built up with high-rise buildings without an air circulation by mountain breeze. Currently, the largest agglomeration in Kazakhstan, where there are more than two million people severely affected by gas pollution and smog, mainly produced by 700,000 cars. The high level of urbanization provides Almaty first place in breast cancer morbidity. Study of environmental factors' influence on the incidence of malignant neoplasms occurring at a certain spatial basis, i.e., geographical area, does not always take into account the ethnic heterogeneity of the population living in the area. At the same time, each nation is different with its own way of living, nutrition, family lifestyle, that is, everything that directly or indirectly may affect the incidence of cancer of specific body organs. Thus, in the *Kyzyl-Orda* region for example high incidence of esophageal cancer is due to eating a lot of all kinds of salted fish and smoked meat. Despite the availability of all the variety of food in the traditional fishing areas, people prefer to use not fresh or freshly frozen but salted fish.

The current way of life of many nations is a combination of old, historical traditions accompanied with modern lifestyle elements. Traditional Kazakh cuisine is mainly fatty boiled meat food (accompanied with traditional noodles) usually washed down with a very hot meat broth or tea. Permanence of a high share of stomach cancer and colon cancer in both men and women groups is connected with preserved national food traditions. Arising under these conditions carcinogenic situation develops in constant interaction of both old and new elements. As a result of this interaction, there is a significant change in the incidence of malignant neoplasms.

For instance, Kazakhs high increase in the incidence of skin cancer is perhaps due to the change of type of clothing—the transition from traditional to modern European. The low incidence of cervical cancer is due to the procedure of male circumcision, which is mandatory for Muslims, who constitute the majority of the population.

Individualized Oncology in Focus

Kazakhstan tends to support current trends in oncology development. As one of that trends—there is an individualized approach to the treatment of cancer patients that now strengthening its positions. As part of the development of this sector in Kazakhstan, "Cancer Registry" (electronic register of cancer patients) combined with a unified database was created in 2012 and successfully operates since then. In addition to general data, it contains the time of occurrence of the disease, the stage of the therapy, and further observation of the patient. It allows maintaining a personalized approach to each patient regardless of the place of treatment. Besides that, in order to address the issue of the appointment of treatment, multidisciplinary committees are being established. Each such committee is composed of oncologist, surgeon, radiologist, and chemotherapist. Each regional oncology center has immune-histochemical laboratory that allows individual approach to the treatment assignment. Also in 2012, free targeted therapy was implemented for patients with breast, colon, lung, kidney, and liver cancer.

Critical Clinical Issues

Insufficient use of modern technologies of diagnosis and treatment of cancer contributed to the slight increase in 5-year survival of patients over the past 5 years from 50.2 % (2009) to 50.4 % (2013). The minimum 5-year survival rate is observed for cancer of the liver, pancreas, and lung. Relatively low 5-year survival rate is because 46 % of patients with cancer are diagnosed and begin treatment too late, in advanced stages (III–IV stage).

The national screening program that is being implemented in our country allows diagnosing malignant tumors at early stages. However, international experience shows that radical healing as well as increase of 5-year survival rate of cancer patients identified at early stages (up to 80 %) is possible only in combination with such high-tech methods (that do not exist in Kazakhstan as of today) as proton therapy, radionuclide diagnostics and therapy, external beam radiotherapy (gamma knife, cyber knife, tomotherapy, stereotaxis, conformal therapy), intraoperative radiation therapy, vertical positron emission tomography, bio-transplantation of organs and tissues, minimally invasive surgery, use of various biological markers in clinical practice—oncogenes, estrogen and progesterone receptors, markers of apoptosis, growth factor, and other receptors. Determination of all these factors gives an opportunity for more detailed study of molecular-biological features of malignant tumors. This allows treatment considering the degree of differentiation of tumor, its sensitivity to therapy, and it allows affecting the course and prognosis of the disease in each case.

Interstitial radiation therapy (brachytherapy), implementation of which could save about 1500 lives a year, is at the initial stage of development in our country. In addition, due to the lack of equipment such method of treatment as intraoperative radiation therapy is not being used; however, this method can highly improve the results of treatment of some localizations (breast cancer, gastric cancer, and colorectal cancer).

Radionuclide diagnostics, single photon emission computed tomography (hereinafter—SPECT), positron emission tomography (hereinafter—PET)—diagnostic and treatment methods that are based on the identification of differences in the metabolism of normal and tumor cells (rather than on the size of the tumor) and which allow identification of signs malignancy in the absence of any anatomical changes. Kazakhstan has only one unit of PET in the capital city Astana, and, of course, this does not cover all the needs of the country. According to international data, on each 1.5 million of population one PET center is created. The use of nuclear medicine and radionuclide therapy can improve the results of treatment of cancer of the thyroid and prostate and increase the 5-year survival rate to 90 %. Besides that, radionuclide therapy allows successful treatment of patients with metastatic lesions in the bones and internal organs. Successes in cancer treatment are majorly determined by the implementation of modern methods of radiosurgery, but the situation in our country is so that due to the absence of high-tech equipment none of the oncology clinics (even a Republican one) uses such techniques.

In developed countries, the mini-invasive diagnosis and treatment of cancer patients is being used widely, and mostly it was predetermined by the improvements in early diagnosis area.

Lack of equipment that could allow conduction of video-endoscopic operations as well as the absence of simulation center and robotics resulted in that mini-invasive diagnostic and treatment methods are not being used in our country. Thus, there is a big number of operations where significant parts of affected body organs are removed and patients become disabled.

The peculiarities of drug therapy in malignant tumor treatment are duration and continuity of treatment that involves the use of drugs in the hospital and continuous treatment on an outpatient basis. Another specific feature of this therapy is the so-called targeted drugs that affecting only tumor cells. Provision of "targeted" drugs is on a steady level of 70 % of the needs. Starting in 2012, patients are provided with "targeted" drugs at the expense of from the state budget.

Due to insufficient use of modern methods of early diagnosis and treatment and, lack of cancer care availability, only 51–52 % of patients with cancer get specialized treatment nowadays.

Availability of cancer care to the population still does not meet current requirements. By the end of 2013, there were 331 cancer offices operating within primary health care organizations, which is only 84 % of the norm required. A shortage of qualified personnel persists: only 48 % of region oncologists (126 specialists) represent the core staff, other doctors—specialists in another area, working part-time.

Number of hospital beds in health care organizations with oncological profile does not meet the standards (2.5 beds per 10,000 population). As of January 1, 2012, this number was 2996 hospital beds, while the required amount is 4130.

In Kazakhstan, palliative care service is still in its development stage. Today, there are six hospices in the country, out of which only one—City Center of Palliative Care in Almaty—is state owned. Rehabilitation assistance to cancer patients is not developed.

Government Involvement

The importance and significance of the contribution that government makes in its effort to preserve either the health of its citizens or treatment of such sophisticated group of patients as cancer one are undeniable. Crucial issue here is the implementation of state programs, initiated by the President Nursultan Nazarbayev. Within these programs, the preservation and improvement of the nation's health, cancer prevention, and reduction of mortality are crucial parts of state policy.

The first in this list are such large-scale nationwide programs as National Healthcare Development Program called "Salamatty (Healthy) Kazakhstan" for 2011–2015 and Cancer Care Development Program in the Republic of Kazakhstan for 2012–2016.

The main objective of Cancer Care Development program for 2012–2016 is to increase the length and quality of life of Kazakhstani people by reducing the mortality from malignant neoplasms.

National Healthcare Development Program for 2011–2015 "Salamatty Kazakhstan"

National Healthcare Development Program for 2011–2015 has following key features:

- Life expectancy increase to 69.5 by 2013, to 70 by 2015
- Total mortality decrease to 8.14 per 1000 people by 2013, to 7.62 per 1000 people by 2015
- Maternal mortality decrease to 28.1 per 100,000 people by 2013, to 24.5 per 100,000 people by 2015
- Infant mortality decrease to 14.1 8.14 per 1000 people by 2013, to 12.3 per 1000 people by 2015
- Tuberculosis disease decrease to 98.1 per 100,000 people by 2013, to 94.7 per 100,000 people by 2015

- Maintenance of the HIV spread in 15–49-aged group at 0.2–0.6 % level (average world rate is 1.1 %)

It is worth noting, that in terms of the magnitude of the above tasks, strategic importance and volume of allocated funds, these development programs are unique among CIS countries and many countries in Europe and Southeast Asia.

In particular, the development of cancer care program provides creation of five powerful regional radiation oncology centers in Astana, Almaty, Semey, Aktobe, and Karaganda.

These centers are planned to be equipped with modern facilities in order to implement such treatment technologies as high-energy external beam radiotherapy, intraoperative radiation therapy, radionuclide therapy, as well as mini-invasive surgery and interventional radiology. On the basis of the National Medical Holding in Astana and the Kazakh Scientific Research Institute of Oncology and Radiology in Almaty (hereinafter—KSRIOR), there is a plan for implementation of proton therapy, which is one of the latest developments in medical technology. By 2016, it is planned to create two nuclear medicine centers, again, on the basis of KSRIOR and Semey city regional oncological dispensary. Implementation of this program will lead to a modern patient-oriented model of cancer care, and thus will help to reduce cancer mortality and improve the length and quality of life of Kazakhstani citizens.

However, "Salamatty Kazakhstan" prescribes financing of external training of professionals.

Today, it is clear that the objectives of the "Salamatty Kazakhstan" and Cancer Care Development programs work, and they work for the future while its target indicators have proven to be realistic and significant for practical health care system.

Institutional Involvement

In accordance with Kazakhstani legislation, treatment of cancer is free of charge and can be held only at specialized oncology centers. Kazakhstan has six medical universities with departments of oncology which perform training of oncology specialists. Private clinics are prohibited to conduct treatment of cancer patients. It is expected that in 2017, within the frames of health care reformation and implementation of mandatory health insurance, oncology sphere will not be only state based. However, the conditions and forms of private clinics involvement are not defined yet.

Insights on Palliative Care

Mortality at the late stages of cancer is unavoidable and practically has no trend for decrease. Moreover, the process of disease on later phases and process of dying of cancer patients go together with highest stress level of stress, simply speaking—with torment. In practice, this shows that oncologists often have to deal with patients with life-threatening condition caused by the nature and stage of the disease, comorbidity, and depletion of organism reserves. Many of them are in need of palliative care that is aimed not to ease the "last days" much, but to provide full and complete assistance in situations when special cancer therapy is not helping anymore. In this situation, the problem of chronic pain syndrome comes to the forefront since almost 100 % of patients with advanced forms of cancer suffer from pain.

Also, though there are WHO recommendations "freedom from pain should be seen as the right of every cancer patient, and the availability of painkillers—as an expression of respect to this right"—in practice, there is a problem with provision of our patients with some types of analgesics. Thus, the issue with the availability of fentanyl transdermal therapeutic system—"analgesic patches" that have been adopted worldwide as the standard for chronic pain treatment and which can substitute many injections—is not solved yet.

Concerning other pain pills, it is worth noting that only injections of opioids, tramadol, promedol, and morphine are registered in Kazakhstan. Tablets are not registered. However, injections are available and prescribed by family physician after consultation with oncologist. Then, relatives or nurses make injections.

So, the issue of expanding the list of permitted opioids is being raised to the Ministry of Health. Deputies are also dealing with it. Also, in addition to this problem, we are to raise quota for narcotic drugs available for treatment purposes.

Another unresolved problem in Kazakhstan is that it is still unclear how and where palliative care should be performed. Despite many discussions and recommendations developed to date, practically palliative assistance does not always correspond with needs and wishes of cancer patients. The problem is that this approach cannot be freely implemented in current conditions of health care systems of post-Soviet countries.

In this regard, system of home-based services is crucial, but it is just on its initial stage. There is still much room to do. Lack of experience of practitioner and family physicians causes that teams include only oncologist, nurse, and psychologist so far.

So, usually specialists do not have an expertise in palliative care and do not have sufficient experience in this field. The essential point in this situation is a close professional relationship and cooperation between general practitioner, medical oncologist, a specialist in the treatment of chronic pain (or anesthesiologist) and hospital doctors assisting cancer patients. Representatives of local authorities from social security service and home care should also be included to this cooperation link, which will help guaranteeing a decent life for the patient.

It should be noted that this approach helps to reduce social burden on the patient and his family, it eases complex and difficult way of struggling with the disease. Although about 70 % of terminally ill patients prefer to be at home until the very end, the model of treatment and home care developed in our country, as well as in other countries of the Commonwealth, is still relatively poor.

Development of these models requires the full support of the medical community and government representatives. Recent innovations in communication technologies (telemedicine, "virtual visits") provide new opportunities for palliative care at home.

Just 2 years ago, the situation with the provision of palliative care in oncology reflected deficit in almost all directions: the total number of hospice beds was not more than 300; there were only three mobile teams, number of doctors, trained in palliative care was not more than 30 with nearly 50 nurses. And there was only one medical university that trained palliative care specialists.

Also trainings are provided by nongovernmental organizations members of which had been trained abroad. Trainings for social workers and psychologists are stipulated within the oncology program. However, these trainings are not everywhere, so the coverage is not full. Though, European colleagues are being invited for the purpose of trainings and sharing experience; it is still insufficient.

There has been positive dynamics over the past 2 years. There is a plan for the development of modern rehabilitation and palliative care to patients. There are palliative care centers with best clinical guidelines, adopted by world oncology practice. At the present moment, these centers operate in Almaty, Pavlodar, Karaganda, Ust-Kamenogorsk, Kostanay, and Semey on the basis of former hospices.

The area of state-private partnership is developing. As a proof of this cooperation, there is a successful operation of public funds that assist oncology patients—"Credo" (Karaganda) and "Together Against Cancer" (Almaty). These funds have organized many educational and humanitarian projects for patients, their families, and oncologists.

There is a planned opening of palliative care center on the basis of hospital in Taldykorgan and opening of oncological dispensary in Aktau. Also, it is expected that work of Uralsk and Atyrau palliative care centers will be started. In 2016, the center of palliative care will be opened on the basis of oncology dispensary in regional centers of South and Zhambyl regions.

Beside governmental direct support, medical community has started working very actively. As a result, there was a creation of the Kazakhstani Association of Palliative Care, initially uniting four public companies: Karaganda NGO "Credo," the Youth Volunteer Center of palliative and social care "Adamgershilik" (Karaganda), Taraz Fund of support to cancer patients, and the Foundation "Together Against Cancer."

The objectives of the Association are to promote the ideology of palliative care at all levels of Kazakh society, participation in the improvement of the legislation. Amendments in legislation include improvements in availability of opioid analgesics and promote the development and implementation of national standards of palliative care and the representation of Kazakhstan in terms of palliative care area on the international arena. One of the most important events organized by the Association of Palliative Care in collaboration with the Foundation of the First President of the Republic of Kazakhstan, the Eurasian Federation of Oncology and Almaty Cancer Center was Eurasian Forum "Predictions, prevention and palliative care" held in October 2013 in Almaty and gathering oncologists from 13 countries.

We believe that it is more than realistic to continue to develop positive changes, and we see "Map of palliative care in Kazakhstan" in 2016 as follows: the total number of hospital beds for palliative care—300 items, not less than 60 mobile teams, trained doctors—not less than 300. The same amount of trained psychologists and social workers will be required, and according to experts of the Association, the number of institutions that are to prepare all these specialists should reach at least 30, including colleges. But most importantly—for those who provide and will provide palliative care, there should be no such saying as "there's nothing more we can do."

We can and will do more.

Local Innovations

As Kazakhstan matures as a country and national economy strengthens, more funds are being allocated for health care. Kazakhstan is the only among former Soviet Union where medical treatment for cancer patients is conducted for free, totally at the expense of national budget. During the recent decade, it has allowed implementation of various innovations in oncology based on the experience of some foreign countries.

Thus, in 2008, first pilot screening program for cervical cancer detection was adopted in 2 of 16 regions. Currently, there are six screening programs in Kazakhstan.

National Cancer Screening Programs

Current screenings programs include cervical cancer since 2008, breast cancer since 2009, and colorectal cancer since 2011.

Starting since 30–60 years old women are recommended to start cervical cancer screening on biannual basis within PAP-test by fluid cytology.

Since 50 years old, women would have charged free breast cancer screening on the biannual basis till the age of 60. There is an analogous mammography equipment in every clinic, and digital equipment is in each oncology center. Mammograms are sent to regional oncology center for the second look. Biopsy and histology are conducted further.

Colorectal cancer screening is recommended for both women and men since 50 years old by I FOB Test, which is being sent to colonoscopy in case of positive reaction.

Esophagus and stomach cancer screenings are for both men and women of 50, 52, 54, 56, 58, and 60 years old. Endoscopy and biopsy in case of pathology.

Liver cancer screening is for those with cirrhosis caused by viral/nonviral etiology: AFP level four times a year, ultrasound and CT-screening, and biopsy (in case of tumors).

Prostate cancer screening for men of 50, 54, 58, 62, 66 years old is being conducted once in 4 years. Level of PSA and proPSA (-2), ultrasound and biopsy.

Since 2013 such practice has been referred to human papilloma virus as well. Pilot vaccination program is being conducted in three regions.

The joint memorandum that was signed by the Ministry of Health of Kazakhstan and Institute of Oncology named after Gustav Roussy (Paris, France) in 2012 enabled more than 30 oncologists of different specialties to be trained modern methods of diagnosis and treatment. Besides that, with thanks to the telepathology, Kazakhstani pathomorphologies can consult with their European colleagues.

The experience of South Korean surgeons allowed launch of mini-invasive surgery for the stomach and intestines cancer.

The experience of the European Oncology Institute (Milan, Italy) allowed implementation of reconstructive plastic surgeries of breast cancer patients and launch of intraoperative radiation therapy.

It should be noted that continuous cooperation with specialists from Western countries has shifted the understanding about the role of palliative care. Today, there are staff psychologists and social workers in all state clinics and oncological centers. Parliament Deputies raised the question to the Ministry of Internal Affairs and the Ministry of Health regarding the increase of state quota for narcotic drugs.

Society Reaction Towards Cancer Patients

Since Soviet period cancer is being considered as a disease which is not to be talked about openly in society. Cancer patients and their relatives conceal the diagnosis, close on themselves and try to deal with it on their own. This is compounded by the Kazakh national mentality that considers this disease as something bad, sometimes leading to such cases when the real cause of death is being kept in a secret. Moreover, there are situations when relatives of the patient ask doctors not to inform the patient about his diagnosis. Close relatives (spouse, kids) take active role in decision making regarding necessary treatment while patient is often not aware of the seriousness of diagnosis and treatment.

Fortunately, our society is becoming more open with positive changes in its reaction to the disease. Open discussion of cancer issues in Western countries is gradually changing attitude to cancer as not to a death verdict, but as to a chronic disease, which is quite possible to resist to. Especially in cases of early diagnosis when 100 % healing is very likely to be reached.

This has caused a creation of public funds and organizations to support both patients and oncology service as a whole. Unfortunately, such notable shifts in society consciousness have appeared just recently, therefore, public organizations do not even have a 10-year history.

For instance, public social fund "Together against Cancer" was established in 2008. This is a noncommercial, nonprofit, nongovernment organization that supports various activities in the fight against cancer.

The strategic goal of the organization is to realize the desire for each citizen in every distant quarter of Kazakhstan, to have access to high quality, world standard cancer treatment at every level, including prevention, diagnostic and laboratory services, excellent professional care, a wide range of the most rigorously tested and approved medications, the necessary psychological, legal and social support, along with rehabilitation and palliative care.

The fund's main activities include raising the professional level of Kazakhstan oncology specialists by hosting scientific and medical practice conferences, organizing seminars and master classes and participating in exchange programs with specialists from vanguard world clinics. Public awareness campaigns, "Open Door Days" and free screenings at various workplaces are being conducted on a regular basis with the aim of cancer prevention and early diagnostics, as well as promotion of a healthy lifestyle. The first specialized Kazakhstan-based Internet resource dedicated to oncology www.oncology.kz is the source of information for both doctors and patients. The toll-free hotline provides consultations on breast cancer prevention for Kazakhstan women while a special cervical cancer prevention cabinet offers vaccination against HPV for girls.

Money gathered through various fundraising campaigns are also used for purchasing essential diagnostic and therapy equipment for cancer treatment facilities, training specialists and caregivers, and facilitating the work of a mobile palliative care team for terminal cancer patients in Almaty city.

Summary and Recommendations

The analysis revealed a number of major challenges and helped to solve current problems in cancer care system.

Challenges

- Insufficient use of modern clinical guidelines/protocols on the prevention, diagnosis, treatment, and rehabilitation of cancer patients
- Low level of implementation of innovative technologies in diagnosis and treatment of malignant tumors, including kids' bone marrow transplantation
- Acute deficit of medicine workers that are prepared in terms of early diagnosis and treatment of cancer (radionuclide diagnosis and therapy, nuclear medicine, mini-invasive technology, brachytherapy, etc.) and the absence of training centers for their preparation
- Lack of nuclear medicine specialists (medical physicists, chemists, engineers) and the absence of centers for their training
- Lack of physical facilities and technical base of cancer organizations, oncology clinics are located in adapted buildings
- Number of hospital beds in oncological organizations does not meet required normative amount
- Number of oncological mammography and proctologic offices is lower than it is required
- Lack of palliative and rehabilitative care for patients with cancer
- The absence of an integrated service providing medical, social, and psychological assistance to cancer patients

Advantages

- Good experience from national screening programs for early diagnosis of malignant tumors
- The presence of a hierarchically constructed network of cancer care, from the district (oncology offices in the organizations of primary health care), and regional (city oncology centers) levels up to the national level (KSRIOR)
- Centralized provision of medicines for the treatment of malignant neoplasms, material and technical equipment of oncological organizations at the expense of the national budget

Opportunities

- Improving the quality of services with patient's ability to choose freely among oncological centers, attraction of patients from abroad
- Transfer of modern technologies from abroad and conduction of fundamental and applied researches
- Priority government funding for prevention and treatment of cancer, which is a socially significant disease
- Improving early diagnosis of malignant tumors by increasing population awareness and its reactions
- Reduction in mortality from cancer by strengthening inter-sector collaboration
- Development of our own technical center and specialists for production of radiopharmaceuticals, realization of project on establishing the Center for Nuclear Medicine and Biophysics

References[1]

1. Indicators of Oncology Services in Kazakhstan, 2013 (statistical data), Kazakh Scientific Institute of Oncology and Radiology.
2. Salamatty Kazakhstan, Decree of the President of 29 November 2010.
3. Program for Oncology Services Development in Kazakhstan for 2012–2016, Decree of the Government of Kazakhstan, 29 March 2012 #366.

[1] All data have been taken from the following official sources.

Chapter 19
An Overview of Cancer Care in Societies in Transition: Global Perspectives—UAE Experience

Mohammed Jaloudi, Jihad Kanbar, David.M. James, and Haytham El-Salhat

Introduction

Cancer is not a modern disease but has clearly existed for many centuries. It is however a more common phenomenon nowadays than previously due to the increase of the world's population and the relatively advanced age to which people now live, since it is a disease that is more common in elderly ages than in younger ages [1].

The burden of cancer worldwide is continuously rising largely because of the aging and growth of the world population alongside an increasing adoption of cancer-causing behaviors, particularly smoking, physical inactivity, and "westernized" lifestyle in economically developing countries. Based on the GLOBOCAN 2008 estimates, about 12.7 million cancer cases and 7.6 million cancer deaths are estimated to have occurred in 2008; of these, 56 % of the cases and 64 % of the deaths occurred in the economically developing world. Cancer is the leading cause of death in economically developed countries and the second leading cause of death in developing countries [2]. Breast cancer is the most frequently diagnosed cancer and the leading cause of cancer death among females, accounting for 23 % of the total cancer cases and 14 % of the cancer deaths. Lung cancer is the leading cancer site in males, comprising 17 % of the total new cancer cases and 23 % of the total cancer deaths. Breast cancer is now also the leading cause of cancer death among females in economically developing countries, a shift from the previous decade during which the most common cause of cancer death was cervical cancer. Further, the mortality burden for lung cancer among females in developing countries is as high as the burden for cervical cancer, with each accounting for 11 % of the total female

M. Jaloudi, M.D. (✉) • J. Kanbar, M.Sc. • D.M. James, M.Sc.
Department of Oncology, Tawam Hospital, Abu Dhabi, UAE
e-mail: mjaloudi@tawamhospital.ae

H. El-Salhat, M.D.
Al Noor Hospital, Abu Dhabi

M. Silbermann (ed.), *Cancer Care in Countries and Societies in Transition*,
DOI 10.1007/978-3-319-22912-6_19

cancer deaths. Although overall cancer incidence rates in the developing world are half those seen in the developed world in both sexes, the overall cancer mortality rates are generally similar. Cancer survival tends to be poorer in developing countries, most likely because of a combination of a late stage at diagnosis and limited access to timely and standard treatment. A substantial proportion of the worldwide burden of cancer could be prevented through the application of existing cancer control

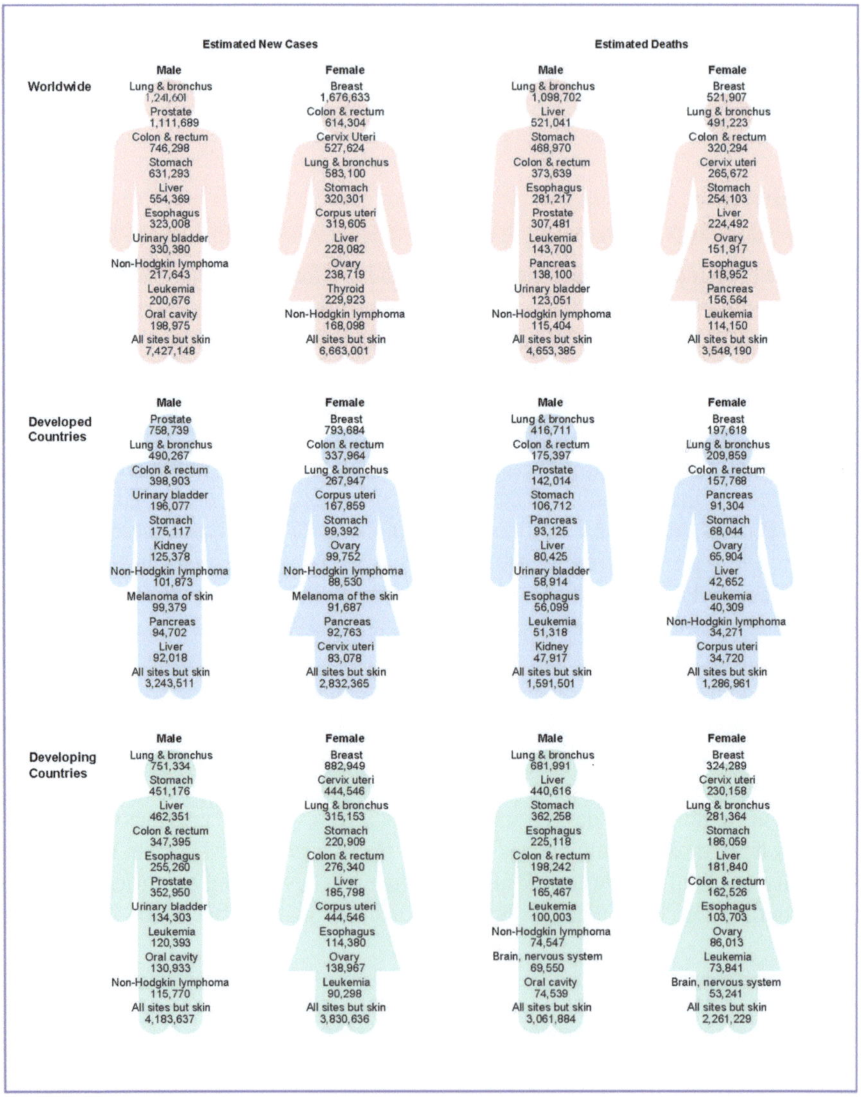

Fig. 19.1 Estimated new cancer cases and deaths worldwide for leading cancer sites by level of economic development. *Source*: GLOBOCAN 2012

knowledge and by implementing programs for tobacco control, vaccination (for liver and cervical cancers), and early detection and treatment, as well as public health campaigns promoting physical activity and a healthier dietary intake. Clinicians, public health professionals, and policy makers can play an active role in accelerating the application of such interventions globally [2] (Fig. 19.1).

The World Health Organization (WHO) projected that by 2030, the cancer figures could increase to 26.4 million new cases and 17 million cancer-related deaths. The majority of the global cancer burden is shifting from the more developed world to economically disadvantaged countries. Nearly 70 % of cancer incidence will occur in economically disadvantaged countries, where survival rates are less than half of those in developed countries. Population growth and aging are the largest contributors to the increasing numbers of cancer cases in low- and middle-income countries. The population aged 65 and over in low- and middle-income countries is expected to increase from 247 million to 982 million between 2000 and 2050, due to increased attention and resources to combat HIV/AIDS and other infectious diseases [2].

The United Arab Emirates (UAE) is a rapidly developing country composed of a multinational population with varying educational backgrounds, religious beliefs, and cultural practices, which pose a challenge for population-based public health strategies. A number of public health issues significantly contribute to morbidity and mortality in the UAE.

The UAE has a highly developed health service, including a sophisticated physical infrastructure of well-equipped hospitals, specialized clinics, and primary care centers. Health care is free for all nationals, and there is a compulsory health insurance scheme in place in Abu Dhabi to cover all residents. The scheme will be extended country-wide.

Currently, there are 65 hospitals in the UAE, 15 of them federal institutions, and over 150 primary health care centers and clinics, in addition to 11 school health centers, 10 centers for mothers and children, and 110 special units for mothers and children in hospitals and primary health care centers. This is compared with 7 hospitals and 12 health centers when the Federation was established in 1971.

Nevertheless, as the population increases and health care demands burgeon, Government policies and strategies, such as Emirates Vision 2021 and the Strategy of the Government of the United Arab Emirates 2011–2013, are committed to make continuing improvements to health care, including remote areas.

UAE Demographics and Population Growth

In Abu Dhabi; one of the seven UAE emirates and the capital; every individual is entitled access to health care and health insurance is mandatory in all emirates, and many elements are being implemented to provide world-class quality health care. Population growth is the product of natural growth and net migration [2]. Migrant workers are recruited from all over the world to satisfy the manpower demands of the fast-paced economic and industrial developments in the UAE [3].

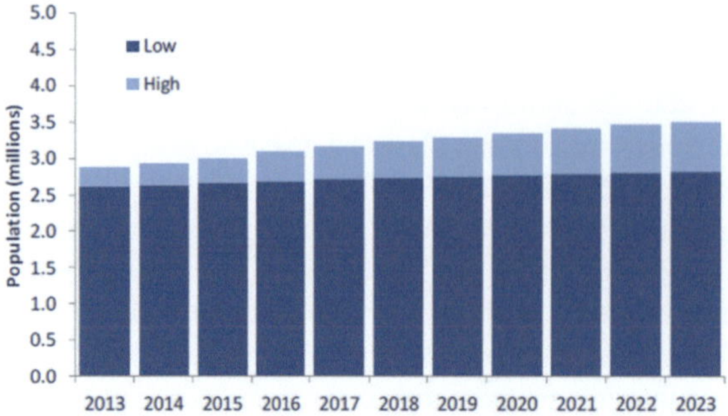

Population growth, scenarios

	National	Expatriate	
Year		Low	High
2013	491'300	2'117'000	2'233'500
2014	505'600	2'128'500	2'279'500
2015	519'600	2'140'000	2'341'500
2016	533'200	2'150'500	2'407'500
2017	546'500	2'160'500	2'466'500
2018	560'000	2'170'000	2'520'000
2019	572'500	2'179'000	2'570'000
2020	585'000	2'187'000	2'617'000
2021	597'500	2'195'000	2'660'000
2022	609'000	2'201'000	2'701'000
2023	620'500	2'206'000	2'739'000

Fig. 19.2 Population estimates here are based on raw insurance data; projections are rounded to the nearest 2.5 % variance between high and low, and those for expatriates at 5 %. *Source*: Health Statistics 2013; HAAD (Health Authority—Abu Dhabi)

Consequently, the UAE population has increased substantially primarily due to the high inward migration of expatriate workers (4.1 million in 2005, 8.3 million in 2010) [4]. Indeed, mass recruitment of migrant workers has created an unusual population structure; with the total UAE population composed of approximately 11 % (950,000) Emiratis, and the rest are expatriates of varying nationalities [5]. Similarly, the total population of Abu Dhabi (the largest emirate in the UAE) is estimated to be 2.3 million, with over half of the population being expatriate males' aged 20–59 years [5].

As a result of expatriate workforce recruitment for industrial projects, males outnumber females 3:1 in the overall UAE population (nationals and non-nationals); however, there are approximately equal numbers of male and female UAE nationals. Among non-nationals, the ratio of males to females is 3.7:1 due to the imbalance between the number of expatriate males employed in construction compared with migrant females working in hospitality, health care, or domestic service [2]. As such, the UAE is composed of a multinational population, with varying educational backgrounds, religious beliefs, and cultural practices, which pose a challenge for population-based public health strategies.

In 2013, HAAD has presented estimates of population growth in Abu Dhabi emirates for both the nationals and expatriates as seen in Fig. 19.2.

Cancer Status in UAE

Cancer is the second leading cause of death worldwide and in all regions of the world. Historically, the UAE had a much lower incidence of cancer than Western countries; however, over the last 40 years, it has undergone a period of dramatic economic, social, and demographic change, resulting in increased life expectancy and prosperity. This epidemiological transition has led to significant increases in the incidence of all chronic noncommunicable diseases, including cancer, which

Table 19.1 Summary of age standardized incidence and mortality rates from cancer in males and females in the UAE and US 2012

	United Arab Emirates			USA		
	Male	Female	Both sexes	Male	Female	Both sexes
Population (thousands)	5619	2486	8105	156,002	159,788	315,791
Number of new cancer cases (thousands)	1.5	1.4	2.9	824.7	778.9	1603.6
Age-standardized rate (W)	83.8	127.2	92.5	347.0	297.4	318.0
Risk of getting cancer before age 75 (%)	9.1	13.6	10.2	34.1	28.5	31.1
Number of cancer deaths (thousands)	0.7	0.5	1.3	323.9	293.4	617.2
Age-standardized rate (W)	57.9	64.9	58.0	123.9	91.7	105.8
Risk of dying from cancer before age 75 (%)	6.0	7.2	6.3	12.8	9.8	11.2
5 years prevalent cases, adult population (thousands)	3.9	5.0	8.8	2402.2	2373.0	4775.2
Proportion (per 100,000)	78.6	271.4	131.1	1943.9	1842.5	1892.1

is now the third leading cause of death in the UAE (after cardiovascular disease and injury) causing 10 % of all deaths in 2010 and 16 % of all deaths in the emirate of Abu Dhabi during the same year [6]. At present, there is no national or regional population-based cancer registry in the UAE, which means there is no reliable information available on the incidence of cancer in the UAE. However, the Ministry of Health collected some cancer registration data for the UAE, which has been submitted for inclusion in the Globocan database [7] and Gulf Cooperation Council-wide cancer registry report, "Ten Year Cancer Incidence Among Nationals of the GCC States 1998–2007," published by the Gulf Centre for Cancer Registration [8].

The Globocan data from 2008 shows that the age-standardized rates for the incidence and mortality from all cancers in the UAE is lower compared to Western countries, such as the United States (Table 19.1). The incidence of all cancers is projected to double by 2020, primarily due to aging and also possibly due to increased exposure to risk factors for cancer. Breast cancer is the most common cancer among Emirati females, lung cancer is the most common cancer among Emirati males but is extremely rare in females, which reflects the prevalence of smoking (23.0 % vs. 0.5 %, respectively), and colorectal cancer is the second most common cancer in both sexes combined (Table 19.2) [7–9]. However, rates for all three types of cancer are much lower than most Western countries and are also lower than in Qatar, Bahrain, and Kuwait [13]. This is likely to be due to the younger age of the population, less exposure to some risk factors, lower levels of screening compared to Western countries, and possibly incomplete registration. Cancer rates are also projected to increase by the year 2030 as the UAE population ages, total fertility declines, exposure time to lifestyle risk factors increases, the prevalence of obesity and diabetes increases, and due to the long latency period between starting

Table 19.2 Five most frequent cancers by gender in the UAE and US 2012

	United Arab Emirates			USA		
Ranking	Male	Female	Both sexes	Male	Female	Both sexes
1	Colorectum	Breast	Breast	Prostate	Breast	Prostate
2	Lung	Thyroid	Colorectum	Lung	Lung	Breast
3	Non-Hodgkin lymphoma	Cervix uteri	Leukaemia	Colorectum	Colorectum	Lung
4	Leukaemia	Colorectum	Lung	Bladder	Corpus uteri	Colorectum
5	Prostate	Ovary	Non-Hodgkin lymphoma	Melanoma of skin	Thyroid	Melanoma of skin

Note: Ranking defined by total number of cases

smoking and developing lung cancer. Population-based education and awareness campaigns are urgently required to increase screening rates for at-risk individuals and to facilitate early diagnosis and prompt treatment, thereby reducing morbidity and improving survival.

In 2009, UAE's population stood at about 5.7 million, of which approximately 21.9 % were nationals and the rest foreigners. As a consequence, UAE nationals form a minority of those who reside in the country. UAE has one of the most diverse populations in the Middle East. 23 % of the population is non-Emirati Arabs or Persians and the majority of the population, about 50 %, is from South Asia.

The population of the UAE also has a skewed sex distribution consisting of more than twice as many males as females. The 15–65 age groups have a male/female sex ratio of 2.743. The average life expectancy is 78.24 years, higher than any other Arab country. The breast cancer in UAE is considered the number one cancer among females and constitutes almost 23 % of all cancer cases and 43 % of all female cancers annually and that is similar to international ratios.

Cancer rates are set to increase at an alarming rate globally as well as locally. Cancer is set to become the fifth disease in UAE and GCC region. A difference can be made by taking action today and use the opportunity to stem this increase. Governments, health practitioners, and the general public need to take urgent action; actions as cost-effective treatment plans, provision of financial support to people, screening awareness, and tobacco cessation (see Figs. 19.3 and 19.4).

Age-standardized rate (W): A rate is the number of new cases or deaths per 100.000 persons per year. An age-standardized rate is the rate that a population would have, if it had a standard age structure. Standardization is necessary when comparing several populations that differ with respect to age because age has a powerful influence on the risk of cancer. Risk of getting or dying from the disease before age 75 %: The probability or risk of individuals developing dying from cancer. It is expressed as the number of new born children (out of 100) who would be expected to develop die from cancer before the age of 75. If they had cancer rates observed in the period in the absence of other causes of death.

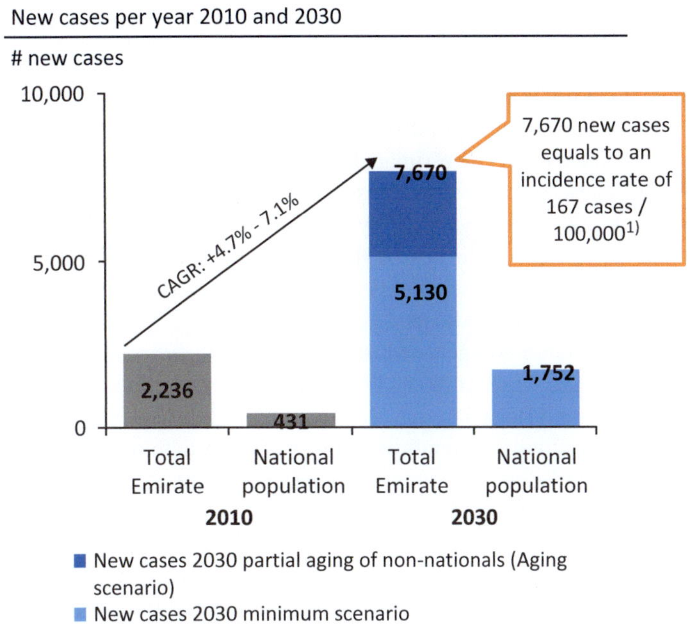

Fig. 19.3 Estimated projection of new cancer cases in UAE amongst national and expatriates based on population growth and market labor needs

Fig. 19.4 Projected level of cancer cases in the UAE and GCC countries showing cancer cases are increasing at an alarming rate. *Source*: McKinsey & Company

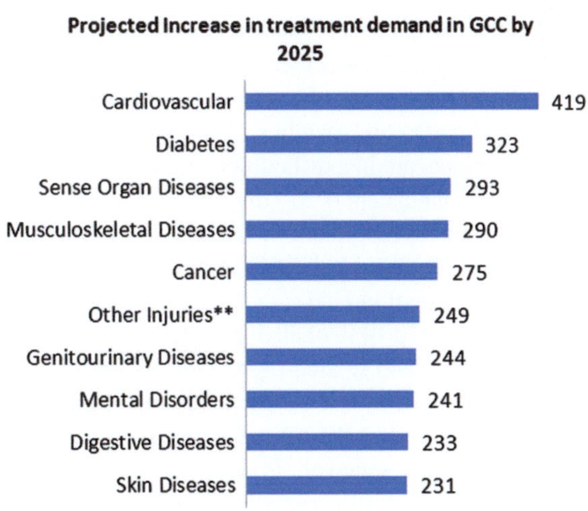

Uptake of Oncology Drugs Costs on Selected Cancers in UAE

UAE hospitals are not unique in the struggle to coping with the existing and further increasing financial burden caused by cancer and its treatment. Worldwide, drugs associated with cancer care are estimated to cost approximately $40 billion per year. In the United States, cancer drugs represent the biggest category of overall pharmaceutical sales, in 2007 sales increased by 14 %. Seventy percent of these sales came from products introduced in the last 10 years and 30 % in the last 5 years [10]. These new drugs have improved the quality of life, delayed disease progression, and helped prolong survival for patients.

New molecular targeted agents introduced in recent years include well-known agents such as Rituximab (1997), Trastuzumab (Herceptin in 1998), Imatinib (Gleevec in 2001), and Bevacizumab (Avastin in 2004) therapies that caused excitement among the oncology community. However, such therapy comes at considerable cost, just recently new agents were released such as Regarofenib (2012) and Pertuzumab (2012) and we know that there are many other new agents under development.

It is widely recognized that the across tumor sites, mean net costs of care are highest in the initial and last year of life phases of care and lowest in the continuing phase [11, 12].

The significant increase in costs of initial cancer treatment reflects more patients receiving surgery and adjuvant therapy and rising prices for these treatments. These trends are likely to continue in the near future, although more efficient targeting of costly therapies could mitigate the overall economic impact of this trend [13].

The costs of cancer care are substantial and vary by tumor site, phase of care, stage at diagnosis, and survival.

Patterns of care have been reported to be more aggressive for younger cancer patients compared with elderly cancer patients in many health care settings. In addition, as the prevalence of comorbid conditions and levels of medical care increase with age, health care spending also typically increases with age [14].

Oncologists are in a difficult position, on the one hand, as prescribers they can be asked to be gatekeepers; on the other, they are advocates for their patients. These issues are well recognized in the oncology community and as such organizations such as ASCO through their Journal of Clinical Oncology publish many studies on economic evaluation [15].

Cancer caused 14 % of all deaths in the Emirate of Abu Dhabi in 2011. Lymphoid, hematopoietic, and related tissue cancers are the dominant cancers in Abu Dhabi. Late detection of breast cancer leads to significant increases in mortality. Female adult nationals aged 40–69 are being screened for breast cancer as part of their Thiqa insurance renewal. Education and awareness campaigns have increased screening rates for all nationalities [16].

The American Society of Clinical Oncologists (ASCO) issued a guidance statement affirming the "critical role of oncologists in addressing costs of care." Since in the United States the high cost of cancer care can be financially devastating to patients and their families, oncologist communicate with their patients and discuss costs of their therapy and implications on the quality of care [17].

Outside of the United States, many counties use a formal process to evaluate new technologies before deciding whether they should be broadly adopted.

Published estimates for the treatment costs of breast cancer vary widely in methodology, perspective, patient populations, and time horizon.

Breast cancer represents the most drug-intensive area when it comes to treatment of solid tumors. Tamoxifen, a costly treatment launched in 1975 has established itself as the most cost-effective cancer treatment to date. Its broad indication for the treatment of advanced disease and adjuvant treatment represents a major breakthrough in the treatment of breast cancer. Newer, innovative drugs (aromatase inhibitors; anastrozole, exemestane, and letrozole) are now replacing, fully or in part, tamoxifen, both in the treatment of advanced disease but also in the adjuvant setting. In addition, anthracyclines and taxanes have established themselves as very valuable palliative and adjuvant treatments.

Trastuzumab, an HER2 receptor antibody, has become a cornerstone of treatment for patients with advanced breast cancer over-expressing HER2, in the adjuvant setting.

The lifetime treatment Estimates per-patient costs of breast cancer ranged from US$ 20,000 to US$ 100,000. (Campbell and Ramsey 2009) [18]. While disease stages I and II were emphasized, the costs of initial and terminal therapy were greater than continuing care on a per unit time basis, but continuing care accounts for the largest share of lifetime cost due to the relatively long survival of breast cancer patients.

Costs of different surgeries were relatively similar (breast-conserving surgery vs mastectomy) but, all else equal, significant costs (US$ 23,000–31,000) were observed for patients who received adjuvant chemotherapy compared with those who did not.

In the 1980s, colorectal cancer remained a therapeutic area in which medical treatment was considered to have little or no effect. Developments in diagnostic and surgical techniques were major contributors to outcome improvement. With the publication of the adjuvant data on modulated 5-fluorouracil (S-FU)-based therapy, colorectal cancer rapidly became an area of focus for further drug development. Recently, two new innovative drugs, Bevacizumab and cetuximab, have also been used for the treatment of advanced colorectal cancer; representing a more cost incurred in the treatment of the disease. Bevacizumab is an anti-angiogenesis drug with its indication in the first-line treatment of advanced colorectal cancer. Cetuximab, which interacts with the epidermal growth factor (EGF) receptor, is indicated in the second or third-line treatment of metastatic disease. The prevalence of colorectal cancer was projected by Mariatto et al. (2006) [19] to increase in the United States from 1,002,786 (0.36 %) patients to 1,522,348 (0.46 %) patients between 2000 and 2020. Their review of SEER data they project that colorectal cancer prevalence will increase more rapidly than the US population, largely due to the aging of the US population. This suggests that considerable resources will be needed in the future for initial, continuing and last year of life treatment of colorectal cancer patients unless notable breakthroughs in primary prevention occur in the future years.

Table 19.3 Top 20 antineoplastic drug expenditures in clinics in 2011

Drug	2010 expenditures ($ thousands)	Percent change from 2009	2011 expenditures ($ thousands)[a]	Percent change from 2010[b]
Bevacizumab (Avastin)	2,455,275	2.9	1,567,494	−16.8
Rituximab (Rituxan)	1,969,996	3.2	1,553,477	6.0
Trastuzumab (Herceptin)	1,243,799	7.6	974,251	4.7
Oxaliplatin (Eloxatin)	665,857	−34.3	806,999	58.9
Pemetrexed (Alimta)	762,243	16.5	594,267	2.6
Docetaxel (Taxotere)	904,063	−6.0	568,714	−17.3
Bortezomib (Velcade)	447,729	21.4	335,141	17.8
Cetuzimab (Erbitux)	437,944	−2.8	335,118	1.8
Bendamustine (Treanda)	287,046	73.0	274,775	32.3
Gemcitabine (Gemzar)	581,067	−1.2	263,104	−43.1
Leuprolide acetate[c]	295,003	−2.7	223,913	1.7
Paclitaxel-albumin (Abraxane)	312,011	19.3	223,347	−7.2
Azacitidine (Viclaza)	201,507	20.8	167,726	13.5
Fulvestrant (Faslodex)	122,988	32.4	157,588	95.0
Ipilimumab (Yervoy)	0	0.0	140,886	100.0
Cabazitaxel (Jevtana)	78,407	100.0	118,566	215.2
Decitabine (Dacogen)	124,454	16.1	105,169	14.7
Liposomal doxorubicin (Doxil)	175,450	6.7	98,385	−24.3
Panitumumab (Vectibix)	94,227	22.7	73,706	5.9
Capecitabine (Xeloda)	69,620	9.7	62,775	26.2
All others	892,444	−5.2	715,074	6.5
Total	12,121,130	2.4	9,410,475	3.2

[a]Based on data collected between January 1 and September 30, 2011
[b]Percent change compared with same period in 2010 (data not shown in table)
[c]Leuprolide acetate includes the following formulations: Lupron, Lupron Depot, Lupron Depot-3 Month, Lupron Depot-4 Month, Lupron Depot-6 Month, Lupron Depot-Ped, and Lupron Dep-Ped 3 Month

Oncology drugs account for a significant proportion of drug expenditures in the clinic setting in the United States (Hoffman et al. 2012) [20].

The top 20 cancer drugs based on expenditures for chemotherapy drugs consumed in UAE in 2011 are listed in Table 19.3. Bevacizumab, Trastuzumab, and Rituximab represent the top three oncology drugs based on expenditures in 2010 (Table 19.3).

Hoffman et al. (2012) go on to describe the top ten therapeutic classes of drugs, with antineoplastic and hemostatic modifiers (such as those used in the treatment of hemophilia) being the top two, with blood growth factors (e.g., Filgrastim, Pegfilgrastim, Lenograstrim) the top four all comprising some 34 % of total expenditure (Table 19.4).

Table 19.4 Top 10 therapeutic classes by expenditures in nonfederal hospitals in 2011 in UAE

Therapeutic class	2010 expenditures ($ thousands)	Percent change from 2009	2011 expenditures ($ thousands)[a]	Percent change from 2010[b]
Antineoplastic agents	3,804,480	6.4	2,994,336	5.7
Hemostatic modifiers	3,932,781	7.6	2,702,472	−3.9
Anti-infectives, systemic	3,079,337	−3.5	2,152,871	−8.0
Blood growth factors	2,051,611	0.2	1,492,320	−3.4
Hospital solutions	1,692,245	−7.3	1339,415	−5.0
Gastrointestinal agents	1,235,580	3.1	954,674	3.1
Diagnostic aids	1,11,433	−8.0	935,857	−3.9
Respiratory therapy	1,099,800	4.7	882,778	*76*
Psychotherapeutics	1,100,536	2.3	874,085	*53*
Biologicals	1,046,946	17.2	860,201	13.6
All others	7,718,213	−0.1	5,845,586	2.0
Total	28,072,962	1.5	21,034,595	0.3

[a]Based on data collected between January 1 and September 30, 2011

[b]Percent change compared with same period in 2010 (data not shown in table)

Opportunities and Challenges to Health Care Systems in UAE

The United Arab Emirates (UAE) is a rapidly developing country composed of a multinational population with varying educational backgrounds, religious beliefs, and cultural practices, which pose a challenge for population-based public health strategies.

Cancer is a cause of a comparable less burden of disease in the Middle East countries compared to Europe and the United States. However, in the Middle East, the burden of illness is expected to change from communicable diseases toward more expensive to treat noncommunicable diseases and injuries over the next decades—it is estimated that these will account for 60 % of the disease burden in 2020, compared to 45 % today, which will have consequences for health system configurations and health spending. Diagnosis and treatment of noncommunicable diseases and acute injuries are often complex and costly, which will put increased pressure on health care budgets. It is therefore increasingly important that investments are well managed and directed toward cost-effective technologies. Challenges for the health systems in these countries are to analyze what the costs and benefits of treating noncommunicable diseases are, and how to adopt the health care systems for treatment of such diseases in the optimal way [21].

The generally high standards of health care in the United Arab Emirates are a result of decades of high levels of public spending since the oil boom. There is a developing private health sector, several small private hospitals have been set up over the past few years, and however wealthy people still tend to travel abroad for medical care. Health expenditure was almost 3 % of GDP in 2004. Health care used to be free to all, but in 2001 the government introduced charges for expatriates, a

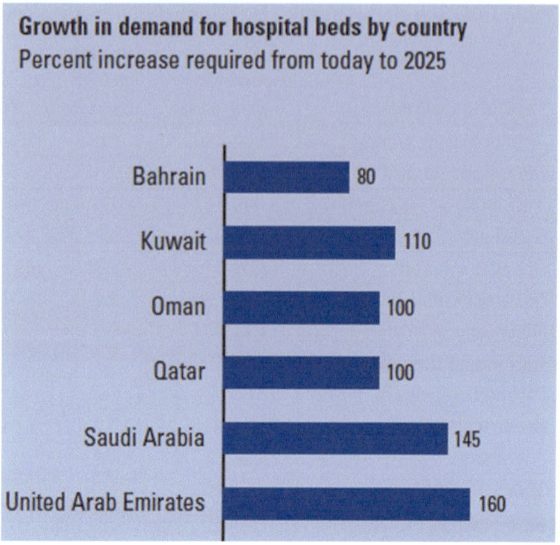

Fig. 19.5 Projected level of hospital beds in UAE and GCC countries showing an increase in the required number of beds to meet the local population needs. *Source*: McKinsey & Company

move that partly sought to reduce the draw of health care on public funds, but also aimed to increase the employers' cost of expatriate labor (which now requires health insurance) and thus encourage the employment of local staff. Since the policy was introduced, visits to government hospitals have fallen sharply, with some reports suggesting a 50 % reduction.

UAE also faces some elements that will dramatically increase health care demand in the area:

Population growth: Until 2025, the size of the population will increase at a compound annual growth rate (CAGR) of around 3.0 %, one of the highest in the world. By then, GCC population in 2025 will be almost twice the size it is today.

Hospital beds: By 2025, demand for hospital beds in UAE will be more than double, requiring almost 162,000 beds to meet this demand. Saudi Arabia and the United Arab Emirates will register the greatest percentage increase in demand for hospital beds (Fig. 19.5).

Oncology Division: Cancer Center

Tawam Hospital has been established as a Regional Center of Excellence for Cancer Care in Al-Ain since 1980. The center is a dedicated facility providing a range of Medical Oncology and Hematology services for all forms of cancers and blood disorders, with a dedicated team of Certified Hematologists/Oncologists. In addition to traditional cancer treatment options of Surgery, Chemotherapy, Radiotherapy, and Palliative care, the Center is continuously offering new therapies, which are creating exciting new treatment possibilities. The oncology program spans from prophylactic check-ups in patients with an increased hereditary risk of developing cancer through to adjuvant treatment for metastatic diseases and palliative treatment.

The Division of Oncology offers highly specialized treatments with antibodies and tyrosine kinase inhibitors, chemotherapy and endocrine therapy for both inpatients and outpatients.

The oncology team consists of highly experienced and trained professionals who treat all kinds of cancers in breast cancer, colorectal tumors, lung cancers, as well as other types.

Health Care Demand in UAE and the World Comparison

Over the past several decades, discoveries in molecular biology have significantly improved cancer care. Biomarkers based on mutation status or over-expression of specific genes is now commonly used to guide treatment, and drugs targeting these biomarkers have helped extend the lives of many patients.

Considerable debate has therefore arisen over the affordability of cancer care, especially in light of the efforts many countries are making to control or reduce health care spending. In fact, cancer is now becoming the most expensive disease. In the European Union alone, insurance companies will spend about €49 billion annually on health services for cancer patients, and it is estimated that total health care spending in the region will reach US$ 60 billion in 2025, up from US$ 12 billion today.

The United Arab Emirates—part of GCC region, will face an unparalleled and unprecedented rise in demand for health care over the course of the next two decades. No other region in the world faces such rapid growth in demand with the simultaneous need to realign its health care systems to be able to treat the disorders of affluence.

The UAE faces some elements that will dramatically increase health care demand in the area:

Population growth: Until 2025, the size of the population will increase at a compound annual growth rate (CAGR) of around 3.0 %, one of the highest in the world. By then, GCC population in 2025 will be almost twice the size it is today. Furthermore, there is demand for more clinical staff; government can help make jobs more attractive to students by creating professionally and financially rewarding career paths for them to stay in the region. Better salaries, substantial investments in professional training and development (such as residencies), and more flexible careers made possible by a greater degree of private-sector participation in the health care system should all help to attract nationals and keep expatriates. Cancer rates are set to increase at an alarming rate globally as well as locally [22].

Screening

Screening is the process of looking for cancer in people who have no symptoms of the disease. Regular screening for some types of cancer can detect changes in cells before they become cancerous. Screening in UAE is currently available for breast, cervical, prostate, and colorectal cancer.

Despite breast-screening services being widely available under health insurance in the UAE, with many facilities offering free checks, many women do not get checked; much still needs to be done in terms of affordability to public as the cost of screenings can often be a constraint for individuals who wish to screen themselves for cancer risk. On average, a mammogram costs about Dh300 and a PAP test to check for cervical cancer costs Dh100. Colonoscopies to test for colorectal cancer cost between Dhs. 2000 to Dhs. 3000, but a fecal exam can also be used as an alternative, and this costs about Dhs. 100 [23].

The fight to raise awareness of this disease is ongoing here in the UAE. Breast cancer accounts for 13.7 % of all cancer deaths in women across the globe and is the most common cause of cancer in women in the UAE. Furthermore, studies have shown that women in the Gulf region are more likely to develop breast cancer at least a decade earlier than their counterparts in Western countries. There is as well the fact that the majority of women in the UAE comprise expatriates on lower incomes—such as maids and nannies—which makes the tests unaffordable to them and this where governments support comes in, by providing and/or bearing the costs of breast screening for all women residing in UAE to help combat the disease locally and globally and also to provide breast cancer education to public to raise awareness to a higher level among people by promoting workshops, seminars, and exhibitions.

There is the psychological factor as well in some Arabic countries, for example, there is a belief that once a woman is diagnosed with breast cancer, she may be divorced by her husband and possibly rejected by the community, or that following a breast cancer diagnosis her breast will be cut off and she will die. As a result of such misconceptions and unfounded beliefs, women may tend to hide their breast cancer symptoms at the early stages when treatment is most likely to be effective.

To further decrease the number of deaths from breast cancer in UAE for instance, there is an extreme need to reemphasize the facts that women must begin screening at age 40 years and continue annually. Health systems as well as insurance plans have to be developed to increase the proportion of the population receiving high-quality screening and treatment when needed, support programs to improve and standardize the quality of screening.

A remarkable milestone in the process of developing health care services in the UAE is the establishment of the National Breast Screening Program (NBSP) in 1995, operated by central department of maternal and child health, a division of the health policy affairs sector at the Ministry of health in UAE. The program's mission is to reduce mortality from breast cancer by delivering high-quality breast-screening service to UAE women as part of the overall spectrum of women's health. The program has been accredited by the WHO and the Nottingham Breast Institute in the United Kingdom in 2005 [24].

The Health Authority Abu Dhabi (HAAD) works with public, private, and community partners to create and implement strategies to help people in the Emirate of Abu Dhabi who live with, though, and beyond cancer. HAAD Cancer Control Plan aims at reducing the risk, incidence, and deaths from cancer, as well as enhancing the quality of life for cancer survivors. They have also issued recommendation for cancer screening and have initiated a 3-year-plan for cancer control in Abu Dhabi emirate (Fig. 19.6; Table 19.5) [25].

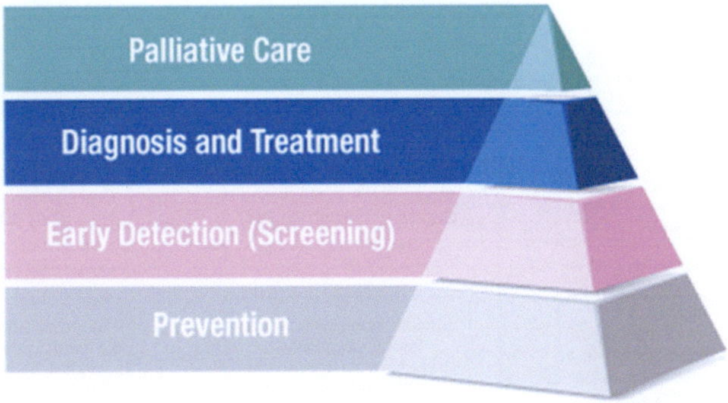

Fig. 19.6 The main cancer control strategies of HAAD, Abu Dhabi; 2012

Table 19.5 HAAD recommendation for cancer screening is described in the table below

Cancer type	Primary population group	Screening test and frequency
Colon and rectum cancer	Men and women	Colonoscopy, every 10 years; Or
	Age: 40–75 years	Stool test, every 2 years
Breast cancer	Women	Mammogram
	Age: 40 years and above	Every 2 years
Cervical cancer	Women	Pap test
	Age: 25–65 years	Every 3–5 years

The main cancer control strategies are:

- Establish evidence-based cancer prevention programs
- Improve quality of cancer care: screening, diagnosis, treatment, and palliative care
- Promote healthy living and early detection on priority cancers: breast, colorectal, lung, and cervical
- Enhance community support services and increase access to screening services
- Strengthen cancer surveillance

HAAD Cancer Control plan is a comprehensive approach that addresses all aspects of cancer care: prevention, early detection, diagnosis and treatment, and palliative care (Fig. 19.7).

Hematopoietic Stem Cell Transplant Program

Hematopoietic stem cell transplant (HSCT) is a new but rapidly expanding field in medicine since the first successful HSCT was performed in 1968. The procedure is utilized to treat medical conditions, previously lacking any treatment options, such as leukemia, myeloma, lymphomas, immune disorders, and some solid tumors.

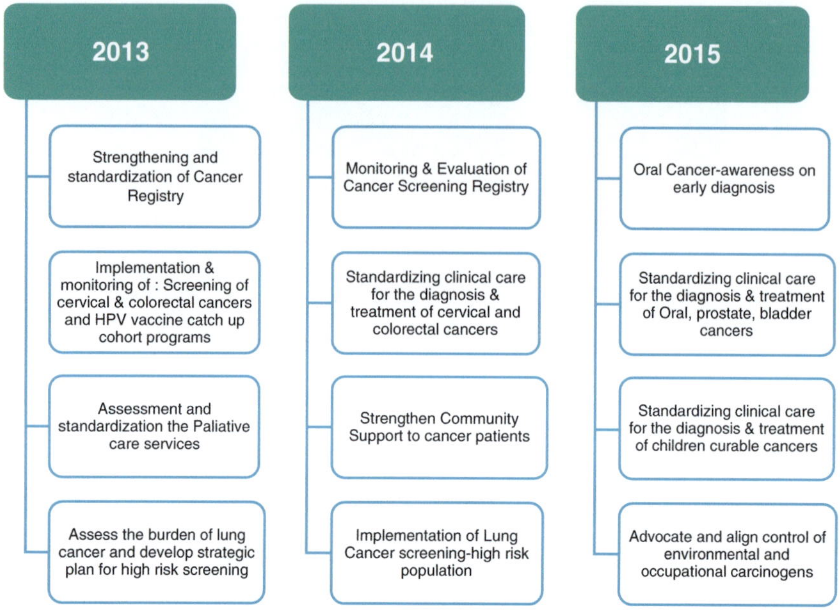

Fig. 19.7 Summary of the 3-year plan for cancer control in Abu Dhabi

The government of Abu Dhabi has requested Abu Dhabi Health Services Authority (SEHA) and Tawam Hospital to submit proposals to host an HSCT program.

At this point in time, there are only a few established HSCT programs in the Middle East region, principally in the Kingdom of Saudi Arabia. Patients residing in the UAE have little option but to seek treatment abroad. The cost of this treatment is very high, compounded by the associated travel, accommodation, and family member expenses.

The number of UAE-based patients sent abroad for treatment is difficult to establish, as there are several means of sponsoring their treatment. Costs are covered by nationwide organizations such as Defense and Police, local government within each Emirate, philanthropic individuals, and charitable organizations as well as self-pay.

There must be no doubt that to establish a successful program significant upfront and ongoing operational investment will be required. Tawam and SEHA have developed a comprehensive Financial Model for the HSCT program.

HSCT is a program that is associated with very high treatment mortality. However, an HSCT program can be successful and can generate significant revenue, provided that the hospital can develop a good reputation. In order to achieve this, many patients must be successfully treated. There should be no limit in the initial years on access to care restricted by insurance; otherwise, the necessary volume required to gain experience will not be available.

To date, SEHA are in the final planning stages having sought input from experienced external advisors.

Palliative Care

Palliative care—treating the pain, symptoms, and stress of serious illness—is vital for patients, but it is still misunderstood among health professionals, cancer sufferers, and the public at large. This type of treatment is also still not recognized as an essential component of health care and is not just for patients who have terminal illnesses.

Tawam Hospital has the distinction of being the only hospital in UAE with an established Palliative Care Program. Palliative care was started as a consultation service in 2007 and was developed into a complete division within oncology providing outpatient clinics and inpatient consultations with a dedicated inpatient unit. The number of outpatient visits and inpatient consultations in Palliative Care are increasing at a steady rate.

Palliative care is an important component of comprehensive cancer care in the developed world. The patients with advance terminal cancer are provided with efficient pain and symptom management with the aim to improve their quality of life. This is achieved by multidisciplinary approach with the involvement of various support staff such as social workers, psychiatrists, dieticians, physiotherapists, speech and language therapists, clinical pharmacists, home health care nurses and physicians, and pain management physicians. This multidisciplinary approach reduces the physical psychological and social suffering of the cancer patients and their families.

The Palliative Care Unit in Radiotherapy building was specially designed for easy access to the families of the terminal patient and is close to green lawns, where patients can go out and view the scenery outside the hospital bedroom. Many patients reach the stage of palliation due to the late presentation and diagnosis of cancer in this region. The Palliative Care Division is proud to have such service in the UAE serving the people of Emirates as well as the other GCC Countries.

While progress has been made in cancer diagnosis and treatment, much remains to be done to improve palliative care, which has emerged as an important subspecialty in high-income countries [26]. The expanding need for palliative care is now recognized, both medically and geographically, with the Worldwide Palliative Care Alliance recommending that governments integrate palliative care into each country's health care system [27].

Approximately 80 % of patients requiring palliative care live in low- and middle-income countries; 96 % are adults, the remainder children. Although childhood cancers are not among the six leading causes for palliative care, 98 % of all children needing palliative and end-of-life care belong to low- and middle-income groups. The highest rates for children needing palliative care for cancer are in eastern Mediterranean countries (WHO-EMRO region) [28].

While relative overall cancer survival rates are greater than 60 %, in less developed countries it is only 30–50 % [29]. The International Agency for Research on Cancer reported that the percentage of patients dying of cancer in 2012 varied between developed countries (40.4 %) and developing countries (66.4 %) [30]. Palliative care needs of a population can be estimated by number of deaths, a valuable reference for service planning and development [31].

Palliative care needs to be integrated into the health care system and added to the curriculum of medical schools through the means of a proper national educational program.

Cancer Registry in UAE

Tawam Cancer Registry (TCR) is a cancer information system for the collection and analysis of information on all cancer patients diagnosed and treated at the hospital. Tawam Hospital Cancer Registry is committed to decreasing the morbidity and mortality caused by cancer, through accurate and complete data collection that can be used to monitor, analyze, and report cancer incidence, treatment, and survival. The Registry covers about 80 % of the country, including all of Abu Dhabi. Its data is still published every year, but is less useful than a complete, UAE-wide record.

Tawam Cancer Registry is the oldest registry in the country, with cases dating back to 1998 and was the first and the only Cancer Registry in the United Arab Emirates which aims to follow Commission on Cancer (CoC) "Facility Oncology Data Standards" for cancer data recording and cancer care at a facility.

Within Tawam Hospital, TCR is considered to be an integral part of the hospital's cancer program which serves the needs of the hospital administration, the hospital's cancer program, and above all the individual patient by maintaining their follow-up

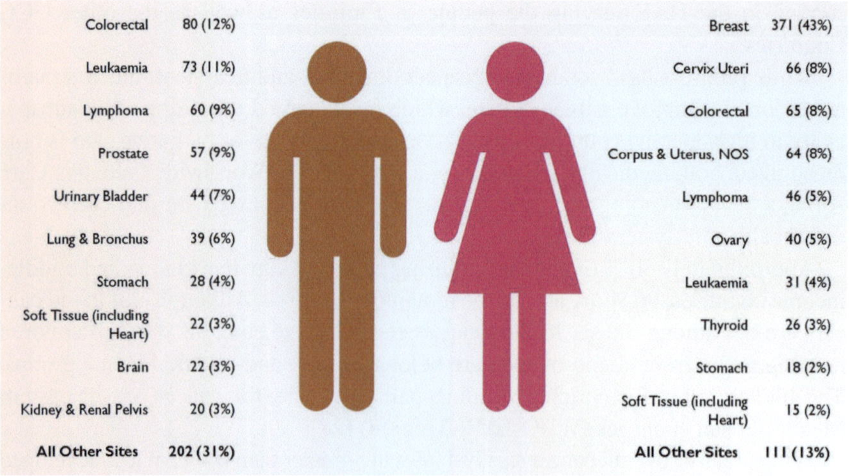

Fig. 19.8 Newly registered/diagnosed cancer cases at Tawam hospital in 2012 showing breast cancer amongst the top ten diagnosed cases (43 %) followed by CRC (12 %)

in a passive manner. TCR plays an important role in measuring cancer care delivery and supports quality improvement studies at Tawam. No other facility across the country has established a systemized and comprehensive approach to monitor and evaluate cancer care.

In 2012, a total of 1500 new cancer cases were registered at Tawam Hospital. Out of this, 43 % of the cases were diagnosed with breast cancer and 20 % were colorectal (Fig. 19.8).

Recommendations

Cancer Care in the Emirate of Abu Dhabi is facing a significant increase of new cases per year and to meet future demand, additional capacities for cancer treatments have to be established. The growth in demand for health care services associated with the prevention and treatment of cancer, cardiovascular disease, diabetes, respiratory conditions, emergency medicine, and neuropsychiatric conditions is expected to be particularly high in the coming years as the population ages. Health care particularly in Abu Dhabi faces growing demand for services arising from an expanding population. The current population is young and has a rate of chronic diseases that is set to increase as it ages. The need for additional capacities is getting more evident as cancer incidents is expected to increase significantly due to changing demographics and morbidity patterns. With a yearly growth of 4.7–7.1 %, the number of new cancer cases is expected to be more than double in the near future.

Bed Capacity

Significant additional capacity is required to meet growth in demand for health care services as the population grows and ages. In existing developed areas, the emphasis is on growing existing facilities to facilitate specialization and scale. Future development plans should be focused on the areas where there is new residential and commercial development and planned population growth.

Cancer Centers

HAAD has recommended the establishment of an optimized delivery model for oncology patients which is based on international standards of cancer care to increase capacities and balance the access to service providers within the Emirate. And based on the expected caseload in 2030 and approved minimum maximum patient volumes for efficient cancer centers, a demand for two integrated cancer centers have been derived and is underway.

Clinical staff: Government can help make nursing and other medical professions more attractive to local students by creating professionally and financially rewarding career paths for clinicians who stay in the region. Better salaries, substantial investments in professional training and development (such as residencies), and more flexible careers made possible by a greater degree of private-sector participation in the health care system should all help to attract nationals and keep expatriates.

Screening

It plays an increasingly important role in determining outcomes in many forms of cancer. However, the high cost of the new tests is not affordable by many patients and although the improved outcomes may not be seen for several years. In some cases (e.g., bladder cancer), evidence is emerging that new diagnostic methods may reduce recurrence rates and lower long-term treatment costs. Methods should be planned and implemented where access to screening for all groups is available and affordable, and to ensure referring doctors have access to tools for training, information, and inclusion in screening programs.

References

1. World Cancer Report 2008.
2. Jemal A, Bray F, Center MM, Ferlay J, Ward E, Forman D. Global cancer statistics. CA Cancer J Clin. 2011;61:69–90. Article first published online: 4 Feb 2011; doi:10.3322/caac.20107.
3. Blair I, Sharif AA. Population structure and the burden of disease in the United Arab Emirates. J Epidemiol Global Health. 2012;2:61–71.
4. Loney T, Cooling RF, Aw TC. Lost in translation? Challenges and opportunities for raising health and safety awareness among a multinational workforce in the United Arab Emirates. Saf Health Work. 2012;3:298–304. doi:10.5491/SHAW.2012.3.4.298.
5. United Arab Emirates National Bureau of Statistics. United Arab Emirates: United Arab Emirates National Bureau of Statistics; 2011. National population by emirate and sex (2010 mid-year estimates). http://www.uaestatistics.gov.ae/ReportDetailsEnglish/tabid/121/Default.aspx?ItemId=1914&PTID=104&MenuId=1 [cited 15 November 2012].
6. Statistical Yearbook of Abu Dhabi. United Arab Emirates: Abu Dhabi Statistics Centre. 2011. http://www.scad.ae/en/Pages/StatisticalYearBook.aspx. [cited 15 November 2012].
7. International Agency of Research on Cancer, GLOBOCAN. Incidence and mortality date for the United Arab Emirates; 2008.
8. Statistics Centre Abu Dhabi. Health statistics 2010. http://www.scad.ae/SCAD%20Publications/Health%20English.pdf.
9. Gulf Centre for Cancer Control and Prevention. Saudi Arabia: Riyadh; Ten-year cancer incidence among national of the GCC states, 1998–2007.
10. Gavel S. The oncology pipeline: maturing, competitive, and growing. Oncol Business Rev. 2008;9:14–6.
11. Yabroff R, Lamont E, Mariotto A, et al. Costs of care for elderly cancer patients in the United States. J Natl Cancer Inst. 2008;100:630–41.

12. Oliviera C, Bremner K, Pataky R, et al. Understanding the costs of cancer care before and after diagnosis for the 21 most common cancers in Ontaria: a population-based descriptive study. CMAJ Open. 2013. doi:10.9778/cmajo.20120013.
13. Warren J, Yabroff R, Meekins A, et al. Evaluation of trends in the cost of initial cancer treatment. J Natl Cancer Inst. 2008;100:888–97.
14. Mariotto A, Yabroff R, Shao Y, Feuer E, Brown M. Projections of the cost of cancer care in the United States: 2010–2020. J Natl Cancer Inst. 2011;103:117–28.
15. Levine M, Ganz PA, Haller D. Economic evaluation in the journal of clinical oncology: past, present, and future. J Clin Oncol. 2007;25:614–6.
16. HAAD Statistics 2001. http://www.haad.ae/HAAD/LinkClick.aspx?fileticket=JY0sMXQXrOU%3d&tabid=1243. Accessed 10 April 2013.
17. Meropol NJ, Schrag D, Smith TJ, et al. American Society of Clinical Oncology guidance statement: the cost of cancer care. J Clin Oncol. 2009;27:3868–74.
18. Campbell J, Ramsey S. The costs of treating breast cancer in the US: a synthesis of published evidence. Pharmacoeconomics. 2009;27:199–209.
19. Mariotto B, Yabroff R, Feuer J, et al. Projecting the number of patients with colorectal carcinoma by phases of care in the US; 2000–2020. Cancer Causes Control. 2006;17:1215–26.
20. Hoffman J, Li E, Doloresco F, et al. Projecting future drug expenditure-2012. Am J Health Syst Pharm. 2012;69:405–21.
21. Patient access to cancer drugs in nine countries in the Middle East; Frida Kasteng; Nils Wilking; Bengt Jonsson.
22. Altekruse SF, Kosary CL, Krapcho M, et al, eds. Surveillance, Epidemiology, and End Results Cancer Statistics Review, 1975–2007. Bethesda, MD: National Cancer Institute; 2010. http://seer.cancer.gov/csr/1975_2007/, based on November 2009 SEER data submission, posted to the SEER Web site, 2010.
23. http://gulfnews.com/news/gulf/uae/health/free-cancer-screenings-in-abu-dhabi-1.1237981.
24. Shaheen R. An overview on breast cancer in Abu Dhabi and United Arab Emirates: barriers & opportunities; 2013.
25. http://www.haad.ae/simplycheck/tabid/127/Default.aspx.
26. Silbermann M, Fink RM, Min S-J, Mancuso MP, Brant J, Hajjar R, Al-Alfi N, Baider L, Turker I, ElShamy K, Ghrayeb I, Al-Jadiry M, Khader K, Kav S, Charalambous H, Uslu R, Kebudi R, Barsela G, Kuruku N, Mutafoglu K, Ozalp-Senel G, Oberman A, Kislev L, Khleif M, Keoppi N, Nestoros S, Abdalla RF, Rassouli M, Morag A, Sabar R, Nimri O, Al-Qadire M, Al-Khalaileh M, Tayyem M, Doumit M, Punjwani R, Rasheed O, Fallatah F, Can G, Ahmed J, Strode D. Evaluating palliative in middle eastern care needs countries. J Palliat Med. 2015;18(1):18–25. doi:10.1089/jpm.2014.0194.
27. Palliative care: a peaceful, humane global campaign is needed. Lancet 2014;383:487.
28. Connor SR, Bermedeo MCS (eds). Global atlas of palliative care at the end-of-life. London: Worldwide Palliative Care Alliance, 2014. http://www.Global-atlas-identifies-unmet-need-for-palliative-care/. Accessed 13 May 2014.
29. Silbermann M, Epner D, Charalmbous H, et al. Promoting new approaches for cancer care in the Middle East. Ann Oncol. 2013;23:5–10.
30. International Agency for Research on Cancer: GLOBOCAN 2012: Estimated cancer incidence, mortality, and prevalence worldwide in 2012. http://globocan.iarc.fr/Pages/fact_sheets_cancer.aspx. Accessed 13 May 2014.
31. Hligginson IJ. Health care needs assessment: palliative care and terminal care. In: Stevens A, Raftery J, editors. Health care needs assessment. Oxford: Oxford Radcliffe Medical; 1997. p. 1–28.

Chapter 20
Cancer Care in Countries in Transition: The Islamic Republic of Iran

Maryam Rassouli and Moosa Sajjadi

Introduction

Patients with cancer are prone to experiencing countless problems in all the personal, family, and social aspects of their life. In order to prevent the adverse effects of disease from setting in and to improve the patients' quality of life as the main purpose of cancer treatment and care, a comprehensive system of both cancer care and palliative and supportive care needs to be established. According to a recent study by the World Health Organization, many countries do not have a cancer control plan that includes the prevention, early detection, treatment, and care of cancer; this study then reveals the urgent help required in these countries to reduce cancer-related mortality and provide long-term treatments and proper care to prevent pain and suffering in humans.

This chapter aims to introduce and present the status of both cancer care and palliative and supportive care in the Islamic Republic of Iran, that is, a country that has recently started devising plans for providing this type of care as well. Cancer is the third leading cause of death in Iran, and the increasing number of cancer patients in the country has turned this disease into a major challenge posed to the national health system. This chapter attempts to explain the current status of cancer in Iran, the present challenges of cancer care, the cultural factors associated with cancer care, the educational and academic challenges, the share and participation of the state and other organizations in cancer care and in providing palliative and supportive care.

M. Rassouli, Ph.D., R.N. (✉)
Nursing Department, Nursing and Midwifery School, Shahid Beheshti University of Medical Sciences, Vali-e Asr Street, Niyayesh Cross, Tehran, Iran
e-mail: Rassouli.m@gmail.com; mrassouli@sbmu.ac.ir

M. Sajjadi, Ph.D., R.N.
Department of Medical-Surgical Nursing, Faculty of Nursing and Midwifery, Gonabad University of Medical Sciences, Beside Asian Road, Gonabad, Iran
e-mail: sajjadi1975@gmail.com

M. Silbermann (ed.), *Cancer Care in Countries and Societies in Transition*,
DOI 10.1007/978-3-319-22912-6_20

The Current Status of Cancer Care in Iran

Iran is located in Southwest Asia, and, as a developing country, it is in an epidemiological transition from communicable to noncommunicable diseases, and is therefore faced with a doubled burden of diseases [1].

As a chronic disease, cancer is the second leading cause of death after cardiac diseases in western countries and in the USA [2], and the third leading cause of death after cardiac diseases and accidents in Iran [3]. According to the latest statistics, the annual incidence rate of cancer in Iran is about 107 per 100,000 people. Given the country's population of nearly 75 million, more than 80,000 people get afflicted with cancer every year. Due to the increasing environmental pollutions and the growing elderly population, cancer is expected to be on the rising trend and to become a major health problem of Iran in the next decade [4]. As a result of the high incidence rate of cancer in Iran and the reducing age of affliction with this difficult and costly disease, some cancer specialists are now using the term "cancer tsunami" to illustrate the severity of the human and financial damages caused by this disease in the country [5]. At the present time, more than 30,000 people die of cancer in Iran every year [6]. The World Health Organization predicts that, by 2020 in Iran, the incidence of cancer will reach 85,653 cases and cancer mortality rates, too, will reach 62,897 cases. It is our hope that, with proper scientific planning for the prevention of the incidence of controllable and preventable cancers, these numbers will decline [7].

In 2009, of the total 74,067 registered cases of cancer, 41,160 (55.58 %) were men and 32,898 (44.41 %) were women. The gender ratio of cancer incidence was therefore 125 during this year which means that 100 female patients existed for every 125 male patients. In Iran, breast cancer still ranks first among women, with the peak age of incidence being around 50–55 years. The five most common cancers in women include breast, skin, colorectal, stomach, and esophagus cancer, in descending order of prevalence; and in men, they include skin, stomach, prostate, bladder, and colorectal cancer, in the same order. The five most common cancers in Iran irrespective of gender include skin, breast, stomach, colorectal, and bladder cancer (Table 20.1) [8].

These statistics are somewhat similar to statistics provided for the various types of cancer in the USA and across the world. However, stomach and esophagus cancers are relatively more prevalent in Iran compared to the global statistics of common cancers. Stomach cancer is highly prevalent in northwestern Iran and esophagus cancer is more common in northeastern Iran, while both less prevalent in central Iran. For instance, the Age-Standardized Rate (ASR) of the incidence of stomach cancer in Ardebil province in northwestern Iran is 49.1 for men and 25.4 for women. Esophagus cancer is highly prevalent in Golestan province in northeastern Iran, which is attributed to habits such as drinking hot tea, not consuming fresh food, and drug use [1].

As the most common cancer among Iranian women, and given that it involves women in their reproductive ages and has a lower age distribution in Iran compared to other countries, breast cancer has always been a major concern for the national

Table 20.1 Ten most common cancers in Iran (2009)

Cancer type	*N*	%
Skin	9114	12.3
Breast	7822	10.6
Stomach	6886	9.3
Colon and anal canal	6210	8.4
Bladder	4601	6.2
Prostate	3856	5.2
Leukemia	3461	4.7
Esophagus	3297	4.5
Lung, bronchus and trachea	2992	4.0
Non-Hodgkin lymphoma	2345	3.2
Others	23,483	31.7
Total	74,067	100

Adapted from annual report of cancer cases. http://www.ircancer.ir/Default.aspx?tabid=95#

health authorities. With an incidence rate of 25 in 100,000 people and nearly 8000 new patients per year, this disease imposes a great degree of negative economic, social, and mental consequences on the individual, the society, and the health system [9]. According to a cancer registry report of 2009 in Iran, 7582 cases of breast cancer were diagnosed in Iranian women, with a peak incidence age of 50–55 years and an ASR of 28.25 in 100,000 women. According to the report data, about 49.4 % of the breast cancer population is in the age group of 50 and older, 31.2 % in the 40–49 age group, and 19.4 % are younger than 40 [8].

Although implementing breast cancer prevention and screening programs are highly efficient tools for the early diagnosis of this cancer, they have yet to be seriously adopted by women and advised by most physicians. Poverty, the lack of health insurance coverage and the absence of regular prevention and screening programs are barriers to the control of cancer. It appears that the poor awareness of women in Iran about the risk factors, symptoms and signs and benefits of screening programs and the functional deficiencies of health clinics in relation to cancer, in particular breast cancer, are due to the absence of prevention programs [10].

Cancer Care and Critical Clinical Issues

Problems of the health system of the Islamic Republic of Iran can be summarized in nine subgroups, some of which challenge the cancer care system and, consequently, the provision of palliative care. Some of them include equity in offering service providing systems (health costs, lack of insurance coverage), efficacy and quality (the absence of a system for evaluating the cost-effectiveness of services), structure (a centralized structure, lack of a defined status for the nongovernmental sector, ineffectiveness of the existing structure faced with new impositions such as cancer), health information system (non-registration of actions, lack of statistics on admitted cases, bed occupancy, etc.), service providing workforce (preference of physical resources over human resources, disproportionate workforce), funding resources, payment systems, and rules and regulations (law deficiencies and conflicting laws) [11].

According to experts of the field, much less attention is being paid to cancer in Iran than in advanced countries, as the public health care status and efforts for culture-building and informing the public have not been emphasized. Cancer registration is not carried out meticulously, and the oncology curriculum is still left unattended by the Ministry of Health and Medical Education, which is in charge of making policies on and executing medical education programs [12].

A number of challenges in the field of cancer care in Iran are discussed in the following section.

Cancer Registry

The prevention and reduction of cancer cases require cancer control programs to be implemented. A cancer registry system is considered a major component of cancer control programs. Iran's Cancer Registry was approved in 1984 and published its first cancer registry report in 1986 with 18,435 cases of cancer. The second cancer registry report of 1996 was published in 1999 with 11,025 cases of cancer. This report had registered only 18 % of all the new cases of cancer. Until 2007, cancer registration was based only on pathology reports. However, due to the system's failure to diagnose cancers that are diagnosed without biopsy, such as brain cancer, a population-based registration system was established across 20 universities of the country in 2008 to complement the pathology-based registration. The statistics rose to 74,067 cases of cancer in 2009. Tehran has qualities that make it perfect for being the center of cancer registry, for example, being home to 10 % of the country's population, to diverse ethnic groups and also to various centers [13].

The National Cancer Registry of Iran covers the whole area and the entire population of the country. Cancer registry is administered centrally by the Ministry of Health and Medical Education. Collected cancer data are sent to the Cancer Office by the health deputies to be published in the form of national reports after thorough statistical analysis. Although the first comprehensive registry report was published in 2004, no such reports have yet been published in the book "Cancer incidence in five continents." The registry is entirely funded through state budgets by the Ministry of Health. There are no independent registries or registrars at the provincial level; instead, data is collected by health deputies [14]. This 5-year program is intended to achieve the desired results in pilot provinces over the next 5 years, and then, if required and if the necessary infrastructures are in place, to be extended to the entire country [15].

Pain and Pain Management

Pain caused by cancer itself or the complications arising from its treatment procedures affect 50–90 % of the patients with cancer. Uncontrolled cancer pain sometimes pushes patients toward suicide [16]. Pain and its management comprise a crucial aspect of cancer care. Pain is a global phenomenon that affects quality of life in people across all cultures. Culture affects all the aspects of the experience of cancer in the patients, their family caregivers, and professional healthcare providers, including the perception, expression, and treatment of pain by the patient and their family. Cultural background has long been recognized as an influential factor in understanding the perception of and the reaction to pain. Findings of studies have shown that family culture, beliefs, and religion play a decisive role in the perception and management of pain by patients and their caregivers. All members of the multidisciplinary oncology team who provide care for the patient should be attentive to the patient's cultural beliefs associated with his health and take advantage of them in their care [17].

There are different cultural and belief perspectives about pain. In some cultures where religion plays a strong role, pain is believed to have been granted by God, and it is a human obligation to tolerate pain; in these cultures, pain is an accepted and anticipated form of life; in other words, pain and disease are human fate and should be tolerated, or else result from the evil deeds of humans [17]. In Islam, pain and suffering is regarded as the patient's atonement for sins [18]. That is why most people consider cancer similar to the tolerating of pain and suffering [19].

In a study conducted with the purpose of determining the relationship between attitude to pain relief and receiving analgesics in patients with cancer, most patients were of the attitude that analgesics are addictive, which might owe to their poor information. Yet, at the end stages of disease, the patient's pain relief and comfort take priority. According to results, patients with the attitude that analgesics are addictive used significantly less amount of opioids than others. Patients with fewer false beliefs and attitudes about pain and the management of pain received sufficient analgesics and were thus able to effectively and adequately control their pain [20].

According to statistics provided by the International Narcotics Control Board (INCB) on the use of opioid analgesics, Iran ranked 115 in the world, 25 in Asia, and 15 in the region, therefore grouped among the low-consumption countries. Nevertheless, Iran is a rich country in terms of raw materials and manufacturing technology required for the production of opioid analgesics, and Mehrdarou, Exir, Shadarou, Daroupakhsh, and Tofighdaru companies produce drugs such as methadone, codeine, oral oxycodone, and morphine injection. The drug formulary used in Iran for opioid analgesics, in particular non-synthetic analgesics, complies in part with the World Health Organization's approved list. These drugs are also so inexpensive that require almost no economic support system at all [21]. A report published in February 2013 assessing the method of opioid use in palliative care attributes the low consumption of these drugs to the lack of proper access to opioid drugs and also, in some cases, the negative attitudes of physicians, patients, and their families to opioid drugs [21].

In a study conducted by Mohagheghi et al. (2003) on 304 cancer patients, the patients' most frequently used opioid drug included morphine injection, oral opium, and methadone (injectable and oral). These researchers also noted the inadequate variety of opioid drugs in Iran and the unfamiliarity of most physicians and almost all patients with the inadequate medical and administrative route for the prescription and preparation of the opioids. The available prescription drugs are also not used in a systematic fashion, and inappropriate use, including abuse, low or high dosage, improper administration route and sequence and carelessness about drug interferences, is widely witnessed. Standard instructions issued by university committees in partnership with the Ministry of Health might be helpful in resolving the current problems [22]. Stringent rules govern the use of opioids in Iran, and due to the absence of statistics on the level of opioid use in cancer patients, this data can only be accessed through a patient registration system in universities of medical sciences across different regions of the country. In Iran, the Food and Drug Department stationed in every university of medical sciences is responsible for providing the opioid drug demands of the medical centers within its area of coverage. The office of Controlled Drugs and Substances of each deputy is responsible for filing separate records for all patients demanding these drugs. Patients who have been using opioids for over a year should be examined by a medical committee, and should be able to refill their prescriptions after their disease and their opioid demands are confirmed once more. After this step, patients can refill their prescriptions for one more month [21].

Cost of Cancer Care

All the health systems across the world are faced with the rising costs of health care threatening high quality care. Health care costs have also sharply risen during the past few years in Iran, posing challenges to the state, insurance companies, and patients. In Iran, there are three sources for budgeting health care, including public state funding, health insurance payments, and individuals' out-of-pocket expenses [23]. Although the country's health budget has been constantly increasing in recent years, and thought it has now three times its previous amount, out-of-pocket expenditure on health remains as high as 55 % [24].

The treatment of cancer is a vital medical obligation. Treatments performed on cancer patients are often invasive and severe and require large expenditure of resources. Treating cancer is a costly affair that not only threatens life and welfare, but also puts the patient's financial security at risk [25]. In Iran, patients with cancer have to travel long distances to receive proper treatment, which increases the financial burden imposed on them or their families. The demand for the treatment of cancer and its associated financial pressures can be a strong source of stress for the patients and their families, particularly in the case of low-income patients. The early estimation of the costs of care for cancer patients is an important component of the development of national cancer policies and programs. Cancer costs of patients are at their peak during the first 6 months after diagnosis and the last 12 months before death, and they significantly reduce between these two stages [25].

A major challenge posed to the treatment of patients with cancer is the discriminate distribution of specialists across the country, which somehow increases costs incurred by patients. For instance, it appears that the dense concentration of more experienced specialists and stronger diagnostic services in Tehran, the country's capital city, allows the patients to be diagnosed with fewer doctor's visits and diagnostic services. The high costs of treatments such as chemotherapy and surgeries incurred by patients in Tehran are attributed to the stronger, more active presence of the private sector in Tehran, while in other cities, patients usually use the cheaper services of the public sector [25].

Adopting new policies to cover the costs incurred by cancer patients, particularly by insurance companies, receiving funding through institutions such as banks or charities, the indiscriminate distribution of specialized cancer centers or providing temporary accommodation to patients traveling from other cities can reduce the financial burdens imposed on cancer patients and help them in their management of the disease, in addition to also realizing health equity indicators [25].

Academic Education Challenges

Many studies have been conducted on the inadequacy of palliative care training in various medical groups, mostly targeting nurses and physicians. Some of these studies have suggested that nurses are still inadequately skilled and not very efficient in providing palliative care and that they require better training for this particular concept and type of care [26].

The main problem of the nursing system in Iran in relation to palliative care for cancer patients is that no clear framework exists for this type of care for nurses and that it does not have a strict presence in the official curriculum. One reason for this problem appears to be the lack of comprehensive studies on this subject in the country, which limits the applicability of the concept of palliative care to these patients [27]. Findings of a study conducted for "examining the attitude and motivation of nursing students for finding work in cancer departments" showed that nursing students did not have a positive attitude toward working in cancer departments, and showed their mean overall score for attitude toward working in cancer departments and all of its components to be low. The incompatibility of the content of theoretical courses on cancer and the real needs in cancer departments ranked lowest among all motivational factors. The lack of adequate communication and care skills for patients at end-of-life stages and the incompatibility of the content of theoretical courses on cancer and real-life needs had contributed greatly to the students' negative attitudes [28].

In many countries, General Practitioners (GPs) are the main responsible authorities for providing patients with medical care, in particular palliative care. In Iran, given the extension of the role of GPs to family doctors, it appears that they will also play the main role in this area. However, there is no formal palliative care training in Iran during the course of general practice education [6]. Results of a study show that, in Iran, only 12 % of GPs have excellent or very good knowledge of palliative care and more than half of them have poor or no knowledge in this area. Only 22 % of participating physicians knew about the WHO pain control guidelines and were well acquainted with the management of patients' physical symptoms. More than half admitted their poor knowledge of pain control, the principles of end-of-life care and palliative care. It appears that the deficient knowledge of physicians on palliative care is rooted in the medical education system in place in Iran, which is mostly symptom based rather than holistic [6].

Despite the guidelines provided by the World Health Organization on the management and treatment of pain in cancer patients, pain is still not well managed in these patients. A main barrier to the control of pain in these patients is the physicians' deficient knowledge. In a study conducted on this subject, the main barrier to the proper management of pain was the absence of pain control specialists and the personnel's lack of knowledge on pain management. The majority of physicians who participated in this study asserted that they were unhappy about the pain management training they had received during their medical education [29, 30].

Given the importance of a well-established, specialized workforce for providing this type of care, and in response to the shortage of human resources at both general and specialized levels, educational planning for the required disciplines has been given priority in the National Bylaw for the Development of Palliative and Supportive Cancer Care (2012), and it has been proposed to develop an educational curriculum, as well as short-term and long-term course requirements, and to issue certificates by the deputy and office of continuing education in the health professions [21].

The Interrelationship Between Cancer Care and Local Culture and Society Reactions to Cancer Patients

In every society, cancer care is affected by the prevailing culture of that society, and the attitude of people in that society toward health and disease affects how that society treats and regards patients. Some of the cultural challenges present in the Iranian society in treating cancer patients are discussed in the following section.

Telling the Truth to the Patient

Cultural elements affect the patients' reactions to being diagnosed with serious diseases such as cancer and the decisions they make about end-of-life care. Studies conducted on this subject identify three fundamental dimensions for end-of-life care and treatment as affected by cultural issues, including the manner of breaking "bad news," the locus of decision-making about treatment procedures, i.e., resort to the available options or discontinuing treatment, and people's attitudes toward end-of-life care [31].

Contrary to the emphasis in Western culture on truth-telling, in some cultures (such as in the Middle East, and more specifically, in Iran), it is not uncommon to hide the cancer diagnosis from the patient, and disclosure of cancer might be misconstrued as bad manners, disrespect, or even detrimental [31, 32]. For example, in Iran, in some cases, the patient might only learn about his disease long after his definitive diagnosis of cancer, and even then only indirectly through chancing upon his medical file, talking to other patients, starting treatments such as chemotherapy; under most circumstances, the diagnosis is not directly disclosed to the patient [33].

Although in many societies, decision-making is based on the patient's autonomy and freedom to act, in some cultures, medical decisions are still doctor-oriented or doctor-family oriented, which might violate the patient's autonomy. Some cultures (such as most Asian cultures) value the principle of productivity and usefulness more than autonomy and freedom to act. Consequently, in many of these cultures, care providers tend to hide cancer diagnoses from the patients. In such cultures, physicians obscurely express the severity of the patient's condition by using medical jargon, and only disclose the information to the patient's family members [31, 34]. In these cultures, the majority of people believe it a pointless cruelty to tell the patient directly that he has cancer [35]. In some Asian cultures (such as in Pakistan), the patient's family members deliberately and actively protect him from the burden of finding out about his end-of-life conditions. In these cultures, disease is mostly a family event rather than a personal one, and it is often preferable if the family takes care of the patient (particularly during the end-of-life stage) [36].

There are major reasons for which cancer is not disclosed in these cultures. In some cultures, for example, talking about death and serious diseases is considered disrespectful and a form of bad manners. Some believe that freely discussing cancer and serious diseases causes unnecessary depression and anxiety in the patient. Some believe it to lead to the loss of hope in the patient. In some cultures, there is even the belief that hypothetical discussions about death and terminal illness might turn them into reality [31]. Moreover, the common belief is that if the patient learns about his diagnosis, his condition will worsen [19].

As a general rule, the less people know about a subject, the more infused with myths and mysteries will be their interpretation of it. Cancer is one such subject. False beliefs and myths are not merely a wrong notion that sticks in minds; they also affect people's tendencies in life. For years, cancer was considered an inevitable cause of death. It is therefore not surprising that there are so many myths about it. Some of the myths that are more common among the general public are that a cancer patient has a tragic fate, or that cancer surgery spreads cancer throughout the body [19].

Such points of view are also observed in the structure of health systems. For example, cancer departments are often located in the worst areas of hospitals and in old, dark, dingy places with no particular design and beauty, while a beautiful, green architecture can significantly improve healing in these patients [37].

Death and Dying

Iran is a country where 98 % of the population is Muslim. Death is a well defined and essential concept in Islam. In Iran, death is culturally well defined and dying is considered a rebirth as part of the stages of life [38]. In the Iranian Islamic culture, pain or painful death are considered atonement for sins committed in life. This view of death leads to the more devoted performing of religious rituals and practices during times of critical illness and end-of-life stages. From a cultural and religious perspective, placing the Quran above the patient's head or by his bedside is one thing that brings the patient peace, even in the form of a peaceful death [18]. Given the increased emotional and spiritual needs of patients in end-of-life stages, which brings intense psychological reactions in them, care providers try to support the patients and their families both emotionally and spiritually so that they can be better prepared and adapted to their conditions [39]. Most people turn to religion to improve the patients' psychological health for facing tensions caused by disease and potential death [40]. In religious societies like Iran, death is deemed "the Will of God," which is a consolation that might result in the acceptance of fate. In other instances, the well-known metaphor "the Will of God" is only used when every hope in medicine is lost [41].

Given what has been said about Eastern and Asian cultures, the common opinion in Iran emphasizes the providing of care for cancer patients in their own homes (particularly for those in end-of-life stages). However, there is still no research-based evidence to suggest what the preferences of cancer patients are in Iran [42].

Local Innovations and Palliative Care

Because of the complexities in the diagnosis, treatment, and symptoms of the disease, cancer patients have complex care needs through all the stages of the disease, from diagnosis to treatment and during the follow-up to the end-of-life stage. Because of its vast scope of effects on the various aspects of the patients' (and their families') life, including the physical, psychological, spiritual, and social aspects, cancer requires a holistic care [4].

Holistic care considers all the needs of the patient and requires a coordinated multidisciplinary care team. In holistic care, extensive services are provided for the patients and their families, including treatment and management of symptoms, training, counseling, support groups (emotional, psychological, financial, etc.), and other special programs designed to help improve quality of life in the patients and their families [43].

The early diagnosis and treatment of cancer can significantly reduce cancer mortality rates. For achieving this goal, it is necessary for countries to make proper use of each others' experiences and innovations in fields concerned with cancer care, such as medications, diagnostic and treatment techniques, and modern care models [44].

A large proportion of cancer care is provided to patients in the form of palliative and supportive care. In Iran, palliative and supportive care is a relatively new concept and providing such services to cancer patients is in its infancy. In terms of providing palliative care, Iran is classified under group A3. In countries of this group, palliative care is provided sporadically and is not well supported; for the most part, it is a type of care provided at the patients' home, and the ratio of available service centers to the population is very low [30].

The need for providing palliative and supportive care in Iran is a well-perceived need [30], and the absence of the documented providing of these services has created countless problems for both patients and the Ministry of Health, including patients' frequent visits to emergency departments for the management of symptoms, their frequent admissions to ICU and other departments and the increased rate of nosocomial infections. However, only 20 % of cancer patients require specialized services to manage their symptoms, and 80 % can manage their problems through primary care. At the present time, palliative and supportive care services are only provided in a limited number of centers across the country [45]. Following the implementation of the plan for the development of a Comprehensive National Supportive and Palliative Cancer Care Program, which was carried out in 2012 under the supervision of the Department of Non-Communicable Diseases, the Cancer Department of The Ministry of Health and the Iranian Cancer Research Network and in partnership with associated science associations and research centers, the "National Bylaw for the Development of Supportive and Palliative Cancer Care" was complied in seven chapters. This bylaw defines the levels of supportive and palliative care providing as composed of the hospital unit, the counseling team, the clinic and the home care team [21].

Modified and localized models commonly used in other countries at the regional and international levels can also be considered suitable models for Iran that can be adapted from their successful programs in this area. For example, in these countries, palliative care is provided in various centers such as palliative care departments in hospitals, hospice facilities, and community care centers [46]. As for Iran, considering the available resources, the health system and the different composition of the Iranian society, appropriate systems of providing care for cancer patients can be effectively adapted from western care systems and instituted in such areas as the establishment of palliative care departments, providing home care, day-care clinics, and hospice facilities (if practical). The NHS has developed a stratified support and care model for patients with cancer, which is helpful in providing holistic care and meeting patients' other needs in addition to needs associated with the disease and its effective treatment. This care model is an innovation in cancer care, and adapting it can be effectively helpful in providing care for cancer patients in Iran [47]. Based on the investigations conducted by a panel of experts on the structures of providing palliative care in Iran, which take into consideration criteria such as health infrastructures, social, cultural, and economic conditions and the availability of equipment and facilities in the country, it appears that the techniques for providing hospital care, home care, and hospital counseling are higher priorities. Providing palliative care is not a priority or a necessity in day clinics across Iran. Hospice facilities are centers in which providing palliative care is of the lowest priority [48].

A helpful and seemingly essential action in providing proper holistic cancer care is to record the medical history of patients, to utilize information technologies, and to create electronic files for patients. Electronic filing is very helpful in coordinating the providing of care among different members of the care providing team [49]. Modeling our country after western health care systems with their valuable experiences in this area can help improve cancer care in Iran. Cancer care requires close interdisciplinary teamwork. Interdisciplinary care does not have a long history in Iran. Using the positive experiences of western countries with long histories in this area also helps accelerate the improvement of palliative care in Iran.

Undoubtedly, an important point to consider in the providing of care for cancer patients is the availability and accessibility of medical resources that can be used along with financial support and better payment methods for the patients. The cost of cancer care and treatment is too high (in Iran and also in many other countries), which deprives many low- and middle-income patients from proper care [50]. One of the measures that have been taken in the Iranian health system to improve this deficiency is the Healthcare Transformation Plan that launched last May. According to this plan, patients with refractory diseases such as cancer are to benefit from major help and support from the state (in particular the low-income patients), so that they do not encounter problems during the course of their treatment. This plan has increased the patients' satisfaction, reduced part of their costs, and provided the means for better care. If the plan turns out to be successful, the health system of other countries can also perhaps adopt it for their own benefit [51].

Government's Share in Cancer Patients' Care

Before addressing the government's share in cancer patients' care, it is essential to provide a brief overview of the health system in Iran. Article 29 of the Constitution of the Islamic Republic of Iran states that every Iranian citizen has the right to benefit from the highest possible level of health. To accomplish this level of health, in Iran, the Ministry of Health and Medical Education is given responsibility for the design and implementation of national health policies. The Ministry of Health has delegated the implementation of these programs to universities of medical sciences throughout the country. Each province of Iran has at least one university. The head of the university of medical sciences is the highest responsible authority in each province and reports to and is accountable toward the Ministry of Health and Medical Education. He is also responsible for the public health, for providing facilities for the public health and for medical education. Health care and public health services are provided through a national network, from primary to tertiary health services [24] (Fig. 20.1).

Over the past two decades, the government has placed a greater emphasis on public sector primary care services. Some health care services, such as vaccination and prenatal care are provided free of charge. The public sector also provides a significant proportion of secondary and tertiary health care services in provinces [24].

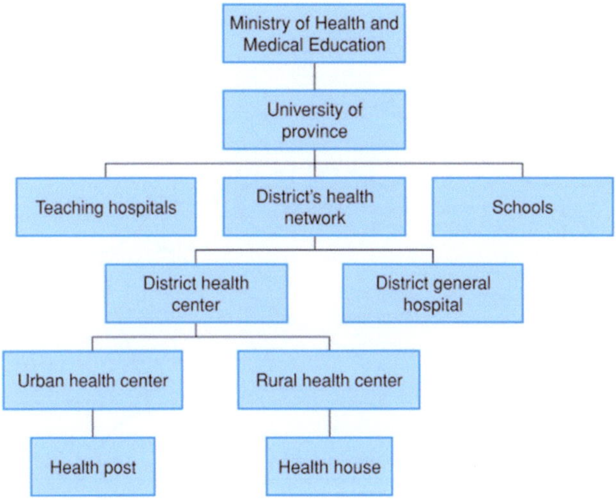

Fig. 20.1 The health system network in Iran (adapted from: Mehrdad R. Health system in Iran. JMAJ 52(1): 69–73, 2009.)

The private sector plays an important role in providing health services in Iran. Most private sectors are located in urban areas and focus on providing secondary and tertiary health care services. There are many nongovernmental organizations (NGOs) in Iran that are active in the health sector. NGOs are often active in specific fields such as children with cancer, breast cancer, diabetes, and special diseases like thalassemia and hemodialysis patients. The Ministry of Health and Medical Education is responsible for planning, monitoring, and supervising the health activities of both the public and the private sectors [24].

Iran's ministry of health has a unique structure that distinguishes it from ministries of health in other countries. In 1986, the integration of the ministry of health and the higher education system created the present ministry, referred to as the Ministry of Health and Medical Education. The proponents of this integration believe it to have strengthened the quality of health services throughout the country, while its opponents believe it to have adversely affected medical education. However, in the absence of systematic studies for proving the standpoints, the controversy over the integration remains unresolved [24].

According to the official data, over 90 % of the population of Iran are covered by at least one type of health insurance. The main health insurances include Social Security Insurance, Iran Health Insurance, Armed Forces Insurance, and Imam Khomeini Relief Foundation [24]. Public state funds and health insurance payments are the main sources for health financing in Iran. The state fund is proposed by the Ministry of Health and is confirmed and approved by the Parliament. Insurance payments are provided by four health insurance organizations and are somewhat state dependent and variously supported by the state. However, the Iranian health system

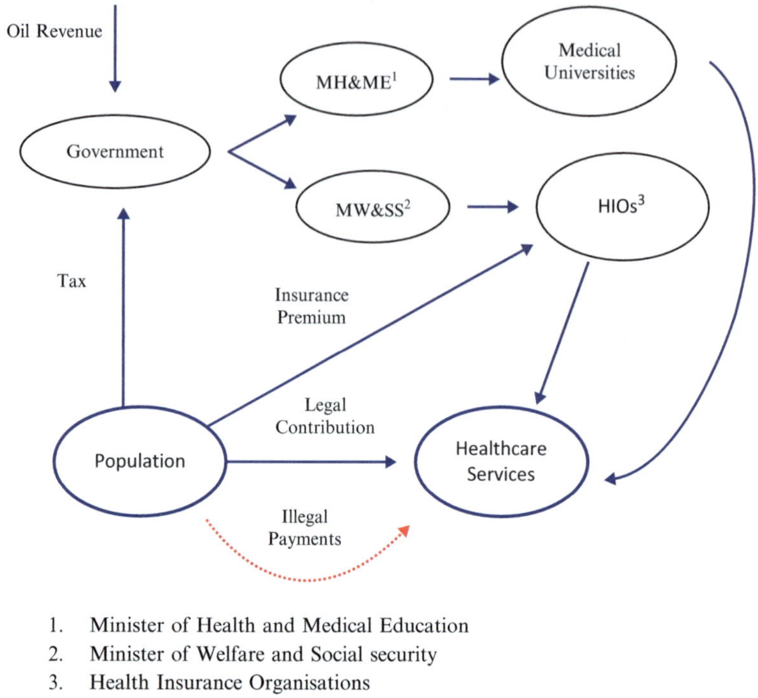

Fig. 20.2 Money cycle within the Iranian health care market (adapted from: Davari M, Haycox A, Walley T. Health care financing in Iran; Is privatization a good solution? Iran J Public Health: 2012,(7) 41.14–23)

aims to reduce payments made by people (out-of-pocket payments) to 30 % in the next few years [23].

To better understand the system, the process of money circulation in the Iranian health care market is shown in Fig. 20.2.

Given the stated points about the health care system in Iran, the extensive share and interference of the state in patients' health care is inferred. In Iran, care services provided to cancer patients are generally hospital based. In other words, the majority of patients receive their health care in hospitals and centers providing home care are rare and hospice facilities are simply nonexistent in the country. These patients can receive the care they need in hospitals and public centers (in most cases) or hospitals and private centers (in fewer cases). As indicated by the role of the state and the Ministry of Health in planning, monitoring, and supervising care services provided to patients in public and private hospitals and even nonprofit hospitals and charities, the government's substantial share and interference in providing every aspect of care to cancer patients, including diagnosis, treatment, and rehabilitation, is prominent [23, 24].

Institutional Involvement

In the prevention of and fight against cancer, early diagnosis, proper treatment, and after-treatment care, public institutions and NGOs contribute greatly with their cooperation and coordination. The costs of diagnosis, treatment, and controlling of cancer are outrageous and become even more so by day, to the extent that even middle-income patients cannot afford the cancer care they need. In all countries, including developed ones, nongovernmental charity organizations vastly contribute to the supporting of cancer patients and governments do not consider themselves well-to-do without the help of these institutions. Governments therefore try to provide the appropriate framework for the establishment, growth and prosperity of NGOs and for their providing of services to patients [50]. NGOs active in the field of cancer can play a major role in the development and implementation of government policies, including the Comprehensive Cancer Control Plan, and can also undertake a significant share of the state responsibilities through promoting good life habits and warning about bad health behaviors and providing inclusive support to the patients and their families.

In the Islamic Republic of Iran, with the rich national and religious culture it boasts, several charities have been organized in the majority of provinces to help support cancer patients and provide care to them. Some of these organizations have a long, illustrious history of supporting cancer patients and their families and provide valuable diagnostic, palliative, and treatment services to cancer patients through their establishment of medical centers such as radiation therapy centers, hospitals and physical and mental rehabilitation centers. Some of these charity organizations have undertaken remarkable activities toward the prevention of cancer and its early diagnosis through providing financial support or through informing and educating the public and promoting awareness in the community [50].

There are nonprofit medical institutions in the form of hospitals or radiation and chemotherapy centers for cancer patients in major cities of Iran, including Tehran, Isfahan, Mashhad, Shiraz, Hamadan, and Urmia, bearing a significant share of the government's responsibility. Charity associations for supporting cancer patients also exist in many other cities of Iran; however, they may not be as extensive as the institutions existing in major cities, and might not be well equipped with treatment and diagnostic centers; yet, they provide notable financial and spiritual support to cancer patients and contribute effectively to their care [49]. These institutions are not merely about providing financial help; rather, they have always directly cooperated in providing care. Examples include Mahak Charity, which provides palliative and treatment care for children with cancer, and Sepas Charity, which provides psychosocial support for cancer patients. Seyed-Al-Shohada palliative care center of Isfahan is another example of charity centers that are active in providing completely free of charge care to cancer patients. The expenses incurred by patients are fully paid for by people's donations [30].

A non-extensive list of NGOs participating in cancer care in Iran follows: Mehraneh Cancer Care Charity in Zanjan, Kurdistan Cancer Patients Supporting

Society in Sanandaj, Iranian Cancer Society in Babul, Aria Breast Cancer Society, Iranian Lung Cancer Society (ASRA), Behnam Daheshpour Charity in Tehran, and many others.

Other than charity organizations, some centers in affiliation with universities and a number of public organizations also play a major role in providing care to cancer patients. The National Cancer Institute, which is under the coverage of the Charity Foundation for Special Diseases, began its activities with an independent charter in 2009, aiming to prevent cancer and help improve cancer patients' health through a network of specialists and volunteers at the national level and the cooperation of relevant organizations. This institute aims to establish a medical center in the next few years [52].

Among other official organizations affiliated to universities of medical sciences and playing an active role in providing care for cancer patients in Iran are the designated cancer research centers that provide significant care services for cancer patients. For example, the Cancer Research Center affiliated to Shahid Beheshti University of Medical Sciences performs extensive activities in applied research for cancer prevention, for the proper treatment of cancer patients and for their care and rehabilitation. These research centers carry out screening projects for some cancers (breast and cervical cancers) in the form of research projects that have proved very useful in the early diagnosis and treatment of cancer and reducing its mortality rates. This center also provides free counseling services for cancer patients. For instance, this center holds free "stress reducing techniques" seminars for patients and is launching palliative and supportive care services for cancer patients visiting this center [53]. Other research centers of the type also exist in other major universities and cities of Iran.

Although charity and nongovernmental centers and institutions and nearly independent centers and institutions affiliated to universities are more or less active in providing care for cancer patients, their share is still negligible compared to the government's share. Further developing the means for the expansion of these institutions in providing care to cancer patients requires the government's assistance, the removal of the legal barriers against the activities of these institutions, and simplifying legislations on matters such as customs and tax [50].

Conclusion

All countries should deploy the core essentials of the health system and information systems required for monitoring and evaluating planned epidemiological data, and should then use these data for a better decision-making. Countries with low to moderate resources such as Iran should consider the key priorities of their region. With any degree of resources at one's disposal, taking a stage-by-stage approach allows every priority to be considered in both the plan's content and the geographical field. Furthermore, cost-effective sustainable technologies should be used in conditions where resources are limited. For Iran, inexpensive and effective maintenance care is the start point that will gradually lead to the adoption of a holistic approach entailing early detection and primary prevention. The priority for actions in maintenance care should be based on the resources of the country, and should target the implementation of comprehensive maintenance care programs in order to improve quality of life in numerous cancer patients or to improve other life-threatening states of theirs and their families'. These programs should improve pain, control other symptoms and provide psychosocial and spiritual support. Under such circumstances, it is essential to ensure that the minimum standards of pain improvement and maintenance care are progressively in place at target areas and at all levels of care; high levels of health service coverage is mainly achieved in the form of home care at these stages. In countries with strong family support systems and poor health infrastructures, home care is the best way to achieve a good quality of care and is the best form of health coverage [54].

Palliative and supportive cancer care has recently become the main focus of attention in Iran as part of the country's National Cancer Control Program. Priorities set by the World Health Organization in this area include increasing sensitivity to the need for palliative services at all levels, providing services and introducing palliative services to physicians and nurses, providing pain reducing palliative services, controlling other symptoms, providing psychological and spiritual services and ensuring that minimum standards for palliative care are in place. As for increasing sensitivity to palliative care, effective actions have been taken, such as holding conferences and workshops among policy makers and introducing palliative care services to physicians and nurses and other groups concerned. Although there is still a long way to achieving desired services, activities that have recently begun, and the position of palliative care as one of the priorities of the National Cancer Control Program, promise the development of these services in Iran in a future not too far away.

References

1. Kolahdoozan S, Sadjadi A, Radmard AR, Khademi H. Five common cancers in Iran. Arch Iran Med. 2010;13(2):143–6. Epub 2010/03/02.
2. Siegel R, Ma J, Zou Z, Jemal A. Cancer statistics, 2014. CA. 2014;64(1):9–29. Epub 2014/01/09.
3. Rasaf MR, Ramezani R, Mehrazma M, Asadi-Lari M. Inequalities in cancer distribution in Tehran; a disaggregated estimation of 2007 incidence by 22 districts. Int J Prev Med. 2012;3(7):483–92. Epub 2012/08/15.
4. Sajjadi M, Rassouli M, Abbaszadeh A, Alavi Majd H, Zendehdel K. Psychometric properties of the Persian version of the Mishel's uncertainty in illness scale in patients with cancer. Eur J Oncol Nurs. 2014;18(1):52–7. Epub 2013/11/05.
5. Mousavi S. Executive guideline for registering and reporting cancer cases; 2007, Cancer Office and the Research fellowship of Cancer Research Center of Cancer Institute: Tehran. p. 122.
6. Asadi-Lari M, Madjd Z, Afkari ME, Goushegir A, Baradaran HR. The concept of palliative care practice among Iranian General Practitioners. Iran J Cancer Prevention. 2009;2(3):111–6.
7. Iran's Cancer Registry System [Persian]. http://www.ircancer.ir/Default.aspx?tabid=95#. Accessed 8 Nov 2013.
8. Iran's Cancer Registry System. Country Reports on cancer (2009) [Persian]. http://www.ircancer.ir/default.aspx?tabid=88&ArticleId=350. Accessed 8 Nov 2014.

9. Zare M, Zakiani S, Rezaie A, Najjari A. Designing and establishment of information and treatment management system of breast cancer in Iran. Iran J Breast Dis. 2011;4(1 and 2): 35–41.
10. Haji-Mahmoodi M, Montazeri A, Jarvandi S, Ebrahimi M, Haghighat S, Harirchi I. Breast self-examination: knowledge, attitudes, and practices among female health care workers in Tehran. Iran Breast J. 2002;8(4):222–5.
11. The Policy of Improving Primary Health Care, Health Policy Council and Health System Reform, 2007. http://www.pdffactory.com/.
12. Islamic Republic News Agency, Interview with the Head of the Clinical Oncology Association of Iran, 2013. http://www.irna.ir/fa/News/81341648/.
13. Mohagheghi M, Zendehdel K, Sheikhtaheri A, Nahvijou A, Sedighi Z, Gilmahi M. Guideline of population- based cancer registry (abstractors' and coders' guideline). Tehran University of Medical Sciences, Cancer Research Center, Department of Cancer Registry, 2012. www.crc.tumsac.ir/portals/0/cancer-registry/education/chapter2_canReglntro.pdf.
14. Zendehdel K, Sedighi Z, Hasanlou ZH, Nahvijou A. Improving quality of cancer registration in Iran. Part 1: evaluation and comparison of cancer registration results in the country. HAKIM. 2010;12(4):42–9.
15. The Ministry of Health and Medical Education, Research and Technology Development and Coordination Center of Iran, the National Cancer Registry Program across 11 Provinces of the Country. http://www.hbi.ir/forms/Special.aspx?hbsId=788&category=1&templateid=1&hdlId=61.
16. Asghari MA, Karimzadeh N, Emarlow P. The role of pain-related beliefs in adjustment to cancer pain. Clin Psychol Personality. 2005;1(13):1–22.
17. Juarez G, Ferrell B, Borneman T. Influence of culture on cancer pain management in Hispanic patients. Cancer Pract. 1998;6(5):262–9. Epub 1998/10/10.
18. Abedi M. Palliative care within the Iranian Context: re-defining palliative care, deploying spirituality as a support measure and need for cultural sensitivity, 2012. http://www.inter-disciplinarynet/wp-content/uploads/2012/02/abedisppaperpdf.
19. Khabar Online. 9 myths about cancer, 2012. http://www.khabaronline.ir/detail/274618/society/health.
20. Najafi GT, Hosseini AF. Attitudinal barriers to effective cancer pain management. HAYAT. 2012;18(1):89–101.
21. Cancer Research Center. Development of a comprehensive national program for palliative and supportive cancer care project [Persian]. http://crc.tums.ac.ir/Default.aspx?tabid=519. Accessed 8 Nov 2014.
22. Mohagheghi MA, Sedighi Z. Pain control in cancer patients by opiate use. Tehran Univ Med J. 2003;61(2):95–102.
23. Davari M, Haycox A, Walley T. Health care financing in Iran: is privatization a good solution? Iran J Public Health. 2012;41(7):14–23. Epub 2012/11/01.
24. Mehrdad R. Health system in Iran. JMAJ. 2009;52(1):69–73.
25. Bazyar M, Pourreza A, Harirchi I, Akbari FE, Mahmoudi M. Medical and non-medical direct costs of cancers in patients hospitalized in Imam Khomeini cancer institution-2010. J Hospital. 2012;11(1):39–50.
26. Sadat HA, Memarian R. The effect of employing synectic model of teaching in teaching palliative care in children on nursing student's writing creativity and academic performance. Iran J Med Educ. 2010;9(3):239–48.
27. Hamooleh MM, Borimnejad L, Seyedfatemi N, Tahmasebi M. Perception of Iranian nurses regarding ethics-based palliative care in cancer patients. J Med Ethics Hist Med. 2013;5(17):141–64.
28. Zakerimoghaddam M, Ghiyasvandian S, Noorikermanshahi S, Haghani H. Nursing students' attitude and motivation towards working in cancer settings. Iran J Nurs Res. 2013;8(3):27–36.
29. Eftekhar Z, Mohaghegh MA, Yarandi F, Eghtesadi-Araghi P, Moosavi-Jarahi A, Gilani MM, et al. Knowledge and attitudes of physicians in Iran with regard to chronic cancer pain. Asian Pac J Cancer Prev. 2007;8(3):383–6. Epub 2007/12/28.

30. Rassouli M, Sajjadi M. Palliative care in the Islamic Republic of Iran. In: Silberman M, editor. Palliative care to the cancer patient: the Middle East as a model for emerging countries. New York: Nova; 2014.
31. Searight HR, Gafford J. Cultural diversity at the end of life: issues and guidelines for family physicians. Am Fam Physician. 2005;71(3):515–22.
32. Candib LM. Truth telling and advance planning at the end of life: problems with autonomy in a multicultural world. Families Syst Health. 2002;20(3):213.
33. Valizadeh L, Zamanzadeh V, Rahmani A, Howard F, Nikanfar AR, Ferguson C. Cancer disclosure: experiences of Iranian cancer patients. Nurs Health Sci. 2012;14(2):250–6. Epub 2012/04/03.
34. Holland JC, Geary N, Marchini A, Tross S. Psychosocial issues: an international survey of physician attitudes and practice in regard to revealing the diagnosis of cancer. Cancer Invest. 1987;5(2):151–4.
35. Matsumura S, Bito S, Liu H, Kahn K, Fukuhara S, Kagawa-Singer M, et al. Acculturation of attitudes toward end-of-life care: a cross-cultural survey of Japanese Americans and Japanese. J Gen Intern Med. 2002;17(7):531–9. Epub 2002/07/23.
36. Moazam F. Families, patients, and physicians in medical decision-making: a Pakistani perspective. Hastings Cent Rep. 2000;30(6):28–37. Epub 2001/07/31.
37. Fars News, interview with head of Imam Hussein Hospital, 2014. http://www.farsnews.com/newstext.php?nn=13930703000526#sthash.TNPrRnzB.dpuf.
38. Zahedi F, Larijani B, Tavakoly Bazzaz J. End of life ethical Issues and Islamic views. Iran J Allergy Asthma Immunol. 2007;6 Suppl 5:5–15.
39. Zamanzadeh V, Rassouli M, Abbaszadeh A, Nikanfar A, Alavi-Majd H, Ghahramanian A. Factors influencing communication between the patients with cancer and their nurses in oncology wards. Indian J Palliat Care. 2014;20(1):12–20. Epub 2014/03/07.
40. Heidarzadeh M, Rassouli M, Shahbolaghi FM, Majd HA, Karam A-M, Mirzaee H, et al. Posttraumatic growth and its dimensions in patients with cancer. Middle East J Cancer. 2014;5(1):23–9.
41. Karimi M. Death and dying as a cultural category. Res Culture Art. 2009;1(1):91–101.
42. Asadi-Lari M, Madjd Z, Akbari M. The need for palliative care services in Iran: an introductory commentary. Iran J Cancer Prevention. 2008;1(1):1–5.
43. http://www.cancer.org/treatment/childrenandcancer/whenyourchildhascancer/childrendiagnosedwithcancerunderstandingthehealthcaresystem/children-diagnosed-with-cancer--understanding-the-health-care-system-comprehensive-care.
44. Murray A. IMS Institute for Healthcare Informatics. Innovation in cancer care and implications for health systems, 2014. Accessed 2 Aug 2014.
45. National Cancer Research Network. Scoping of comprehensive program for supportive and palliative care of cancer in Iran. 2012. http://www.crc.tums.ac.ir/Portals/6/mostanadat/scoping.docx.
46. Cancer Research Center. Development of a comprehensive national program for palliative and supportive cancer care project [Persian]. http://crc.tums.ac.ir/Default.aspx?tabid=550. Accessed 8 Nov 2013.
47. National Cancer Survivorship Initiative (NCSI). Innovation to implementation: stratified pathways of care for people living with or beyond cancer. http://www.ncsi.org.uk/wp-content/uploads/howtoguide.pdf. Accessed 2 Aug 2014.
48. Strategy document on supportive and palliative care. http://crc.tums.ac.ir/Portals/6/rahbord/Jalase_5_Bahman/Final.pdf.
49. Zakieye P. Determinants of the acceptance and advancement of implementation of EHR. http://ihima.behdasht.gov.ir/uploads/279_983_NO2_S84_Maghboliat.htm. Accessed 4 Nov 2014.
50. kheshabi J. Abstract book of first national cancer seminar. Sanandaj [Persian]. http://www.iausdj.ac.ir/research/DocLib10/%D8%A7%D9%88%D9%84%DB%8C%D9%86%20%D9%87%D9%85%D8%A7%DB%8C%D8%B4%20%D9%85%D9%84%DB%8C%20%D8%B3%D8%B1%D8%B7%D8%A7%D9%86%2090/%D9%85%D9%82%D8%A7%D9%84%D8%A7%D8%AA%20%D8%A7%D8%B1%D8%A7%D8%A6%D9%87%20

%D8%B4%D8%AF%D9%87%20%D8%A8%D9%87%20%D8%B5%D9%88%D8%B1%D8%AA%20%D8%B3%D8%AE%D9%86%D8%B1%D8%A7%D9%86%DB%8C.pdf. Accessed 30 July 2014.
51. Ministry of Health, Health sector evolution. http://tahavol.behdasht.gov.ir/. Accessed 1 Nov 2014.
52. Cancer research, treatment and education institute[Persian]. http://www.ncii.ir/page.aspx?id=14. Accessed 30 July 2014.
53. Cancer Research Center. Shahid Beheshti University of Medical Sciences. http://crc.sbmu.ac.ir/?siteid=148&pageid=9757&siteid=148. Accessed 28 July 2014.
54. National Cancer Control Programs of the Ministry of Health and Medical Education, the Health Deputy of the Center for the Management of Diseases, Cancer Office, 2007. http://fhc.sums.ac.ir/files/gh-vagir/…/NationalCancerControlPrograms.pdf.

Chapter 21
Cancer Care in Regions/Societies in Transition in the Gulf States: Sultanate of Oman

Zakiya M.N. Al Lamki

Oman, like its neighboring Gulf Cooperation Council (GCC) States of the Arabian Peninsula in the Middle East region, has been transformed in the last four decades, from an underdeveloped country dominated by infections to a modern welfare state in which noncommunicable diseases pose a great challenge. It enjoys a stable political, economic, and social system with good relationships with neighboring countries. The country is a middle-income economy that is heavily dependent on revenues from its oil sector. There is a strong commitment by the government to provide wide access to free basic services including health care to its citizens. On average 2.6 % of the GDP of US$80.57 billion at current prices is spent on health care at a rate of US$690 on health care expenditure per capita [1, 2]. The organization of health care delivery is based on a primary health care approach with clearly delineated referral pathways between three levels of care namely primary, secondary, and tertiary. Since the concentration of the population (71.5 %) live in the urban areas and half live in the capital Muscat and the coastline (Al-Batinah) regions, it makes the accessibility of services easier for a large portion of the population [3].

The diagnostic and therapeutic services for cancer patients all over Oman are provided at the two main tertiary public centers, namely the Royal Hospital and the Sultan Qaboos University Hospital. The National Oncology Center at the Royal Hospital which was established in 2004 has divisions of medical oncology, radiation oncology, and pediatric oncology. The Center has been granted accreditation by international organizations such as International Union against Cancer (UICC) and European Society of Medical Oncology (ESMO) [4]. The university hospital has divisions of medical oncology, pediatric hematology–oncology, and the Bone Marrow Transplant Unit. Palliative care services are still not fully implemented at

Z.M.N. Al Lamki, F.R.C.P., F.R.C.P.C.H. (✉)
Department of Child Health, Haematology/Oncology Unit, College of Medicine and Health Sciences, Sultan Qaboos University, Al Khoudh P.C. 123, P.O. Box 47, Muscat, Sultanate of Oman
e-mail: zakiya.allamki@gmail.com

M. Silbermann (ed.), *Cancer Care in Countries and Societies in Transition*,
DOI 10.1007/978-3-319-22912-6_21

the two centers. Although small pain management teams are established, their operational functions are limited and complicated with the strict regulations of narcotics control by the regulatory authorities. However, various steps to provide comprehensive service including palliative care at a national level are under way. A sizeable portion of the health care workforce is expatriate population, but this is beginning to change as a result of an aggressive policy of omanization. So far 65 % of the nurses and allied health staff including laboratory technicians are Omanis and only 30 % of the total doctors are Omanis. In 2014, UNDP in its Human Development Index report ranked Oman 56th out of 187 countries, positioning it the highest of the Arab states [5].

In addition to the equitable quality of health care provision in the country, a patient support group, the Oman Cancer Association (OCA) officially registered in 2004; work hand in hand with the health care providers in the field of cancer management. Its mobile mammogram unit launched in November 2009 covers all regions and aims to reach all the women population of Oman. About 8000 subjects were screened so far through this program and around 17 cases were identified to date.

Besides the developed infrastructure of its health care system, Oman is well recognized for the reliability of its data from the department of Health Information and Statistics. There has been a mandatory notification of all cancer cases to its population-based Cancer Registry established in 1996 with its first data published in 1998. As a result of the completeness and quality of its data, Oman is one of only two countries in the region whose data appeared in Cancer Incidence in Five Continents, a result of the work of the International Agency for Research on Cancer (IARC) and the network for cancer registries worldwide [6, 7].

Significant reduction of communicable diseases has been brought about based on sound planning and implementation of vertical and horizontal health programs and community-based initiatives. The economic prosperity has led to a shift in the epidemiological patterns of diseases with noncommunicable diseases including cancer, constituting more than 75 % of the disease burden. As observed in other regional countries, Oman is challenged by its aging population and growth together with unhealthy lifestyle changes such as physical inactivity, unhealthy diet, and smoking. Life expectancy has increased from 50 years of age in 1970 to currently 77 years of age. Over the next 25 years, the elderly population of Oman is expected to increase sixfold. There is a growing concern that a large numbers of the population across all ages are living sedentary lifestyles. Oman is experiencing nutrition transition, with a double burden of prevailing micronutrient deficiency states and rising trend of obesity. The current prevalence rates of adult obesity and overweight are estimated at 20 % and 30 %, respectively. Use of tobacco in the form of cigarette and water pipe smoking (shisha) is increasingly popular among the youth population. The Global Youth Tobacco survey conducted in 2007 revealed smoking in 17.8 % and 13.3 % of boys and girls, respectively. A national tobacco control committee was established in 2005, and the country has ratified framework convention on tobacco control. With the changing structure of the population and these new emerging challenges, cancer prevalence is therefore inevitable [3, 8, 9].

Furthermore, exposure to occupational and environmental carcinogens due to industrialization might pose significant health risks. About 1–4 % of all cancers worldwide accounts to pollution of air, water, and soil. Due to the limitations in measuring the accurate exposure, the precise contributing environmental risk factors and their interaction with genetic factors in our region are difficult to elucidate. Total CO_2 emissions in Oman are minimal due to its small population; however, per capita emissions are comparable with high-income countries which may be as a result of socioeconomic development, industrialization, and motorization. Although pollution monitoring is undertaken by the government, but stronger strategy for prevention is required in addition to implementation of the existing national preventive strategies into health services [3].

Even though cancer is considered a universal problem, the patterns and related causes differ markedly by countries in the region. This heterogeneity has important implications and can be translated into different priorities for national cancer control programs. The Gulf Center for Cancer Registration (GCCR) which was established in 1998 collects data from each of the gulf state's cancer registry and publish periodic incidence reports every 5 years [10]. The pattern of cancer in Omani women is dominated by cancer of the breast followed by thyroid cancer whereas in men stomach cancer was a major contributor to the cancer burden in morbidity and mortality [11]. More recently, there has been a decline over time in the trend of stomach cancer incidence. The changing trend could be explained by the changes in the environmental risk factor, namely the high content of salt used in preserving foods, a practice that is now replaced by storage method of refrigeration [12]. Stomach cancer has thus been replaced by the increasing incidence of prostate and colorectal cancer while non-Hodgkin lymphoma and leukemia remain top of the list of common cancers in both males and females. In other GCC countries, the top common cancers are lung and colorectal followed by the non-Hodgkin lymphoma (NHL). As in developed countries, leukemia is the most common cancer reported among children below 15 years of age [10]. Studies have demonstrated that about half of the patients with Breast Cancer in Oman present in advanced stages (III and IV) at a younger age and with aggressive clinic-pathologic variables compared with data in western countries. Although this has a negative impact on survival and a significant cost burden, there is an overall improvement in survival due to optimization of surgical and medical management [13–15]. The scarcity of comprehensive review of the completeness and quality of cancer registrations in the other GCC countries limits the conclusion that can be drawn from the comparative analyses (Tables 21.1 and 21.2).

A significant feature of the demographic transition, therefore, is the change in disease epidemiology. The age adjusted annual incidence rates of cancer range from 80 to 110 per 100,000 population which is lower than some other countries in the region as well as globally [11]. By 2030, the number of new cancer cases worldwide is projected to rise by about 70 % [16]. In the region, the estimated increase is 68 % in just over a decade. According to GLOBOCAN estimates, Oman is facing an almost twofold increase in cancer incidence in the period 2008–2020. It is one of the most common causes of death in the Arab countries, ranking third in Oman. It

Table 21.1 Ten most common cancer among Omani 2011

Male			Female		
Topography	Frequency	Percentage	Topography	Frequency	Percentage
Leukemia	58	9.8	Breast	147	24.8
Prostate	57	9.6	Thyroid	67	11.3
Colorectal	53	8.9	Non-Hodgkin lymphoma	37	6.2
Non-Hodgkin lymphoma	51	8.6	Colorectal	34	5.7
Stomach	49	8.2	Leukemia	30	5.1
Trachea, bronchus, lung	39	6.6	Cervix uteri	29	4.9
Bladder	29	4.9	Uterus	27	4.6
Liver	24	4	Stomach	23	3.9
Other skin	21	3.5	Hodgkin lymphoma	22	3.7
Hodgkin lymphoma	20	3.4	Other skin	20	3.4

Table 21.2 Five most common cancer among nationals of GCC states (1998–2007)

	Oman	UAE	Bahrain	KSA	Qatar	Kuwait
Male	Stomach	Lung	Lung	Non-Hodgkin lymphoma	Lung	Colorectal
	Non-Hodgkin lymphoma	Colorectal	Colorectal	Colorectal	Colorectal	Non-Hodgkin lymphoma
	Leukemia	Non-Hodgkin lymphoma	Prostate	Liver	Liver	Liver
	Prostate	Prostate	Bladder	Leukemia	Leukemia	Leukemia
	Lung	Leukemia	Leukemia	Lung	Bladder	Prostate
Female	Breast	Breast	Breast	Breast	Breast	Breast
	Thyroid	Thyroid	Colorectal	Thyroid	Thyroid	Colorectal
	Cervix uteri	Leukemia	Lung	Colorectal	Colorectal	Thyroid
	Leukemia	Colorectal	Thyroid	Non-Hodgkin lymphoma	Non-Hodgkin lymphoma	Non-Hodgkin lymphoma
	Stomach	Cervix uteri	Ovary	Leukemia	Corpus uteri	Leukemia

accounts to 10.5 % of Ministry of Health (MOH) hospital deaths and is the top morbidity in noncommunicable diseases based on MOH hospitals' discharges [17]. The sound health policies and strategies based on the primary health approach have led to significant changes of the morbidity and mortality patterns which show clear signs of transition in Oman, similar to those observed in the west. Based on the

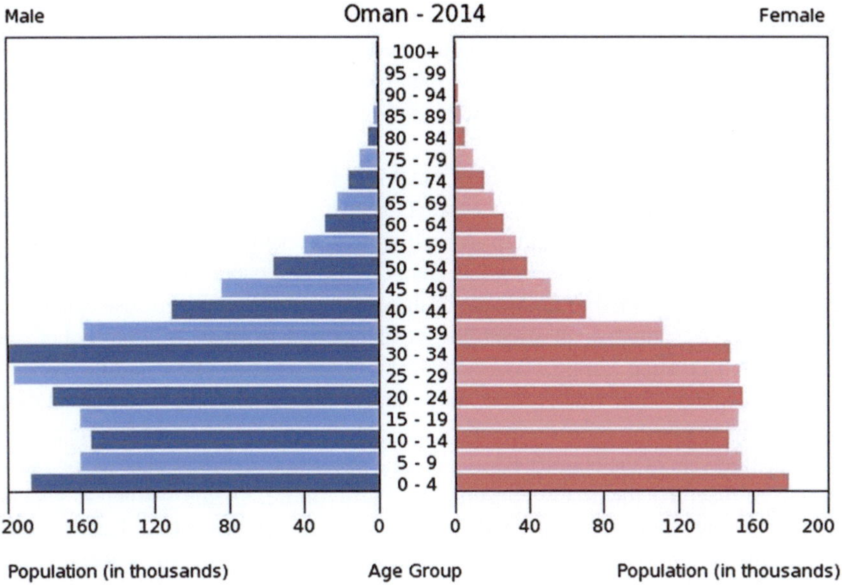

Fig. 21.1 Oman population pyramid 2014

changing patterns and the anticipated rising numbers, Oman requested a WHO-IAEA joint Program of Action for Cancer Therapy (imPACT) in 2013 to effectively and efficiently address the cancer burden [18] (Fig. 21.1).

Cancer patients in the country continue to present with advanced disease despite the universal coverage of health care services, availability of hospitals, and treatment facilities with utilization of the most advanced treatment modalities that includes surgery, chemotherapy, radiotherapy, hormonal, and targeted therapies. The delayed presentation can be a result of patient delay, a prolonged interval from the onset of the initial symptoms to seeking medical advice or can occur from a delay on the part of the health care provider or system itself resulting in a prolonged interval from patient presentation to initiation of treatment. Within the countries in transition, many personal, sociocultural, and economic factors cause late patient presentation. This has been attributed, namely to lack of awareness, cultural barriers, and limited screening programs. Understanding these barriers is crucial to optimizing interventional measures. Studies on breast cancer care have shown strong evidence that inferior or poor education level and less income status contribute to patient delay. In Oman, it is difficult to ascertain the level of poverty however the health gaps in level of education and income that existed in the past have been somehow narrowed. In some of those studies, the evidence for sociocultural variables is less strong. Other studies showed contradictory results in the association of personal characteristics (such as age, marital status, family history, presenting symptoms) and patient delay. There could be a reflection of the varying risks of bias in the studies or geographic variation in barriers to care due to multidimensional heterogeneity of the countries whose society, culture, and systems differ to some extent [19]. Breast cancer studies conducted in United Arab Emirates and other countries in the Middle East such as Qatar have generally shown below average knowledge scores on risk factors, warning signs, and methods for early detection [20, 21].

Research is therefore required in Oman through validated questionnaire to obtain baseline information on the current status of awareness that includes patients with and without delayed presentation as well as in identifying unknown risk factors. Although the literacy rates in Oman has gone up to 86 %, sociocultural context delays can be attributed to ignorance of initial signs and symptoms, use of alternative treatments, and fear of social consequences and stigma. Spiritual belief and religious observance can be a source of strength for patients and entail the concept of acceptance of God's will which may prevent the patient from seeking medical advice thus hindering access to medical care. Inadequate numbers of female professional caregivers in the country restrict female patients with breast cancer, for example, from reaching for timely consultation. Furthermore, Omani women in general tend to neglect their problems, and concern for their health is at the least priority. Their duty is first to their husbands and children. Some have the misconception that surgical treatment may lead to loss of their femininity. Islamic healing is frequently sought as a choice by Omani women and their children who are afflicted with cancer. Traditional healers may in some occasions be the first "port call." As in other Arab and Muslim countries, faith healing is one of the received forms of traditional treatment. This could be in the form of certain spiritual rituals or recitation of Quran verses and prayers in healing water as well as ingestion of herbs. One of the popular herbs which is grown and marketed in the region is the black seeds originating from the common fennel flower plant, the Nigella Sativa. This has been used historically from the time of the Christian era, by the ancient Egyptians and Greeks as an ailment for general health problems. Prophet Muhammad (peace upon him) has recommended its use by being quoted as saying "The Black Seed is a cure for all diseases except death" (Sahih Bukhari; 7–591). Drinking milk and urine of camels is a recognized practice for cancer treatment in Oman as well as in some of the neighboring countries. Cupping is also sought as a traditional form of treatment for cancer pain. Another type of pain therapy that was commonly practised in the past and still occasionally applied is the cauterization or burning of the skin at the site of pain or swelling called *wassam*. Frankincense oil, a resin from the bark of trees growing in the south of Oman has been used for years as treatment of anti-inflammatory and skin conditions as well as cancer. Recent research conducted in Oman showed promising results for its use as an anticancer drug [22, 23].

Most Omanis view Islam not only as a religion but as part of their cultural attitudes, values, and behavioral norms. Islam reminds them that humans have their limits at times and put their trust in God to guide the course thus accepting illness such as cancer with patience. They prefer to live with uncertainty rather than definitive prediction of disease outcome and defer end-of-life decisions to the physician. Unlike the western world, where individual autonomy and open communications are the core of ethical practice, family members tend to contribute significantly to the decision making process in the care of the patient and sometimes actively protect the patient from complete disclosure on the true nature of the condition. While holding Islamic principles, Omani patients embrace the socioeconomic transition, and thus traditional beliefs and social taboos are slowly and gradually broken while following the health care transformation. Complementary and alternative medicine is thus being replaced by modern medicine. However, Oman faces a significant challenge to keep its citizens from travelling abroad to seek to what is believed, better treatment options. Some patients have lack of confidence in the locally available facilities for cancer treatment. Sometimes, they choose to go away for treatment as they want to keep their diagnosis a secret. In these patients, safety is at risk due to poor or no follow-up care. Some return home with complications of surgery and treatment. In such instances, there is limited ability to complain about poor medical care as some of those treatment centers have weak malpractice laws.

Current evidence suggests that interventions such as education to both patients and all health care providers together with enhancing cancer awareness will reduce delays in diagnosis and treatment as well as its complications. The situation in Oman relates more to education and culture rather than accessibility and availability of services. Diagnosis and treatment modalities are improving while education and public awareness are still lacking, and there is a low uptake of screening especially among women. Focus therefore should be made on implementation of primary and secondary prevention programs. Awareness programs should therefore be directed towards tackling obesity and physical inactivity as well as education and awareness of causative factors such as tobacco control, screening, and early detection programs. Such educational programs should involve health care providers working in primary care settings, namely doctors, nurses, and community health workers. Strengthening the capacity of primary care services in providing affordable early detection tests such as clinical breast examination and timely referral of patients with suspected lesions are important, given the fact that majority of the patients contact occur at this level. In Oman, there is a growing concern related to health lifestyle issues, and so efforts have been introduced in the last few years to implement strategies that increase awareness. Initiatives have been undertaken to implement the WHO Framework Convention on Tobacco Control and vaccination against Hepatitis B virus covered in the childhood immunization programs and those at risk. Concerning the emerging health issues related to lifestyle, the MOH is active in promoting health initiatives in schools. However, it needs to strengthen these efforts by tuning to the important cancer control comprehensive measures in the domain of primary prevention through WHO Action Plan for the prevention and control of noncommunicable diseases 2013–2020. The OCA and other national associations help in creating public awareness and education through community-based programs and to some extent the media and social networks which can be further utilized as important sources of information for the public and also help to eradicate some of the myths about cancer. Much remains to be accomplished in order to provide the evidence base for public health decisions on cancer control [24, 25].

Recent evolved political conflicts and instability in Arab countries of the region, causing mass displacement and human migration flow in addition to the high ongoing labor migration rates, result in reappearance of certain infectious diseases and emergence of new ones. Like other GCC countries, Oman continues to host a large expatriate labor population of around one-third of its total midyear population [17]. Although medical checks are conducted routinely, the increased risk of return of the communicable diseases and the growing burden of noncommunicable ones might therefore result in lack of preparedness of the current health system to cope. Since oil is the mainstay of economy, high oil prices have continued to feed growth. However, being a modest producer compared to its neighbors is a fact that poses a major challenge to meet its developmental needs. Oman's main structural challenge lies in the transition from a country with an over-reliance on oil revenues to a diversified economy by promoting non-oil industries, gas sector, privatization, tourism, and foreign investment. The health care system is therefore challenged by sustainability of achievement of health reform in Oman [26, 27].

The spiral costs of cancer care and treatment due to increased use of new and advanced technologies as well as high pharmaceutical costs, coupled by the rising public demand for better quality care are difficult to sustain with the volatile oil prices which might hamper the development efforts. According to estimates, only 30–50 % of cancers are preventable. There remain a number of common cancers for which the causes are poorly understood and are barely related to economic transition and thus less amenable to prevention. Studying the molecular and cellular underpinnings of cancer towards a better understanding of both causes and prevention, identification of risk factors as well as screening programs and early detection would make a considerable contribution in cancer prevention. There is thus a need to foster new science of personalized medicine. So far, participation in clinical trials is very limited and biomedical research is usually physician driven. Oman should therefore take the opportunity and encourage a leadership role in value-based research especially that the financial investment of this is being met by the newly established National Research Council. Knowledge of the genomic variation of individuals and subpopulations will usher a new era of personalized medicine for more accurate abilities to predict, prevent, and promote diseases such as cancer. Currently, Oman uses treatment protocols for the various cancers, imported from the west. It is recognized that cancer care guidelines developed in high-income countries have limited application in developing countries. To create realistic and sustainable cancer care strategy, efforts are undergoing in collaborative studies with countries in the region to develop personalized treatment regimens. Instead of relying on the altruism of western interests to address specific health needs of its population, Oman should establish a critical mass of researchers and domestic capacity in emerging genomic sciences in efforts to improve national health. Despite the appreciable achievement in health workforce development, the changing health needs of the population and the health services' expansion put tremendous pressure for additional health manpower with a large scope of specialties. Given the shortage of specialist oncologists as in low and middle-income countries, greater priority should be given to clinical oncology specialization in order to address this shortage [28, 29].

Conclusion

Oman has achieved an impressive progress and a dramatic transformation in cancer care in a remarkably short time and therefore stands as a model for other countries in transition state.

However, the rapidly changing disease profile poses a potential threat of increasing health costs and a dramatic impact on its economy. Oman might not be able to sustain a high-income country model of cancer management but only through complementary efforts to improve the cancer continuum of prevention, risk assessment, early diagnosis, and patient-centered treatment and follow-up would the impending epidemic of this disease be addressed. Oman's advances in the delivery of primary health care services have given the country extensive experience in health promotion and disease prevention. The WHO has provided technical support to Oman since the renaissance and major strides are further being undertaken by professional organizations such as the Middle East Cancer Consortium among others. The commitment of the Government of Oman to prevent and treat noncommunicable diseases and improve health care is evident in its 2050 vision for health. It sets out a strategic framework for health development and a growing interest of improving infrastructure such as medical centers of excellence. Unless reforms are introduced to the current health care system, namely improving cost-efficiency and quality of care and prevention there could be a major drain on Oman's human and financial resources threatening the advances in health achieved so far. These interventions should be implemented with ongoing evaluation [30, 31].

References

1. Health expenditure total (% of GDP): 2010–2014. Oman data.worldbank.org.
2. Annual report. Central Bank Oman. 2013. www.cbo-oman.org/annual/CBOAnnualReport Accessed Jun 2014.
3. Country cooperation strategy for WHO and Oman 2010–2015. WHO Document EM/ARD/036/E/12.10. Geneva: WHO.
4. ESMO designated centers of integrated oncology and palliative care. Lugano: ESMO. http://www.esmo.org/Patients/2014-ESMO-Designated-Centres.
5. UNDP human development report: sustaining human progress: reducing vulnerabilities and building resilience explanatory note on the 2014 human development report composite indices Oman. http://hdr.undp.org/sites/all/themes/hdr_theme/country-notes/OMN.
6. Nooyi SC. The Oman national cancer registry—every case counts. Special issue on "non communicable disease surveillance and control". Newsletter. 2008;17(3):1–7.
7. Curado MP, Edwards B, Shin HR, Storm H, Ferlay J, Heanuem M, Boyle P. International cancer incidence in five continents. IARC Scientific Publications Preventive Chronic Diseases Public Health Research, Practice and Policy #160. Edited by Association of Cancer Registries. Lyon: IARC. ISBN 9789283221609.
8. Al-Lawati JA, Mabry R, Mohammed AJ. Addressing the threat of chronic diseases in Oman. Prev Chronic Dis. 2008;5(3):A99.

9. Hajjar R, Atil T, Al-Mandhari Z, Balducci L, Silbermann M. Prevalence of aging population in the Middle East and its implications on cancer incidence and care. Ann Oncol. 2013;24 Suppl 7:vii11–24.
10. Al-Madouj AN, Eldali A, Al-Zahrani AS. Ten-year cancer incidence report among nationals of the GCC states. 1998–2007 (Cancer Incidence Report of the Cooperation Council States) 2011; Executive Board of Health Ministers' Council for the Gulf Cooperation Council States, Research Centre Scientific Information Office.
11. Department of non communicable disease surveillance and control. Trends of cancer 1999–2011, Cancer incidence in Oman. Oman Cancer Registry, Directorate General of Health Affairs, Ministry of Health.
12. Al-Mahrouqi H, Parkin L, Sharples K. Oman incidence of stomach cancer in Oman and the other gulf cooperation council countries. Oman Med J. 2011;26(4):258–62.
13. Al-Moundhri M. The need for holistic cancer care framework: breast cancer care as an example. Oman Med J. 2013;28(5):300–1.
14. Kumar S, Burney IA, Al-Ajmi A, Al-Moundhri MS. Changing trends of breast cancer survival in Sultanate of Oman. J Oncol. 2011;2011:316243.
15. Mehdi I, Monem EA, Al Bahrani BJ, Al Kharusi S, Nada AM, Al Lawati J, Al LN. Age at diagnosis of female breast cancer in Oman: issues and implications. South Asian J Cancer. 2014;3(2):101–6.
16. Franseschi S, Wild CP. Meeting the global demands of epidemiologic transition—the indispensable role of cancer prevention. Mol Oncol. 2013;7(1):1–13.
17. Health facts. Department of Health Information and Statistics, Directorate General of Planning; Ministry of Health. 2013.
18. imPACT: assessing cancer burden: Sultanate of Oman faces the growing cancer burden report by World Health Organization (WHO), International Agency for Research on Cancer (IARC) and other partner organizations. 2013.
19. Sharma K, Costas A, Shulman LN, Meara JG. A systematic review of barriers to breast cancer care in developing countries resulting in delayed patient presentation. J Oncol. 2012;2012:121873.
20. Al-Sharbatti SS, Shaikh RB, Elsheba M, Al-Biate MA. Assessment of breast cancer awareness among female university students in Ajman, United Arab Emirates. Sultan Qaboos Univ Med J. 2014;14(4):493–500.
21. Brown R, Kerr K, Haoudi A, Darzi A. Tackling cancer burden in the Middle East: Qatar as an example. Lancet Oncol. 2012;13(11):501–8.
22. Abukhader MM. Thymoquinone in the clinical treatment of cancer: fact or fiction? Pharmacogn Rev. 2013;7(14):117–20. Department of Pharmacy, Oman Medical College, Muscat, Sultanate of Oman.
23. Oman researchers find cancer treatment in frankincense—Gulf News. http://gulfnews.com/news/gulf/oman/oman-researchers-find-cancer-treatment-in-frankincense-1. Accessed 6 Nov 2013.
24. Aggarwal A, Sullivan R. Achieving value in cancer care—the case of low- and middle-income countries. http://www.ajmc.com/publications/evidence-based-oncology/2014/the-american-society-of-clinical-oncology-annual-meeting-2014#sthash.XpnLrvsE.dpuf.
25. WHO. Global action plan for the prevention and control of non-communicable diseases 2013–2020. Geneva: WHO. ISBN 9789241506236.
26. Wild CP. Cancer control: a reminder of the need for a balanced approach between prevention and treatment. East Mediterr Health J. 2014;20(6):340–62.
27. Al Dhawi AA, West Jr DJ, Spinelli RJ, Gompf TA. The challenge of sustaining health care in Oman. Health Care Manag (Frederick). 2007;26(1):19–30.
28. Al-Mulla NA, Chandra P, Khattab M, Madanat F, Vossough P, Torfa E, Al-Lamki Z, Zain G, Muwakkit S, Mahmoud S, Al-Jassmi A, Tuncer M, Al-Mukharraq H, Barsaoui S, Arceci RJ, Howard SC, Kulozik AE, Ravindranath Y, Reaman GH, Farranoush M, AlNasser AA. Childhood acute lymphoblastic leukemia in the Middle East and neighboring countries: a

prospective multi-institutional international collaborative study (CALLME1) by the Middle East Childhood Cancer Alliance (MECCA). Pediatr Blood Cancer. 2014;61(8):1403–10.

29. Silbermann M, Epner DE, Charalambous H, Baider L, Puchalski CM, Balducci L, et al. Promoting new approaches for cancer care in the Middle East. Ann Oncol. 2013;24 Suppl 7:vii5–vii10.
30. WHO regional office for the Eastern Mediterranean. Scaling up non communicable disease prevention and control in Oman. 2012. http://www.emro.who.int/media/news/scaling-ncd-oman.html.
31. Al-Riyami A. Health vision 2050 Oman: a committed step towards reforms. Oman Med J. 2012;27(3):190–1.

Chapter 22
Challenges and Prospects in Cancer Care in Georgia

Tamar Rukhadze

Introduction

Georgia is a sovereign state in the Caucasus region of Eurasia, situated in the South Caucasus and is bounded to the west by the Black Sea, to the north by Russia, to the south by Turkey and Armenia, and to the southeast by Azerbaijan.

Historical Introduction

After the collapse of the Soviet Union, Georgia's population decreased by nearly a fifth, the economy rapidly moved from a communist regime to a market system. Real per capita public expenditures on healthcare rapidly declined from around US$13.00 in 1990 to less than $1.00 in 1994. Planning for healthcare reform began in 1993 and was led by the Ministry of Health and was undertaken during the post-independence shift towards a market economy. In the 1990s, social health insurance as a mandatory was introduced and has been abandoned and private health insurance is being promoted as the main mechanism for the prepayment of health services in Georgia. Private insurance coverage for households living below the poverty line is paid from public funds [1–6].

The first major changes took place as a result of the 1995 Georgian Health Care Reform Package that introduced new concepts, including social insurance, official user fees, and new provider payment mechanisms like co-payments. In 1999, the Georgian National Health Policy, which outlined objectives to improve the equity, accessibility, and affordability of health services, was developed [1–7]. Georgia has

T. Rukhadze, M.D., Ph.D. (✉)
Oncology and Palliative Medicine, Faculty of Medicine of Iv. Javakhishvili Tbilisi State University, Tbilisi, Georgia
e-mail: tamar.rukhadze@tsu.ge

M. Silbermann (ed.), *Cancer Care in Countries and Societies in Transition*,
DOI 10.1007/978-3-319-22912-6_22

made a significant effort to adapt health policy and the health system to the new environment. Mandatory social health insurance was introduced after independence, but was abolished after the 2003–2004 Rose Revolution, which brought about fundamental change in the role of government in providing, financing, and managing public services like healthcare, but those were not the last changes in healthcare system [1, 2, 6, 8, 9]. In February, 2013 by the new Government the Universal Healthcare (UCH) Program was introduced by Government of Georgia for more than two million citizens without medical insurance. Financial availability of basic medical service became guaranteed for every citizen through universal healthcare or state and private insurance programs [10–12].

Current Status of Cancer Care

From 7000 to 8000 people are diagnosed with cancer in Georgia annually. Every year nearly 4500 patients die from cancer. Cancer is a second leading cause of death and main priority in Georgian Health Care System. The leading cancer for the female is the breast and lung cancer for males. The leading cancer pathologies between female and male are presented in Fig. 22.1.

Unfortunately, about half of newly revealed cancer cases are diagnosed at stage III–IV. The big number of the cases are resistant to treatment and rest require long term, costly treatment, medical, social, and psychological rehabilitation. Many cancer patients became disabled, abandon active lifestyle and often need a caregiver, what constitutes a heavy burden for their families and the public (Fig. 22.2).

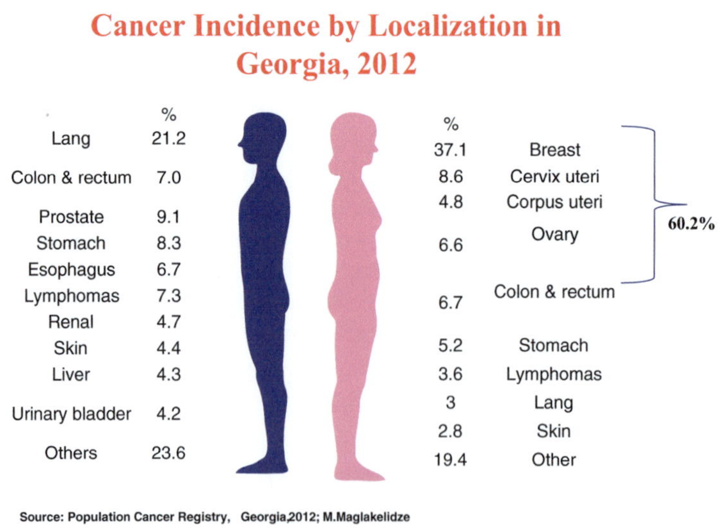

Fig. 22.1 Cancer incidence by localization and sex in Georgia (2012)

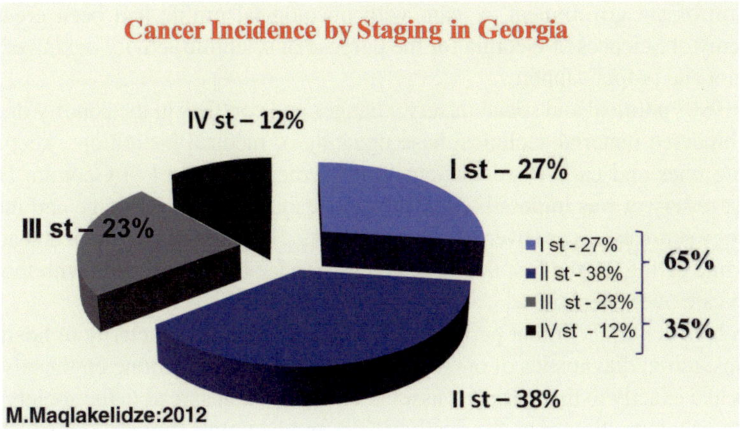

Fig. 22.2 Cancer incidence by staging in Georgia (2012)

The destruction of registration process in recent years and the lack of statistical data on the distribution of real image distortion can be bases of missing clear date for cancer pathologies. To accomplish this, the incidence and mortality of malignant tumors in Georgia in recent years was significantly lower than in the CIS and European countries, which might not shows the real picture. According the date provided by NCDC, in 2012 the 94 new cases were registered in Georgia in malignant tumors per 100,000 inhabitants, including women—51.7 % [11–13].

In 2006, the Ministry of Labour, Health and Social Affairs in Tbilisi, first introduced in breast cancer and cervical screening programs using mammography and PAP (smear test). Since 2010, the 13-year-old girls in the country are carried out by the human papillomavirus (HPV) immunization program.

Since 2011, cancer screening programs in the country are as follows:

- Breast cancer screening for women 40–70 years old
- Cervical cancer screening for women 25–60 years old
- Prostate cancer screening for men 50–70 years old
- Colorectal cancer screening for 50–70-year-old population [11–13]

Oncology Service in Georgia

Creation of oncology service in Georgia outsets from the beginning of the twentieth century. The first oncology dispensary throughout the country was opened in 1946, and oncology research institute started functioning in 1958. Thus, oncology service used to function in Georgia during the soviet period constantly aiming to improvements. In 1960s, scientific, research, educational and most active practical activities were conducted at the scientific institute of oncology; collection of articles had been issued; workshops and conferences used to be arranged. Since 1959 under the decision of the government, a team with oncological profile had been created in Academy of Sciences of Georgia for the purpose of scientific activity organized management and proper support.

In 1990s political and social misery, changes and conflicts in the country dramatically hindered material–technical base updating of medical institutions, keeping of existing ones and caring over patients and medical personnel in Georgia. Due to utmost misery, it was impossible to distribute resources and to manage and monitor oncology services or care over oncology patients. However, during impeded activity and while caring for the first needs, oncology service tried to proceed with the work and to care over the patients.

Archive materials of that period show that during impeded activity of healthcare systems, initial diagnostics of oncology diseases were mainly done on the advances stages and exactly to that period is associated the opinion spread in the society interpreting oncology disease as the death verdict and incurable disease.

Unfortunately, abovementioned stigma appeared to be too strong and continuous struggle needed to be conducted. Such opinion still exists in certain part of the population till today; however, technological and medical achievements greatly altered this opinion.

Reimbursement of Cancer Service

Financial support of oncology and cancer diseases always existed in Georgia in very different ways. Co-financing had been performed with certain proportion. During the overhaul economic misery, oncological diseases, diagnostics, and treatment expenses had been reimbursed only for socially unguarded population and children (1990s/2000s years). Along with the private insurance sector development in the country oncological patients financing was initiated in Georgia by private insurance companies; however, this process was the reason for constant conflicts due to multiple limits existing in patients financing by the insurance companies. Since 2010s state share in co-financing had been increased and oncology service reimbursement became available for teachers and afterwards, for students [11, 13].

It should be noted that notwithstanding the state support and co-financing, there always had been certain limit and methods of diagnostics and treatment not subjected to financing. In case, if methods were not self-financed by the patient, effect of the care was reflected on the patient as the low quality of cancer care. For example, during a lot of years, in case of chemotherapy limit of reimbursement constituted GEL 600 (under the different currency rate it was US$250–300), it means that due to patients insufficient funds, it was impossible to conduct treatment in accordance with international standards and acknowledged clinical guidelines. It should be mentioned that, hormonotherapy did not financed and still is not financing currently (not by the state neither by the most of private insurance companies), palliative in patient service financing was also limited and it should be also noted, that none of the private insurance companies acknowledged necessity of palliative care and respectively didn't finance cancer patients [11, 13].

State vision had been changed from 2013; state healthcare programs had been centrally implemented and the transition to state insurance system was conducted; cancer patients' care (diagnostics, treatment, palliative care) became available for each citizen of Georgia; however, limits still exist and nowadays financing doesn't apply to hystomorphology and endoscopy methods of diagnosis of patients, surgical and radiological treatment is still limited, targeted therapy is still not financed, inpatient palliative care is under the limitation of daily costs (inpatient limit for patient per day is 75 GEL, which means about US$40), and outpatient palliative care services are limited (only allowed for physician for visit reimburse; the reimbursement for physician cost for a visit is 11 GEL by the state program (about US$7 per visit); the maximum visits per month is eight and no other team members are paid, including the nurse) [11, 13].

NCCP of Georgia

The cancer professional community and policymakers spent a lot of time developing a comprehensive cancer control plan (NCCP). Between September and October 2010 there was an open public debate. Later, during November 2010 additional consultations on the Plan took place. In 2011, after permanent public debates and consultations, final version was adopted by Health Council. This enables to enact certain programs and activities already in 2011. With input from more than 20 professional, academic, and community-based organizations that worked together ten major goals were identified in the field of cancer control. The objectives of NCCP were promoting cancer data collection; rising public cancer awareness and healthy lifestyle popularization; enhancing healthy behaviors; increasing screening rate; improving access to the full spectrum of cancer diagnosis and care; implementing national diagnostic and treatment guidelines; increasing patient, caregiver, and healthcare professional awareness about issues of quality of life; increasing access to palliation and pain control; improving reporting quality of cancer incidence, mortality, and staging data; improving oncology service at each level.

NCCP sets out comprehensive strategy in fight against cancer. It's the first time government adopted major program of action linking prevention, diagnosis, treatment, care, and research. As a result of reviewing the several governmental programs were implemented and have been funded so far, there is no the full, comlete implementation of NCCP and exact steps of development for it are exist yet.

Insights on Palliative Care

Approximately, 42,000 death cases are registered annually in Georgia, with a population of 3.5 million. According to international experience, approx. 60 % of deceased that means approx. 25,000 patients require palliative care (PC) and pain relief, including the use of opioids like morphine. Given that at least two family members provide care for terminal stage patients, significant improvement of approximately 75,000 people overall can be achieved through PC service annually.

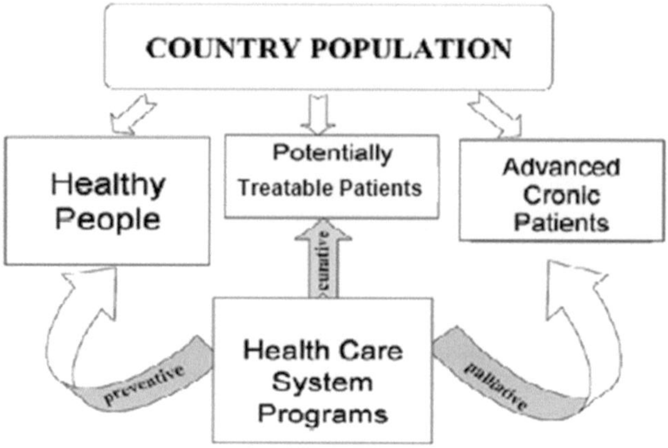

Fig. 22.3 Model of health care system planning

Most patients prefer to die at home in Georgia—this is their will and right, firmed through traditions. First, diagnosis usually is established on advanced stages in a big number of patients with cancer in Georgia, where 7000–8000 newly diagnosed cases are annually registered. For this reason, these patients pertain to untreatable category. Therefore, delivering of pain relief a PC to cancer patients refer to the most humane measures [11, 14].

"*What the Palliative Care means for Country?*"—to answer this question, the pioneers of palliative care and National Coordinator for PC of the Country advocated that the population of every country generally can be divided into three main groups: "Healthy People," "Potentially Treatable Patients," and "Advanced Chronic Patients." Taking into account the abovementioned groups, evidently, the healthcare system must also have three principal directions: (1) Preventive (aimed at healthy people), intending the maintenance of healthy status and decreasing morbidity; (2) Curative (for potentially treatable patients), aimed at the patient convalescence and rehabilitation; (3) Palliative (for Advanced Chronic Patients), intending the maintenance of maximally available life quality. If any of the listed directions is omitted, the healthcare system cannot be considered as perfect, for in this case, the corresponding part of the society becomes deprived of the healthcare service. Principally, the same outcomes are ensued if any of the listed directions are realized through incorrect strategies and methods, e.g., incorrectly planned and performed preventive programs fail to avoid and/or effectively prevent the development of certain diseases. Similarly, the incorrect PC is unable to provide an adequate life quality [11] (Fig. 22.3).

Practical implementation of PC (in pilot project) was initiated from 2004 since this period several successful steps were made: Healthcare professionals were trained in PC by invited international PC experts; home-based and inpatient services were organized; the amended legislation, supporting and promoting PC development had been approved; Georgian-language educational-methodical material in PC were prepared and issued; several PC pilot programs for advanced cancer and AIDS out- and inpatients in Capital and three different regions of Georgia were implemented with financial support of Governmental Budget and Global Found; The Georgian National

Association for Palliative Care and the Office of Coordinator of PC National Program (at the Health Care Committee of Parliament of Georgia) were established; PC subspecialty and continuing medical educational programs were elaborated and implemented; healthcare professionals from former soviet countries were trained; two PC services were granted as an ESMO PC designated centers for 2009–2014 period; Georgian-language educational-methodological material in PC were prepared and issued; PC pilot programs were implemented with financial support of Governmental Budget; The Georgian National Association for PC and the Office of Coordinator of PC National Program were established; PC National Plan for 2010–2015 was prepared and approved by the Government of Georgia; National Guideline for Cancer pain was elaborated and approved in 2012 [11].

Not with standing organizational, educational, practical legislative changed and successful steps done in 2004–2011 years, further development of cancer patients' PC was hindered since 2012 due to bureaucracy changes in the program management and program beneficiaries identification tools. Thus, National PC program acknowledged by the Parliament of Georgia did not realized. It was resulted by outpatient palliative care program modification in 2013 meaning canceling the nurse's service, limiting of home visits. In addition, it should be noted that palliative service rendering at home officially doesn't request respective knowledge and education necessity, and its implementation is directly imposed on primary healthcare and the latter made this program formality.

All the abovementioned resulted in program devaluation and factual canceling. To date, the program is implemented only officially and most of practical implementers have no minimal educational skills and knowledge.

For the purpose of state finances saving, program beneficiaries had been limited as follows: State undertook as responsibility to render the service only to the patient being in terminal condition and in alternative case, state defined obligatory life expectancy not exceeding 3–6 months as the program inclusion criteria and in case of life expectancy exceeding sanction is imposed on the doctor as he/she incorrectly defined life expectancy and included the patient in the PC program early notwithstanding existing diagnosis and needs; after 6 months of physicians (no any nurse is allowed) care, the patent's service needs to be disconnected notwithstanding the hard condition [11, 13].

Thus, existing system of PC is devastated and trained medical personnel in this field who cared over the patients prior to the reform cannot perform this unimaginable demand implying nurse service canceling in PC and obligatory death of beneficiary in 3–6 months or care disconnection.

Human Resources in Health

There is an extremely high number of doctors per capita in Georgia compared with other European countries. In Georgia, the number of physicians is higher than the European average, where there are 462 doctors per 100,000 people, compared to 327 in European countries. At the same time, the country faces an acute shortage of nurses, both in urban and rural areas (Fig. 22.4). The country's educational institutions produce far more doctors than needed. Approximately, 1200 doctors

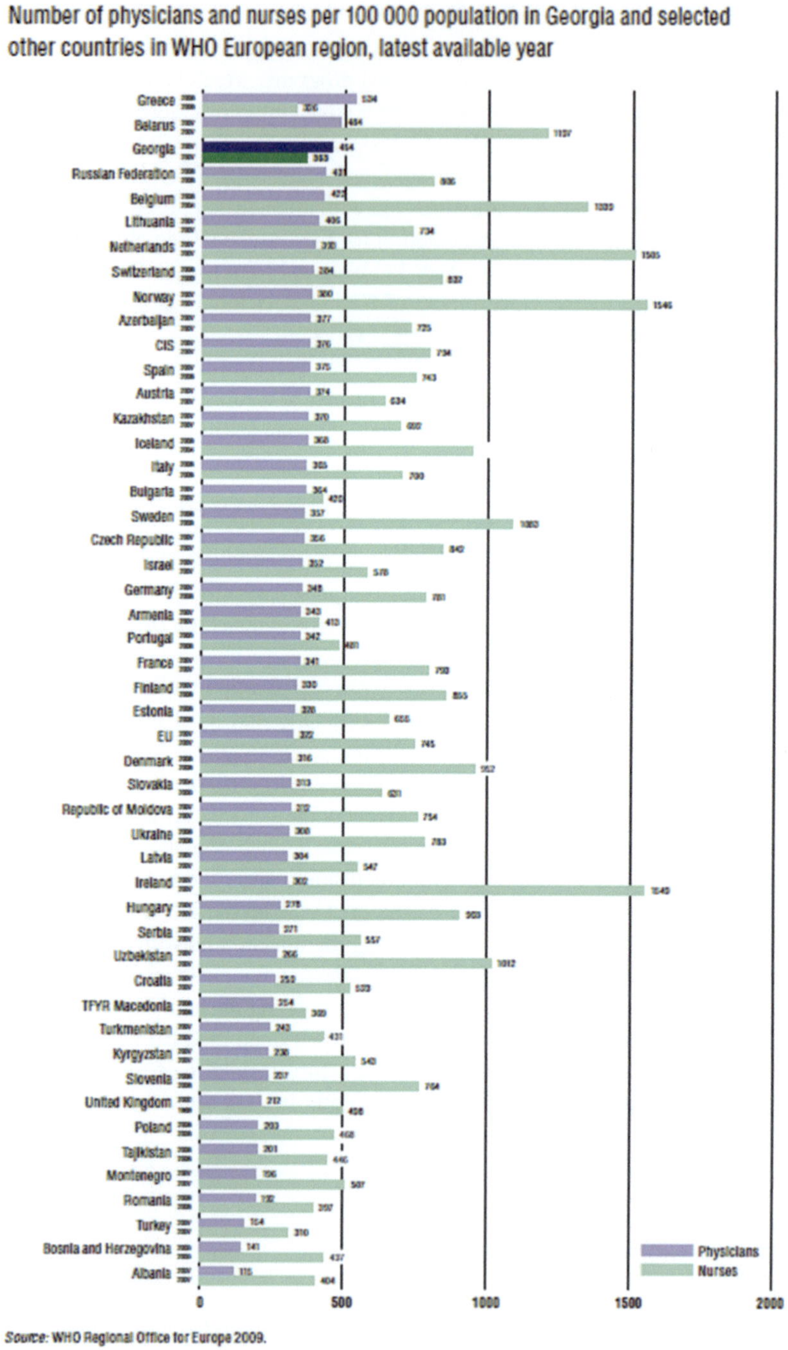

Fig. 22.4 The ratio of health care professionals in Georgia and European region presented by WHO (2009)

(excluding dentists) enter the labor market every year, whereas only about 100 nurses graduate every year from nursing schools. Therefore, Georgia's annual physician production count per 1000 inhabitants is 3 times higher than the European average, while the number of nurses produced by educational system is more than 10 times less than observed in Europe [6–8, 10, 15].

Nowadays, there are up to 350 licensed oncologists in Georgia, and most of them are middle and young age specialists. Most of young specialists know foreign language, share, and apply in practice internationally acknowledged clinical practice guidelines and try to supply qualitative medical service to patients. There is motivation and readiness for knowledge improvement and active participation in constant medical educational process.

Critical Clinical Issues

It should be noted that since 2010 with the initiative and assistance of European Society for Medical Oncology (ESMO), 33 clinical practical guidelines had been translated and adapted by Oncology Association of Georgia with the participation of ESMO national representative that shall greatly improve quality of patients' service. Abovementioned protocols had been reviewed and acknowledged by the Ministry of Health, Labour and Social Care of Georgia; however, they still remain to be nonobligatory (optional) manuals and are not mandatory guidelines, as their acknowledgment to be mandatory equals to the responsibility to ensure patient with proper technologies, medicines, and costs reimbursement that today cannot be provided by the healthcare system.

Absence of the abovementioned limits necessity of protocols mandatory application in practice and reduces possibility of qualitative service supply to the patients. This creates the provision resulting in stressing minor bureaucracy issues instead of importance while evaluating medical service quality towards the patients by regulator that shall by all means be followed by punitive measures against medical personnel.

Summary and Recommendations

The quality care and service for cancer patients in Georgia is under the transition period. Lot of changes were done during the difficult socioeconomic period of the country, but there are lots of important and urgent issues needed to be improved to progress the patients' care and their quality of life.

For the improvement of care of cancer patients, the following are important:

1. To release the multidisciplinary approaches of the patient care in real medical practice

2. Constant education of medical personnel and active cooperation with western leading clinics and educational institutions
3. Evaluation by the state of the burden resulted by cancer disease, recognition, and allocation of adequate funds in this field
4. Necessity and need of acknowledged clinical guidelines application
5. To analyze the necessity of palliative care and not to separate part of the healthcare (and cancer care) and not only verbal but also business support; proper evolution of successful steps in palliative care development and concern about the field surviving
6. To educate and evaluate the primary healthcare net medical staff, introduse the primary/basic skills and elements before the delivery of care, which will make possible to perform patients' care in reality
7. To understand more about "cancerophobia" and "opioidophobia" in the society and strategic planning of its improvement in the country
8. Urgent revision of palliative care program and obligatory modification of program design according to the international experience
9. To analyze oncological patient multidisciplinary care model and its adoption in practice that shall considerably improve life and living quality of patients
10. To be objective, critical, and honest, see the gaps and try to find the ways of improvement.

References

1. Rukhadze T. An overview of the health care system in Georgia: expert recommendations in the context of predictive, preventive and personalized medicine. EPMA J. 2013;4:8. doi: 10.1186/1878-5085-4-8.
2. Rukhadze T. An overview of the healthcare system in Georgia. In: Costigliola V, editor. Healthcare overview: new perspectives. New York: Springer; 2012. p. 133–52.
3. Gamkrelidze A, Atun R, Gotsadze G, MacLehose L. Health care systems in transition: Georgia, vol. 4. 2nd ed. Copenhagen: European Observatory on Health Care Systems; 2002.
4. Gotsadze T, Schouten E. Healthcare reforms in Georgia: an analytical overview. Tbilisi: UNICEF & Health Net International; 1997.
5. Chanturidze T, Ugulava T, Durán A, Ensor T, Richardson E. Georgia: health system review. Health Syst Transit. 2009;11(8):1–116.
6. Sakvarelidze L, Center for Disease Control and Public Health. Health care in Georgia compared with the European region countries. 2008. www.ncdc.ge/Eng/Health/Georgia¬%20vs%20International.pdf. Accessed 12 Oct 2011.
7. Saclarides CP. Developing a nursing registration system in the Republic of Georgia. TuftScope. 2010;10(1):32–3.
8. National Centre for Disease Control and Public Health of Georgia. Health and health care in Georgia: statistical yearbook. 2008. http://www.ncdc.ge/W1/cnobari 2008_en.htm. Accessed 13 Oct 2011.
9. USAID. 2002–2009. Country health statistical report: Georgia. http://permanent.access.gpo.gov/lps107486/. Accessed 12 Oct 2011.
10. Universal healthcare (UHC) program evaluation from 'beneficiaries' and 'service providers' perspectives final report. http://www.moh.gov.ge/files/JAN-USID/2.pdf.
11. MoLHSA. www.moh.gov.ge.

12. National Center of Disease Control and Public Health, Department of Statistics. www.ncdc.ge.
13. Social Service Agency. www.ssa.gov.ge.
14. Kordzaia D. Georgian national program for palliative care. Action plan for 2011–2015.
15. Access to Quality Health Care; Georgia-National Health Care Strategy 2011–2015. www.moh.gov.ge.

Chapter 23
Romania, Attempting to Catch up the European Standards of Care for Cancer Patients

Alexandru Eniu, Dan Dumitraşcu, and Marius Geanta

A Recent History of Cancer Treatment in Romania: Before and After 1989

Cancer is the second cause of death in Romania, following cardiovascular diseases. The latest data from Globocan [2] shows that breast cancer is currently the most common cancer among women and the number one cause of cancer mortality in women. Furthermore, the mortality rate for cervical cancer in Romania is the highest in Europe. In men, the most frequent causes of cancer deaths are lung, colorectal, and gastric cancers. Life expectancy in Romania appears to be increasing, and the number of patients with malignant tumors is also expected to rise. Currently, the majority of malignant tumors that oncologists see present in the late stages of disease. For example, more than half of the new breast cancers diagnosed in 2004 at the Cancer Institute Ion Chiricuţă in Cluj-Napoca were locally advanced. Lack of patient-oriented information and regional screening programs are some possible explanations for such late-stage presentation.

With a population of 21 million people inhabiting a country roughly the size of Great Britain, Romania is the youngest member of the European Union. The country inherited the former "state-owned" health system of the former Eastern European communist bloc, characterized by centralized organization, limited resources such as equipment and drugs, and trained but underpaid health professionals. The lack of national or regional cancer registries still hampers the evaluation of health interven-

A. Eniu, M.D., Ph.D. (✉)
Department of Breast Tumors, Cancer Institute Ion Chiricuta, Republicii 34-36, Cluj-Napoca 400015, Romania
e-mail: aleniu@iocn.ro

D. Dumitraşcu, M.D. • M. Geanta, M.D.
Center for Innovation in Medicine, Bucharest, Romania
e-mail: marius.geanta@kolmedia.ro

M. Silbermann (ed.), *Cancer Care in Countries and Societies in Transition*,
DOI 10.1007/978-3-319-22912-6_23

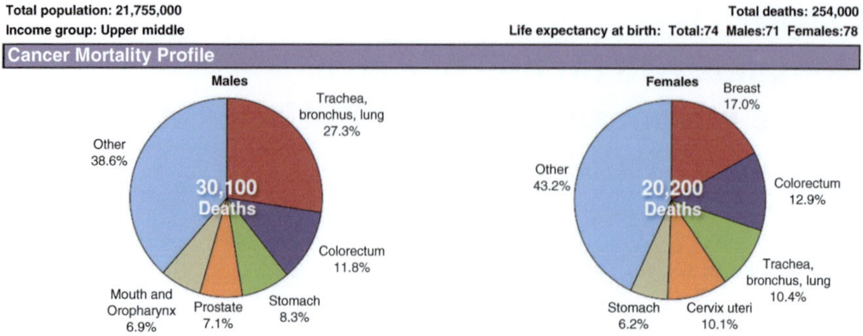

Fig. 23.1 Cancer mortality profile (*Source*: World Health Organization—cancer country profiles; Romania, 2014)

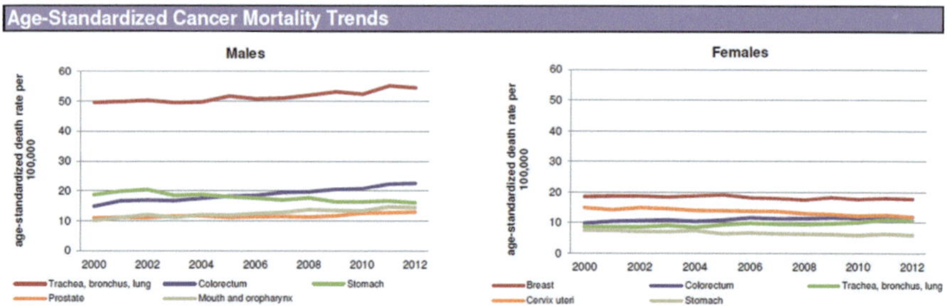

Fig. 23.2 Age-standardized cancer mortality trends (*Source*: World Health Organization—cancer country profiles; Romania, 2014)

tions. According to WHO [1], for a population of about 21 million, in 2014 Romania had an estimated 254,000 deaths due to cancer, with a distribution quite similar to most of the countries in this European region. With a life expectancy at birth of 71 years for men and 78 years for women, the cancer mortality profile shows lower airways (27.3 %), colorectum (11.8 %), and stomach (8.3 %) cancers—for male individuals, and breast (17 %), colorectum (12.9 %), and lower airways (10.4 %)—for females, being the main causes of death due to cancer in Romania, with a special mention that other, undefined specific causes still keep a large percentage, of 38.6 % and 43.2 %, respectively (Fig. 23.1). The age-standardized cancer mortality trends keep this order for females, while in males, in recent years colorectum cancers overtook the gastric cancers (Fig. 23.2).

Among all types of cancer, lung cancer has the greatest incidence in men (with 9317 cases), followed by colorectum (5760) and prostate cancer (4532), while in women breast cancer has an incidence of 8981 cases, double than colorectum (4496) and cervical cancer (4343) that follows (Fig. 23.3).

When looking back in time, before 1989, during the communist era, the Party's health program appraised health as an essential "factor for social and economic

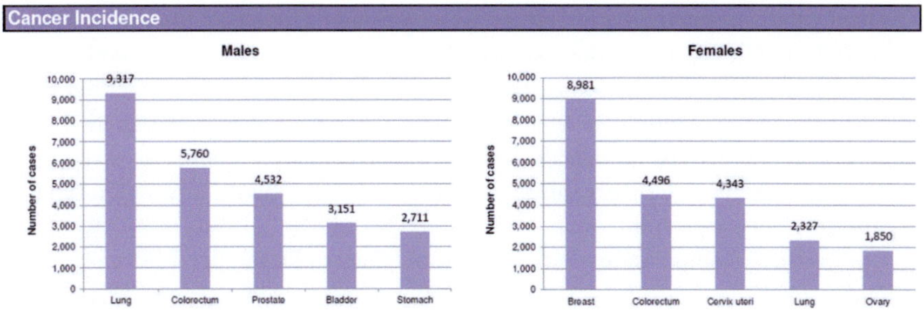

Fig. 23.3 Cancer incidence (*Source*: World Health Organization—cancer country profiles; Romania, 2014)

development […] to satisfy in the best conditions the population life requirements, harmonious development, physical, intellectual and moral capacity, to ensure a full work and creative of every member of society." [6] Despite the communist slogans, health wasn't a real priority of policy makers. Thus, the only legal provision regarding population healthcare provision during this period was a law issued in 1978.

Healthcare services were provided by a centralized state system and the full costs were covered by the state. There were also healthcare services requiring direct out-of-the-pocket payment, but also belonging to the government-owned units. Therefore, one of the communist heritages is the common belief that the state should provide healthcare for free and for all.

The medical education was quite well developed, provided through vocational and high schools for undergraduate training, while five universities offered graduate medical studies. The universities are still operating. Basic public education for health was offered in schools and through communist organizations meetings.

There was no program for public health screening to provide a yearly public health evaluation. People were addressing the doctor only when they got sick. There were no national cancer screening program and no public awareness campaigns. However, the industry provided some health checking screening for the workers. The number and type of health checks per year depended on the workplace health risks. One example was the yearly gynecological examination. This examination aimed to prevent the abortion, which was prohibited by law. In fact, the purpose was to identify the pregnant women, to register and supervise them. The gynecologists had confessed after 1990 that through this system were detected most of cervical cancers as well as some of other gynecological cancers, thus representing a form of screening. After 1990, the abortion prohibition was cancelled together with the yearly gynecologic examination, which was considered a communist practice, but it was not replaced by a cervical cancer screening program.

Doctor–patient relation during that period was difficult: patients used to offer money or goods to doctors and nurses thinking that they will receive better healthcare. This is another communist heritage, a matter of mentality, still occurring today.

During the communist regime, there were two main Oncology Institutes, one set up in 1929 in Cluj and the other one in 1949 in Bucharest, cities with well-known medical schools. During that time, there was little investment in the cancer field, nor in early diagnosis, neither in treatment, because cancer was considered a fatal disease [7]. There were no cancer patient organizations or groups, as, except for unions, communist youth organization, and communist party, any other type of organizations were prohibited.

The eventful Romanian revolution that took place in December 1989 meant that Romania paid the democracy with many unnecessary deaths. In the early 1990, NGOs from all over the world offered a lot of support in goods or money without asking anything in change. Therefore, the role of NGOs is, to some extent, still seen to be simply to support people in difficulties and the larger scope of an NGO is still today misunderstood. Volunteering during the communist regime was actually a compulsory involvement required by the party in different activities called patriotic work. Therefore, there is not much tradition in this field and still a misperception of what volunteering and charity mean.

The Impact of Political Changes

After 1990, policy makers and public were focused more on the economic reform of the country, failing to improve the social services and healthcare.

A young democracy, with young politicians, without much or any political education characterized the initial political landscape in the early 1990 that soon led to a multitude of different parties. Politicians' vanity and personal interests, rather than national/population interest and well-being led step by step to current political instability and poor trust of the voters in Romanian politicians. Health is unfortunately not considered a priority by the authorities, and the civil society is still shy in acting publicly, due to poor solidarity among the constituents.

The Romanian healthcare policy is incoherent due to the following main issues:

(a) Lack of national long-term healthcare strategy in place: the health ministers changed so often, that Romania can apply for Guinness Book of Records for having 19 health ministers and 20 terms during the last 22 years. For instance, in 2012 Romania had three health ministers. Each minister almost cancelled all what the previous did and attempted to draft its vision but did not have the time to implement it;

(b) Too much involvement of politicians and lack of technocrats: main positions in the healthcare system, starting from the minister of health down to local health authorities and hospital managers are mostly appointed on political criteria. Most of the healthcare legal provisions were issued without public debate, usually "over the night" without any implementation tools (criteria, norms, etc.) that were issued afterwards quite late, after several months. This situation changed since 2007, when it became mandatory to allow public debates regarding the drafts of legal provisions. Draft of new regulations is posted on the websites of the Ministry of Health and/or National Health Insurance Agency to be consulted by interested stakeholders and public debates are organized.

The healthcare legal provisions are regulating more or less everything in this field (the organization and operation the national health authorities, healthcare national program, etc.). Most of EU recommendation and directives were transposed in national regulations, including the cancer screening Directive, cross-border healthcare Directive, patient rights according to European Charter and most of them are also implemented to the extent that our limited budget allowed.

Romania has a national healthcare social insurance system. Only a part of the population pays the healthcare insurance, but in practice everyone benefits of healthcare services. There is no transparency regarding the amount collected for healthcare insurance, and the amount is collected in a common fund with other taxes and fees, under the administration of the Ministry of Public Finances that decides the amount of the budget allotted to each national activity, including healthcare.

There is a decrease in the number of payers/contributors to the national healthcare insurance found, due to the decline of national economy and the bankruptcy of the large industry. Currently, there are an estimated 3.5 millions payers to national fund of healthcare insurance out of about 18 million beneficiaries of healthcare services.

The Healthcare National Programme

Romania had developed a National Health Programme that also includes the National Programme of Cancer Prevention and the National Programme of Cancer Treatment. The National Programme of Cancer Treatment was implemented in 2002 only after the intense lobbying and advocacy campaign of some of the cancer patients' organizations existing at that time. These programs were always subfinanced, due to the limited budget available.

In 2007, a reform of the healthcare system was initiated, through a law issued that year. This law has been several times modified. Regarding cancer screening, this law implemented what can be called an opportunistic screening program. Upon request by the individual or by the general practitioner, insured citizens have access to yearly mammography, Pap Test, and PSA testing. People with cancer history in the family can also access additional health checks. These investigations are partially or fully covered by the health insurance depending on the contract with service provider and the available budget. In 2012, a new healthcare law was drafted that is still subject to public consultation.

The budget forecast is drafted at the end of each year for the next year. Usually, the budget is approved in March of each year for the year that was already started. The budget is then distributed for each county and then to each hospital more on political criteria that on evidence base. This leads to inequalities in cancer diagnosis and treatment across the public healthcare system.

With all these very complex regulation in force and in place, the healthcare system is not operating properly, affecting cancer patients; due to the high direct cost of certain interventions for cancer diagnosis and treatment, there are severe limitations in access to high-performance examinations (such as PET-CT or MRI scanning), radiotherapy, or expensive anticancer medications. The radiotherapy equipment is outdated and insufficient. It is estimated that only one third of the patients requiring radiotherapy actually receive it. For certain expensive medications such as monoclonal antibodies or tyrosine kinase inhibitors, the patient needs to receive a special, case-by-case approval for treatment from the National Insurance House—which leads to delays in initiating treatment; not all patients requiring such medications actually receive it.

The Involvement of the Civil Society

The Romanian Cancer Society, the first cancer patient organization in Romania, was set up in 1993 by physicians from Oncology Institute Cluj City and their patients [3]. This is an umbrella cancer patient organization aiming at increasing public awareness, cancer patient education and supports initiatives geared towards improving outcomes for cancer patients, as well as lobbying and advocacy.

The "Common Destinies" Association, the first breast cancer organization, was started in 1996 by doctors and cancer patients as a support group within the professional organization "Romanian Cancer Association." Other cancer patient organization were initiated in different area of Romania, either as breast cancer support groups, either as umbrella organization most focused in lobby and advocacy. Most of cancer patient organizations were gathered in 2005 under a national umbrella, called Federation of Cancer Patient Associations, the interface between the cancer patients groups and relevant stakeholders [5].

The aggressive advocacy led by these organizations was successful at the beginning. Later, the fact that most groups are 100 % sponsored by pharma industry and because of inappropriate partnership in advocacy campaigns (e.g., national associations of pharma industry), besides the internal disagreement and the fights among the patients' groups publicly disclosed, had led to lost of the trust of the public and relevant authorities (e.g., Ministry of Health, National Health Insurance Agency, Oncology Commissions, etc.) towards the activity of the cancer patients organizations.

Unfortunately, most of cancer patient organizations didn't improve enough their capacity to be able to advocate in the same manner as the European Cancer Patient Coalition, to be a real dialog partner and to help strengthen the healthcare system. The communist mentality among the beneficiaries of the health system still persists, expecting the Ministry of Health and National Health Insurance Agency to solve everything over the night [4].

There are however a few cancer patient organizations managed according to the good governance code and ethics of the NGOs. These are accessing non-pharma financing and help develop most of public awareness, organize opportunistic screening programs and are partners of relevant authorities in solving certain issues related to cancer policy.

Unfortunately, due to the misperception of the role that the NGOs can play, many of cancer patients or caregivers requesting help from patients' organizations are seeking either financial support, support like treatment abroad or speeding of some processes such as special approvals for expensive medications. Due to the fact that breast prosthesis are expensive for most of breast cancer patients and unfortunately are not covered by healthcare insurance, neither by social protection, many patients are expecting the NGOs to provide them.

Cancer Diagnosis and Treatment in Romania

Cancer diagnosis and treatments are delivered through two national cancer institutes—one in Bucharest and the other one in Cluj-Napoca—as well in regional centers throughout Romania's 41 counties. Of those centers, 29 have radiotherapy facilities. However, a recent analysis performed by the National Subcommission on Radiotherapy revealed that the equipment is outdated and insufficient: only 16 centers have high-energy radiotherapy machines (11 linear accelerators and 15 telecobalt machines) and the rest of the centers have brachytherapy and/or conventional radiotherapy machines. It is estimated that only one-third of all the patients that require radiotherapy have access to treatment, mostly because of a lack of facilities for such treatment.

Patients with cancer in Romania are served by about 270 medical oncologists and 110 radiation therapy specialists. Although medical oncology has existed in our country since 1997 as a separate specialty with a 5-year residency training requirement, reformatory measures in 2007 led to the withdrawal of medical oncology from the list of medical specialties in Romania. However, with the help of strong official protests from the national medical oncology societies and crucial support from ESMO and ASCO, medical oncology was successfully reinstated as a specialty in 2008.

Patients with cancer receive free medical treatment through the National Cancer Program, which ensures funding for oncologic and supportive medication. Because of limited resources, expensive drugs (targeted therapies including monoclonal antibodies and tyrosine kinase inhibitors) are reimbursed only after the individual patient's file has been approved by a national commission; this process leads to delays and waiting lists for certain pathologies. In 2008, the lists of drugs reimbursed by the National Cancer Program was updated to include new medications that have demonstrated benefits in several tumor types; also, protocols for several drugs have been proposed to offer guidance and to ensure that their use is limited to approved indications. However, the list has not been updated since 2008, which means that the new drugs approved in the last 5 years are not available to our patients.

The concept of personalized medicine is not yet ready for prime time even in very developed countries. We are practicing stratified oncology—in the sense that for certain diseases we know there are several clinical and molecular subtypes that have different prognosis and respond differently to certain targeted agents. We are able to identify certain subtypes (such as her-2 positive breast cancer or EGFR-mutated non-small cell lung cancer) that benefit extensively form some targeted agents. However, testing for these mutations is not explicitly reimbursed in Romania. Moreover, the newer targeted drugs are not always reimbursed. Because of all these difficulties, personalized cancer care is not yet a reality in Romania.

There are more than 100 units in Romania providing cancer diagnosis; therefore, the waiting time for accessing cancer diagnosing is usually between 3 days and maximum 3 weeks.

To illustrate better the limitations and the complexity of the situation in Romania, we will discuss in brief the breast cancer care scenario. This pathology is the quintessential example of multidisciplinary cooperation across many specialties—therefore putting at test the functionality of the health system as a whole. As we have shown in the first part of this chapter, for a population of around 21 million people, the WHO estimated a number of around 9000 new breast cancer yearly, positioning breast cancer as the most frequent cancer in women. Due to around 3400 breast cancer death each year, this tumor kills more women than any other cancer in Romania, accounting for roughly 17 % of cancer death in females (World Health Organization—Cancer Country Profiles; Romania, 2014). The other big cancer killers in Romania are colorectal cancer (13 %) followed by lung cancer (10.3 %)—almost as frequently as cervical cancer (10.1 %). The lack of a functional national cancer registry does not allow to present detailed data regarding age or stage at diagnosis for breast cancer. Limited studies performed in some institutions such as the Cancer Institute Ion Chiricuta provided some data on stage distribution of breast cancer in 2004 (A. Eniu, personal communication)—Fig. 23.4. The low frequency of stages 0 (0 %) and I (9 %) reflect the absence of a national/regional screening program. Most patients will seek medical help for a lump in the breast, usually when the tumor is at least 2 cm in diameter (stage II—41 %). Also, a large

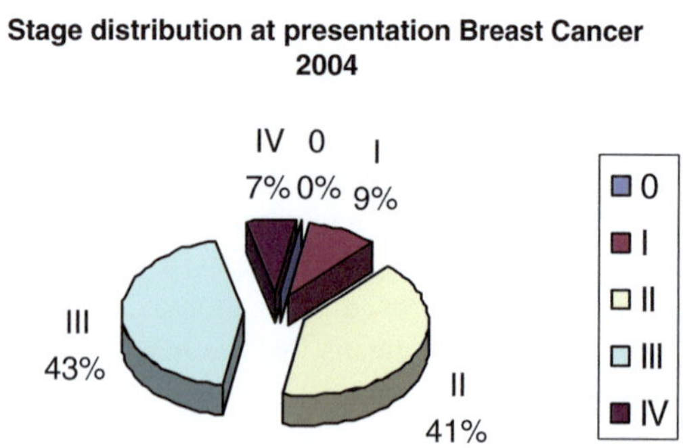

Fig. 23.4 Breast cancer stage distribution at presentation at the Cancer Institute Ion Chiricuta, Cluj-Napoca, in 2004 (A. Eniu, personal communication)

number of patients will neglect their tumors until some symptomatology appears or the dimension of the tumor increases. This leads to the high prevalence (43 %) of stage III breast cancer. A number of patients (8 %) will already have overt metastatic disease at presentation. Overall, over 50 % of the patients will present with stage III and IV disease. Compared with the treatment of early breast cancer, the treatment of advanced breast cancer is more resource intensive and generally has poorer outcomes, highlighting the potential benefit of earlier detection and diagnosis, both in terms of conserving scarce resources and in terms of reducing morbidity and mortality. The efforts were undertaken in the past 10 years to increase women's awareness regarding breast cancer; this situation is likely to have improved; an analysis is currently underway to compare this early data with the actual situation in 2015. However, most women do not routinely undergo screening mammography. At the national level, women have access to "opportunistic" mammographic examination—which means that this examination is covered by the insurance, but there is no invitation to participate in a controlled screening program. Therefore, women can elect to perform or—as is much more frequently the case—to not perform a yearly mammogram. As women face many difficulties in their daily life—struggling to maintain their job in an economic crisis environment, while at the same time caring for their families—they tend to neglect themselves as other priorities are considered. For the older generations, cancer is still considered a stigma—something that has to be hidden away, even from other family members; this leads to situations where these women will only seek medical advice in case of bleeding or severe pain—usually in a late stage of the disease.

The all-too-frequent scenario at the Breast Cancer Unit of the Cancer Institute Ion Chiricuta is that women will show for a breast cancer examination because they felt a lump in their breast. They will usually wait 2–3 months before seeking medical advice, "hoping" that the lump will disappear. This leads to a situation in which most tumors have a diameter of more than 2 cm at presentation. Effective awareness campaigns directed towards early detection of breast cancer, coupled with the implementation of regional screening programs, are needed to change this situation.

Screening and Palliative Care

As mentioned before, Romania has the highest mortality rate caused by cervical cancer among European countries. This situation is caused by late diagnosis: due to lack of national screening programs, and possibly also linked to a lack of information and education of the public regarding cervical cancer, combined with the cultural resistance to address the physician for gynecological problems, the majority of patients present with advanced disease at diagnosis. Over the past 2 years, plans have been devised to expand regional and national pilot screening programs for cervical cancer deployed by the Cancer Institute Ion Chiricuţă from Cluj and to develop screening programs for breast and colorectal cancer. To complement the screening program, a vaccination program is underway for the prevention of cervical cancer. As it was mentioned above, the cancer patient organizations developed public awareness campaigns together with offering opportunistic screening for breast cancer, cervical cancer, and prostate cancer to low income and rural area population through mobile facilities (mammovan, Pap smear van, etc.). The difficulty faced during these campaigns is to change the cultural beliefs of the population, as cancer is still associated with stigma, and the population is not willing to voluntarily take advantage of these provided services.

On the other hand, the availability of palliative care in terminal phase is limited, mainly provided by NGOs in partnership with local healthcare authorities. Unfortunately, the reimbursement for these services is covered by the insurance for a limited period in time; therefore, still today many terminally ill patients do not have access to proper care. As in many former communist countries, there were no palliative services organized during that period. After the revolution, the palliative services began to appear in connection with the few hospices created mainly in collaboration with Anglo-Saxon NGOs. Following the intense lobbying and campaigns undertaken by "Casa Sperantei" hospice in Brasov, led by Dr. Daniela Mosoiu, palliative care began to be recognized as an important service for terminally ill patients. Their first success was to change the old laws that regulated very strictly the prescription of morphine for these patients; following the introduction of "European-like" prescription rules, access to pain-controlling medication improved substantially, helping numerous patients. As a result, the opioid consumption in morphine equivalents, as reported by the International Narcotics Control Board (World Health Organization population data, The Pain & Policy Studies Group, University of Wisconsin/WHO Collaborating Center, 2014) increased after 1995 when the new regulations were introduced, from a low level of 2–3 mg per capita to 7.5–10 mg per capita. Another area of improvement was the reimbursement of palliative care services by the national health insurance system. Although imperfect, the system covers services for palliation, for a limited period of time; this led to the establishment of several palliative care units (even if still insufficient for the existing demand) in several cities (Bucharest, Alba-Iulia, Cluj-Napoca, Iasi, Lugoj, Oradea, etc.). Currently, the Ministry of Health, together with Casa Sperantei Hospice, is developing a National Program for Palliative Care. Nowadays, palliative care is recognized as a special competence; more than 300 physicians acquired this competence until 2013.

Clinical Research

Clinical research has been growing steadily in our country. Many patients are treated in areas with limited resources, and although heterogeneity exists in the level of care, some centers qualify for participation in clinical studies. Well-designed, controlled trials are a means of delivering state-of-the-art diagnosis, treatment, and follow-up care. They lead to improvement of care quality through education and implementation of Good Clinical Practice principles, while patients enjoy free access to standard-of-care treatment (e.g., targeted therapies). According to the Romanian National Drug Agency, the number of phase II and phase III studies to which Romanian centers are contributing patients doubled in the last 2 years.

Table 23.1 Cancer plans, monitoring, and surveillance

Has an operational cancer policy/strategy/action plan	Yes
Has a cancer registry	Yes
Scope	Population-based
Coverage	Subnational
Last year of data	2010

Table 23.2 Cancer primary prevention policies

Tobacco control	
Has an operational policy, strategy, or action plan to reduce the burden of tobacco use	Yes
Smoke-free legislation	Up to two public places completely smoke free
Tobacco dependence treatment	National "quit smoking" line, and both NRT and some cessation services cost—covered[a]
Warning labels	Medium size warnings with all appropriate characteristics OR large warnings missing some appropriate characteristics
Bans on advertising, promotion, and sponsorship	Bans on national television, radio, and print media as well as on some but not all other forms of direct and/or indirect advertising
Tobacco taxes	51–75 % of retail price is tax
Overweight and obesity prevention and control	
Has an operational policy, strategy, or action plan for reducing overweight/obesity	No
Physical inactivity prevention and control	
Has an operational policy, strategy, or action plan to reduce physical inactivity and/or promote physical activity	No
Harmful use of alcohol prevention and control	
Has an operational policy, strategy, or action plan to reduce the harmful use of alcohol	No
National immunization	
Human Papillomavirus vaccination schedule	No
Hepatitis B vaccination schedule	Birth
Hepatitis B vaccination coverage, infants	96 %

[a]Indicates highest possible level of achievement

Table 23.3 Cancer screening and early detection

Cervical cancer	
Cervical cytology (PAP)	Not generally available at the public primary healthcare level
Acetic acid visualization (VIA)	Not generally available at the public primary healthcare level
Breast cancer	
Breast palpation/clinical breast exam (CBE)	Generally available at the public primary healthcare level
Mammogram	Not generally available at the public primary healthcare level
Colorectal cancer	
Fecal occult blood test or fecal immunological test	Not generally available at the public primary healthcare level
Bowel cancer screening by exam or colonoscopy	Not generally available at the public primary healthcare level

Table 23.4 Cancer treatment and palliative care

Radiotherapy	Generally available in the public health system
Total high-energy teletherapy units/million inhabitants	1.2
Number of radiotherapy centers	22
Number of radiation oncologists	82
Chemotherapy (medicines not specified)	Generally available in the public health system
Oral morphine (formulation not specified)	Not generally available in the public health system
Non-methadone morphine equivalent consumption per cancer death (mg)	…
Community/home care for people with advanced stage cancer and other NCDs	Not generally available

… = No data available

National Health Strategy for 2014–2020 [9]

Taking into account the current status of oncologic diseases, the drawbacks and advances made in monitoring and surveillance, primary prevention, screening and early detection, and also in treatment and palliative care (summarized in the Tables 23.1, 23.2, 23.3, and 23.4 below; source: World Health Organization), a national strategy was developed for the next years, aimed to allow an "up-to-date" to the European context and towards "Strategy Europe 2020" (Health 2020) of WHO for Europe Region. This strategic document/policy is issued in the context of the planning process for European funds, being also justified by the necessity to follow the country recommendations of European Commission concerning the health sector. Also, the general development framework takes into account the measures suggested in the "Functional analysis of the health sector in Romania" of the World Bank experts [8].

Romania performs suboptimally in prevention (Table 23.2), including early detection of cervical cancer (Tables 23.3 and 23.4), the mortality in this type of cancer increasing or maintaining a constant level, at most. The recent established national program for screening in cervical cancer requires a few good years to be implemented, and also a sustained funding and an improved performance according to the specific standards before the first significant signs of a stable impact on mortality. The high rates of morbidity and mortality make the primary prevention of this type of cancer, through the vaccination for Human Papilloma Virus (HPV), an intervention highly relevant and necessary in Romania, also because the types 16 and 18 are responsible for about 70 % of cervical cancers and the benefits of vaccination are already well documented [9]. There is an urgent need to implement the so-far delayed interventions for early detection by population screening for the other two common types of cancer (colorectal and breast), according to the European recommendations. Table 23.2 also shows that on the background of the unconfined circulation of hepatitic viruses B and C and of the high risk behaviors (smoking, alcohol consumption), the incidence of liver cancer in Romania is high—the third highest rate in Europe for men.

Summary and Recommendations

Over the past two decades, Romania has traveled a long road in its attempt to become a true European Union country. In the field of cancer care, measures attempting to reduce the disparities among Romania and the other European countries in cancer outcomes have provided benefit to the patients, but we are still facing a context lacking a national strategy for cancer control. Doctors and hospitals are overwhelmed by a large number of patients, many with advanced disease stage. Because of resource limitation, some patients still do not have access to certain interventions such as radiation therapy or targeted therapy.

To improve on the long term the outcome of cancer patients, the consolidation of the National Cancer Registry is crucial to be able to assess the current situation and to monitor progress. With the current trend of escalating costs of cancer treatment in general it is foreseeable that no country, even the most developed ones, will be able to cover all interventions. Therefore, countries like Romania should implement an evidence based, health technology assessment system to prioritize the use of the limited resources to fund the most relevant interventions that are essential for cancer control.

References

1. WHO. World Health Organization—cancer country profiles Romania. Geneva: WHO; 2014. http://www.who.int/cancer/country-profiles/rou_en.pdf?ua=1.

2. The Globocan project. Population fact sheet—Romania. http://globocan.iarc.fr/Pages/fact_sheets_population.aspx
3. IPRI. The state of oncology. 2013. http://www.i-pri.org/oncology2013/
4. Boyle P, Sullivan R, Zielinski C, Brawley OW, editors. State of oncology 2013. Lyon: iPRI; 2013.
5. Ene S. Cancer in Romania: patient perspective. In: Boyle P, Sullivan R, Zielinski C, Brawley OW, editors. State of oncology 2013. Lyon: iPRI; 2013.
6. LEGEA Nr. 3 din 6 iulie 1978 privind asigurarea sanatatii populatiei. EMITENT: Marea Adunarea Nationala a Republicii Socialiste Romania, aparuta in Buletinul Oficial nr. 54 din 10 iulie 1978
7. Silvia Ionescu-Goga M.D., Ph.D. In loc de Prafata Intre Umbre si Lumini. Rev. Hipocrate, 2014.
8. World Bank, Romania, Functional Review Health Sector, Final report 2011
9. OMS, Immunization, vaccines and biologicals, Human papillomavirus (HPV). http://www.who.int/immunization/topics/hpv/en/. Accessed 28 Feb 2014.
10. Ministerul Sănătăţii. Strategia Nationala de Sanatate 2014–2020. http://www.ms.ro/upload/Anexa%201%20-%20Strategia%20Nationala%20de%20Sanatate%202014-2020.pdf.

Chapter 24
Recent Challenges and Achievements in Cancer Care in Latin American Societies

Eduardo Cazap

Overview

Today, an individual's odds of surviving cancer are strongly correlated with where that person lives. Whereas in the USA the 5-year survival rate for patients with breast cancer is 84 %, in the Gambia, breast cancer survival is just 12.5 %. Interestingly, gains in survival have not always been due to very expensive treatments. Frequently, increased survival has been achieved by cancer treatments that are relatively low cost.

Considered for many years, a problem almost exclusive of rich countries, cancer is rapidly becoming a leading cause of death and disability in poor countries. Currently, low-income countries have just 5 % of resources to deal with 80 % of the global burden [1].

In addition to this, the existing treatments and new therapies are accessible to less than 10 % of the world population.

Cancer and noncommunicable diseases are now recognized by the United Nations and World Health Organization as a major public health crisis. Because of this, cancer care in low- and middle-income countries (LMICs) is now acknowledged as a global health priority [2]. As urbanization and conversion of the low-income populations to a western style economy continues, the cancer rate continues to increase and will need to be matched by strengthening of the health systems of the Low-Income Countries (LICs). In)Middle Income Countries (MICs), good cancer treatment centers are to be found but most of them are located in urban populations.

E. Cazap, M.D., Ph.D., F.A.S.C.O. (✉)
Latin American and Caribbean Society of Medical Oncology (SLACOM), Buenos Aires, Argentina

Union for International Cancer Control (UICC), Geneva, Switzerland

National Cancer Institute (INC), Buenos Aires, Argentina
e-mail: ecazap@slacom.org

M. Silbermann (ed.), *Cancer Care in Countries and Societies in Transition*,
DOI 10.1007/978-3-319-22912-6_24

The disparity in access to care and outcomes between)High-Income Countries (HICs) and LMICs are staggering. The reasons for this disparity include cost, access to care, manpower and training deficits, and a lack of awareness in the lay and medical communities [3]. Many people (particularly in LMICs) have little understanding of cancer, and in some cultural environments, women are loath to admit to their husbands that they have noticed a lump in the breast or vaginal bleeding. This, coupled to the cost of transportation and treatment, and frequently too, the failure of the primary health care provider to recognize the possibility of cancer results in an unknown fraction of cancer patients dying before reaching a treatment facility. Because of these barriers, diagnosis is usually late (80 % stage III and IV), such that the assumption that cancer is almost invariably fatal becomes a self-fulfilling prophecy. Before developing strategies to improve cancer care, however, it is essential to first establish what cancer health services exist on a country-by-country basis [4].

Argentina

In 1816, the United Provinces of the Rio Plata declared their independence from Spain. After Bolivia, Paraguay, and Uruguay went their separate ways, the area that remained became Argentina. The country's population and culture were heavily shaped by immigrants from throughout Europe, with Italy and Spain providing the largest percentage of newcomers from 1860 to 1930. Up until about the mid-twentieth century, much of Argentina's history was dominated by periods of internal political conflict between Federalists and Unitarians and between civilian and military factions. After World War II, an era of Peronist populism and direct and indirect military interference in subsequent governments was followed by a military junta that took power in 1976. Democracy returned in 1983 after a failed bid to seize the Falkland Islands (Islas Malvinas) by force, and has persisted despite numerous challenges, the most formidable of which was a severe economic crisis in 2001–2002 that led to violent public protests and the successive resignations of several presidents. In January 2013, Argentina assumed a nonpermanent seat on the UN Security Council for the 2013–2014 term.

Located in the south part of South America (Figs. 24.1 and 24.2), Argentina's population continues to grow but at a slower rate because of its steadily declining birth rate. Argentina's fertility decline began earlier than in the rest of Latin America, occurring most rapidly between the early twentieth century and the 1950s and then becoming more gradual. Life expectancy has been improving, most notably among the young and the poor. While the population under age 15 is shrinking, the youth cohort—ages 15–24—is the largest in Argentina's history and will continue to bolster the working-age population. If this large working-age population is well-educated and gainfully employed, Argentina is likely to experience an economic boost and possibly higher per capita savings and investment. Although literacy and primary school enrollment are nearly universal, grade repetition is problematic and secondary school completion is low. Both of these issues vary widely by region and socioeconomic group.

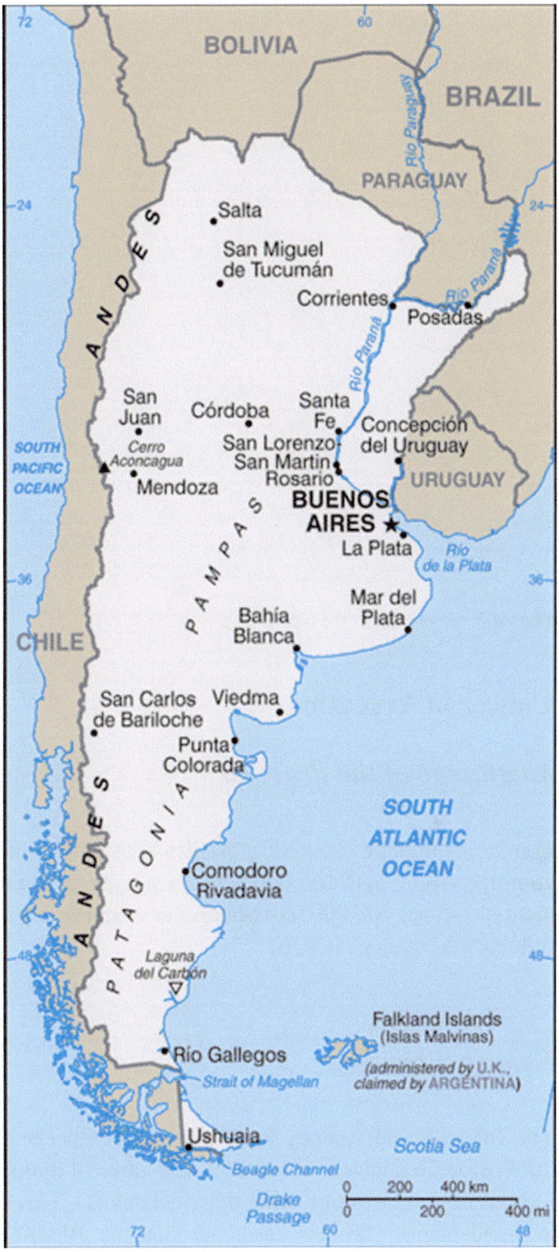

Fig. 24.1 Map of Argentina

The total population (2013) is 41,446,000 inhabitants, with a life expectancy at birth m/f (years, 2012) of 73/79 years (2012). The probability of dying between 15 and 60 years m/f (per 1000 population, 2012) is of 152/84. The total expenditure on health per capita is US$1551 (2012) and the total expenditure on health as % of GDP (2012) is 8.5 % [5].

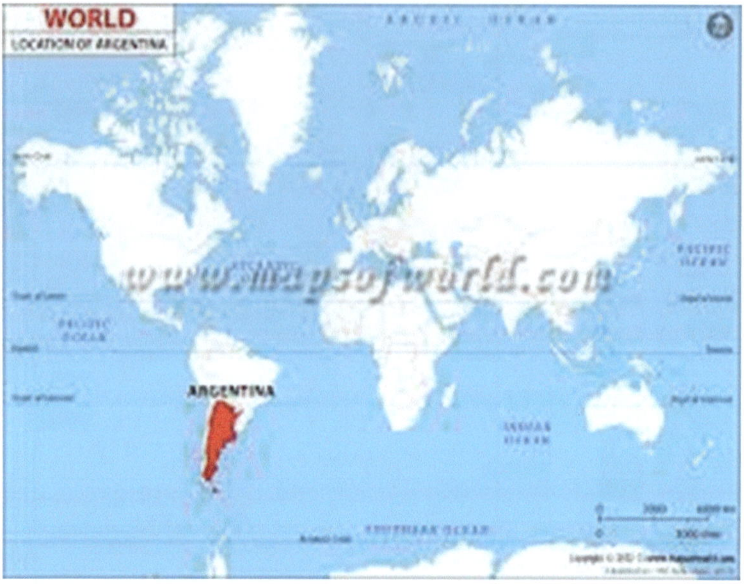

Fig. 24.2 Argentina in the world map

Cancer in Argentina

Magnitude of the Problem

Cancer is the main cause of mortality between 45 and 64 years in the country and comprises more than 100,000 new cases and close to 60,000 deaths per year; equivalent to 145 per 100,000 individuals per year. Poverty and educational level strongly influence mortality rates [6].

Cancer Incidence

The International Agency for Research on Cancer (IARC) has estimated that in 2008 Argentina have had 104,859 new cases of malignant tumors (excluding those located in skin histology other than melanoma). This estimate is for both genders to an incidence of 206 new cases per year per 100,000 population. These estimates determine that, in relation to the rest of the world, Argentina has a medium–high cancer incidence. In magnitude, the larger volume of cases corresponds to breast cancer with more than 18,000 new cases per year (18 % of total), followed by prostate cancer (13,000 cases, 13 %). The incidence of cancer, considering all sites except skin non-melanoma is higher in men. However, the incidence of breast cancer in women is higher than that of prostate cancer in men [7] and Fig. 24.3.

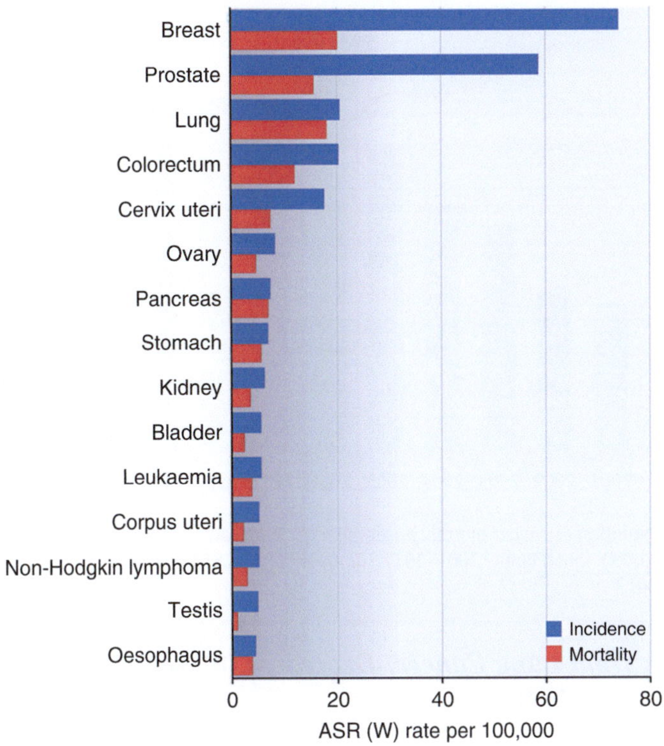

Fig. 24.3 Argentina: estimated age-standardized incidence and mortality rates: both sexes (Globocan 2008-IARC-)

Cancer Mortality

The number of deaths from cancer has increased approximately 9 % in the last decade due to population growth and aging. However, the behavior of mortality was exactly the opposite; Standardized Mortality Rate (SMR) for cancer has decreased 10 %; from 118.82 cases per 100,000 inhabitants in 2001 to 107.49 cases per 100,000 inhabitants in 2011 (Fig. 24.4).

In 2011, cancer killed almost 58,000 men and women in Argentina. The Central region of the country, being the most populated, reported more than 70 % of these deaths. Lung cancer is observed in the first place of importance in all regions. Next, in order of frequency are colorectal cancer and breast cancer, except in South and North-West, where third and fourth are prostate cancer and stomach, respectively. Cervical cancer is registered in tenth place in the country and is among the five leading causes of cancer death in the North-East region [8].

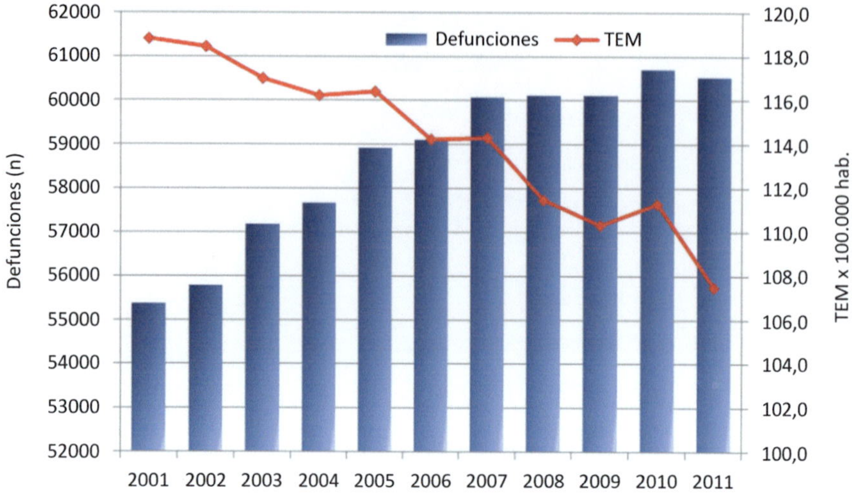

Fig. 24.4 Evolution of cancer mortality—number of deaths and SMR according to world population per 100,000 inhabitants, 2001–2011. *Source*: SIVER/INC according to DEIS database. Argentina, 2013

Mortality from Lung Cancer: Decreased in Men and Increased in Women

In Argentina, lung cancer mortality in men has declined since 1980 at a sustained rate of 1.3 % annually. However, it increased in women—even at a steady pace—of nearly 2 % (Fig. 24.5). In this way, while in 1980 the gap between the genders was 37.7, in 2010 decreased to 19.7 deaths per 100,000 population.

Mortality from Colorectal Cancer: Decreased in Women and Increased in Men

Colorectal cancer mortality decreased in women since 1980 at a sustained rate of 0.8 % annually. However, in men this cancer mortality increased in the period 2002–2010 with an estimated annual change of 1 % (Fig. 24.6).

National Cancer Institute of Argentina

The National Cancer Institute of Argentina (INC) is a body dependent on the Ministry of Health. Created on September 9, 2010 by Presidential Decree 1286, is responsible for the development and implementation of health policies and the

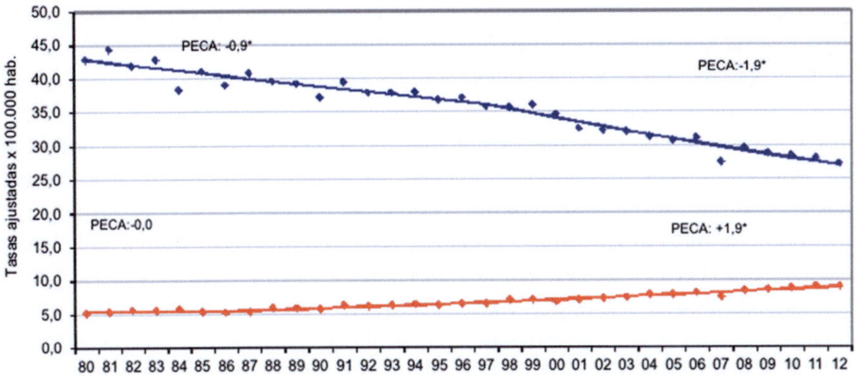

Fig. 24.5 Specific mortality by lung cancer in man (*blue line*) and women (*red line*) standardized rates by age according to the world population per 100,000 inhabitants. Argentina, 1980–2012. *Source*: SIVER/INC–Ministry of Health, based in mortality registries from DEIS-Argentina, 2014

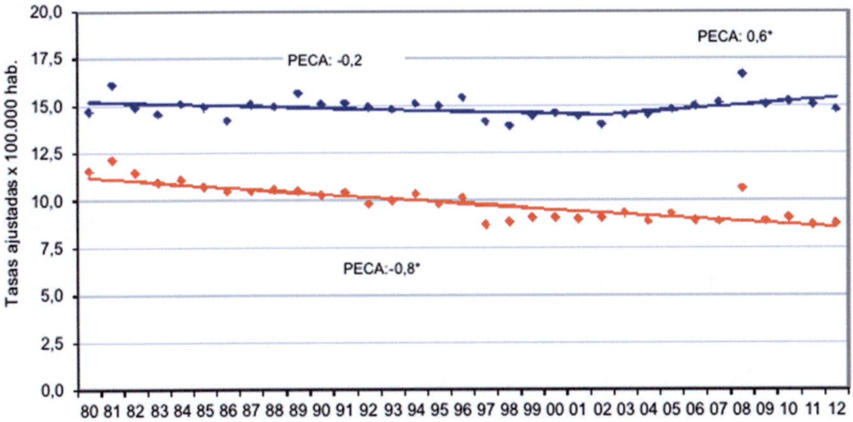

Fig. 24.6 Specific mortality by colorectal cancer in man (*blue line*) and women (*red line*) Standardized rates by age according to the world population per 100,000 inhabitants. Argentina, 1980–2012. *Source*: SIVER/INC–Ministry of Health, based in mortality registries from DEIS-Argentina, 2014

coordination of integrated prevention and cancer control actions. Its main objective is to reduce cancer incidence and mortality in Argentina, as well as improve the quality of life of those affected by the disease.

Among its functions, the INC is responsible for coordinating promotion and prevention of cancer, early detection, treatment, and rehabilitation, as well as cancer research and human resources training in the country. The scope of activities include the development of standards for the comprehensive care of patients with cancer, promoting health and reducing risk factors, defining strategies for prevention and early detection, training of professionals, and the establishment of surveillance systems and epidemiological analysis.

The creation of the INC in Argentina was a decision of great significance in the health agenda of the government, and the main reason was to promote cancer control at the policy level, with the coordination of all actions nationwide, according to the available resources, culturally adapted and taking advantage of the existing resources of the Health System of the country.

Main programs of INC are: National Program for Cervical, Colon, and Breast cancers, together with a National Plan for Familiar and Hereditary Tumors, whose primary mission is "to improve the detection, management and prevention of high-risk groups in the Argentinean population," contributing to the development of a hereditary tumor registry and the national development of a comprehensive network of care. The pediatric area aims to improve the morbidity and mortality of children and adolescents with childhood cancer and their social rehabilitation after specific treatment, through equitable access to quality health care. The Palliative Care program promotes continuous and integrated care for all cancer patients throughout their .disease, with particular emphasis on reducing their suffering and improving their quality of life for patients and families. Getting pain relief and access to opioid medication is an effective reality for all patients in the country, removing barriers to drugs access. The Tobacco Control Program general objective is to promote the production of scientific knowledge for the formulation of public policies planned to protect people from the effects of tobacco and the exposure to smoke snuff.

Fellowships and Educational Workshops .are also part of the activities, together with the Departments of Cancer Research, Epidemiological surveillance, Evaluation of Health Technologies, and Communication and Cancer Registries.

INC maintains continuous .collaboration with national, regional, and international organizations such as the Pan American Health Organization (PAHO), National Cancer Institute-US (NCI-US), IARC, International Atomic Energy Agency (IAEA) through the Program for Action for Cancer Therapy (PACT), the Network of Latin-American Cancer Institutes (RINC), and others [9].

Breast Cancer

National Breast Cancer Program

Breast cancer is a major health problem of Argentine women, since it is the leading cause of cancer deaths in women. Annually, 5400 deaths from this disease and it is estimated that 18,000 new cases occur each year, representing 17.8 % of total cancer incidence in Argentina (Fig. 24.7).

The overall objective of the National Breast Cancer Program is to reduce morbidity and mortality associated with the disease. This program is based on the findings of

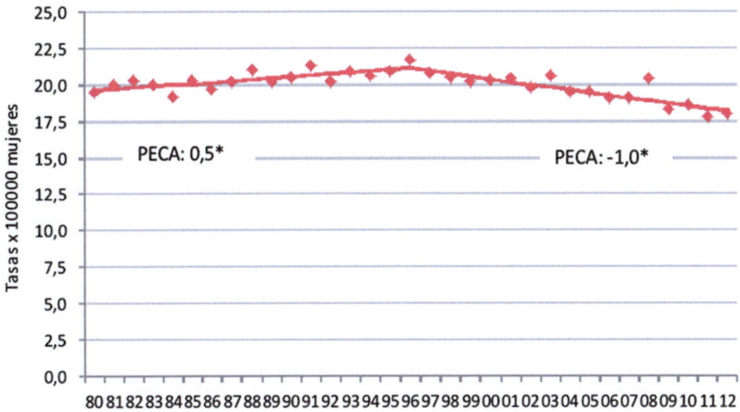

Fig. 24.7 Specific mortality by breast cancer in women (*red line*) standardized rates by age according to the world population per 100,000 inhabitants. Argentina, 1980–2012. *Source*: SIVER/INC–Ministry of Health, based in mortality registries from DEIS-Argentina, 2014

a Situational Diagnosis of the National and Provincial Programs, conducted between 2009 and 2010 in the area of the Secretary for Community Health of the Ministry of Health, with technical and financial support from the PAHO.

Current Actions

The three axes of the National Breast Cancer Program are quality control, coverage, and monitoring.

Quality control procedures imply that the detection, diagnosis, and treatment of women at risk, or with suspected or confirmed cancer, have the required quality services to ensure the best results.

Coverage is the ability of a program to reach people in need. Most of the population knows he has to stay healthy, but not everyone has the same opportunities to do so. In this sense, the program must work towards removing barriers that prevent access to coverage as lack of information, lack of time, overcharging for work, children, dependents, lack of money to get to hospital, and various complications to access the benefits of the health service. During 2012, the program generated social research inputs in order to build an appropriate strategy.

The third axis of the program is the implementation of a monitoring system to provide data on program performance as well as how many mammograms were performed, number of women screened, age of presentation, and how many cancers were diagnosed. This information is essential to achieve quality in mammography studies. Thus, the program has implemented a breast cancer computerized system (SITAM) for data collection and follow-up of the screened population.

The program has also developed manuals, guidelines, educational material for general population, patients, and health care providers as well as a newsletter.

Cervical Cancer

Cervical cancer is an indicator of health inequity. In Argentina, approximately 4000 new cases are diagnosed each year and 1800 women die from the disease. The mortality rate adjusted for age is 7/100,000 women (Fig. 24.8). The burden of disease and mortality varies by province, being higher in populations with lower socioeconomic development. Argentina defined as a priority a comprehensive approach to prevent cervical cancer, with the aim of reducing mortality from the disease, which includes incorporating HPV vaccine for girls 11 years and the strengthening of the prevention strategy through secondary screening based on cytology, and the introduction of the HPV test as a primary screening.

The implementation of actions to control the disease is part of the National Cancer Institute strategy, through the National Program for Cervical Cancer Prevention (PNPCC). Current programs ongoing include:

(a) Implementation of the project to incorporate the HPV test as a primary screening in the province of Jujuy, in conjunction with the PNPCC and the Ministry of Health of the province of Jujuy.
Main activities: workshops in counseling and communication strategy for health teams; refresher training in colposcopy for cervical pathology).specialists; establishing circuits for finding women with positive HPV results and abnormal PAP; development of communication materials for the introduction of the HPV Test.

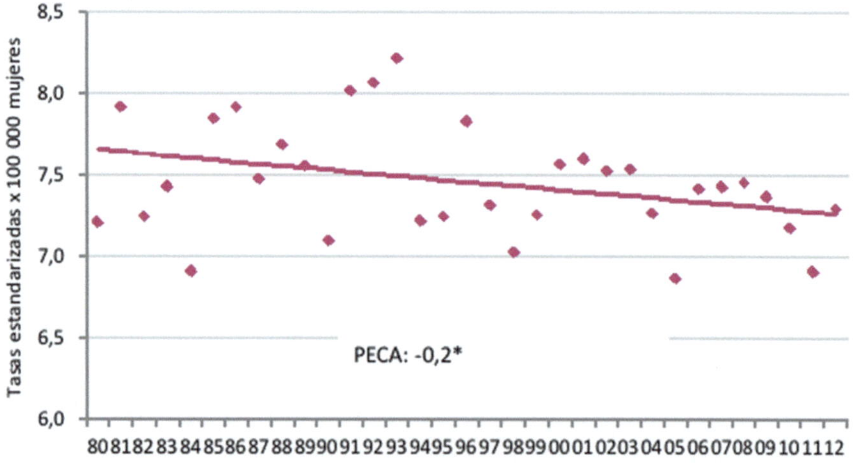

Fig. 24.8 Specific mortality by cervical-uterine cancer in women. Standardized rates by age according to the world population per 100,000 inhabitants. Argentina, 1980–2012. *Source*: SIVER/INC–Ministry of Health, based in mortality registries from DEIS-Argentina, 2014

(b) Development of scientific evidence and technical assistance for incorporating HPV test as primary screening.
Main activities: development of a Manual for the inclusion of the HPV Test; development of a communication strategy based on HPV Test;).activities to support the PNPCC; research development "Welcome, circulation, and assessment of media communications: the HPV test campaign."

(c) EMA Implementation Project (evaluation of self-sampling test mode HPV), in conjunction with the PNPCC, Ministry of Health of the province of Jujuy, and IARC-WHO, in order to assess the performance test by self-sampling method and its effectiveness to increase coverage of screening programs.
Main activities: development of the protocol;).development of communication materials; ongoing training workshops with health workers and primary health care teams involved in the project; monitoring of project development.

(d) Establishing quality criteria for the operation of cytology laboratories.
Main activities: development of quality control for).cytology laboratories; study about the correlation of cytology and histology.

HPV Vaccination

In Argentina, human papillomavirus (HPV) vaccination was approved in 2006, but not included in the National Immunization Program (NIP). In 2008, a mass media campaign was carried out by a cancer Non-Governmental Organization (NGO), but it was stopped due to criticisms about the publicity. In October 2011, the Ministry of Health (MoH) has introduced HPV vaccination in the NIP. It is mandatory and free to all girls, 11 years old and according to data from the NIP the compliance to the vaccine is currently over 90 % [10].

Pediatric Cancer

In the population under 15 years, according to information provided by the Argentine Oncology Pediatric Registry (ROHA), the annual incidence rate in Argentina is about 124 cases per million in children of this age. The cancers most frequently observed in the period 2000–2007 were: leukemia (30–40 %, about 470 cases annually), brain tumors (20 %, about 240 cases annually), and lymphomas (13 %). The chance of survival of these children in developed countries has been increasing to rates of 70 and 80 % due to early diagnosis, proper treatment, and comprehensive care. However, in Argentina the survival of children with cancer is around 65 % due to various conditions, including loss of opportunity for proper diagnosis, lack of timely referral, treatment complications, and in some cases, lack of comprehensive patient care [11].

It is important to underline that all new cases of pediatric cancer are registered at the country level by ROHA. With respect of access to treatment, the best care is available in big cities (Buenos Aires, Cordoba, Santa Fe, and Mendoza). In several provinces or cities that lack of pediatric oncology care, the patients must be transferred to specialized centers in the main cities.

National Plan of Family and Hereditary Tumors

The Hereditary and Family cancers constitute a clear challenge in today's cancer care, as they involve a population exposed to greater risk of cancer that requires to be approached appropriately. This involves the complexity of molecular techniques and requires a multidisciplinary preventive management that covers various aspects of the individual, not only organic but also emotional, social, and cultural.

The National Plan of Family and Hereditary Tumors (PROCAFA) was created in August 2011 in response to a clear need for early detection strategies and integrated management of the high-risk population of cancer in Argentina.

The primary mission of the Plan is to "improve the detection, management and prevention of groups at high risk of cancer in the Argentinean population" contributing to the national development of a comprehensive network of registration and care of family hereditary tumors.

Besides the overall objective, there are also planned specific objectives and main lines of action:

- Identify the epidemiological profile of hereditary cancers in our country
- Train multidisciplinary groups of detection, management, and counseling of high-risk populations in different regions of the country
- Create guidelines and unified algorithms for prevention of high-risk groups, developed through national consensus
- Promote and encourage the implementation at national level of molecular studies of frequent Hereditary Cancer Syndromes, prioritizing rational use of resources and accessibility for patients, both in public and private institutions
- Disseminate the matter in the community and educate about the relevance
- Promote epidemiological analysis and research projects
- Establish collaborative regional networks at South American–Latin American level

Palliative Care

The vision of the Palliative Care Program at the *Instituto Nacional del Cáncer*—INC (National Cancer Institute) is to develop a comprehensive program of palliative care for cancer patients, prioritizing quality of life and symptom relief. Among the values and principles that govern this view is the notion of considering quality of care as a human right in which the patients' beliefs and preferences are preserved.

The mission was defined as the promotion of continuous and integrated care for all cancer patients throughout their disease, with particular emphasis on reducing their suffering and improving their quality of life as well as of their families. Getting support and access to opioid medication and removing barriers to access to these drugs.

General Objectives

To implement a model of assistance for palliative care in the continuum of care of cancer patients, according to their specific needs as well as of their families at every stage of the disease, through various intervention strategies.

Specific Objectives

1. To promote the coordination and joint actions between different levels and resources, in order to improve care and satisfaction of patients, families, and professionals
2. To design networks of care according to the general objective all over the health system
3. To promote a model of interdisciplinary and comprehensive work in response to the needs of the patient and their family, to reduce the impact of the disease in the continuum of care
4. To install the continuous training of health teams involved in the care of cancer patients at different levels
5. To provide families with the knowledge and tools needed to sustain the process of care at home
6. To establish mechanisms to ensure a continuous supply and proper distribution of essential palliative drugs and opioids
7. To implement a system of quality assessment indicators to measure the performance of the different levels of palliative care

The current situation of cancer patients in our country is very different from one another. In the poorest provinces, there is a high proportion of patients with late diagnosis and, consequently, with bad treatment results. Oncology services receive, then, an important proportion of patients in advanced stages of the disease. Although these patients are "incurable," they are "treatable" and present various clinical challenges due to the physical, social, psychological, and spiritual impact the treatment and illness carry out.

Within this context and along with the aging of the population, it is evident that in a few years Argentina will have an aged oncological population that will require caring, attention, and follow-up. These patients will only be taken care of, in a good level of quality if there is a comprehensive and effective integration of oncological centers and palliative care teams within a system of networks at all a level of care.

In this direction is heading INC's Palliative Care Program.

Current Situation of Palliative Care

According to estimates published by WHO in 2011, there had been approximately 54.6 million deaths. Of these, 66 % were due to noncommunicable diseases. Globally, more than 29 million people (29,063,194) died due to diseases that would have been benefited from palliative care [12].

The estimated number of people who need palliative care at the end of life is about 20.4 million at worldwide level. Taking these estimates as a basis, we could say that, globally, approximately 377 people over a population of 100,000 people older than 15 years and 63 children over every 100,000 people younger than 15 years will require palliative care at the end of their lives.

The following map (Fig. 24.9) shows the global distribution of rates of palliative care needs for cancer patients at the end of life, grouped by regions, classified by WHO.

In this kind of grouping, Americas is considered as a whole region (WPR western pacific region). The INC has estimated 65,000 people as the minimum number of cancer patients in need of palliative care nationwide [13].

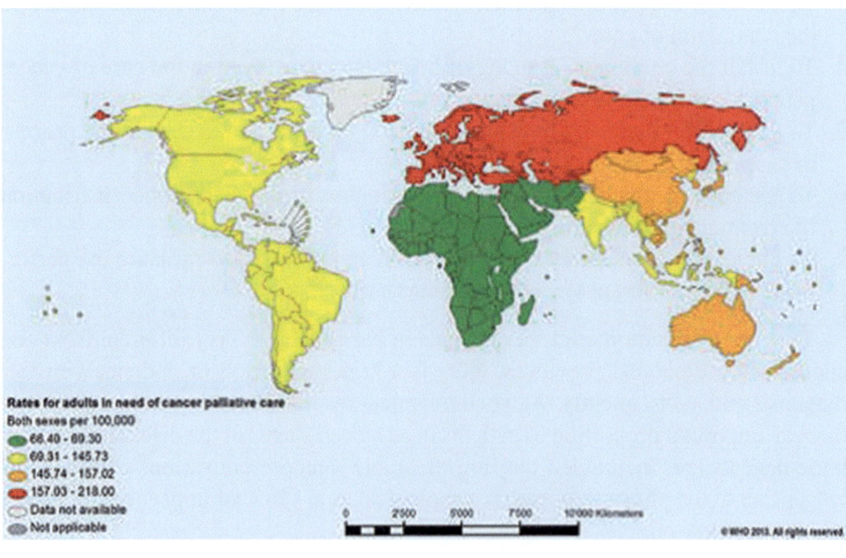

Fig. 24.9 Rates for adults in need of cancer palliative care. *Source*: WPCA

Within this context, Argentina is situated among the countries with intermediate level of Palliative Care development (categorized as 3b in the WPCA map), which means that even though there is a certain level of palliative care development in the country, palliative care teams are not included or even systematically integrated within the national health programs of the country (Fig. 24.10).

As it is shown, the relationship between the number of palliative care services, and the population is 4 times less in Argentina than in the USA or Canada. While the USA/Canada have 1 service every 48,000 inhabitants, Argentina has 1 service every 200,000 [14] inhabitants concentrated mainly in big cities.

However, despite the fact that Argentina does not have a National Program of Palliative Care, it has a significantly better performance than the rest of Latin American countries insofar as:

- Palliative care is guaranteed at PMO level (mandatory medical program) since 2000.
- There are terms of references for palliative care services approved by the Ministry of Health (MoH).
- Is recognized as subspecialty for physicians and pediatricians since 2014 and for nurses since 2012
- There are national standards for treatment of pain (MoH) and handbook specific for palliative care for primary health care (INC).

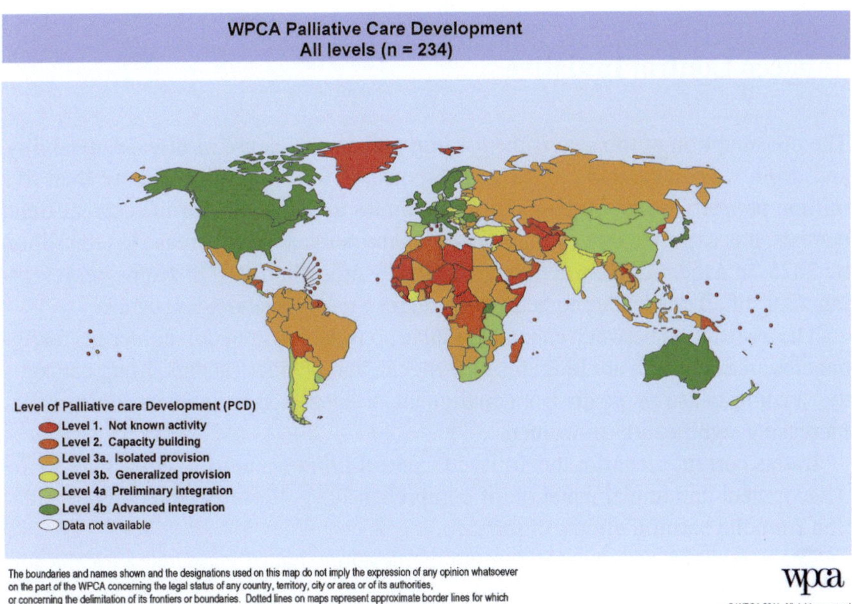

Fig. 24.10 Level of palliative care development. *Source*: WPCA

- There is a public pilot program of opioids production (2014) with free distribution to all patients within public hospitals since 2015 (Palliative Care Program—INC/MoH/ANMAT).
- It is registered an opioid consumption by 2010 (expressed in equivalence of morphine) of 13,068 g/per capita/per year with a tendency towards sustainable growth.
- Argentina has a high availability of opioids which includes all recommended by WHO, but it has accessibility issues especially in the poorest provinces of the country.

Training of Professionals on Palliative Care

Regarding training of professionals, there are postgraduate programs for physicians, nurses, and psychologists through a scholarship system from the INC.

There are also distance education courses such as a Degree in Palliative Care given by NGOs of recognized prestige. A Master on Palliative Care given at Universidad del Salvador and a 2-year long post-basic multidisciplinary residence, organized by the Ministry of Health of the City of Buenos Aires. Undergraduate education on Palliative Care in universities of medicine is still underdeveloped (elective subjects in the last year of Medicine).

Tobacco Control Initiative

The consumption of tobacco is the leading preventable cause of disease, disability, and death worldwide and annually is responsible for the deaths of more than five million people. The tobacco epidemic continues to spread and, if the current trend persists, it is expected that the number of deaths per year will increase to ten million by 2025. In Argentina; tobacco causes annually more than 40,000 deaths, representing 13 % of all deaths due to heart disease, respiratory disease, and cancer.

The association between cancer and tobacco is demonstrated in numerous malignancies among which are lung, oropharyngeal, and bladder cancers. Lung cancer is the leading cause of death from malignant disease in men, and its incidence is increasing significantly in women.

In this current scenario, the Tobacco Control Initiative aims to contribute to the development and implementation of comprehensive policies to protect the population from the harmful effects of tobacco.

The general objective is to promote the development of knowledge for the formulation of public policies to protect the population from the effects of smoking.

The initiative is providing to the community and policy makers numerous reports with information and data on the health and economic impact of the tobacco addiction.

Health System

Argentina's health system is financed by three sectors: public health, social security, and private insurance. A fourth subsystem, known as the National Institute of Social Security and Retirement Fund (INSSJP-PAMI), specifically covers retirees, similar to Medicare in the USA. Although this matrix structure is intended to provide universal coverage, its multiple independent systems lack vertical and horizontal integration, resulting in inadequate coverage for many. In the social security and private systems, health care can be contracted from different sources, some of which own their health care facilities. In the public sector, financing is provided by the provincial or municipal government. The national government has an oversight role, including specific programs to reduce provincial differences. Financing of the public system comes from national and provincial taxes, and coverage is open to all; however, it is mainly used by people who lack any other type of health coverage. It is mandatory for employers to provide health insurance for all workers. Additionally, social insurance is mandatory for all government employees and is usually provided by workers unions. This insurance is funded by employers' contributions and can include copayments. The system includes the National and Provincial Social Security and the INSSJP-PAMI. By contrast, the private system consists of direct contributions and prepayments to medical companies. Both the social security system and private insurance are regulated by the Superintendent of Health Services, reporting to the Ministry of Health, and by the Compulsory Medical Program (PMO). Any resident of Argentina has, according to the law, the right to medical care for catastrophic diseases, including cancer. Funding sources for cancer differ according to the health sector responsible for the patient. If a patient does not have private or social security insurance, the patient's province must cover costs. The national government also has resources to provide coverage for patients, including non-residents, located anywhere in the country. High-cost medications and treatments are covered by a special fund as part of the Special Programs Administration, supported by the Superintendent of Health Services [15].

Costs and Financing of the Health Sector

In 2007, the total health expenditures in Argentina were estimated at 10 % of GDP, which represented a per capita expenditure of approximately US$663. The largest external funding come from loans for projects funded by the Inter-American Development Bank and the World Bank [16].

It is important to mention that cancer costs are included in the total budget of the different subsystems, making very difficult to know the real costs of cancer treatment in the country.

Cancer is a public health problem in Argentina, influenced by poverty and educational levels and is the main cause of mortality between 45 and 64 years in the country. Breast, prostate, colorectal, and lung are the most relevant cancers in the country while cervical cancer has high incidence in the poorest provinces, usually in the north part of Argentina. Pediatric cancers are fully covered by a National Pediatric Cancer registry (ROHA). The National Cancer Institute of Argentina was created in 2010, and it is the governmental body responsible for the development and implementation of health policies in cancer and the coordination of integrated prevention and cancer control actions. HPV vaccination is mandatory since 2011 through the NIP. It is mandatory and free to all girls 11 years old. Argentina's health system is financed by three sectors: public health, social security, and private insurance. A fourth subsystem, known as the National Institute of Social Security and Retirement Fund (INSSJP-PAMI), specifically covers individuals aged 65 and older, younger people with disabilities and war veterans. The system is fragmented and many persons have double or even triple affiliations. In 2007, the total health expenditures in Argentina were estimated at 10 % of GDP, which represented a per capita expenditure of approximately US$663. The specific costs for cancer care are unknown.

Challenges and Achievements in Argentina

It is complex to describe the different challenges and achievements in cancer in Argentina due to several factors which include, between others, variability in the epidemiological picture, regional variations, fragmentation of the health care system, and sociocultural and economic components.

If we consider the case of breast cancer, for example, mean age at diagnosis is close to 35 years old, an older population in comparison with other Latin American countries. In the last years, data obtained from different sources indicate that the mean age of diagnosis is affecting younger populations in our region (Fig. 24.11) Regarding stage at diagnosis early stages are frequent in big cities or main provinces, while in poor regions of the country late diagnosis is a common situation.

The country has not a National Breast Cancer Screening Program, but mammography is quite available around the country. The National Breast Cancer Program of the National cancer Institute includes quality control of mammography and training of technicians.

It is important to mention that the rate mortality/incidence is acceptable and similar to some developed regions of the world (Fig. 24.12).

Due to better information and education, many women are aware about breast and cervical cancer facilitating prevention campaigns. There are also a growing number of breast cancer survivors participating in patients nongovernmental breast cancer organizations.

Recent achievements are the creation in 2010 of the National Cancer Institute of Argentina. It is true that the country has, since 1921, the Roffo Cancer Institute, a prestigious cancer hospital, depending on the University of Buenos Aires but without the necessary governmental support that must have a National Cancer

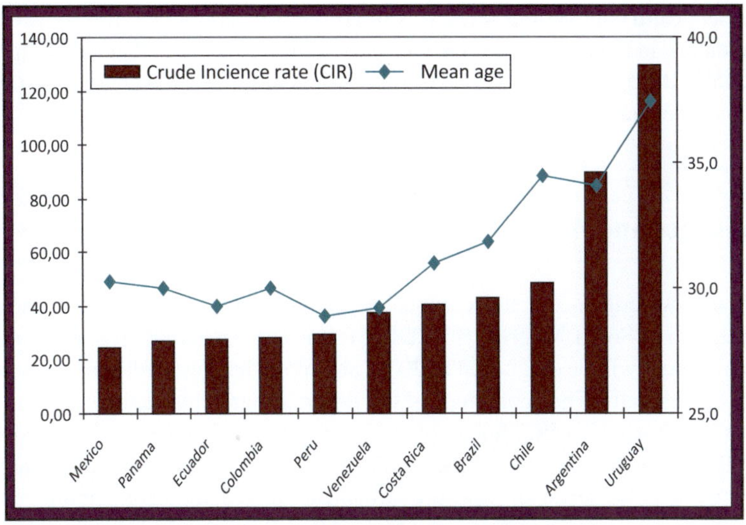

Fig. 24.11 Breast cancer incidence and age in Latin American countries (*Source*: Justo N, Wilking N, Jönsson B, Luciani S, Cazap E. The Oncologist. 2013;18(3):248-56)

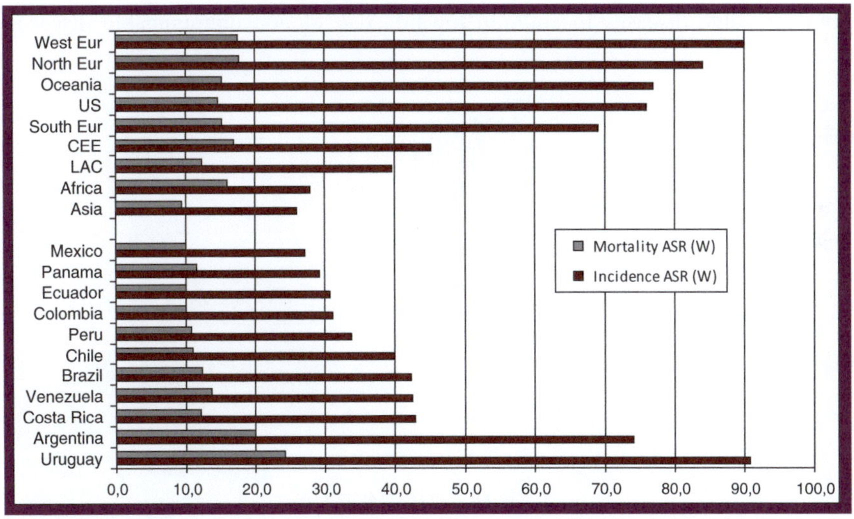

Fig. 24.12 Mortality-to-incidence ratios, world and Latin American countries (*Source*: Justo N, Wilking N, Jönsson B, Luciani S, Cazap E. The Oncologist. 2013;18(3):248-56)

Institute (INC), mainly in the area of public policy and national guidelines. Recently, the IARC from Lyon established the regional Latin-American hub of the Global Initiative for Cancer Registries (GICR) in Buenos Aires, at the National cancer Institute. Another significant achievement has been the participation of INC as founder member of the Network of Latin American Cancer Institutes (RINC).

At the health care system level, it is important to mention that the HPV vaccine is mandatory in the country, for girls 11 years old, for free, and that the compliance to the third dose is over 90 %, due to the success of the implementation within the National Vaccination Program.

Challenges and Achievements in Latin America

The Latin American and the Caribbean region comprise Central America, the Caribbean, and South America (Fig. 24.13). It is estimated that around 1.7 million cases of cancer will be diagnosed in 2030, and more than one million cancer deaths will occur annually. The economies of the region are growing rapidly, and the standard of living is increasing. Such growth is accompanied by increases in sedentary lifestyles, unhealthy dietary habits, smoking, alcohol consumption, environmental carcinogenic pollutants, sun exposure, urbanization, and population aging.

By 2020, it is estimated that more than 100 million people older than 60 years will be living in Latin America and the Caribbean, and that more than half of this group will live beyond 80 years. Worldwide, the contribution of different risk factors to disease burden has changed substantially, with a shift away from risk of communicable diseases in children towards risk of noncommunicable diseases,

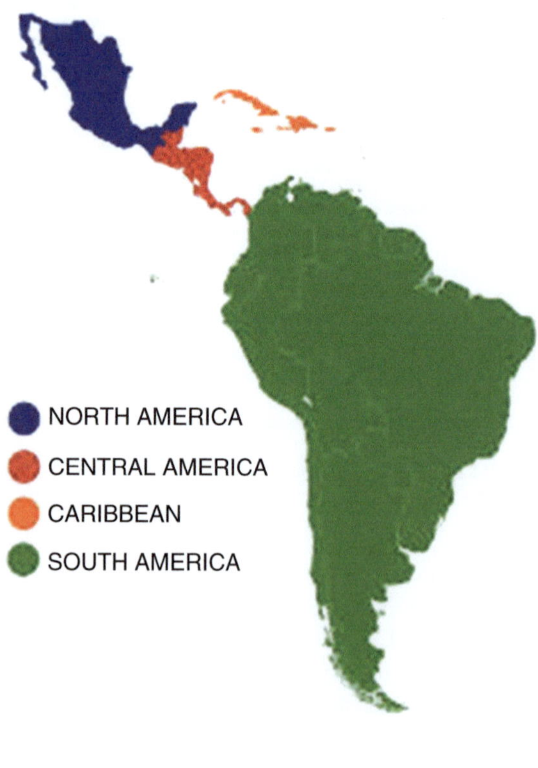

Fig. 24.13 The Latin American region

including an increasing burden of cancer, in adults. In 2010, the leading risk factors for global disease burden were high blood pressure, tobacco smoke (including secondhand smoke), alcohol use, household, air pollution, diets low in fruits and vegetables, and high body-mass index. Apart from household air pollution, these risk factors are the main causes of chronic disease in adults, particularly cardiovascular disease and cancer. For most of Latin America, the leading risk factors for disease are alcohol use and high body-mass index, whereas tobacco smoke is the leading risk factor in North America and Western Europe. A major problem with interpreting these data is that they are generally extrapolated from local hospital or regional databases, and only 6 % of the Latin American population is covered by national cancer registries, by contrast with 96 % in the USA and 32 % in Europe.

Although the overall incidence of cancer is lower in Latin America (age-standardized rate of 163 per 100,000) than in Europe (264 per 100,000) or the USA (300 per 100,000), the mortality burden is greater. This is mainly due to presentation at more advanced stages, and partly related to poorer access to cancer care. In the USA, 60 % of breast cancer cases are diagnosed in the earliest stages, whereas in Brazil only 20 % and in Mexico only 10 % are diagnosed at an early stage. The all-cancer mortality-to-incidence ratio for Latin America is 0:59, compared with 0:43 for the European Union and 0:35 in the USA. All cancer mortality-to-incidence ratios (MIR) also vary within Latin America, from 0:39 in Puerto Rico to 0:65 in Belize, Honduras, and Guatemala. Breast and cervical cancer are the most common cancer types in women in Latin America, and prostate, stomach, and lung cancer are most common in men.

Analyzing the example of breast cancer in the region, in a majority of countries breast cancer mortality is raising and only in Argentina and Uruguay rates seem to be flat but at a high level [17] (Fig. 24.14). It is estimated that these figures will double in 20 years, and also with an increasing economic cost for families and governments.

Breast cancer is the most frequent cancer and kills more women than any other cancer in the region.

Aging is the principal risk factor and, due to demographic transition in the region, will approach epidemic proportions.

The burden of the disease has different shapes. In Peru, Mexico, Colombia, and Brazil, younger age at diagnosis and death deprives societies of numerous productive years; as does the high occurrence of the disease in Argentina and Uruguay.

The economic burden is also relevant, and it can be clearly observed that countries today allocate insufficient resources to tackle the disease. Women go undiagnosed, uncared for or treated with suboptimal therapies; which results in high morbidity with the associated costs for the societies.

Universal health care coverage is still not the rule in the region and, even in those countries where the entitlement to breast health services is guaranteed by law; it is not accompanied by the necessary resources.

There are vast inequities in access to health which translates in unequal results in cancer outcomes.

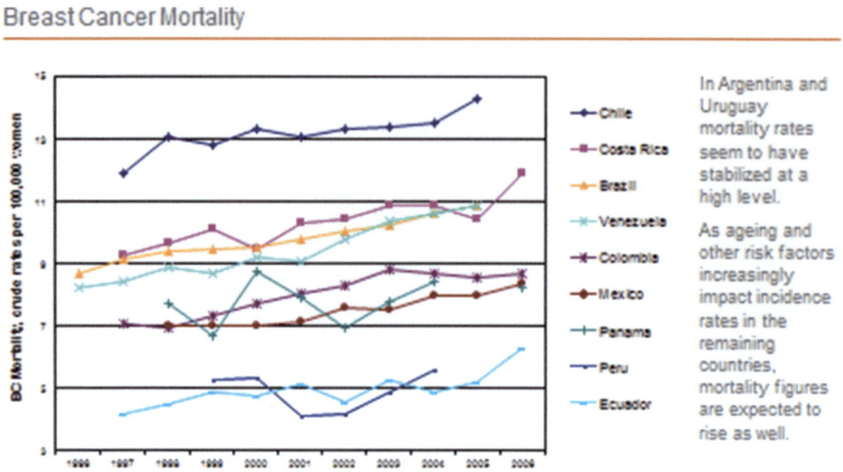

	Number of deaths		DALYs lost	
2004/2008	36 952	Change: 99%	612 816	Change: 38%
2015	57 782		726 480	
2030	73 542		848 665	

OPTUMInsight™ Data sources: PAHO, Mortality Series and WHO The global burden of disease: 2004 Summary Tables. October 2008 update.

Fig. 24.14 Breast cancer mortality in Latin American countries (*Source*: Justo N, Wilking N, Jönsson B, Luciani S, Cazap E. The Oncologist. 2013;18(3):248-56.)

Regrettably, data on survival is scarce and fragmented and what is available shows a wide dispersion across and also within countries. Yet, the evidence signals that only in a few countries 5-year survival surpasses 70 %.

Breast cancer outcomes have improved during the last decade, as evidenced by comparison of the MIR between 2002 and 2008. Costa Rica is the country where most progress is seen, while Brazil, Mexico, and Panama have not been able to significantly improve MIR ratio over the past years (Fig. 24.15).

The reduced survival is partly due to the fact that around 30–40 % of patients are only diagnosed in metastatic phases III and IV while in Europe late diagnosis is only 10 % of the cases.

Nowadays, the majority of cases are detected when women seek care following symptoms onset. Initiatives to increase the awareness are very important so that women are attentive and do not postpone seeking care until the symptoms have reached a critical stage.

One big challenge is how to develop better and more effective prevention strategies. It is difficult to apply a one-suit-all prevention strategy for the region given the outstanding epidemiological contrasts in terms of disease occurrence, risks, and available resources both across and within countries.

It is true that population-based mammography has been shown to improve outcomes as it leads to a larger share of breast cancers being diagnosed at an early stage

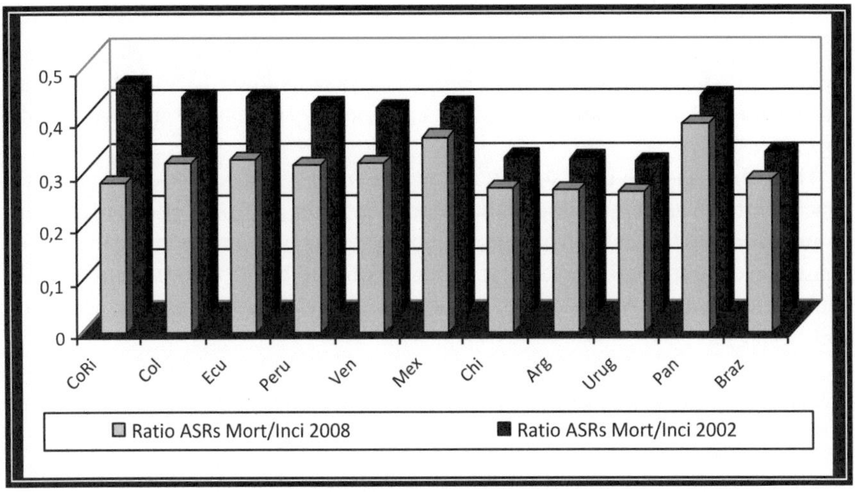

Fig. 24.15 Mortality-to-incidence ratios in breast cancer in the Latin American region (*Source*: Justo N, Wilking N, Jönsson B, Luciani S, Cazap E. The Oncologist. 2013;18(3):248-56)

but in some countries with limited resources and low incidence, the best screening strategies differ. In poor countries awareness, clinical examination and breast self-examination may provide better outcomes trough down-staging of the disease. Since affordability remains a limiting factor in the region, recommendations from the Breast Health Global Initiative (BHGI) and World Health Organization (WHO) highlight the role of prevention but contemplating several additional measures like health education, behavior modification, breast self-awareness, and clinical breast examination.

It is recognized that most LAC countries count with medical care standards but, the challenge in the region is to implement policies and control mechanisms to ensure compliance and their applicability to the whole population.

National Cancer Control Plans (NCCP) are the fundamental building blocks to an organized governance, financing, and health delivery of cancer. There is a marked absence of NCCP in countries of the region, so deviating from 2005 World Health Assembly resolutions.

A recent initiative ongoing in the region is the International Cancer Control Partnership, a group of international organizations engaged in cancer control planning efforts and leaded by the NCI-US. The group is seeking to create synergies in a united approach to maximize collective resources and efforts to support NCCP development, implementation, and evaluation; and several Latin-American organizations are part of the project [18].

Complementing health care systems and governments, Latin American patient groups realize an important task, there where systems cannot or do not sufficiently assist cancer patients. Additionally, it is also necessary to mention that faulty patient information services and governmental failure to include them in policy-decision making need further improvements.

Our vision on the future on cancer care in the region is optimistic. Latin America is well organized with institutes and networks working together, several governments are taking the lead in promoting diverse actions towards better cancer care and health systems, despite their fragmentation, are promoting universal health coverage.

The public and the civil society as a whole are now more conscious about the cancer problem and requesting to the authorities better and more effective actions.

In addition to this, human and economic development is improving so the natural consequence of this will be better and more organized health care systems with the natural consequence of less cancer incidence (mainly of late stages) and better curability and survival.

Acknowledgement The author would like to thank Dr. Graciela Jakob for her contribution in the topic of Palliative Care.

References

1. Farmer F, Frenk J, Knaul FM, et al. Expansion of cancer care and control in countries of low and middle income: a call to action. Lancet. 2010;376:1186–93.
2. http://www.who.int/nmh/events/un_ncd_summit2011/en/
3. Baroness Jenkin. Non-communicable diseases in the developing world. Cancer Control 2014, INCTR.
4. Cazap E, Magrath I, Kingham P, Elzawawy A. Structural barriers to diagnosis and treatment of cancer in low-middle income countries (LMIC's). The urgent need of scaling-up. J Clin Oncol. 2015 (in press).
5. http://www.who.int/countries/arg/en/
6. http://www.msal.gov.ar/inc/index.php/acerca-del-cancer/estadisticas
7. http://globocan.iarc.fr
8. Abriata G. Análisis de Situación en Salud—ASIS-Cáncer en Argentina. 2011.
9. http://www.msal.gov.ar/inc/
10. Arrossi S, Maceira V, Paolino M, Sankaranarayanan R. Acceptability and uptake of HPV vaccine in Argentina before its inclusion in the immunization program: a population-based survey. Vaccine. 2012;30(14):2467–74.
11. http://www.msal.gov.ar/inc/index.php/investigacion-y-epidemiologia/registro-/roha
12. Global Atlas of palliative care at the end of life. Worldwide Palliative Care Alliance. 2014. http://www.who.int/nmh/Global_Atlas_of_Palliative_Care.pdf
13. Updated data based on own elaboration upon data taken from the Atlas de CuidadosPaliativos en Latinoamérica—ALCP. http://cuidadospaliativos.org/uploads/2013/12/Atlas%20of%20Palliative%20Care%20in%20Latin%20America.pdf
14. Diagnóstico Epidemiológico y Situación de los Cuidados Paliativos en la Argentina INC. Draft doc. from INC Palliative Care Program. 2015.
15. Goss PE, et al. Planning cancer control in Latin America and the Caribbean. Lancet Oncol. 2013;14(5):391–436.
16. Report of World Health Statistics, World Health Organization (WHO). 2010.
17. Justo N, Wilking N, Jönsson B, Luciani S, Cazap E. A review of breast cancer care and outcomes in Latin America. Oncologist. 2013;18(3):248–56.
18. http://www.iccp-portal.org/

Chapter 25
Caring for Refugees with Cancer: A Case for Training of US Oncology Professionals

Lidia Schapira

Introduction

It is sobering to reflect on our individual and collective responsibilities towards immigrant patients who, having already suffered so greatly due to war and subsequent displacement, must then confront a diagnosis of cancer. The United States has always been a country of immigrants, and from its early history through present day, it has provided a safe haven for war refugees, from individuals seeking asylum to children fleeing violence and gang warfare. Unfortunately, however, medical care for refugees and asylum seekers is distributed across a variety of healthcare systems and networks across the country, without standard protocols or national guidelines, and referrals for specialist care, including oncology and palliative care services, are typically provided by generalist clinicians working in primary care settings or neighborhood clinics. Specialists have expertise in their respective fields, but typically no training at all in meeting the complex physical and psychological needs of this vulnerable population. Ultimately, clinicians have no developed, structured framework with which to address the multiple needs of these patient populations who have suffered such a wide range of atrocities. The psychological repercussions of their experiences have long-term effects on their mental health, and it is imperative that clinicians handle the emotional, as well as physiological, needs of these patients with sensitivity and care. Furthermore, given the multitude of language and cultural barriers between Western trained clinicians and immigrant patient populations, the challenge remains to provide personalized care that is both culturally attuned and clinically beneficial, and addressing this challenge will require partnerships with professional interpreters and social workers who are trained to meet these needs.

L. Schapira, M.D. (✉)
Department of Medicine, Massachusetts General Hospital,
Harvard Medical School, 55 Fruit St., Boston, MA 02114, USA
e-mail: lschapira@partners.org

M. Silbermann (ed.), *Cancer Care in Countries and Societies in Transition*,
DOI 10.1007/978-3-319-22912-6_25

Growing Interest in Global Health

American physicians have a long history of involvement in global health, serving on volunteer missions and performing complex surgeries in poor countries or providing primary care, acting as consultants to offer remote opinions on complex cases, or through committed service to help build capacity in countries with limited resources. In 2002, the number of cancer deaths worldwide was estimated at 6.2 million, 55 % in the developing world [1]. In 2013 the number rose to 13 million, 69 % in developing world [1]. In 2011, the United Nations recognized noncommunicable diseases such as cancer as problems that concern the global community. In response to the UN call for action, the National Cancer Institute (NCI) established the Center for Global Health [2]. This agency was created to help coordinate the global portfolio and support the open exchange of scientific and clinical knowledge, and to provide a framework to encourage bilateral cooperation in addressing issues and problems in public health, medicine, science, and cancer research. There are several NCI designated Cancer Centers with an active presence in Africa, among them the Fred Hutchinson Cancer Center and its program in Uganda, the University of North Carolina's program in Malawi, the University of Maryland's program in Nigeria, the University of Michigan's program in Ghana, Indiana University's program in Kenya, and Harvard's programs in Botswana, Rwanda, and Haiti (the last two in collaboration with Partners in Health).

Although these programs have different priorities, they share a common goal of establishing cancer control programs that address the fundamental needs of their respective partner countries. Each of these programs has ties to local governments and institutional support in the United States. They focus on prevention, public education campaigns to raise awareness of cancer, establishing databases, and the provision of clinical services for patients with cancer, ranging from anticancer therapy to palliative measures. US oncologists involved in global work are currently confronting the morally complex issue of how best to advise physicians and governments in areas with high prevalence of cancer but without the infrastructure, trained personnel, and medications needed to meet the needs of all patients [3]. Among US oncologists involved in global health, there is a growing sense of urgency to step up national efforts to help reduce global disparities in outcomes for patients with cancer and attend to the suffering of those afflicted with the disease.

A Country of Immigrants

In the United States, 57 million people, 20 % of the US population, speak a language other than English at home. Approximately 25 million people, 8.6 % of the US population, are defined as having low English proficiency, or LEP, and a considerable number of those with LEP have low literacy in their native languages as well [4, 5]. Together, these factors place this population at a distinct disadvantage when seeking medical assistance. Immigrants with LEP are at risk for longer hospital stays and readmissions after discharge simply because they did not properly understand instructions, and they are also at greater risk for infections and falls during hospitalizations [6, 7]. Immigrants and Americans from ethnic minorities diagnosed with cancer have poorer outcomes than comparable nonimmigrant groups, with lower screening and survival rates, more adverse effects, poorer quality of life, and greater distress due to multiple factors including barriers to care and misunderstandings [8–11].

The safety and welfare of patients with low English proficiency depends on the availability of trained interpreters, and consequently, medical interpreters are fast becoming key members of clinical care teams [12]. Some are born overseas and are native speakers of the languages for which they interpret, others were raised in bilingual households, and still others are English speakers who acquired a second language while studying or working abroad [13]. However, despite the growing need for medical interpreters, many healthcare institutions across the United States still lack formal interpreter services and, as a result, rely on informal interpreters such as nonclinical staff, relatives, and friends of the patient. Research suggests that using ad hoc interpreters—as opposed to professional interpreters—can lead to an increase in clinically consequential errors [5, 14]. To complicate matters, medical interpretation remains an unregulated industry, without nationally recognized professional standards. There is no accepted curriculum for interpreter training, no recognized certification at a national level and no single model that defines and demarcates the interpreter's role [13, 15].

Multiple metaphors have been used to characterize the ideal role of the medical interpreter, from conduit to detective, illustrating the range of opinion as to the appropriate extent of the interpreter's involvement in the clinical triad [13]. Some institutions expect professionals to play a strictly technical role, emphasizing the need for accuracy, restraint from additions, editions, and omissions, and, most important, neutrality [13]. At Massachusetts General Hospital, in addition to having trained medical interpreters, each inpatient care unit houses a mobile interpreter phone, which can be rolled into a patient's room and hooked up to a wall jack to provide telephonic interpretation on demand in any language. Some hospitals provide patients with an "interpreter requested card" in their language and in English that can be used throughout the care process to notify clinicians and other staff that the patient requires an interpreter. This strategy visually reminds staff of the patient's LEP status and helps encourage patients to participate in their own care. Other models and healthcare institutions lean towards a co-constructive dimension of the interpreter role that emphasizes the need to understand not only the linguistic content, but also the cultural context [13]. Programs dedicated to caring for refugees typically favor a model that extends the role of the interpreter beyond that of a language and cultural broker, adding a third component of advocacy. Examples of advocacy might involve speaking up when a patient appears not to have understood an explanation, escorting patients to their appointments and tests, making phone calls on the patient's behalf, or engaging in community level activities to raise awareness of cancer-screening services.

The Role of the Medical Interpreter

Medical interpreters have expressed the view that they are not always allowed to provide context or meaning and are sometimes marginalized as a consequence [16]. Interpreters are also sensitive to relationships and power dynamics in clinical settings. They may perceive a clinician as brusque and disinterested, or pick up on time pressures requiring doctors to rush through the interview, basically quizzing or interrogating the patient without allowing sufficient time to explore their answers or concerns.

A Thai interpreter shares a patient's narrative outside the exam room after she was told to not eat rice. The order provokes the opposite of the clinician's intent:

> *... You have to understand, they were surviving through war, lots of family members, where they have nothing, ... but for you to say "don't eat rice," it's almost like telling them, hey, I'm going to cut one of your arms off ... "wow,* [patients will say] *I lived off from nothing for me to be here to have food! food! food!; and now you want to tell me I can't eat this?... no, I'm going to eat before I'm going to die!!"* [16].

This rapid fire exchange requires the interpreter to think very quickly about how to present concepts in a way that will allow the listener in either direction to better understand the meaning and intent of the speaker and calls for a three-way relationship of trust, interest, and respect.

Clinicians are growing more familiar with the professional interpreter role. Some remain disdainful of patients with limited English proficiency but, on the whole, physicians are more cognizant of the need to involve trained interpreters to minimize errors, to promote clarity, and to engage patients and families in decision-making regarding cancer treatment. Oncologists are sometimes frustrated by the interpreter's lack of knowledge of basic terms and expressions used commonly in cancer medicine, and are sometimes reminded by interpreters that there are actually no words in the native language that describe the concept the doctor seems keen to discuss. Programs designed to increase the interpreter's knowledge of basic cancer terminology and to train cancer clinicians to work collaboratively with interpreters are sorely needed [12, 17].

Oncologists need to bear in mind that even professional interpreters can make mistakes that have direct clinical consequences. Butow and colleagues analyzed audiotapes of oncology consultations mediated by both ad hoc and professional interpreters [14]. They found multiple types of errors, ranging from (1) the interpreter either omitted, corrected, or editorialized the information, (2) the message was simplified in order to reduce the emotional impact on the patient, (3) the interpreter introduced more or less certainty than what was conveyed in the original message, (4) the interpreter used euphemisms, (5) the interpreter appeared more authoritative or paternalistic than the oncologist, and (6) the interpreter simply provided misinformation. These errors occurred more frequently when family or ad hoc interpreters translated than when professional interpreters were involved [14].

A particularly difficult situation for oncologists occurs when a patient refuses to have a professional interpreter, citing concerns about confidentiality. This typically occurs when a community of immigrants is rather small and all members know each other socially, and the interpreter belongs to that particular community. In such cases, patients may prefer to rely on family members, such as an adult child who is more fully acculturated than the patient and a fluent bilingual speaker. The trusted family member may have little or no medical knowledge and will likely feel personally involved and may wish to protect the patient or insert his or her point of view. If the patient then seeks an appointment without allowing for a professional interpreter and the relative cannot accompany him or her, the patient and clinician may easily misunderstand each other, which can have meaningful repercussions for the patient's care.

Refugees with Cancer

The United Nations High Commissioner for Refugees [18] defines a refugee as someone who has been forced to flee his or her country because of persecution, war, or violence [19]. Most refugees cannot or will not return to their countries of origin. The UNHCR also reported that in 2012, 45 million people were forcibly displaced worldwide as a result of persecution, conflict, violence, and human rights violations, the highest number since 1994. This figure includes ten million refugees, and half of these are women and children [18]. The major source countries of refugees were Afghanistan, Somalia, Iraq, Syria, Sudan, Democratic Republic of Congo, Myanmar, Colombia, Vietnam, and Eritrea. The major refugee hosting countries were Pakistan, Islamic Republic of Iran, Germany, Kenya, Syria, Ethiopia, Chad, Jordan, China, and Turkey [18, 19].

In a scholarly review, Spiegel notes there is little epidemiological data about the impact of war and displacement on the outcomes of cancer treatment [20]. Studies of cancer have not been undertaken in many countries affected by humanitarian emergencies, even before conflict. In many locations where there are refugees, there are few data for cancer surveillance, cancer registries, or cancer patterns and outcomes in populations at risk. Spiegel identified six peer-reviewed articles published between 1993 and 2013 of cancer diagnoses in refugees. These presented limited data for cancer in Afghan, Tibetan, and Iraqi refugees [20]. Countries in the Middle East have welcomed, and continue to welcome, millions of refugees, first Iraqis and now Syrians, but this massive influx of refugees to these countries has stressed their national health systems at all levels, particularly tertiary care in the public sector. For example, in 2013, the Jordanian Ministry of Health spent an estimated $53 million on care for refugees from January to April. Even in the private sector, some treatments, diagnostic equipment, and medical technologies might be insufficient [20].

Since 1975, the United States has resettled more than three million refugees. The technical difference between a refugee and asylum seeker relates to the timing and location of the application to resettle in the United States. Refugees apply for processing in other countries before reaching the United States. Asylum seekers apply for processing in the United States after they have entered the country or are at the border. Torture survivors are allowed to arrive under forms of immigration status that were necessary to get out of the country (i.e., visitor's visa) and later apply for political asylum once they are safe in the United States. The distinction between refugees and asylum seekers is critical to understand, given the implications for healthcare: asylum seekers may be undocumented and ineligible for public benefits including health insurance, housing, and food stamps. Once asylum is granted to asylum seekers, they are afforded the same protection and benefits as refugees. From a clinical perspective, asylum seekers may have lived in the host country for a prolonged period prior to seeking any medical care, whereas refugees arriving through the resettlement program are referred for screening shortly after arrival. In 2012, 62,000 refugees and 40,000 asylum seekers were admitted to the United States. The countries of origin for refugees were Bhutan, Myanmar, Cuba, Iraq, Democratic Republic of Congo, Iran, Eritrea, Sudan, and Ethiopia. Refugee demographics vary from year to year [19] and annual statistics for refugee numbers are available at the UNHCR website.

The Boston Center for Refugee Health and Human Rights (BCRHHR) provides healthcare coordinated with social services and legal aid for asylum seekers, refugees, survivors of torture, and their families [21]. BCRHHR provides direct assistance as well as training for professionals who are caring for these patients, while at the same time sponsoring research with the ultimate goal of improving the quality of life for survivors of torture and their communities [21]. In 2012, this agency assisted 446 persons, the majority (83.6 %) from Africa, the rest from the Middle East, Eastern Europe, Asia, Latin America, and the Caribbean. More than 80 % of those served had a personal or family history of torture, defined as an assault of a person's mind, body, and sense of security that may cause lasting effects [19, 21]. Among the different forms are blunt trauma, penetrating injuries, burns, asphyxiation, electric shocks, forced human experimentation, extreme physical conditions, and sexual and mental torture [19]. National estimates of the prevalence of torture among refugees vary widely, estimated to be around 36 % among Somalis resettling in Minneapolis-St. Paul, Minnesota, and 55 % among the Oromo in the same area. Rape is increasingly being used as a weapon during times of conflict to cause fear, shame, and demoralization of victims as well as members of the community [19]. The prevalence of sexual violence is difficult to document nationally and internationally. The BCRHHR estimates that for the year 2012, about 44 % of females and 12 % of males were victims of sexual violence. Sexual and gender-based violence, a global problem, affects children and adults of both sexes and may have serious consequences on sexual, reproductive, physical, and psychological health that only become apparent months or years after the assault [21]. Civilians who fled war torn areas may have witnessed murder or rape of members of their own families or communities, also with lasting psychological consequences.

These data demonstrate that refugees have often been exposed to various traumatic events that leave permanent marks on their physical and emotional health. Their prior experience of displacement, humiliation, torture, or violence may affect the way they relate to medical professionals and their ability to tolerate procedures that rekindle fears and feelings of vulnerability.

From Routine Follow-up to End-of-Life Care

Clinicians working with refugees face the challenge of attempting to engage with patients who may be distrustful of those in positions of power, or who may have suffered from trauma inflicted by physicians. Inviting the patient to tell his or her story of emigration and trauma can help the clinician to formulate a differential diagnosis that may assist in explaining symptoms and helps to build trust [19]. Sadly, in the experience at the BCRHHR, 85 % of refugees and asylum seekers who had a primary care physician and 60 % who had contact with some healthcare professional were *never asked about human rights abuses* [21] One study found that when physicians did not ask about trauma, refugee patients did not believe it appropriate to initiate conversations about their experiences [22]. Physical trauma goes hand in hand with psychological trauma, so it is not surprising that an estimated 30 % of refugees meet the diagnostic criteria for post-traumatic stress disorder (PTSD) and another 30 % for depression.

Academic teaching hospitals serving the greater Boston area have established neighborhood clinics in areas serving impoverished and immigrant populations. At the Chelsea Healthcare Center, an affiliate of the Massachusetts General Hospital, clinical teams typically meet 10 new refugees and 50 new immigrants every month. A number of these patients are functionally illiterate and harbor deep fears associated with the diagnosis of cancer. Many have never seen a mammography machine and require an escort—a community health worker who also serves as interpreter—in order to complete the most basic examinations. Clinicians recall a case of an Iraqi woman with grown children who insisted on interpreting for her, and ensured that all communication was conducted with the patient's husband and male children. The medical team was not allowed to converse directly with the patient and the doctor could not build rapport. This became problematic when the patient missed two appointments for her annual mammogram, and returned to clinic only when she palpated a lump in her breast.

At the Chelsea clinic, the most common cancer is breast cancer among Iraqi women. Many received their cancer treatment in Iraq or in the country to which they first fled, and now require longitudinal follow-up. Primary care physicians recount that many of these women worry constantly about a recurrence and cope poorly with uncertainty. They may present to clinic with multiple somatic complaints that require investigation. Some are hypervigilant and very scared of physical sensations that remain unexplained. These patients require frequent visits and consistency with staff and are encouraged to build relationships with all the staff working in the clinic to make them feel at ease and welcome. They are often reluctant to accept referrals for mental health assessments and treatment, fearing the stigma attached to mental illness.

It is unusual for a refugee or asylum seeker to present directly to a hospital emergency department and when this occurs, it typically leaves the staff unprepared to handle all aspects of care. One recent example was that of a patient who presented with swelling of her left arm to the emergency room of the Massachusetts General Hospital. The cause of her massive arm swelling was discovered during her exam when she was found to have a mass in her left breast. Her cancer had also metastasized to the brain and her care required a multidisciplinary cancer care team. Although the medical aspects were relatively straightforward, the clinical team was unprepared to meet her complex social and legal needs. The team learned the patient had fled her war torn country and was seeking asylum, without the financial resources to secure a lawyer. With the help of free legal services from Harvard Law School, the patient was able to obtain her legal residence and her family able to visit and provide care and support. This case was quite dramatic and the patient's needs required a very dedicated and specialized team. More frequently, oncologists are asked to intervene on an immigrant patient's behalf in order to prevent deportation or to request visas for family caregivers.

Conclusion

Refugees and asylum seekers face cultural, language, literacy, and economic barriers that may result in negative experiences with the healthcare system and may interfere with the provision of state-of-the-art care. Refugee medicine is an emerging area of specialty care that is mostly confined to academic centers, but refugees are settling and resettling across the country. Oncologists typically have no training for addressing the complex social and psychological needs of this vulnerable population, and specialty clinics and practices are ill equipped to tackle these challenges. For oncologists, the major challenge remains the mental health problems, ranging from post-traumatic stress to depression, that add another level of complexity to treatment plans for patients with both early stage and advanced cancer. Ultimately, efforts to improve the health of refugees and asylum seekers who require specialty care must involve community health workers and interpreters, who can escort and advocate for these patients and shed light on how their life experiences impact on their preferences for care, in order to improve healthcare outcomes for these largely undeserved populations.

References

1. GLOBOCAN. http://globocan.iarc.fr/Pages/fact_sheets_cancer.aspx. Accessed 10 Jan 2015.
2. NCI Center for Global Health. http://www.cancer.gov/aboutnci/organization/global-health. Accessed 10 Jan 2015.
3. Shulman LN, Mpunga T, Tapela N, et al. Bringing cancer care to the poor: experiences from Rwanda. Nat Rev Cancer. 2014;14:815–21.
4. Divi C, Koss RG, Schmaltz P, et al. Language proficiency and adverse events in US hospitals: a pilot study. Int J Qual Health Care. 2007;19(2):60–7.
5. Flores G, Ngui E. Racial/ethnic disparities and patient safety. Pediatr Clin North Am. 2006; 53(6):1197–215.
6. Jiang HJ, Andrews R, Stryer D, Friedman B. Racial/ethnic disparities in potentially preventable readmissions: the case of diabetes. Am J Public Health. 2005;95(9):1561–7.

7. Elixhauser A, Weinick RM, Betancourt JR, Andrews RM. Differences between Hispanics and non-Hispanic whites in use of hospital procedures for cerebrovascular disease. Ethn Dis. 2002;12(1):29–37.
8. Gordon HS, Street Jr RL, Sharf BF, Kelly PA, Souchek J. Racial differences in trust and lung cancer patients' perceptions of physician communication. J Clin Oncol. 2006;24(6):904–9.
9. Bach PB, Cramer LD, Warren JL, Begg CB. Racial differences in the treatment of early-stage lung cancer. N Engl J Med. 1999;341(16):1198–205.
10. Chan A, Woodruff RK. Comparison of palliative care needs of English- and non-English-speaking patients. J Palliat Care. 1999;15(1):26–30.
11. Greenstein AJ, Litle VR, Swanson SJ, Divino CM, Packer S, McGinn TG, et al. Racial disparities in esophageal cancer treatment and outcomes. Ann Surg Oncol. 2008;15(3):881–8.
12. Schapira L, Vargas E, Hidalgo R, Brier M, Sanchez L, Hobrecker K, et al. Lost in translation: integrating medical interpreters into the multidisciplinary team. Oncologist. 2008;13(5): 586–92.
13. Willen S. Pas de Trois: medical interpreters, clinical dilemmas, and the patient-provider-interpreter triad. In: Mary-Jo Delvecchio G et al., editors. Shattering culture: American medicine responds to cultural diversity. New York: Russell Sage; 2011.
14. Butow PN, Goldstein D, Bell ML, Sze M, Aldridge LJ, Abdo S, et al. Interpretation in consultations with immigrant patients with cancer: how accurate is it? J Clin Oncol. 2011;29(20):2801–7.
15. Medical interpreting standards of practice. International Medical Interpreters Association & Education Development Center. 2007. http://www.imiaweb.org/uploads/pages/102.pdf. Accessed 10 Jan 2015.
16. Wahl E. Paper presented at the American Anthropological Association Annual Meeting. 2014. Personal communication.
17. Donelan K, Hobrecker K, Schapira L, et al. Medical interpreter knowledge of cancer and cancer clinical trials. Cancer. 2009;115(14):3283–92.
18. United Nations High Commissioner for Refugees. Convention and protocol relating to the status of refugees. http://www.unhcr.org. Accessed 10 Jan 2015.
19. Crosby S. Primary care management of non-English-speaking refugees who have experienced trauma. A clinical review. JAMA. 2013;310:519–27.
20. Spiegel PB, Checchi F, Colombo S, et al. Health-care needs of people affected by conflict: future trends and changing frameworks. Lancet. 2010;375:342–5.
21. The Boston Center for Refugee Health and Human Rights (BCRHHR). http://www.bcrhhr.org/. Accessed 10 Jan 2015.
22. Shannon PJ, Wieling E, McCleary JS, et al. Exploring the mental health effects of political trauma with newly arrived refugees. Qual Health Res. 2014;2:1–15.

Chapter 26
University of Texas MD Anderson Cancer Center Experience Caring for Patients from Countries Undergoing Political–Social Conflict

Daniel E. Epner and Kathleen M. Schmeler

Brief Overview of the Current Status of Cancer Care in the USA

Cancer care in the USA is highly technologically advanced. Personalized cancer care using molecular diagnostics to guide therapy is now the standard for patients with hematological malignancies, such as lymphoma and leukemia, as well as cancers originating in the breast, lung, colon, and other sites [1]. Personalized, high-tech medicine is expensive. US citizens spend far more per capita on medical technology, such as expensive imaging techniques and intensive care, than citizens of any other country [2]. The USA spends over 17 % of its gross domestic product (GDP) on health care, as compared to other countries in the Organization for Economic Development and Cooperation (OEDC), which spend approximately 8–9 % GDP [3]. Despite spending more, Americans have a life expectancy that is approximately 4 years less than that of citizens of other developed nations [4]. The US cancer burden is projected to increase substantially in future years due to the burgeoning older population, infectious diseases that transmit cancer-causing viruses and other pathogens, and an obesity epidemic. For instance, the population of Texas, the state in which MD Anderson Cancer Center is located, is projected to

D.E. Epner, M.D., F.A.C.P. (✉)
Department of Palliative Care and Rehabilitation Medicine,
University of Texas MD Anderson Cancer Center,
1400 Pressler Street, Unit 1414, Houston, TX 77030, USA
e-mail: depner@mdanderson.org

K.M. Schmeler, M.D.
Department of Gynecological Oncology and Reproductive Medicine,
University of Texas MD Anderson Cancer Center,
1515 Holcombe Blvd., Unit 1362, Houston, TX 77030, USA
e-mail: kschmele@mdanderson.org

M. Silbermann (ed.), *Cancer Care in Countries and Societies in Transition*,
DOI 10.1007/978-3-319-22912-6_26

increase to 29 million in 2030 and to 32 million by 2040 (Texas Data Center and Office of the State Demographer, 2012, Migration Scenario for 2010–2050 in 1-year increments). Texans 65 or older likely will make up 21 % of the state's population by 2050, compared to 12 % in 2014 (Texas Data Center and Office of the State Demographer, 2012. Age, Sex, and Race/Ethnicity Population by Migration Scenario).

Personalized cancer care is much more than just molecular and high-tech medicine. Another important aspect of personalized cancer care is palliative and supportive care integrated throughout the illness trajectory, especially as end-of-life approaches. Cancer care near the end of life should be person centered, family oriented, and evidence based. Education of US health professionals who provide care to people nearing the end of life has improved substantially in the past two decades, and the clinical fields of hospice and palliative care have become more established. Nonetheless, the number of specialists in these fields is too small, and too few clinicians in primary and specialty fields that entail caring for individuals with advanced serious illnesses are proficient in basic palliative care. Availability of palliative care services has not kept pace with the growing demand. Clinicians are often reluctant to have honest and direct conversations with patients and families about end-of-life issues. Patients and families face additional difficulties presented by the health care system itself, which does not provide adequate financial or organizational support for the kinds of health care and social services that might truly make a difference to them [5].

In addition, significant disparities exist in the US health care, since many Americans are either uninsured or underinsured. The Affordable Care Act (ACA) was passed by congress and signed by President Obama in March 2010 with the intention of reducing health disparities and ultimately making health care more affordable. However, the ACA remains politically charged, and debate continues regarding how best to reform the American health care system to optimize clinical outcomes and cost-effectiveness [6].

Populations in Transition

Many undocumented immigrants who are neither citizens nor permanent residents seek health care in the USA. The vast majority of these immigrants come from Latin America, primarily Mexico and the northern triangle of Central America, namely El Salvador, Honduras, and Guatemala. Many are unaccompanied minors. Drug violence, lack of economic opportunity, and poor access to health care have driven massive Latin American migration in recent years. In addition, the worldwide economic recession of 2008 caused many US residents, both citizens and noncitizens of all ethnic backgrounds, to lose private health insurance and seek care in safety net systems. An estimated 5.7 million Texans—22.5 % of the state's population—lack health insurance, the highest percentage of uninsured citizens in the country (U.S. Census Bureau, 2012 American Community Survey). An estimated 17.9 % of

Texans have incomes below the federal poverty level (U.S. Census Bureau, Small Area Income and Poverty Estimates, 2012). Indigent patients are much less likely to seek preventive services. Economic hardship and the recent wave of immigration from Latin America have therefore resulted in a much higher incidence of preventable cancers, such as cervical cancer, and a shift toward higher stage cancers.

MD Anderson Cancer Center Affiliation with Harris Health System to Address Health Disparities Resulting from Migration Shifts and Economic Hardship

MD Anderson Cancer Center is closely affiliated with the Lyndon Baines Johnson (LBJ) hospital, which is a major component of the Harris Health system, the safety net for indigent patients in Harris County, Texas. LBJ is one of the busiest county hospitals in the nation serving one of the largest uninsured populations. LBJ and other Harris Health system facilities serve anyone who can prove they reside in Harris County, but not all such residents are US citizens or permanent US residents. Several are undocumented immigrants, primarily originating from Latin America and to a lesser extent Far East Asia and other countries. However, it is impossible to determine the country of origin or immigration status of LBJ patients. Regardless of this uncertainty, Harris Health System clearly serves many patients who were displaced from other countries by economic hardship and violence.

Since 1995, MD Anderson faculty and fellows have provided innovative and multidisciplinary cancer care for thousands of patients at LBJ Hospital at no expense to Harris County. The service started 20 years ago as one part-time medical oncologist working one day a week. In FY13, MD Anderson funded 11 clinical faculty members, 18 medical oncology fellows, and five research nurses and mid-level providers to staff oncology services at LBJ, without cost to Harris Health. MD Anderson faculty and staff at LBJ provided care for 952 new patients and 9747 follow-up patient visits. The estimated annual value of professional services provided by faculty and staff is $3.6 million. In addition to the medical oncology clinic, MD Anderson faculty and staff run busy gynecologic oncology and urologic oncology clinics. Every day of the week, MD Anderson faculty, physicians in training, and staff care for outpatients make hospital rounds and perform surgery and outpatient procedures at LBJ. Patients at LBJ may also participate in several clinical trials approved by MD Anderson's Institutional Review Board.

MD Anderson faculty members helped lead pivotal gynecological oncology clinical trials and enrolled many patients from the Harris Health System into those trials. Examples include Radiation Therapy Oncology Group (RTOG) 90-01, Gynecological Oncology Group (GOG) 204, and GOG 240. (RTOG) 90-01 was a randomized trial that showed that addition of fluorouracil and cisplatin to radiotherapy as compared to radiotherapy alone significantly improved survival of women with locally advanced cervical cancer without increasing the rate of late treatment-related side effects [7]. GOG 204 was a randomized trial for metastatic and recurrent cervical cancer that compared four cisplatin-based doublets containing paclitaxel, topotecan, vinorelbine, or gemcitabine [8]. GOG 240 was a randomized clinical trial that showed that addition of bevacizumab to combination chemotherapy in patients with recurrent, persistent, or metastatic cervical cancer was associated with an improvement of 3.7 months in median overall survival [9]. MDACC faculty members have helped establish standards of care for cervical treatment by contributing significantly to these pivotal trials. In doing so, they also provided state-of-the-art cancer care to many underserved patients, many of whom were immigrants from Latin America and other regions in conflict who otherwise would not have had access to care.

MD Anderson faculty and staff also provide extensive cervical cancer screening to Harris Health System patients and other underserved patients throughout Texas and in Latin America. Virtually, all cases of cervical cancer are preventable. Cervical cancer is caused by persistent infection with high-risk types of the human papillomavirus (HPV) [10]. Preventive vaccines are commercially available and are recommended for girls and boys between the ages of 11 and 12, before the onset of sexual activity [11, 12]. Although these vaccines hold great promise to further reduce the incidence of cervical cancer, uptake of HPV vaccination in the USA has been poor, with only 30 % of children completing the three vaccine series [13, 14]. In addition, existing vaccines do not cover all high-risk HPV types or treat preexisting HPV infections. There are 2–3 generations of at-risk HPV-positive women who will not benefit greatly from HPV vaccination. Thus, secondary prevention via cervical cancer screening, diagnosis, and treatment will remain necessary for the foreseeable future.

In the USA and other high-income countries, cervical cancer incidence and mortality rates have decreased by 70 % over the last 40 years due to implementation of screening programs based on Pap and more recently, HPV testing [15, 16]. Evidence-based guidelines for cervical cancer screening are consistent between the American Cancer Society, the American Society for Colposcopy and Cervical Pathology, and the American Society for Clinical Pathology [17]. Women who have an abnormal screening Pap and/or persistently positive HPV test are referred to colposcopy for diagnosis. Areas of the cervix that appear abnormal are biopsied and women with precancerous lesions, including cervical intraepithelial neoplasia grade 2 or grade 3 or adenocarcinoma in situ, are recalled for treatment using loop electrosurgical excision procedure (LEEP) or cold knife conization at a third visit.

However, women in medically underserved regions of the USA, including areas along the USA-Mexico Border, experience significant cancer health disparities including a disproportionate burden of cervical cancer [18, 19]. These populations are less likely to receive cervical cancer screening. These disparities have been attributed to economic, social, educational, and geographical barriers. In addition, many of these regions do not provide the necessary preventive services due to a lack of trained personnel, infrastructure, and resources necessary to implement cervical cancer prevention programs. There is often a shortage of locally available trained providers to manage abnormal cervical cancer-screening tests including performing colposcopy, cervical biopsies, and LEEPs. Furthermore, many women with abnormal screening tests do not receive the recommended diagnostic and treatment procedures, as they are unable to travel to central health care facilities for the multiple necessary follow-up visits due to the long distances and high costs associated with travel. Thus, increased participation in screening coupled with navigation services and an expansion in diagnostic and treatment services is needed to decrease cervical cancer rates in underserved areas.

MD Anderson Research Efforts to Improve Cervical Cancer Screening in Underserved Patients

Studies to Evaluate High-Resolution Microendoscopy

MD Anderson faculty recently obtained funding from the National Cancer Institute for cervical cancer-screening trials that address some of these challenges. One such study is a collaborative project between MD Anderson Cancer Center, Barretos Cancer Hospital in Brazil, and Rice University to evaluate high-resolution microendoscopy (HRME) as a novel cervical cancer-screening method. HRME is a low-cost cervical visualization diagnostic technique to evaluate epithelial cell morphology in situ, eliminating the need for cervical biopsies. The technique involves first applying Proflavine, a topical contrast agent, to the cervix. The tip of a small fiber-optic probe is then placed directly onto the cervix, and the fluorescence from the proflavine-stained epithelium is immediately transmitted back to the HRME unit and displayed on a laptop computer or tablet screen. Morphologic features typically evaluated by pathologists including nuclear crowding, pleomorphism, and nuclear-to-cytoplasm (N/C) ratio are assessed in vivo in real time. Image analysis software is then used to quantify nuclear morphology parameters and calculate N/C ratio. This approach allows for real time, point-of-care detection of high-grade precancerous cervical lesions without a biopsy being performed. These lesions can therefore be treated at the same visit with cryotherapy or LEEP. Pilot data strongly suggest that HRME is highly sensitive and specific and therefore a very promising method for detecting and treating cervical cancer in its early stages. MD Anderson investigators and their collaborators are in the process of completing larger studies of HRME involving several thousand participants. If HRME proves to be as accurate and cost-effective as preliminary results suggest, it will have an enormous impact on cervical cancer morbidity and mortality. Furthermore, it will potentially have the greatest impact on underserved populations due to its easy accessibility and low cost compared to current standards of care. Such underserved patients include indigent patients at LBJ hospital, patients in low-income communities along the Texas-Mexico border, and undocumented US immigrants who fled violence or economic hardship in their home countries.

Studies to Evaluate Novel Education and Patient Navigation Programs to Enhance Cervical Cancer Screening

MD Anderson faculty in Gynecological Oncology also recently applied for funding of studies to test effectiveness of two innovative, evidence-based interventions at the Texas-Mexico border to increase public participation in cervical cancer screening and expand the professional capacity for accurate diagnosis and treatment of precancerous lesions. The first is Cultivando La Salud, an educational outreach program designed to teach low-income Hispanic women about cervical cancer screening. This is combined with patient navigation services to facilitate connection with the cervical cancer-screening services offered at participating sites. The second intervention is the implementation of Project Extension for Community Healthcare Outcomes (ECHO) to increase the number of community providers in south Texas who are sufficiently trained and supported to manage abnormal cervical cancer-screening tests, including performing the recommended diagnostic and treatment procedures. ECHO is a well-established telementoring model proven to expand access to specialty medical care for underserved areas using videoconferencing, case-based learning, and patient co-management. The Project ECHO model will be used to train and support local providers in the appropriate evaluation and management of abnormal cervical cancer-screening tests. This proposal is a collaborative partnership involving Su Clínica Familiar (a Federally Qualified Health Clinic serving the poorest segment of the local population), The University of Texas Health Science Center School of Public Health, Brownsville Regional Campus, The University of Texas Medical Branch, and MD Anderson Cancer Center.

The Roles of MD Anderson's Office of Health Policy to Enhance Care of Underserved Patients in Texas

One of the roles of the MD Anderson Office of Health Policy is to guide Uncompensated Care programs at the institution. MD Anderson has a long tradition of providing care for low-income residents of Texas. A patient financial assistance program provides coverage for care delivered at MD Anderson to cancer patients who meet residency and financial eligibility requirements. Additionally, the institution participates in the Texas Medicaid program that provides state and federal support for certain low-income persons.

The key components of uncompensated care reporting include unreimbursed costs of care for patients who either have no insurance or are underinsured, or whose care was not fully covered by government-sponsored health programs such as Medicare and Medicaid. MD Anderson provided $225 million in uncompensated care to Texans with cancer in Fiscal Year 2013. This figure includes unreimbursed costs for Medicare, Medicaid, and indigent patients. A total of 53,222 patients,

42.6 % of all MD Anderson patients, received some level of uncompensated care in FY13. Approximately 29 % of uncompensated care patients were Harris County residents, another 17 % came from the seven surrounding counties, 32 % came from other Texas counties, and the remaining 22 % came from outside Texas.

Another role of the MD Anderson Office of Health policy is to facilitate oversight and manage administration of the health care delivery programs funded by the 1115 Medicaid Transformation Waiver. Section 1115 of the Social Security Act gives the US Secretary of Health and Human Services (HHS) authority to waive provisions of major health and welfare programs authorized under the Act, including certain requirements in Medicaid. Medicaid is a jointly financed partnership between the US government and individual states within the USA. The federal government provides open-ended federal matching dollars for allowable state spending on Medicaid, and states administer the program on a day-to-day basis. To receive federal Medicaid matching funds, states are required to meet federal core requirements, which include covering a specific set of eligibility groups and benefits. Under Section 1115 of the Social Security Act, the Secretary of HHS can allow a state to receive federal Medicaid matching funds to operate its Medicaid program in ways not otherwise allowed under federal rules. The Medicaid 1115 Transformation Waiver matches funds provided by MD Anderson to support the program's six projects, including (1) colorectal cancer screening (co-funded by a grant from the Cancer Prevention and Research Institute of Texas), (2) Tobacco Cessation with Persons Living with HIV, (3) tobacco prevention for youth, (4) breast cancer screening for uninsured, low-income or Medicaid-eligible women, ages 40–69, (5) tobacco cessation for adults without HIV infection, and (6) an evidence-based program to reduce obesity in children in underserved and minority families through better nutrition and physical activity habits. This program gives providers a chance to find new ways to improve quality of care, health status, patient experience, coordination, and cost-effectiveness in regions developed throughout the State to more effectively and efficiently deliver care and provide increased access to care for low-income Texans.

Summary

MD Anderson Cancer Center and its affiliated institutions, such as the Harris Health System, are committed to improving cancer detection and treatment for underserved patients who face economic hardship are displaced from their home countries by violence. Many such international patients enter the USA from Mexico and Central America via Texas and other southern states. MD Anderson's Office of Health Policy has partnered with the US Office of HHS and the Center for Medicare and Medicaid services to develop novel programs to enhance cancer prevention, screening, and early detection for underserved populations. The MD Anderson Office of Health Policy also provides several million dollars of uncompensated care each year. MD Anderson faculty members in the Department of Gynecology Oncology have developed novel federally funded research programs to enhance cervical cancer screening and treatment, which has the potential to dramatically diminish morbidity and mortality from this preventable malignancy.

References

1. Patient-centered cancer treatment planning: improving the quality of oncology care, a National Coalition for Cancer Survivorship and Institute of Medicine Workshop. Washington, DC: The National Academies; 2011.
2. Carroll A. JAMA forum: OECD report offers a contrast in perception vs reality in US health care. 2013.
3. Delivering high quality cancer care: charting a new course for a system in crisis. Washington, DC: The National Academies; 2013.
4. OECD. Health at a glance 2013: OECD indicators. Paris: OECD; 2013.
5. Dying in America: improving quality and honoring individual preferences near the end of life. Washington, DC: National Academy of Sciences; 2014.
6. Schnipper LE, Meropol NJ. Payment for cancer care: time for a new prescription. J Clin Oncol. 2014;32(36):4027–8.
7. Eifel PJ, Winter K, Morris M, Levenback C, Grigsby PW, Cooper J, et al. Pelvic irradiation with concurrent chemotherapy versus pelvic and para-aortic irradiation for high-risk cervical cancer: an update of radiation therapy oncology group trial (RTOG) 90-01. J Clin Oncol. 2004;22(5):872–80.
8. Tewari KS, Monk BJ. Recent achievements and future developments in advanced and recurrent cervical cancer: trials of the gynecologic oncology group. Semin Oncol. 2009;36(2):170–80.
9. Tewari KS, Sill MW, Long III HJ, Penson RT, Huang H, Ramondetta LM, et al. Improved survival with bevacizumab in advanced cervical cancer. N Engl J Med. 2014;370(8):734–43.
10. Walboomers JM, Jacobs MV, Manos MM, Bosch FX, Kummer JA, Shah KV, et al. Human papillomavirus is a necessary cause of invasive cervical cancer worldwide. J Pathol. 1999;189(1):12–9.
11. Future II Study Group. Quadrivalent vaccine against human papillomavirus to prevent high-grade cervical lesions. N Engl J Med. 2007;356(19):1915–27.
12. Paavonen J, Naud P, Salmeron J, Wheeler CM, Chow SN, Apter D, et al. Efficacy of human papillomavirus (HPV)-16/18 AS04-adjuvanted vaccine against cervical infection and precancer caused by oncogenic HPV types (PATRICIA): final analysis of a double-blind, randomised study in young women. Lancet. 2009;374(9686):301–14.
13. National and state vaccination coverage among adolescents age 13–17 years, United States 2012. Centers for Disease Control and Prevention; 2013. Report No.: 62(34).
14. Chou B, Krill LS, Horton BB, Barat CE, Trimble CL. Disparities in human papillomavirus vaccine completion among vaccine initiators. Obstet Gynecol. 2011;118(1):14–20.
15. Schiffman M, Wentzensen N, Wacholder S, Kinney W, Gage JC, Castle PE. Human papillomavirus testing in the prevention of cervical cancer. J Natl Cancer Inst. 2011;103(5):368–83.
16. Papanicolaou GN. A new procedure for staining vaginal smears. Science. 1942;95(2469):438–9.
17. Saslow D, Solomon D, Lawson HW, Killackey M, Kulasingam SL, Cain J, et al. American cancer society, American society for colposcopy and cervical pathology, and American society for clinical pathology screening guidelines for the prevention and early detection of cervical cancer. CA Cancer J Clin. 2012;62(3):147–72.
18. Scarinci IC, Garcia FA, Kobetz E, Partridge EE, Brandt HM, Bell MC, et al. Cervical cancer prevention: new tools and old barriers. Cancer. 2010;116(11):2531–42.
19. Excess cervical cancer mortality: a marker for low access to health care in poor communities. National Institutes of Health; 2005.

Chapter 27
Forty Years Fast Forward: Vietnamese Refugees in the United States with Comments on Their Cancer Care

Phuong L. Nguyen and Aminah Jatoi

The arrival of war refugees from Vietnam into the United States took place in stages [1]. The first stage occurred at the time the Republic of (South) Vietnam fell to communism in April 1975. This stage consisted largely of Vietnamese and their families who had been involved with US military forces in Vietnam. The second stage included the "boat people," who left Vietnam shortly after the fall of the country and continued to depart through the late 1970s. The "boat people" consisted of people fleeing Vietnam largely because of persecution or sociopolitical and economic issues associated with living within the Socialist Republic of Vietnam; these people had relatively limited resources, struggled to exit the country, relied on mostly makeshift seafaring vessels to do so—hence, the term "boat people"—and yet eventually found refuge in the United States or in other parts of the world. This stage was followed by others who were perhaps no longer considered refugees but who had a multitude of other reasons for leaving, including the fact that they were rejoining their US military fathers (the so-called Amerasian children) or husbands. Taken together, the Vietnamese comprise the sixth largest group of Americans who were born outside the United States; the number of people who identify themselves as Vietnamese-Americans has increased nearly sixfold since 1975. In all, this group comprises two million individuals who reside in the United States.

Commenting on the US involvement in Vietnam, Martin Luther King, Jr. once said, "We have destroyed their two most cherished institutions: the family and the village. We have destroyed their land and their crops…. We have corrupted their women and children and killed their men" [2]. Other Americans—as well as some

P.L. Nguyen, M.D. (✉)
Department of Laboratory Medicine and Pathology, Mayo Clinic,
Hilton 8-60 E, 200 First Street SW, Rochester, MN 55905, USA
e-mail: nguyen.phuong@mayo.edu

A. Jatoi, M.D.
Department of Oncology, Mayo Clinic, Rochester, MN 55905, USA

M. Silbermann (ed.), *Cancer Care in Countries and Societies in Transition*,
DOI 10.1007/978-3-319-22912-6_27

other Vietnamese—took a very different view, seeing the United States as the defender against a communist threat of a small country in Southeast Asia and as a champion for this country's sovereignty. It was perhaps the polarizing nature of this war, as well as a strong sense of responsibility and compassion that led the US government and people to open its arms to the waves of Vietnamese described above to provide them refugee status, and then to accelerate their permanent resident status, thus affording these Vietnamese refugees the opportunity to assimilate into their newly adopted homeland and to access healthcare more readily.

The United Nations Commissioner for Refugees describes how "there are 25 such [protracted] situations in 21 countries" and that tertiary care is "still a major problem" [3]. Such circumstances underscore the need to look carefully at other refugee populations in other countries, particularly those who have settled over a span of decades, in an effort to understand what worked and what did not from the standpoint of health and dissemination of healthcare. In addition, the above historical scenario relevant to the Vietnamese raises two questions that pertain to healthcare challenges that other refugee groups might encounter. Do refugee populations manifest illnesses, for example, specific types of cancers, which are relatively less commonly seen in the more dominantly represented populations within a country? This question is important because healthcare providers' awareness of such specific illnesses would need to increase, and screening efforts specific to the refugee population might need to intensify. Second, are refugee populations able to access healthcare and comfortable with accessing healthcare? Assessing whether trust exists within the refugee community is of paramount importance. In the absence of such trust, healthcare efforts would never be able to be successful.

An Educational and Economic Characterization of the Vietnamese in America

First, as one looks back over the nearly 40 years since their arrival in the United States, how has this group of refugees from Vietnam fared? Despite the often taxing and disheartening circumstances surrounding the Vietnamese diaspora in the United States, Vietnamese Americans appear to have added to the "melting pot" of American culture. Admittedly, members of this community have encountered violent, discriminatory acts both from within and externally, including direct assaults from Ku Klux Klan members in the southern United States [4]. Nonetheless, this point of adding to the "melting pot" is important because, in general, not all refugees are able to settle in a country with the financial resources and acceptance of diversity to enable a refugee population to assimilate and yet maintain its cultural identity. Evidence of this acceptance includes the fact that several Vietnamese refugees or their children have achieved prominence within the news media, business, and government: the US Patriot Act was drafted by Viet D. Dinh, a Vietnamese American, who served as Assistant Attorney General of the United States, and Jacqueline Nguyen is the first Asian American woman to serve on the US federal appellate court, as appointed by

President Obama [5]. In general, although rooted as a refugee population in the United States, Vietnamese Americans do not appear to lag markedly behind from an educational standpoint, as evidenced by the fact that 23 % of Vietnamese immigrants age 25 or older have a college degree compared to 29 % in the US born population.

Vietnamese Americans Have Higher Rates of Hepatocellular Cancer, Lung Cancer, and Cervical Cancer Compared to the General US Population

And yet despite such social and economic assimilation, certain healthcare issues remain somewhat unique to this population of Vietnamese Americans. Some Vietnamese Americans were exposed to Agent Orange, a defoliant, which the US military sprayed over agricultural land in Vietnam in an effort to engage in herbicidal warfare [1]. Dioxin was included in the sprayed defoliant. Appearing orange in color and thereby acquiring its moniker, Agent Orange was manufactured by the US Department of Defense in collaboration with a few large US industrial companies. Although the apparent original intentions of herbal warfare were to spare direct bloodshed, individuals who had been exposed to this chemical have higher rates of specific cancers as well as other health problems. Such cancers were observed both among Vietnamese and American servicemen and are widespread in nature, including soft tissue sarcomas, lymphomas, Hodgkin lymphoma, and chronic lymphocytic leukemia/small lymphocytic lymphoma [6].

For reasons that are less clear, Vietnamese Americans are also at a higher risk for chronic hepatitis B and C, which in turn increases their risk for hepatocellular carcinoma. Indeed, the majority of people coming from the western Pacific and Southeast Asia regions—close to 100 million individuals—carry this risk factor, leading to endemic rates of this malignancy in that part of the world and, now, relatively higher rates in the United States as a result of the Vietnamese diaspora [7, 8]. This influx of Vietnamese Americans into the United States has also led to a greater awareness of this malignancy among individuals within this ethnic group. In a recent review on this topic, Nguyen and Nguyen described how many Southeast Asian patients carry few of the risk factors for hepatitis C and for hepatocellular carcinoma as typically recognized within other patient populations by healthcare workers in the United States, and as a result may be underdiagnosed for this virus-related malignancy that could potentially be cured if diagnosed and resected early. These investigators also make the point that, although Southeast Asian patients at risk for hepatitis C tend to be older, they also appear to respond better to antiviral therapy for hepatitis C than other patients. Thus, these investigators go so far as to advocate in favor of screening for hepatitis C among Asian patients with known high rates of hepatitis C, including Vietnamese Americans, regardless of their risk factors. Along similar lines, a greater awareness of hepatitis B infection is perhaps also indicated.

Furthermore, this ethnic group suffers high rates of lung cancer—35 % higher when compared to Asian Americans born in the United States. Although war exposures may in part account for this higher rate of lung cancer, smoking likely also plays a role [8, 9]. McPhee and Nguyen report that 33–56 % of Vietnamese men living in the United States smoke, with much lower self-reported rates among women [8]. Of relevance, Vietnamese Americans who develop lung cancer also suffer poorer overall and disease-specific survival compared to Chinese Americans [9]. These findings underscore the need to increase awareness of lung cancer among Vietnamese Americans to facilitate early detection, and thus to provide these individuals with therapeutic options in a timely manner.

McPhee and Nguyen also indicate that cervical and breast cancers are sizable health issues for Vietnamese women [8]. Although it is challenging, if not impossible, to extract real-time data, the SEER program shows that from 1988 to 1992, the annual average age-adjusted incidence rates for cervical and breast cancer were 43 and 37.5 per 100,000 individuals, respectively, in the United States. Cancer rates among Vietnamese women living in California are comparable to slightly higher. Although such data may suggest at first glance that breast cancer is the more common cancer among Vietnamese women and that cervical cancer is second most common, when viewed against women in the general population, Vietnamese women in fact have a lower breast cancer rate but a disproportionately high rate for cervical cancer. Thus, cervical cancer is a specific health problem among Vietnamese women.

These data on cervical cancer become all the more concerning in light of poor screening rates [10]. Robinson and others recently conducted a cross-sectional survey with questions relevant to cervical cancer, healthcare practices, and human papilloma virus infection [11]. This survey was sent to both Chinese and Southeast Asian women in the United States. The main purpose was to assess patients' knowledge with respect to cervical cancer, screening, and associated risk factors. These investigators reported on 96 Chinese women and 132 Southeast Asian women with some degree of college education in 67 % and 37 %, respectively, an annual household income of greater than $10,000 in 19 % and 3 %, respectively, and health insurance in 90 % and 80 %, respectively. Regardless of ethnic group, 25 % of respondents either never had a Pap smear performed or reported being unsure about its role with poor knowledge about the relationship between cervical cancer development and human papilloma virus infection. These investigators concluded that greater education and awareness of cervical cancer and its risk factors are relevant for not only Vietnamese women but also for Chinese women. These findings also indicate that current efforts can be improved upon and that such efforts likely promise to fill gaps that are by no means specific to a group of individuals whose families arrived in the United States as refugees.

Vietnamese Americans' Perceptions of Healthcare in the United States

Our group had performed a study of former officers of the Army of the Republic of Vietnam (ARVN) who arrived among the first and earlier waves of refugees, as described above [12, 13]. At the time of this survey, some of these individuals had lived in the United States for as long as 35 years. This long duration is an important and valuable aspect of our study, as it sheds light on the compounding issue of aging among older refugees and provides the longitudinal perspective on refugee populations and their healthcare needs over time. In effect, our study was undertaken to explore language barriers among older refugees and how such barriers might influence the acquisition of healthcare; to understand how older Vietnamese Americans view their healthcare opportunities, and how such opportunities might have changed over time; and to glean a general sense of other related issues from their perspective.

With such goals in mind, our group drafted a survey that consisted of 48 items to elicit patient demographics, information on health status, and patients' views and satisfaction levels with healthcare at the time of survey completion as well as upon initial arrival to the United States. We incorporated the Patient Satisfaction Questionnaire-18 (PSQ-18) as part of this survey and also put together a series of relevant questions that we believed were in alignment with our study goals but otherwise not achievable with the PSQ-18 alone. Retired military officers who had served the former Republic of Vietnam and who were then living in the State of Oregon were to focus of this survey. This state was chosen because it is one of many where a large number of Vietnamese Americans has chosen to relocate, with others consisting of California, Texas, Washington State, Florida, Virginia, Ohio, and Oklahoma.

This small pilot survey revealed several important findings, as relevant to Vietnamese Americans in general and their perceptions of healthcare. First, 22 of 49 (45 %) former military officers responded to the survey; this percentage was much higher than expected and appears to show a willingness to participate in research and in other endeavors that may help the community. Second—and more salient still—21 of 22 respondents (95 %) completed the survey in Vietnamese, when given the opportunity to do so in either Vietnamese or English. (The one person who completed the English version was a spouse.) For the write-in comments, most patients described how they still use an interpreter when seeking healthcare, and many described how language is a barrier to acquiring healthcare. And thus, responding to the item, "Language barriers have prevented me from accessing healthcare when I need it," 77 % said that this was "sometimes" the case even at the time of survey completion, 30–35 years after their arrival in the United States. Third, those who completed the survey viewed their healthcare favorably with positive perceptions even over time. It appeared that their healthcare providers were good about explaining test results, that patients felt that all their healthcare issues were carefully and well addressed, and that they were consistently treated in a courteous manner. Contrary to what we had anticipated, many who completed the survey described that their access to a medical specialist had improved over time.

The one exception to the above centered on healthcare costs. The survey indicated concerns about a healthcare crisis in the United States and a need to make healthcare more cost-efficient: 45 % strongly agreed/agreed with the statement, "There is a healthcare crisis in the United States," in contrast to 9 % who said they would have responded in this manner upon first coming to the United States.

Finally, it was noteworthy to observe a high degree of patriotism among these individuals who had come to the United States as refugees but who now apparently had come to see the United States as their home. For example, one person stated, "[We] need to be willing to do whatever it takes to help build this country and to maintain its status as a world superpower." As another example, another said, "Very fortunate to have settled in the United States." This last point suggests that despite the language barriers and despite the concerns for healthcare costs, these former refugees now view the United States as their home, see themselves as Americans, and remain engaged in helping with social problems.

Lessons Learned in Seeking Input from a Refugee Group

Building further on the survey work described above, our group has formulated and published on four strategies to help others conduct similar pilot work in refugee populations [13]. With the hope that others may find our observations to be of relevance in assessing healthcare needs and identifying issues related to accessing healthcare among refugee populations worldwide, we provide this list below.

First, we believe it is important to identify a group who has been displaced and who has real healthcare needs. As alluded to earlier, we focused on Vietnamese Americans because they comprise a growing group in the United States and because they have a disproportionate rate of certain cancers as well as other healthcare issues. Although in today's world, it is likely that all refugee groups have their own real healthcare needs, it remains crucial nonetheless to understand these needs very accurately—and to learn, as is the case with cancer, whether the issues revolve around effective screening for cancer or prevention strategies against the right set of risk factors as opposed to a more downstream set of issues.

Second, although immigrating to a new country can be challenging, we do not believe that these degrees of challenge in any way approach the difficulty of entering a country as a refugee. Upon entry, most refugees are confronted with an absence or disruption of family support, no social networks, limited/no proficiency in English, confusion with regard to customs, loss of social status, financial hardship, unknown job prospects, shifts in family relationships that arise when children adapt more readily than parents, and an abrupt, perhaps uncomfortable reliance initially on the good will of others. In essence, it is hard to understand these issues in the absence of working with someone who has been through such an experience. In surveying refugees or former refugees or in conducting other research within such groups, it appears helpful to partner with someone who is part of the community, as we had done. To our knowledge, while the role of the so-called community partner has been extensively discussed in the literature as relevant to other ethnic populations, it is perhaps somewhat less well-referenced specifically among refugee populations.

It is our opinion that working with someone who is part of the community is of paramount importance to understanding the needs of that community. This community partner can play an important role in language communication but also in helping others, who are not part of the community, understand the customs and needs of that community. For example, initially, our group had one of our contact letters for the community translated to Vietnamese by a company which had been institutionally vetted and required by our IRB for translation. Our community partner picked up on many translated words that would have been poorly received by our target refugee audience had we sent out the unedited version of our survey. The word "officer" became "quân nhân," which really meant "soldier;" "former military officer" became "quân nhân cũ," which literally translated to "old soldier." For the latter, the correct translation should have "cựu sĩ quan." Thus, simple words do not always capture the true essence of meaning and may convey subtle negative connotations that could be easily misconstrued by members of a community with refugee roots. Understanding the cultural and emotional context of the language sometimes occurs only by working with someone who is genuinely a part of that community.

Third, we believe it is also important to accept that working with a population that has refugee roots will likely lead to exploratory observations. Researchers will be unlikely to find validated surveys. They will likely find individuals who are too traumatized to complete a survey or who because of health issues have already passed away. Understanding these possibilities and accepting them is the only way to enable researchers to complete the assigned work of interest. Furthermore, accepting these limitations is a requisite to the initiation of this research.

Fourth, Katz noted that community-based participatory research is most successful when the researchers develop ongoing, trusting relationships with the community and share their observations with that community. Such transparency enhances trust and allows for future work to proceed at a later date. On a related note, while monetary compensation may be commonplace in certain research spheres, it may not always be appropriate from a cultural standpoint. The prevalent consumption of tea in many Asian cultures, coupled with the fact that it is often considered part of the ritual of greeting, appeared to make it a culturally appropriate "gift" to include with our survey as a means to say "thank you." In effect, allowing community to feel vested in the research efforts contributes to the success of such efforts.

Conclusions and Personal Observations

As challenging as the experiences described above may seem, they are, nonetheless, real and remain so for this group of individuals who had fled South Vietnam nearly 40 years ago. The father of one of the authors (and the author herself) was one of these refugees. Similar to all refugees before him and after him, he made the difficult decision to leave behind his birth country when it became evident that he could no longer be assured of his or his family's personal safety under a new form of government. Furthermore, like other refugees during times of great political and world instability, he became a refugee more than once: first when Vietnam was partitioned into its northern Socialist and southern Republic halves in 1954, forcing him to leave his home in the North, and again in 1975 when the Republic of (South) Vietnam fell. And like all other refugees throughout history, despite all of the perils, fears, and uncertainties associated with making a new life in a new country, he became a refugee because of a determination and optimism that life could be better somewhere else. To him, the late ARVN Colonel Dai V. Nguyen, and to all other brave refugees like him, the authors dedicate this chapter.

Finally, in the history of mankind, there has probably never been a time when we have had no refugees among us. We hope that the lessons we have learned from this group of Vietnamese refugees provide helpful information to others as they work to meet the healthcare needs of these displaced individuals—whether such lessons serve to better recognize the risks and disease patterns specific to certain populations, to communicate both linguistically and in a culturally sensitive manner with refugee groups, or to form the appropriate partnership with the community for meaningful and long-lasting outreach. We conclude with words from Martin Luther King, Jr. as expressed during his speech on the Vietnam War and descriptive of Americans who opposed this war [2]:

> Even when pressed by the demands of inner truth, men do not easily assume the task of opposing their government's policy, especially in time of war. Nor does the human spirit move without great difficulty against all the apathy of conformist thought within one's own bosom and in the surrounding world.

We believe that, when taken from their original context, these words also pertain to refugees, who are often brave and bold in their questioning of the political circumstances dealt to them and who are therefore deserving of our respect for leaving their homeland in their quest for a better life for themselves and their families. We believe these people are deserving of society's efforts to provide healthcare in alignment with what is provided to the more prevalent communities and in alignment with their own specific needs.

References

1. Karnow S. Vietnam: A History. New York: Penguin; 1997.
2. http://www.informationclearinghouse.info/article16183.htm. Accessed 31 Dec 2014.
3. http://www.un.org/en/globalissues/briefingpapers/refugees/overviewofforceddisplacement.html. Accessed 31 Dec 2014.
4. http://www.splcenter.org/get-informed/case-docket/vietnamese-fishermens-association-v-knights-of-the-ku-klux-klan. Accessed 31 Dec 2014.
5. http://en.wikipedia.org/wiki/List_of_Vietnamese_Americans. Accessed 31 Dec 2014.
6. Veterans and agent orange: health effects of herbicides used in Vietnam. Institute of Medicine Committee to review the health effects in Vietnam veterans of exposure to herbicides. Washington, DC: National Academies; 1994.
7. Nguyen LH, Nguyen MH. Systemic review: Asian patients with chronic hepatitis C infection. Aliment Pharmacol Ther. 2013;37:921–36.
8. McPhee SJ, Nguyen TT. Cancer, cancer risk factors, and community-based cancer control trials in Vietnamese Americans. Asian Am Pac Isl J Health. 2000;8:18–31.

9. Raz DJ, Gomez SL, Chang ET, et al. Epidemiology of non-small cell lung cancer in Asian Americans: incidence patterns among six subgroups by nativity. J Thorac Oncol. 2008; 3:1391–7.
10. Morash M, Bui H, Zhang Y, Holtfreter K. Risk factors for abusive relationships: a study of Vietnamese American immigrant women. Violence Against Women. 2007;23:653–75.
11. Robison K, Cleark L, Eng W, et al. Cervical cancer prevention: Asian-American women's knowledge and participation in screening practices. Womens Health Issues. 2014;24:231–6.
12. Stephens EK, Nguyen PL, Radecki Breitkopf C, Jatoi A. Former military officers now living in the United States (US): exploring their perceptions of the US healthcare system. J Community Health. 2011;36:992–8.
13. Stephens EK, Nguyen PL, Jatoi A. Practical strategies to circumvent and/or surmount six barriers in health disparities research: observations from a pilot project among Vietnamese Americans. J Cancer Educ. 2011;26:243–7.

Chapter 28
The Current State of Cancer Care in North America

In Cancer Care in Countries in Transition: Individualized Care in Focus

Joseph F. O'Neill and Thomas J. Smith

Introduction

Cancer care is becoming more effective, increasingly more expensive, and both more and less accessible—all at the same time. In this chapter, we will explore the evolving trends in North American cancer treatment, with an emphasis on the United States and Canada as examples of high-income societies that are struggling to maintain services.

Society Reaction Towards Cancer Patients

This has changed remarkably in the last 40 years. Once, we did not tell patients their diagnosis or prognosis, but that has changed to full disclosure in nearly all patients. Fewer than 10 % choose not to know their diagnosis and prognosis. We should still start every discussion with the most important question for an oncologist to know: "What is your understanding of your situation"? For nearly all patients, it boils down to five issues: naming the diagnosis, the natural history of the illness, symptoms, what caused it, and prognosis [1].

J.F. O'Neill, M.D., M.P.H.
Shore Regional Palliative Care Program, University of Maryland Shore Health,
219 S. Washington St., Easton, MD 21601, USA
e-mail: Joseph.oneill@umm.edu

T.J. Smith, M.D., F.A.C.P., F.A.S.C.O., F.A.A.H.P.M. (✉)
Departments of Medicine and Oncology, Sidney Kimmel Comprehensive
Cancer Center of Johns Hopkins, Johns Hopkins Medical Institutions,
600 N. Wolfe Street, Blalock 369, Baltimore, MD 21287-0005, USA
e-mail: tsmit136@jhmi.edu

M. Silbermann (ed.), *Cancer Care in Countries and Societies in Transition*,
DOI 10.1007/978-3-319-22912-6_28

Table 28.1 Communication miscues in modern-day oncology

Information	Facts	Comment
Number of patients with an accurate awareness of their prognosis	16.5 %; 18.5 % IF the most-important doctor discussed prognosis [47]	Patients with metastatic colon or lung cancer who could identify the usual prognosis as <5 and 2 years, respectively
		Accuracy was directly related to the propensity of the doctor to actually discuss prognosis
Number who thought chemotherapy could cure their metastatic disease	69 % of patients with lung cancer and 81 % of those with colorectal cancer	All of these patients had incurable disease
Number who understood that palliative radiation was not going to cure them	Only 36 % of 384 lung cancer patients understood that radiation would not cure them	All of these patients had incurable disease
Number of lung cancer patients who had discussed hospice with *any* doctor, 2 months before death	Only 53 % had discussed hospice with any provider 2 months before death [48]	Having this discussion 2 months before death decreased the in-hospital death rate from 51 to 19 % [49]
Number of lung and colorectal cancer patients with any documented end-of-life discussion	73 % overall	Most terminally ill cancer patients never discuss their death with their oncologist, even though we know such discussions do not increase anxiety or depression, or take away hope
	55 % occurred in the hospital	
	27 % of the time with oncologists	
	Most common time was 33 days before death [50]	
Prognostic awareness or knowing that one has a terminal cancer	74 % [51]	Patients who die in the hospital have more emotional and physical distress, especially ICU decedents, compared with home hospice [52]
Regret about end-of-life care	At least 50 % experience regret about the EOL care their loved one receives	Completion of advance care planning strongly associated with reduced caregiver distress [53]

Despite the emphasis on communication, there are still wide gaps in communication that have yet to be successfully bridged, as shown in Table 28.1. For example, only 17 % of patients with life-ending colorectal or lung cancer could correctly guess their diagnosis (less than 5 and 2 years, respectively), and only one quarter of oncologist's charts had any mention of discussion about planning for death.

Effectiveness of Treatments

First, the good news about enhanced effectiveness is that cancer death rates are falling from a combination of prevention, earlier detection, and treatment, 1.8 % a year for men and 1.4 % a year for women [2]. The main themes are targeted treatments to a specific pathway or ligand, harnessing of the immune system, and combinations of drugs. Table 28.2 lists some of the major advances of the past 10 years and is a harbinger of things to come as we understand both the mechanism of cancer growth, how it escapes immune regulation by masquerading as "self," and how cancer growth can be modulated.

The bad news is the cost of cancer care in both the United States and Canada, and for those who have access to state-of-the-art care in Mexico, is escalating. Drugs make up about 10 % of the cancer care budget but are increasing in price. The most recent small molecules or antibodies to cancer cost over $13,000 *a month*, not including imaging such as PET or MRI scans, and lab tests. The best predictor for the cost of the new drug is the price of the last five drugs that came to market before it, rather than the effectiveness or originality of the new drug [3]. The drug companies that make the new drugs state that the cost of clinical trials is extraordinarily high and that the targeted drugs have a smaller market (for instance, only 1–3 % of lung cancers are anaplastic lymphoma kinase (ALK)-positive for an ALK-targeted drug.). Critics of the high prices point out that the costs of designing new drugs may be substantially less with techniques like X-ray crystallography allowing for easier design that can be used for multiple drugs; the much smaller trials in selected groups of patients with the target; that drug companies are still highly profitable; and that the best predictor of price is not efficacy but the price of the last drug to come to market [4]. With no transparency in the process, this argument will be unresolved for the immediate future. These issues are in all high-income countries, not just the United States and Canada.

There is no good solution to this crisis of high prices, although all parties agree that it needs be fixed [5]. There has been some recent progress in negotiating lower prices by large insurance companies forcing manufacturers to compete when there are alternative drugs, such as the new antivirals for hepatitis C [6]. The successful bidding has decreased the price to that paid in Europe, about one-third less. However, not all situations have competing drugs, especially with novel cancer treatments, and when insurance companies refuse to cover a drug it leads to calls of "rationing" and "death panels" in the United States. In Canada, the coverage of new drugs varies considerably from province to province, but with a mostly one-payer system, there appears to be more buy-in for a communal process. Most drugs approved by the provincial authorities for efficacy have made it belatedly, if at all, to the budget. In the United Kingdom, there have been multiple disapprovals of new drugs based on formal cost-effectiveness, with much public disapproval but not real recourse given a set budget.

Drugs make up only about 10 % of the total cancer budget; the most expensive part of treatment remains hospitalization [7]. This is where palliative care and hospice have become increasingly important as models of concurrent palliative care

Table 28.2 Some representative major advances in cancer treatment

Cancer	Agent	Impact	Comment
Chronic myelogenous leukemia	Imatinib mesylate (Gleevec), followed by other drugs that can circumvent resistance such as nilotunib, dasatinib, and others	Controls the disease in 90 % of more of patients with a daily pill; mechanisms of resistance are well enough described that we can target a second or third drug effectively [54]	Highly effective but costly: the cost of imatinib has risen from $30,000 per year at its introduction in 2001 to $92,000 in 2015 [55], and patient co-pays are reducing compliance [56]
Breast cancer	Trastuzamab [57] (Herceptin), followed by Kadzilla and Perjada	Doubles life-span in metastatic disease with some long-term survivors; doubles the effectiveness of adjuvant treatment (after surgery)	Has met the requirement for cost-effectiveness in most countries
	"Lumpectomy" followed by radiation therapy to remaining breast	Equal or better cure rates than surgery, less surgery, and disfigurement	Initial resistance by surgeons, with demand driven by patients and by specialized breast cancers offering the treatment
	Genetic testing [58], including BRCA 1 and 2	Most mutations allows for more genetic change in the breast DNA, which eventually allows cancer-causing mutations. Accounts for ~5 % of breast cancer cases	Has not changed treatment, but if a mutation is found, the risk of second breast cancer or ovary cancer is much higher. Affected relatives can elect prophylactic mastectomy and oophorectomy or chemoprevention with tamoxifen

Lung cancer	Helical Computerized Tomography screening in patients at high risk of lung cancer reduces the risk of death by 7 %, and the risk of lung cancer death by 20 % [59]	Useful in patients at high risk of lung cancer due to smoking, family history, etc.	Controversial because it identifies so many other non-cancer entities, with attendant complications and costs due to need to biopsy them all. The cost-effectiveness is about $240,000 to save one life from lung cancer [60]
	Targeted agents against Epidermal Growth Factor Receptor (EGFR), anaplastic lymphoma kinase (ALK) [61] that inhibit the cancer cells more than normal cells	Anti-ALK drugs induce remission and disease control in 60–75 % of patients, lasting on average 6 months; EGFR drugs induce responses in 50 %	At present, all cancers develop resistance, usually in 6–12 months, so the impact on survival has been small. The drugs cost $6000–13,000 a month
	Unleashing the immune system to target lung cancer by using antibodies or small molecules to block Programmed Death (PD) 1 or PD Ligand 1 (PDL) pathways. These pathways are used by the cancer to hide from the immune system [62]	About 1 in 4 patients have a dramatic response to PD-1 therapy, often lasting years	The drugs cost $13,000 or more a month and can cause unusual autoimmune side effects such as pneumonitis, colitis, and pituitary failure
Acute or chronic lymphocytic leukemia refractory to usual treatments	Treatment harvests T cells by extraction from the blood, uses a disabled virus vector to carry the CD-19 gene into the T-cells, so the T-cells attack and kill any cell bearing CD 19	Highly effective in adult chronic lymphocytic leukemia and pediatric acute lymphocytic leukemia patients, inducing durable remissions in over 75 % [63]	Still not widely available but will soon be available As the technology advances, available for more cancers including epithelial cancers [64]

along with usual oncology care show improved symptoms, better quality of life, equal or longer survival [8], and lower cost in nearly all trials [9]. As shown in Table 28.3, palliative care has multiple opportunities to reduce the cost of care by at least 10 %, thus saving a substantial amount of money for advances in cancer treatment [10]. These include, but are not limited to—in addition to better care—prevented hospitalizations, lower cost per day if hospitalized, shorter length of stay, and reduced readmission rates.

Table 28.3 Ways in which palliative care can improve care while reducing the cost of care

Mechanism	Study	Savings
Prevent hospitalizations from symptoms, which account for 60 % of cancer admissions [65]	Non-randomized U Wisconsin academic center; 64 % of admissions were due to symptoms and potentially preventable	$$$
Allow hospice transition sooner by introducing concurrent care	Non-randomized Aetna provided enhanced hospice with concurrent care, introducing the hospice team sooner Now being tested by Medicare in the United States	Hospitalizations were reduced from 15 days to 2 per member; ICU days 10 down to 1 per member; doubling of use of hospice and length of stay [66]. Overall savings 22 % in the last 40 days of life [67]
Concurrent interdisciplinary inpatient palliative care team (IPCT) for patients with less than 1 year to live patients	517 Patient randomized trial	Approximately equal survival; markedly better satisfaction; half the rate of ICU use (12 versus 21, $p=0.04$). Costs were $4900 less even including the cost of the IPCT [68]
Concurrent interdisciplinary palliative care for homebound terminally ill patients	Randomized trial of 298 patients, homebound, to usual care versus usual care and IDPCT	Approximately equal survival; almost $8000 savings per person [69]
Recognition of hospice-eligible patients, with enrollment if eligible	U Iowa academic center. 229 decedents identified; 60 % of decedents were eligible for hospice on the penultimate admission, based on National Hospice and Palliative Care Organization (NHPCO) criteria [70]	Only 14 % had any discussion of hospice, despite being eligible; 14 of 17 enrolled, all from ONE service. If they enrolled in hospice the chance of dying in the hospital was 7/14 (50 %) at a cost of $5000. If they were not offered hospice, 202/209 died in the hospital at a median cost of $52,000 [71]
Reducing readmission rates and costs	Non-randomized but carefully controlled study	If patients were seen by the inpatient palliative care team and sent home with hospice or palliative care, the readmission rate in 30 days was ~5 %; if not, about 25 % [72] Not restricted to palliative care: Acute Care for Elders programs have similar savings and reduced readmissions [73]

These difficulties are not unique to the United States. Canada's system has been called "a system in name only" with marked variation in available services [11]. Only half of drug costs are paid by the provinces; the rest by individuals. About 30 % of total health care costs are borne by individuals. There are substantial variations in cancer drug availability even after the drugs have been approved by the federal and provincial governments [12]. The same congestive heart failure patient in different provinces could spend $74–$1332 for $1200 worth of medicines [13]. Canada doubled real-value spending on health care in the last decade but remains tenth of 11 industrialized countries in a respected review by The Commonwealth Fund [14] suggesting that more fundamental reforms in the provision of care will be needed in the future.

Innovations

In all countries, innovations in evidence-based guidelines or practice pathways continue to lead the way to better care and lower costs. A private US firm, US Oncology that provides 15 % of the care to all US cancer patients, has provided the best examples. Using doctor-approved pathways, they have maintained or improved survival in metastatic lung [15] and colorectal [16] cancer patients while reducing the total cost by 35 %. By added nurse phone calls to patients after chemotherapy ("troubleshooting"), they were able to further reduce ER visits and costs [17]. Adding a fixed reimbursement model (the oncologist got paid the same no matter what drugs she prescribed, and got paid more for following an evidence-based guideline) reduced the total cost of care by almost one-third [18], from an expected $98,121,388 for 810 patients in five practices to an actual cost of $64,760,116. Surprisingly, drug costs were triple than expected but the total cost savings to the insurer were still nearly one-third.

Interrelationship Between Cancer Care and Local Culture

In all countries, there are persistent `disparities in care due to race, socioeconomic status, and location. For instance, colorectal cancer screening has been underutilized by African-Americans for decades. The state of Delaware reduced the disparities by making colonoscopy available in patient communities by raising the reimbursement, giving coupons for free colonoscopy, public outreach especially to faith communities, education, and ensuring completion with patient navigators [19, 20]. Whether this can be replicated in larger more diverse states remains to be seen, but it is an encouraging step. Other disparities are a mix of biologic and socioeconomic circumstances. For example, African American women have the highest rates of triple negative breast cancer (negative for estrogen, progesterone, and HER-2 targets) with a rate of 28 % of all cancers, compared to 12 % for age-matched white women [21, 22]. Current evidence suggest that improvements in the care provided can reduce many of these disparities, such as more federally financed health centers to provide screening in low-income areas [23], and patient navigation [24].

Insights on Palliative Care in Cancer Patients

Palliative Care in North America

Modern palliative care and hospice programs trace their origins to the work of Dame Cicely Saunders at St. Christopher's Hospice in London in the late 1960s. Earlier use of the term "hospice" reference (usually religious) homes for the dying—a tradition that reaches far back into the Middle Ages—that did not offer the evidence-based, multidisciplinary approach to suffering and death that characterizes the modern use of the word.

While the countries of North America (Mexico, the United States, and Canada) share a continent and certain cultural and ecologic characteristics (especially in border regions) their health care systems and, hence, their palliative care and hospice programs, have evolved in different ways and with different paces. Comparisons of palliative care between countries is made difficult by several methodological factors including the lack of a theoretical background, lack of information on use of experts as sources of information, use of grey literature, problematic international rankings, and difficulties associated with the nature of data on palliative care provision [25]. In this chapter, we will, therefore, simply describe key aspects of palliative and hospice care in the three countries noting important policy and institutional developments.

Mexico

Health in Mexico is defined as a social right and guarantee in Article IV of the Federal Constitution [26]. Stemming from this, on November 25, 2008 the Senate of the Republic voted in reforms to the General Health Law that were implemented in January 2009 with publication in the *Official Federal Gazette*. These reforms included the right of Mexicans with a terminal disease to be treated with palliative care [27].

A report entitled "Care When There is No Cure: ensuring the right to Palliative Care in Mexico" by the Non-Governmental Group Human Rights Watch and published in October 2014 found however "…that currently only a few dozen public healthcare institutions in the country offer palliative care and even fewer provide it in patients' homes. Most healthcare personnel have received no training in the discipline, and few doctors are licensed to prescribe strong pain medicines that are essential for palliative care. Where palliative care is available it is often due to the efforts of individual physicians or advocates rather than the result of a deliberate policy of the government, health system or insurer" [28]. Human Rights Watch identified a number of specific issues that have made access to palliative care challenging in Mexico. These include lack of availability of opioid analgesics, lack of training of health professionals in palliative care, cumbersome regulations governing opioid prescribing, and overall health resource limitations.

The International Association for Hospice and Palliative Care's Global Directory of Programs and Services identifies 20 palliative care programs in Mexico [29]. These include community-based organizations, academic and hospital-based initiatives. Considering that the World Health Organization Cancer Country Profiles (2014) [30] estimate an annual total of 605,000 deaths (71,900 from cancer) in Mexico, it is clear that there is a substantial unmet need for palliative services.

An important step to meet this need was recently made by the Mexican Ministry of Health in December 2014 when it issued national palliative care guidelines that outline criteria and methods for initiating palliative care and which emphasize the importance of providing palliative care in home settings. Additionally, other reforms related to prescribing analgesics and professional education were announced [31].

Canada

The Canadian Hospice and Palliative Care Association (CHPCA) traces the origins of palliative and hospice care in Canada to the near simultaneous opening in 1975 of palliative care units at St. Boniface General Hospital in Winnipeg, Manitoba, and The Royal Victoria Hospital in Montreal, PQ [32]. A cancer surgeon, Dr. Balfour Mount, led the development of the latter facility. He had occasion to visit St. Christopher's hospice in London and was inspired to create a hospital-based set of similar services for his cancer patients in Montreal. Additionally, he is credited with the first use of the term "palliative" to describe these services as an alternative to the word "hospice" which had already occupied a place in French lexicon [33]. The first research and educational institute for palliative care was created at the University of Ottawa in 1983 [32].

Today, the CHPCA's 2012 directory of programs lists 525 hospice palliative care programs in the country [34]. There organizations are represented at both provincial and national levels through voluntary associations that encourage public policy, nongovernmental and educational initiatives to support hospice palliative care. Significant milestones/achievements include:

- 1983: publication of by Health and Welfare Canada of "Palliative Care Services Guidelines"
- 1994: incorporation of the Canadian Palliative Care Association
- 1995: publication of report by the Canadian Senate "Of Life and Death" that examined legal, social, and ethical issues surrounding euthanasia and assisted suicide [35]
- 2000: publication of "Quality End of Life Care: The Right of Every Canadian" by the Standing Senate Committee on Social Affairs, Science and Technology.

This report followed on the 1995 report and made 14 key recommendations intended to advance hospice and palliative care in Canada[1] [36]
- 2002 and 2013: publication and revision of "A Model to Guide Hospice and Palliative Care: based on National Principles and Norms of Practice" [37]
- 2013: The Royal College of Physicians and Surgeons recognize Palliative Care as a subspecialty of medicine

The United States

Like Canada, early palliative care interest in the United States was inspired by the work of Dame Saunders at St. Christopher's and the writings of Elisabeth Kubler-Ross. A nurse, Florence Wald, founded what is generally recognized as the first hospice palliative care institution in the United States—Connecticut Hospice—in Branford, CT in 1974. Since then, the number of facilities that provide hospice and palliative care has increased dramatically: The National Hospice and Palliative Care Organization estimates that in 2013 there were approximately 5800 hospices operating in the 50 states, the US Virgin Islands, Puerto Rico, the District of Columbia and Guam [38]. The Center to Advance Palliative Care estimated that between 2002 and 2012 the number of hospital-based palliative care programs in the United States increased 148 % to more than 1600 [39], and the US Accreditation Council for Graduate Medical Education (ACGME) now lists 109 programs for physician fellowship training in hospice and palliative medicine [40].

Some significant policy and programmatic milestones highlighted by the NHPCO include:

- 1974: The first hospice legislation is introduced by Senators Frank Church and Frank E. Moss to provide federal funds for hospice programs. The legislation is not enacted.
- 1979: The Health Care Financing Administration (HCFA) initiates demonstration programs at 26 hospices across the country to assess the cost-effectiveness of hospice care and to help determine what a hospice is and what it should provide.
- 1980: The W.K. Kellogg Foundation awards a grant to the Joint Commission on Accreditation of Hospitals (JCAHO) to investigate the status of hospice and to develop standards for hospice accreditation.

[1] Conclusions of the 2000 Senate Report are worth noting: *As set out in the 1960 Canadian Bill of Rights, Canada is founded upon the dignity and worth of the human person. That dignity and worth compels the provision of excellent end-of-life care at a time when each person is at his or her most vulnerable. Quality end-of-life care must become an entrenched core value of Canada's health care system. Each person is entitled to die in relative comfort, as free as possible from physical, emotional, psychosocial, and spiritual distress. Each Canadian is entitled to access skilled, compassionate, and respectful care at the end of life. This Subcommittee sees care for the dying as an entitlement for all…. The Subcommittee believes that such quality end-of-life care will not happen unless the federal government takes a leadership role in developing a national end-of-life care strategy.*

- 1982: Congress includes a provision to create a Medicare hospice benefit in the Tax Equity and Fiscal Responsibility Act of 1982, with a 1986 sunset provision.
- 1986: The Medicare Hospice Benefit is made permanent by Congress and hospices are given a 10 % increase in reimbursement rates. States are given the option of including hospice in their Medicaid programs. Hospice care is now available to terminally ill nursing home residents.
- 2002: The Department of Veterans Affairs launches program to increase veterans' access to hospice and palliative services while providing educational opportunities for clinicians in veterans' health care facilities.
- 2003: A Clinical Guide to Supportive and Palliative Care for HIV/AIDS is released by the U.S. Health Services Resource Administration. The White House sponsors a Conference on Palliative Care and the HIV/AIDS Global Pandemic.
- 2006: The American Board of Medical Specialties (ABMS) recognizes hospice and palliative medicine as a medical specialty.
- 2006: A Guide to Supportive and Palliative Care for HIV/AIDS in Sub-Saharan Africa is released; the publication was funded by the US Government through the HIV/AIDS Bureau, Health Resources and Services Administration, and NHPCO.
- 2009: The Accreditation Council for Graduate Medical Education, a private, nonprofit organization responsible for the accreditation of post-MD medical training programs within the United States, adds hospice and palliative medicine to its list of accredited programs.
- 2010: *NHPCO Standards of Practice for Pediatric Palliative Care and Hospice* Receives American Academy of Pediatrics' Affirmation of Value.
- 2012: An innovative, online advocacy resource, the Legislative Action Center, is created online by the Hospice Action Network. More than 1.5 million people are reached through the six-part online video series, *Basics of Hospice*" [41].

There are three types of care in the United States: outpatient, inpatient, and respite care (to give the family a few day break in caregiving). Some hospices can offer residential care at a hospice home, with the family paying for room and board. Hospice in the United States is truly managed care: the hospice receives about $150 a day for each day the patient is enrolled in hospice. In return, the hospice must provide all the care needed for the terminal illness including physician and nurse visits, home care, oxygen, drugs, and supplies. Hospices are required to provide the same level of service regardless of the ability to pay. This $150 a day is based on inflation adjustments from the expansion of the Medicare hospice benefit from President Reagan in 1986 and was chosen to keep the Medicare budget neutral (or not cost any more). The $150 day payment works well when patients spend 30 days in hospice as the high cost initial enrollment/assessment and final end-of-life days are usually offset by less intense and less expensive middle days. The recent trend to shorter hospice enrollments to <19 days and over one-third of hospice stays being <7 days is troubling. For the patient, this means that important clues to progressive illness were either ignored or neglected, and unhelpful chemotherapy may have made things worse leading to delayed enrollment. Worldwide in developed countries, 10–30 % of patients get chemotherapy in their last 2 weeks of life when it is highly likely to be harmful and not helpful. For the hospices, such short stays are financially bankrupting and emotionally bankrupting to the staff.

Hospice is currently well established as a service in the United States but is undergoing rapid change and turbulence [42]. Once dominated by local, small, nonprofit firms, the growth has been essentially all in large, national, diversified for-profit firms. Medicare now spends over $13 billion on hospice, up from $4.4 billion in 2004. For-profit hospices rose from about 10 % in 1990 to 62 % of all hospices by 2010. They earned margins of 11.2 % on Medicare patients, compared to <2 % for nonprofit hospices. There are some data that for-profit hospices use fewer services per patient, hotly disputed by for-profit hospices. Whatever the ownership status, hospice is currently undergoing significant scrutiny from all quarters. Recent "exposé" articles in the Washington Post document large variations in the quality of care received, high profits, and concentration on the finances [43].

While hospice is certain to survive in the United States, the exact structure will likely change. We anticipate continued financial pressure to reduce costly types of care. We have already seen in our own practice reluctance to cover such important medicines a patient-controlled analgesia (PCA) an octreotide ($15 a dose, 3 doses a day, taken from the $150), and reduced availability of inpatient hospice.

Palliative care has been growing rapidly in the United States with nearly 90 % of medium to large hospitals reporting programs (Fig. 28.1). There are no uniform quality metrics for palliative care programs although they are under development. The benefits of palliative care alongside usual cancer care have been well described and include equal or longer survival, better quality of life and symptom control, less caregiver distress, less depression and anxiety, and equal or lower costs.

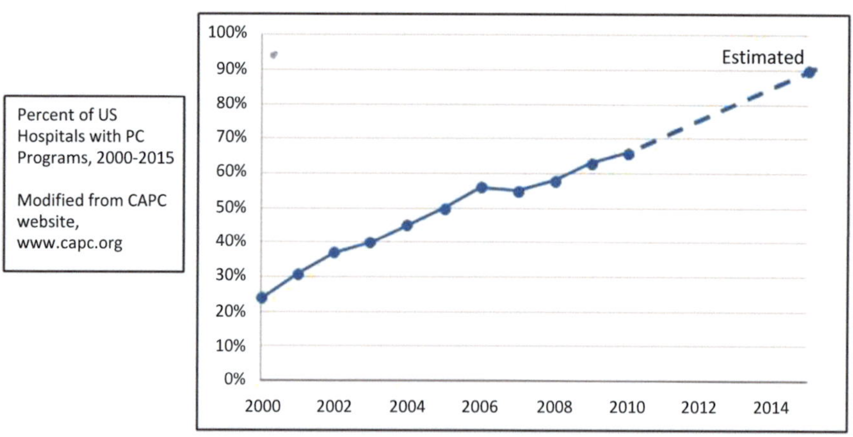

Fig. 28.1 Growth of palliative care programs in the United States

Government Involvement

The federal government has become the largest spender for health care in the United States as the population ages and more people enter Medicare, the guaranteed insurance for people over 65. Access to high quality cancer care has been both increased and more problematic in the last years. In the United States, the Affordable Care Act has given new access to cancer treatment to up to 40 million people by providing affordable insurance. Unfortunately, the cost of cancer care has gotten so high, and so often the primary breadwinner is affected or dies, that medical care is the first or second most common cause of bankruptcy. Patients with cancer have a 2.5-fold higher risk of bankruptcy than those with other illnesses [44]. And, the precursor to the Affordable Care ("Obamacare") started in Massachusetts ("Romneycare") did not reduce the rate of medical bankruptcies [45]. If someone has Medicare B that covers outpatient costs but no supplemental insurance plan, their 20 % co-payment on a $13,000/month drug can be as high as $2600—unaffordable for many.

We have seen differing cancer systems evolve side by side in the United States and in other countries, illustrating how culture influences treatment. For instance, in the government-funded Veteran's Administration (available to those who serve in the military), the VA has a tightly restricted formulary so many of the newest drugs an options are not immediately available, such as multiple lines of tyrosine kinase inhibitors in metastatic renal cancer. However, the results of cancer treatment are as good as in the rest of the United States [46] even with per-person costs that are as much as one-third lower.

Summary and Recommendations

> It was the best of times, it was the worst of times… in short, and the period was so far like the present period that some of its noisiest authorities insisted on its being received, for good or for evil, in the superlative degree of comparison only.
>
> Charles Dickens, A Tale of Two Cities
> English novelist (1812–1870)

These are the best and the worst of times. We have made amazing advances in basic and applied science, and even some of the toughest cancers such as metastatic lung cancer and melanoma can be put into long-lasting remission in some people. We have developed excellent home care and palliative programs and diagnosis-to-cure or diagnosis-to-end-of-life models. At the same time, we are faced with an increased number of people with cancer, their longer survival with many more comorbid illnesses, an unsustainable system of health care financing, and rising public expectations. We are worried that at least in the United States the system will go more to "haves" and "have nots" for some time before we come to some equitable distribution.

Our recommendations are to continue to work on models that advance concurrent palliative and usual care, and to continue to solve difficult symptoms and diseases with scientific advances. We should all be working to develop more of an evidence base for our medical prescribing, including cultural values, personal values, and cost consciousness into the ways we take care of people.

Acknowledgements Supported by the Veterans Administration Medical Center Fellowship Grant, the Lerner Foundation and Rosenthal Foundation HPM Fellowships, and the P30 CA 006973 SKCCC Cancer Center Grant.

References

1. Morris DA, Johnson KS, Ammarell N, Arnold RM, Tulsky JA, Steinhauser KE. What is your understanding of your illness? A communication tool to explore patients' perspectives of living with advanced illness. J Gen Intern Med. 2012;27(11):1460–6. doi:10.1007/s11606-012-2109-2.
2. Siegel RL, Miller KD, Jemal A. Cancer statistics, 2015. CA Cancer J Clin. 2015;65(1):5–29. doi:10.3322/caac.21254.
3. Bach PB. Limits on Medicare's ability to control rising spending on cancer drugs. N Engl J Med. 2009;360(6):626–33. doi:10.1056/NEJMhpr0807774.
4. Epidemiologist Peter Bach discusses high drug prices in an opinion piece for The New York Times. Why drugs cost so much. The New York Times. 15 Jan 2015.
5. Gogineni K, Shuman K, Chinn D, Weber A, Cosenza C, Colten ME, Emanuel EJ. Making cuts to Medicare: the views of patients, physicians, and the public. J Clin Oncol. 2015;33(8): 846–53.
6. http://www.bloomberg.com/news/articles/2015-01-12/prime-covers-both-gilead-and-abbvie-liver-drugs-as-prices-plunge
7. Torio CM, Andrews RM. National inpatient hospital costs: the most expensive conditions by payer. 2011. http://www.hcup-us.ahrq.gov/reports/statbriefs/sb160.pdf
8. Parikh RB, Kirch RA, Smith TJ, Temel JS. Early specialty palliative care–translating data in oncology into practice. N Engl J Med. 2013;369(24):2347–51. doi:10.1056/NEJMsb1305469.
9. Hughes MT, Smith TJ. The growth of palliative care in the United States. Annu Rev Public Health. 2014;35:459–75. doi:10.1146/annurev-publhealth-032013-182406.
10. Kelly RJ, Smith TJ. Delivering maximum clinical benefit at an affordable price: engaging stakeholders in cancer care. Lancet Oncol. 2014;15(3):e112–8. doi:10.1016/S1470-2045(13)70578-3.
11. Lewis S. A system in name only–access, variation, and reform in Canada's provinces. N Engl J Med. 2015;327(6):497–500.
12. Hoch JS, Morgan S, Peacock S, Abbott R, Sullivan T, Chafe R, Culyer A, Dobrow M, Coyte PC, Sawka C, O'Reilly S, Laing K, Trudeau M, Smith S. Access to cancer drugs in Canada: looking beyond coverage decisions. Healthc Policy. 2011;6(3):27–36.
13. Demers V, Melo M, Jackevicius C, Cox J, Kalavrouziotis D, Rinfret S, Humphries KH, Johansen H, Tu JV, Pilote L. Comparison of provincial prescription drug plans and the impact on patients' annual drug expenditures. CMAJ. 2008;178(4):405–9. doi:10.1503/cmaj.070587.
14. Davis K, Stremikis K, Squires D, Schoen C. Mirror, mirror on the wall: how the performance of the U.S. health care system compares internationally. New York: Commonwealth Fund; 2014. http://www.commonwealthfund.org/~/media/files/publications/fund-report/2014/jun/1755_davis_mirror_mirror_2014.pdf.
15. Neubauer MA, Hoverman JR, Kolodziej M, Reisman L, Gruschkus SK, Hoang S, Alva AA, McArthur M, Forsyth M, Rothermel T, Beveridge RA. Cost effectiveness of evidence-based treatment guidelines for the treatment of non-small-cell lung cancer in the community setting. J Oncol Pract. 2010;6(1):12–8. doi:10.1200/JOP.091058.

16. Hoverman JR, Cartwright TH, Patt DA, Espirito JL, Clayton MP, Garey JS, Kopp TJ, Kolodziej M, Neubauer MA, Fitch K, Pyenson B, Beveridge RA. Pathways, outcomes, and costs in colon cancer: retrospective evaluations in 2 distinct databases. Am J Manag Care. 2011;17(Suppl 5 Developing):SP45–52.
17. Hoverman JR, Klein I, Harrison DW, Hayes JE, Garey JS, Harrell R, Sipala M, Houldin S, Jameson MD, Abdullahpour M, McQueen J, Nelson G, Verrilli DK, Neubauer M. Opening the black box: the impact of an oncology management program consisting of level I pathways and an outbound nurse call system. J Oncol Pract. 2014;10(1):63–7. doi:10.1200/JOP.2013.001210.
18. Newcomer LN, Gould B, Page RD, Donelan SA, Perkins M. Changing physician incentives for affordable, quality cancer care: results of an episode payment model. J Oncol Pract. 2014;10(5):322–6. doi:10.1200/JOP.2014.001488.
19. Grubbs SS, Polite BN, Carney Jr J, Bowser W, Rogers J, Katurakes N, Hess P, Paskett ED. Eliminating racial disparities in colorectal cancer in the real world: it took a village. J Clin Oncol. 2013;31(16):1928–30. doi:10.1200/JCO.2012.47.8412.
20. Potera C. Delaware eliminates racial disparities in colorectal cancer. Am J Nurs. 2013;113(7):16. doi:10.1097/01.NAJ.0000431904.27355.62.
21. Turkman Y, Sakibia Opong A, Harris L, Knobf M. Biologic, demographic, and social factors affecting triple negative breast cancer outcomes. Clin J Oncol Nurs. 2015;19(1):62–7. doi:10.1188/15.CJON.62-67.
22. Sturtz LA, Melley J, Mamula K, Shriver CD, Ellsworth RE. Outcome disparities in African American women with triple negative breast cancer: a comparison of epidemiological and molecular factors between African American and Caucasian women with triple negative breast cancer. BMC Cancer. 2014;14:62. doi:10.1186/1471-2407-14-62.
23. Adams SA, Choi SK, Khang L, A Campbell D, Friedman DB, Eberth JM, Glasgow RE, Tucker-Seeley R, Xirasagar S, Yip MP, Young VM, Hébert JR. Decreased cancer mortality-to-incidence ratios with increased accessibility of federally qualified health centers. J Community Health. 2015;40(4):633–41.
24. Braun KL, Thomas Jr WL, Domingo JL, Allison AL, Ponce A, Haunani Kamakana P, Brazzel SS, Emmett Aluli N, Tsark JU. Reducing cancer screening disparities in Medicare beneficiaries through cancer patient navigation. J Am Geriatr Soc. 2015;63(2):365–70. doi:10.1111/jgs.13192.
25. Loucka M, Payne S, Brearley S, Euro Impact. How to measure the international development of palliative care? A critique and discussion of current approaches. J Pain Symptom Manage. 2014;47(1):154–65.
26. https://www.constituteproject.org/constitution/Mexico_2007.pdf?lang=en
27. Bistre S. New legislation on palliative care and pain in Mexico. J Pain Palliat Care Pharmacother. 2009;23(4):419–25.
28. http://features.hrw.org/features/HRW_2014_report/Mexico_Care_When_There_Is_No_Cure/index.html
29. http://hospicecare.com/global-directory-of-providers-organizations/
30. http://www.who.int/cancer/country-profiles/mex_en.pdf
31. http://www.ehospice.com/ArticleView/tabid/10686/ArticleId/13355/language/en-GB/View.aspx
32. http://www.chpca.net/about-us/history.aspx
33. http://www.canada.com/ottawacitizen/story.html?id=896d005a-fedd-4f50-a2d9-83a95fc56464%20
34. http://www.chpca.net/media/314972/annual-report-2012-en_final_-_online_version.pdf
35. http://www.parl.gc.ca/Content/SEN/Committee/351/euth/rep/lad-e.htm
36. http://www.parl.gc.ca/Content/SEN/Committee/362/upda/rep/repfinjun00-e.htm
37. http://www.chpca.net/media/319547/norms-of-practice-eng-web.pdf
38. http://www.nhpco.org/sites/default/files/public/Statistics_Research/2014_Facts_Figures.pdf Page 8
39. http://reportcard.capc.org/pdf/capc-growth-analysis-snapshot-2011.pdf

40. http://www.acgme.org/ads/Public/Programs/Search?specialtyId=153&orgCode=&city=
41. http://www.nhpco.org/history-hospice-care
42. Thompson JW, Carlson MD, Bradley EH. US hospice industry experienced considerable turbulence from changes in ownership, growth, and shift to for-profit status. Health Aff (Millwood). 2012;31(6):1286–93. doi:10.1377/hlthaff.2011.1247.
43. Peter Whoriskey, Dan Keating. Dying and profits: the evolution of hospice. This is the seventh installment in the "Business of Dying" series. Washington Post. 26 Dec 2014.
44. Ramsey S, Blough D, Kirchhoff A, Kreizenbeck K, Fedorenko C, Snell K, Newcomb P, Hollingworth W, Overstreet K. Washington state cancer patients found to be at greater risk for bankruptcy than people without a cancer diagnosis. Health Aff (Millwood). 2013;32(6):1143–52. doi:10.1377/hlthaff.2012.1263.
45. Himmelstein DU, Thorne D, Woolhandler S. Medical bankruptcy in Massachusetts: has health reform made a difference? Am J Med. 2011;124(3):224–8. doi:10.1016/j.amjmed.2010.11.009.
46. Keating NL, Landrum MB, Lamont EB, Bozeman SR, Krasnow SH, Shulman LN, Brown JR, Earle CC, Oh WK, Rabin M, McNeil BJ. Quality of care for older patients with cancer in the veterans health administration versus the private sector: a cohort study. Ann Intern Med. 2011;154(11):727–36. doi:10.7326/0003-4819-154-11-201106070-00004.
47. Liu PH, Landrum MB, Weeks JC, et al. Physicians' propensity to discuss prognosis is associated with patients' awareness of prognosis for metastatic cancers. J Palliat Med. 2014;17(6):673–82.
48. Huskamp HA, Keating NL, Malin JL, et al. Discussions with physicians about hospice among patients with metastatic lung cancer. Arch Intern Med. 2009;169(10):954–62.
49. Kumar P, Temel JS. End-of-life care discussions in patients with advanced cancer. J Clin Oncol. 2013;31(27):3315–9.
50. Mack JW, Cronin A, Taback N, et al. End-of-life care discussions among patients with advanced cancer: a cohort study. Ann Intern Med. 2012;156(3):204–10.
51. Mack JW, Weeks JC, Wright AA, Block SD, Prigerson HG. End-of-life discussions, goal attainment, and distress at the end of life: predictors and outcomes of receipt of care consistent with preferences. J Clin Oncol. 2010;28(7):1203–8.
52. Wright AA, Keating NL, Balboni TA, Matulonis UA, Block SD, Prigerson HG. Place of death: correlations with quality of life of patients with cancer and predictors of bereaved caregivers' mental health. J Clin Oncol. 2010;28(29):4457–64.
53. Garrido MM, Prigerson HG. The end-of-life experience: modifiable predictors of caregivers' bereavement adjustment. Cancer. 2014;120(6):918–25.
54. Mathisen MS, Kantarjian HM, Cortes J, Jabbour EJ. Practical issues surrounding the explosion of tyrosine kinase inhibitors for the management of chronic myeloid leukemia. Blood Rev. 2014;28(5):179–87. doi:10.1016/j.blre.2014.06.001.
55. Kantarjian HM, Fojo T, Mathisen M, Zwelling LA. Cancer drugs in the United States: Justum Pretium–the just price. J Clin Oncol. 2013;31(28):3600–4. doi:10.1200/JCO.2013.49.1845.
56. Dusetzina SB, Winn AN, Abel GA, Huskamp HA, Keating NL. Cost sharing and adherence to tyrosine kinase inhibitors for patients with chronic myeloid leukemia. J Clin Oncol. 2014;32(4):306–11. doi:10.1200/JCO.2013.52.9123.
57. Balduzzi S. Cochrane review—Trastuzumab-containing regimens for metastatic breast cancer. J Evid Based Med. 2014;7(3):229. doi:10.1111/jebm.12119.
58. Shiovitz S, Korde LA. Genetics of breast cancer: a topic in evolution. Ann Oncol. 2015;26(7):1291–9.
59. National Lung Screening Trial Research Team, Aberle DR, Adams AM, Berg CD, Black WC, Clapp JD, Fagerstrom RM, Gareen IF, Gatsonis C, Marcus PM, Sicks JD. Reduced lung-cancer mortality with low-dose computed tomographic screening. N Engl J Med. 2011;365(5):395–409. doi:10.1056/NEJMoa1102873.
60. Goulart BH, Bensink ME, Mummy DG, Ramsey SD. Lung cancer screening with low-dose computed tomography: costs, national expenditures, and cost-effectiveness. J Natl Compr Canc Netw. 2012;10(2):267–75.

61. Kumarakulasinghe NB, Zanwijk NV, Soo RA. Molecular targeted therapy in the treatment of advanced stage non-small cell lung cancer (NSCLC). Respirology. 2015;20(3):370–8. doi:10.1111/resp.12490.
62. Forde PM, Kelly RJ, Brahmer JR. New strategies in lung cancer: translating immunotherapy into clinical practice. Clin Cancer Res. 2014;20(5):1067–73. doi:10.1158/1078-0432.CCR-13-0731.
63. Maus MV, Grupp SA, Porter DL, June CH. Antibody-modified T cells: CARs take the front seat for hematologic malignancies. Blood. 2014;123(17):2625–35. doi:10.1182/blood-2013-11-492231.
64. Levine BL. Performance-enhancing drugs: design and production of redirected chimeric antigen receptor (CAR) T cells. Cancer Gene Ther. 2015;22(2):79–84. doi:10.1038/cgt.2015.5.
65. Rocque GB, Barnett AE, Illig LC, Eickhoff JC, Bailey HH, Campbell TC, Stewart JA, Cleary JF. Inpatient hospitalization of oncology patients: are we missing an opportunity for end-of-life care? J Oncol Pract. 2013;9(1):51–4. doi:10.1200/JOP.2012.000698.
66. Spettell CM, Rawlins WS, Krakauer R, Fernandes J, Breton ME, Gowdy W, Brodeur S, MacCoy M, Brennan TA. A comprehensive case management program to improve palliative care. J Palliat Med. 2009;12(9):827–32. doi:10.1089/jpm.2009.0089.
67. Krakauer R, Spettell CM, Reisman L, Wade MJ. Opportunities to improve the quality of care for advanced illness. Health Aff (Millwood). 2009;28(5):1357–9. doi:10.1377/hlthaff.28.5.1357.
68. Gade G, Venohr I, Conner D, McGrady K, Beane J, Richardson RH, Williams MP, Liberson M, Blum M, Della PR. Impact of an inpatient palliative care team: a randomized control trial. J Palliat Med. 2008;11(2):180–90. doi:10.1089/jpm.2007.0055.
69. Brumley R, Enguidanos S, Jamison P, Seitz R, Morgenstern N, Saito S, McIlwane J, Hillary K, Gonzalez J. Increased satisfaction with care and lower costs: results of a randomized trial of in-home palliative care. J Am Geriatr Soc. 2007;55(7):993–1000.
70. Freund K, Weckmann MT, Casarett DJ, Swanson K, Brooks MK, Broderick A. Hospice eligibility in patients who died in a tertiary care center. J Hosp Med. 2012;7(3):218–23. doi:10.1002/jhm.975.
71. Weckmann MT, Freund K, Bay C, Broderick A. Impact of hospice enrollment on cost and length of stay of a terminal admission. Am J Hosp Palliat Care. 2013;30(6):576–8. doi:10.1177/1049909112459368.
72. Enguidanos S, Vesper E, Lorenz K. 30-Day readmissions among seriously ill older adults. J Palliat Med. 2012;15(12):1356–61.
73. Flood KL, Maclennan PA, McGrew D, Green D, Dodd C, Brown CJ. Effects of an acute care for elders unit on costs and 30-day readmissions. JAMA Intern Med. 2013;173(11):981–7. doi:10.1001/jamainternmed.2013.524.

Chapter 29
Application of Genetic Testing for Childhood Cancers in Emerging Countries

Jamie E. Flerlage, Bhavana Pathak, and Joann Bodurtha

A 10-year-old boy was having pain in his left leg that continued to worsen over the span of a month and keep him up at night. He was seen by a local clinic where he was given a medication for pain and told to come back in a month if it was still there. A month later he returned as the pain was persistent and with edema around his distal thigh. An X-ray revealed a mass and he was sent on a bus 8 hours away to see a pediatrician. After reviewing his case he was sent to a Pediatric Cancer facility where a work up confirmed a diagnosis of osteosarcoma. Thankfully he did not have metastatic disease and after an amputation and chemotherapy he recovered well and remains disease free. Family history was negative for other cancers and the reduced concern about a familial tendency to childhood cancers, the Li–Fraumeni syndrome, was discussed with the family. His experience brought him into a city he had never known and he returned home with resilience beyond words. Many under-resourced countries are at a point where cancer is a leading cause of death in children and deserves attention alongside all of the other resource issues the countries are facing.

J.E. Flerlage, M.D., M.S.
St. Jude Children's Research Hospital, Memphis, TN, 38105, USA
e-mail: Jamie.flerlage@stjude.org

B. Pathak, M.D.
Department of Medicine, Johns Hopkins Medical Institutions,
1800 Orleans Street, Baltimore, MD, 21287, USA
e-mail: bpathak1@jhmi.edu; pathakbhavana@gmail.com

J. Bodurtha, M.D., M.P.H. (✉)
Departments of Pediatrics and Oncology, McKusick-Nathans Institute
of Genetic Medicine, Johns Hopkins Medical Institutions,
600 N. Wolfe St., Blalock 1008, Baltimore, MD, 21287, USA
e-mail: jbodurt1@jhmi.edu

M. Silbermann (ed.), *Cancer Care in Countries and Societies in Transition*,
DOI 10.1007/978-3-319-22912-6_29

Introduction

Contemporary molecular and imaging technologies have increased the accuracy and precision of cancer diagnosis, recognition of residual disease, and treatments in some parts of the world. Global development varies in levels of poverty, education, health system infrastructure, regional hospital networking, work force numbers and training, health care access, national research programs, and cancer services [1]. Optimal individualization of pediatric cancer care requires the resources and organization to have a health care system capable of providing care for all children with focused attention and resources addressing childhood malignancies. Important components that impact the continuum of pediatric cancer care with a genetic lens can include:

- A provider system that can triage by physical exam for cancer susceptibility conditions [2–6] with appropriate surveillance and follow-up
- An administrative system that can incorporate newborn and other genomic screening for high risk conditions in particular subpopulations at increased risk [7–9]
- A health care system that is working toward preventing cancers caused by infections, roughly 23 % in less resourced countries and 7 % of cancers in more developed countries [10]
- Organized cancer registries, research networks clinical trial groups [11]
- Ongoing attention to evidence-based molecular diagnostics especially those tied to therapeutic interventions and pharmacogenomic variation, including clinical trials [12–15].

At least one pediatric cancer hospital has taken a step-wise approach to the integration of clinical genomics in its management of acute lymphoblastic leukemia over the past 30 years (Fig. 29.1) [16].

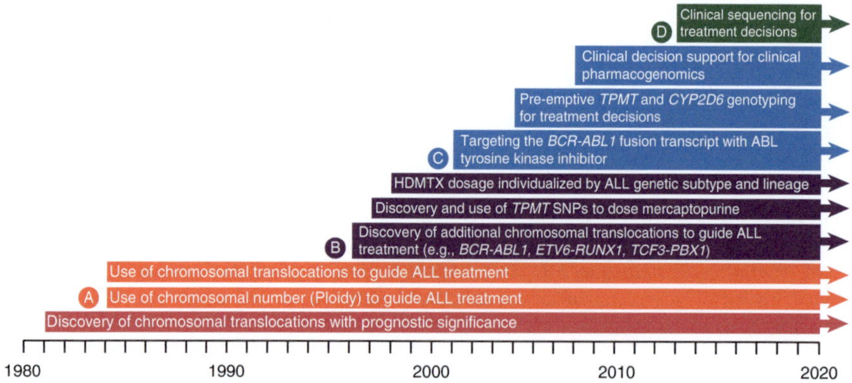

Fig. 29.1 A time line of discovery and clinical implementation of genomics to advance treatment of childhood ALL. *ALL* acute lymphoblastic leukemia, *SNP* single-nucleotide polymorphism, *TPMT* thiopurine methyltransferase

Integration of genetic testing in childhood cancer care occurs across a range that includes variations in available money, price policies, time, evidence, expertise, inertia, advocacy, coordinated electronic health records, and health care systems.

Individualized attention to pediatric cancer receives less or little emphasis in countries where health care resources are limited and other diseases are viewed as more serious public health problems. Campaigns such as the UICC World Cancer campaign, including My Child Matters™ have supported projects to increase awareness and improve coordination of care and training for health professionals who address childhood cancer care in varied countries [17]. Later presentation and likely death without attention to underlying cause occurs in low resource countries, even for tumors with strong genetic etiology, such as retinoblastoma, Wilms tumor, and Li–Fraumeni syndrome [18–20].

Cultural beliefs and stigmas also impact the responses to pediatric cancer across the world with wide variations in illness representations, coping, degrees of disclosure and communication, use of traditional healing, and handling of medical procedures [21]. The complex issues involved in understanding of causation, genetic testing, informed consent, and other ethical issues require continuing dialogue and cultural humility.

Overview of Childhood Cancer Around the World

In resource-rich countries, 80 % cure rates for many childhood cancers are the norm. In emerging countries where cancer detection may be too late for effective treatment and where appropriate treatment may be unavailable or unaffordable, roughly 60 % of children with cancer die [1, 17]. Yet approximately 80 % of children who develop cancer and leukemia live in under-resourced countries. Dispersed rural and overall younger populations, as well as the burden of infectious disease in countries in early or intermediate stages of economic development contribute to the reality that most children with cancer in these countries succumb to their disease [22].

Data on incidence and mortality is robust in high resource countries with recorded incidence rates consistently above 12 per 100,000 [23]. Generally, leukemias and lymphomas are most common with tumors of the brain and central nervous system second. The completeness and quality of data on childhood cancer incidence and mortality varies widely around the world; GLOBOCAN estimates that the annual incidence of childhood cancers ranges from 50 to 200 cases per million children per year in different countries [24] (Fig. 29.2 [1]).

Paucity of data and variations in data methodologies are key issues in any worldwide comparisons. Countries may have relatively robust public health infrastructure and relatively low overall mortality in children under 5 years but low cancer survival because they lack specific professional, technological, and infrastructure resources necessary for pediatric cancer management. In addition, abandonment of therapies may occur. Availability of adequate pediatric cancer units with staffing, supplies,

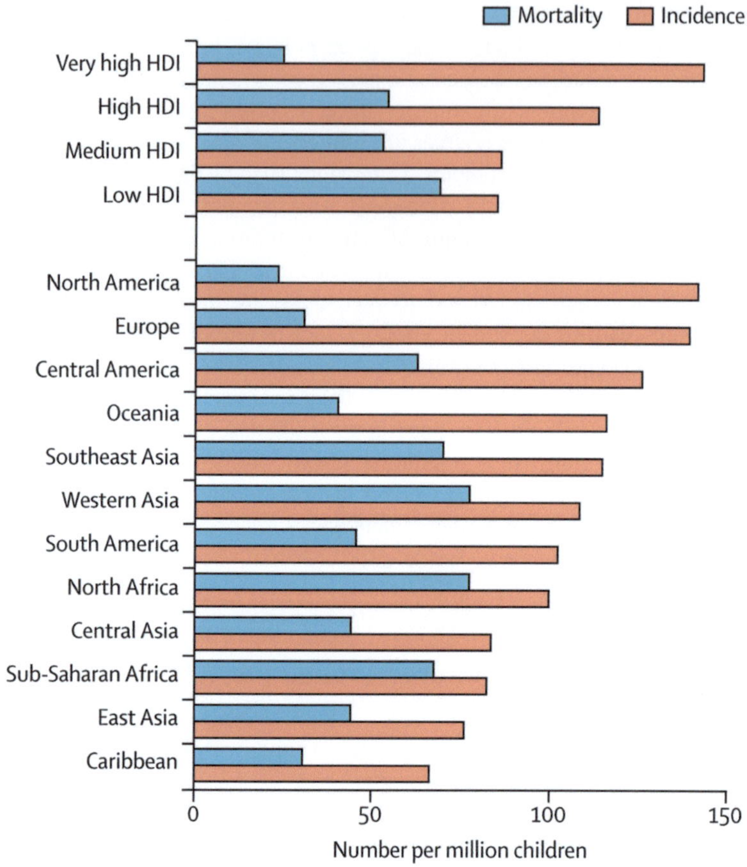

Fig. 29.2 Estimated childhood cancer incidence and mortality in 2008 by Human Development Index (HDI) classification and region. Data from GLOBOCAN

therapies, diagnostic technologies, guidelines, advocacy, palliative care programs, and international partners may impact childhood cancer mortality; however, annual government health care expenditure per capita has been shown to correlate most significantly with postulated 5-year cancer survival [22]. Exemplary questions in which more robust data are needed include:

- Are sick girls less likely than boys to reach specialist care [25]?
- How is the known increased risk of HIV-related cancers—non-Hodgkin's lymphoma and Kaposi sarcoma in some African countries changing?
- Does age affect access to care and cost of care?
- What is the availability of pediatric specialists?

Overview of Genetic Testing for Childhood Cancers

Only a small percentage (<10 %) of all childhood cancer is related to a heritable syndrome, but as the cost of genetic testing falls, screening for genetic syndromes may become available to emerging countries [2]. Population-based studies have demonstrated that there is no increased risk for a sibling of pediatric cancer patient to develop cancer outside of known hereditary syndromes [26]. Therefore, screening for genetic conditions is worthy of the cost if it can be afforded. For families with many siblings, despite the cost there is a potential to save lives if tumors are found early (as in retinoblastoma) or preventive surgeries are performed prior to the formation of cancer.

Several heritable genetic syndromes which predispose children to cancer are:

Syndrome	Gene
Familial retinoblastoma	RB1
Familial adenomatous polyposis	APC
Beckwith–Wiedemann syndrome	CDKN1C, KCNQ10T1, LIT1, H19, IGF2
Li–Fraumeni syndrome	TP53, CHEK2
Neurofibromatosis	NF1, NF2
Ataxia telangiectasia	ATM

As genetic testing becomes available, screening for heritable syndromes is only effective if close follow-up for those whom test positive can be performed. The recommended follow-up varies for each syndrome.

Familial retinoblastoma comprises approximately 3–4 % of all childhood tumors. It is autosomal dominantly inherited with a 90 % penetrance if the affected parent has bilateral tumors. For retinoblastoma, the recommendation is for frequent fundoscopic exams beginning at birth and every 2 weeks after that until the age of 3 months, then every 2 months with a complete exam under anesthesia and then space to every 6 months around 4–5 years of life [2]. Appropriate genetic testing (defining the specific mutation in the family) can alter this follow-up regimen in siblings who are found not to carry the responsible family mutation.

Beckwith-Wiedemann syndrome carries a 10 % cumulative risk cancer by the age of 4 years old. Screening consists of an abdominal ultrasound that is needed every 3 months until the age of 8 years to monitor for tumor development [2].

Familial adenomatous polyposis causes tumors along the GI tract at an early age and morbidity and mortality can be prevented with a colectomy at a young age prior to the development of cancer. Li-Fraumeni syndrome is an autosomal dominant disorder that is associated with the formation of many types of cancer. Surveillance for breast cancer in young females is successful, but there is no clear-cut consensus on how to screen for other associated malignancies [27]. In centers offering genetic testing, access to follow-up services and recommended screening for a given genetic defect should be built at the same locations or at nearby locations in order for the testing to be helpful to the patients and their families.

In addition, access to genetic testing in research and clinical trials will become important in improving global childhood cancer outcomes. The introduction of less toxic and more targeted drugs over time requires partnerships among the pharmaceutical industry, regulators, patients, their families, and researchers. National cancer plans with clear referral and care pathways are needed to improve access to the best standard of care in each country and respect cultural and linguistic diversity [11].

Review of Frameworks for Considering Genetic Testing: Clinical Utility, Ethical, and Social Issues

Countries in transition face many barriers to the implementation of community genetic services: the paucity of trained health professionals, competing curative and preventative priorities (i.e., communicable disease), misconceptions about the costs of such services, low genetic literacy rates, cultural stigmatization of diagnoses, and a lack of data on the actual burden of congenital diseases [28]. These barriers all contribute to the need for a proper framework to assess the utility and feasibility of genetic testing in low and middle income countries. The United States has created one major international genetic evaluation framework, the ACCE model. In Europe, the United Kingdom utilizes the UKGTN (United Kingdom Genetic Testing Network Gene Dossier which is based off of the ACCE framework [29].

The ACCE model can provide a framework to critically appraise genetic testing for countries in transition. The model has four components: analytic validity, clinical validity, clinical utility, and the ethical, legal, and social implications (ELSI) of genetic testing. Analytic validity refers to the ability of an assay to accurately and reliably measure the genotype of interest. It is primarily a measure of the quality of the test performance in a laboratory, as opposed to clinical validity. Clinical validity is the ability of a genetic test to detect or predict the presence of absence of the phenotype of clinical disease. Both analytic and clinical validity require sensitivity and specificity measurements. Clinical utility is the propensity for a genetic test to actually lead to improved outcomes. Patient versus provider opinions on clinical utility may in fact differ, affecting the clinical utility of a test. If an older test is being replaced, a cost-effectiveness comparison is recommended. The integration of resource issues in overall family, community, and national health plans has consequences throughout the world, but is especially challenging in under-resourced countries.)The "ELSI" (ethical, social, and legal implications) of genetic testing require the broadest assessment, necessitating refocus on the purpose and particular population for which the genetic testing was designed. The social, economic, and cultural risks of genetic testing must be outweighed by the potential benefits for improved health outcomes or behaviors. The democratization of low-cost genetic testing in low and middle income countries must be met by an equally widespread critical appraisal process to ensure that these interventions fortify rather than detract from epidemiologic and preventative health efforts [29–31].

Genetic Testing: Family and Cultural Issues

The spread of genetic testing technology provides a unique opportunity for global cancer prevention and control. While genetic testing may allow for early detection and inform prognosis in cancer, there are also many psychosocial consequences and limitations to having this new information. Many cultures have a particularly high degree of stigma associated with cancer. Westbrook et al. found significantly higher degrees of stigma related to cancer in Arabic-, Greek-, and Chinese-Australians compared to Anglo-Celtic Australians [32]. Goss et al. similarly noted that patients in China and India had high degrees of stigma and fatalism attached to their cancer diagnoses, preventing them from pursuing further diagnostic, prognostic, and therapeutic evaluation [33].

Carriers and noncarriers of mutations can undergo significant turmoil with regard to the implications of a certain genetic status. Diversity of kinship systems and genetic literacy can affect how people engage in community genetic resources. Western concepts of bilateral inheritance share a similar backbone to Mendelian patterns of inheritance. In Asia and the Middle East however, patrilineal concepts of kinship can suggest that hereditary diseases may be derived from a singular, shared ancestor—which can impact familial health seeking behavior, particularly those implicating cancer diagnoses, for children [34–36]. Genetic conditions can be perceived as particularly devastating, for they not only may reflect poorly on the child, but on the family as a whole. Receiving counseling, via genetic counselors can be seen as an admission of public shame, and therefore not as freely accepted. Cancer fatalism—the belief that cancer is destined and beyond individual control—further prevents efforts at engaging patients and their families in preventative and therapeutic genetic evaluations [33, 37, 38].

Ethically, the principles of autonomy and beneficence suggest that genetic testing should belong to the subject tested and do no harm. Yet cultures with high concepts of familial and community interdependence may struggle with valuing individual autonomy, directly impacting the confidentiality of genetic testing. As such, the political framework in many low and middle income countries has similarly not reflected the value of individual confidentiality as a priority. This can be particularly problematic for vulnerable populations such as girls and ethnic minorities, who may already face systemized discrimination [39, 40]. Furthermore, the paucity of national cancer registries in low and middle income countries diminishes the awareness of cancer as a preventable and treatable disease, further reducing the participation of parents and children in diagnostic genetic testing for cancers [36, 41].

In addition to an organized public health system, knowledgeable professionals, low-cost technology, and motivated policy makers—culturally sensitive genetic counselors will play a particularly important role in transforming the landscape for genetic testing in developing countries. Health behaviors and decisions, such as sunscreen use for xeroderma pigmentosa and prophylactic colectomies for Familial Adenomatous Polyposis, can ultimately not come without a nuanced understanding of the impact of such decisions within an individual's familial, cultural, and societal constructs [28, 35, 40, 42].

Genetic Testing: Informed Consent and Resource Issues

The balance of autonomy, beneficence, privacy, nonmaleficence, and equity are in ongoing tension in serious pediatric illnesses across a world of widely varying resources. Moving toward global equity in children's health is monitored by the World Health Organization (http://www.who.int/gho/health_equity/en/ [43]). The family and cultural norms for truth-telling in children vary markedly with more attention to assent and consent in countries and institutions that have a focus on childhood developmental issues and family-focused programs, such as child life and family advisory committees. Adolescent autonomy to decide about personal cancer treatments and participate in shared decision-making, whether in line with or different from parental or health care team recommendations, has received increasing attention in countries with more resources [44].

Cancer susceptibility syndromes with varying ages of diagnosis and onset of findings can challenge systems of care, as testing in adults has implications for children. For example, BRCA1/2-positive women aged 18 to their mid-20s may find challenges in reconciling their adult independence with family support needs related to their risks. Family members who have been most directly involved in caring for them as girls may inadvertently apply pressure, complicating family relationships and their autonomous decision-making. The capacity of health care professionals to help insure young women remain informed and receive objective counseling about their risk-management decisions [45] requires enhanced medical education. In under-resourced countries, late diagnosis of cancer and limited treatments in young adults has a major impact on the economy and child-rearing [46]. For example, the variation in worldwide programs and technologies applied to HPV immunization and cervical cancer screening demonstrate the impact of varied resources and beliefs on cancer prevention and deaths [47].

International Approaches

Collaboration is the key to success around the world. Many institutions have adopted "Twinning" programs, where a well-established institution pairs with a site in an emerging country to form a partnership that is mutually beneficial. This has aided in the development of international databases and research protocols relevant to local needs. Awareness of childhood cancer, the need for access to care, and the fact that all children have a fundamental right to receive care for potentially curable diseases increase through these collaborations. Developed countries can assist in the formation of alliances with political leaders, ministries of health, nongovernmental organizations, and lobby for funding and resources [48].

With the ability to consult on challenging cases and a constant train the trainer mentality, the education level is elevated on a regular basis. Additionally, the sharing of information and education provides a transfer of skills and expertise to one another and encourages specialists in emerging countries to develop practices in their home countries and remain there [48]. As specialists increase, the need for medical tourism falls and more children receive the care they need. Genetic specialists can become part of these programs.

Laboratory partnerships have enabled many countries to enhance the care they deliver through the opportunities to use specialized testing that may not exist in their country, such as immunophenotyping [48]. Samples of cancer cells from leukemias to solid tumors can be sent for confirmatory testing and diagnosis through collaborations. This process helps to ensure correct diagnosis are made and provide appropriate prognostic information prior to initiation of therapy.

"Twinning" partnerships are one of the most successful strategies for international cancer care to date [49]. With time, the goal is to elevate the level of care delivered around the world.

Individualized Oncology in Focus

The field of pediatric oncology is changing every day. Once a patient is found to have a cancer, the genetics of the cancer cells themselves carry great prognostic significance. The more we know about the genetics of each person's cancer, the more we can risk stratify treatment and predict outcomes. The survival curves for cancers such as leukemia are categorized into risk groups based on the genetics within the cells. For the same disorder, a patient's response to chemotherapy can be predicted and therapy is risk adapted as various subtypes are found to be refractory [50]. Determining the treatment needed for an individual patient may help avoid unnecessary toxicity in low risk patients and delineates those with a poor prognosis for who comfort measures may be most appropriate [48]. Through laboratory collaborations this testing is becoming a reality in emerging countries (Fig. 29.3) [51].

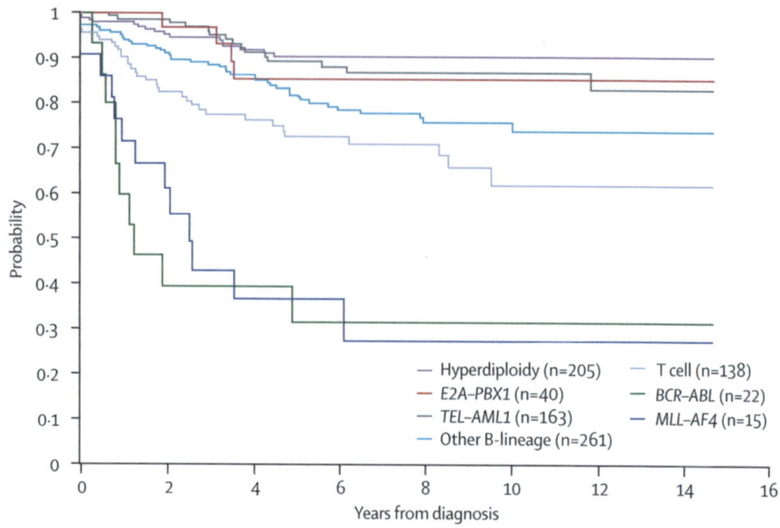

Number at risk

	0	2	4	6	8	10	12	14	16
Hyperdiploidy	205	190	144	108	80	52	25	10	1
E2A–PBX1	40	36	27	19	14	9	6	0	0
TEL–AML1	163	144	105	83	60	46	30	10	0
Other B-lineage	261	221	161	130	92	50	28	13	3
T cell	138	112	75	60	36	22	8	3	1
BCR–ABL	22	15	7	5	3	2	0	0	0
MLL–AF4	15	9	6	4	4	2	1	1	0

Fig. 29.3 Kaplan–Meier analysis of event-free survival according to biological subtype of leukemia

Critical Clinical Issues

Improving care in existing institutions and partnering with genetic laboratories that are addressing adult oncology and infectious disease issues may be a logical step in the development of an overall national cancer control plan that incorporates genetics. Prompt referral and diagnosis by appropriate means coupled with patient management and family supports that are based on protocols adapted to local conditions are important elements in models of childhood cancer control in under-resourced countries. Ultimately with more research in populations worldwide, we will continue to learn that the biology and genetics of tumors can differ [1].

After receiving months of therapy, patients and their families in countries with lower resources may be exposed to new areas of their country they have never seen, educated on science occurring within them and around them to a new level, are able to see city life, hear other languages, and so much more. Despite their predisposition to cancer, it still may be a life-changing experience that impacts them, their relatives and communities. The sustainability of improved individualized medicine includes reduced cancer stigma and improved survivorship with long-term follow-up.

Insights on Palliative Care in Pediatrics

The majority of mortality in pediatric cancers occur in low and middle income countries. With late presentations of diseases such as pediatric CNS tumors, the paucity of treatment resources for critically ill patients, and cultural factors affecting compliance to cancer treatment—palliative care plays an essential role in improving pediatric cancer care globally [36, 52–55].

The World Health Organization has defined pediatric palliative care as the "total care of the child's body, mind and spirit, and also involves giving support to the family. It begins when illness is diagnosed, and continues regardless of whether or not a child receives treatment directed at the disease. It can be provided in tertiary care facilities, in community health centers and even in children's homes" [55, 56]. In a survey of 58 developmentally diverse countries, availability of palliative care programs was proportional to the countries income—with low and middle income countries severely lacking properly developed palliative care programs [36, 57]. Some of the barriers to palliative care delivery include lack of palliative care teams, lack of specialized nursing training, and restricted access to opiates, primarily in government control [36, 58, 59]. Pain control remains a disproportionately outstanding issue in LMIC—with less than 50 % of pediatric oncology units having pain management initiatives and less than 15 % of countries surveyed having access to high potent opiates and neuropathic medications [57]. Higher income countries, in contrast, enjoy access to a majority of the world's opioid analgesic supply according to the International Narcotics Control Board (INCB), with the additional fortitude of established standardized palliative care practices, via organizations such as the National Consensus Project for Quality Palliative Care [36, 60].

Globally, palliative care in pediatric oncology can take note from the similar experience with palliative care in pediatric HIV, where the level of poverty is strongly correlated with prognosis. In sub-Saharan Africa, the Integrated Community-Based Home Care Model utilizes community care givers to link patients with HIV/AIDS to diagnostic counseling, treatment, and palliative care across a spectrum of settings—home, clinics, hospitals, allowing for a sustainable system of palliative care service delivery in a low resource setting [61].

Early integration of pediatric palliative care, regardless of disease outcomes, appears to particularly critical to the success of palliative care programs. In Lebanon, Saad et al. describe their experience with a palliative care program for children with cancer who did not respond to disease-specific treatment protocols. They found that these children and families still experience high rates of symptoms and lack of preparedness for their child's end-of-life issues, suggesting the need for earlier integration of such program, as an integrative strategy of both curative and palliative care in pediatric cancer [62, 59]. In Guatemala members of the pediatric palliative care team meet the patient from the moment of diagnosis, are part of the initial discussions and consents and provide longitudinal care and symptom management for all pediatric patients with cancer [63].

Across the world, it is hard for a parent to deal with the dying child. Feelings of parental failure, cultural expectations of disease course, and variations in communication styles—make broad implementation of Western-style palliative care programs unlikely. Valuing a child's life, in the context of their individual illness, family structure, and belief system requires an adaptive and collaborative approach to succeed. Family-centered programs with early integration provide the best chance to respect individual needs in the context of their collaborative familial, cultural, and socioeconomic environment [64, 65]. The genetic aspects of childhood cancer and its impact on siblings, e.g., testing for a family mutation, in particular may be integrated in palliative care's family focus in the future.

Summary and Recommendations

Public education, more and better-trained health professionals, strengthened cancer services, locally relevant research, regional hospital networks, international collaboration, and health care access are all essential components of enhanced cancer care in childhood. Genetic knowledge and technologies can aid in the screening and prevention of various pediatric cancers as well as in the prognosis and treatment of patients. As Sullivan and colleagues have summarized, "The effective management of children with cancer needs long-term commitment from both health care professionals and federal authorities to support research and care networks. The gains in outcomes should be seen in the context of other major issues, and drawbacks that arise as health care and political systems change. In terms of policy, resource-rich countries still need continuous vigilance and development." ([66], p. e127) We recommend:

- Early integration of culturally sensitive, family-centered palliative care services and the availability of low cost, critically appraised genetic tests should be a priority to level the playing field in morbidity and mortality of pediatric cancer cases in low and middle income countries.
- International partnerships and "twinning programs," as well as broad international collaboration on data collection and use should be supported to insure successful strategies for sharing of resources, education, and drug development that includes genetic understanding and effective technologies.
- International laboratory collaborations in clinical care and genetically aware research are needed for emerging countries to make progress in and sustain their ability to ensure proper diagnoses, risk stratification, and treatments of children with cancers.
- Regular discussions about difficult cases, including their genetic aspects, collaborative clinical trials, and sustained advocacy can enhance ongoing training in emerging countries.

References

1. Magrath I, Steliarova-Foucher E, Epelman S, Ribeiro RC, Harif M, Li CK, Kebudi R, Macfarlane SD, Howard SC. Paediatric cancer in low-income and middle-income countries. Lancet Oncol. 2013;14(3):e104–16.
2. Rao A, Rothman J, Nichols KE. Genetic testing and tumor surveillance for children with cancer predisposition syndromes. Curr Opin Pediatr. 2008;20(1):1–7.
3. Slavin TP, Wiesner GL. Developmental defects and childhood cancer. Curr Opin Pediatr. 2009;21(6):717–23.
4. Hopman SM, Merks JH, de Borgie CA, Aalfs CM, Biesecker LG, Cole T, Eng C, Legius E, Maher ER, van Noesel MM, Verloes A, Viskochil DH, Wagner A, Weksberg R, Caron HN, Hennekam RC. The development of a clinical screening instrument for tumour predisposition syndromes in childhood cancer patients. Eur J Cancer. 2013;49(15):3247–54.
5. Hopman S, Merks J, Eussen H, Douben H, Snijder S, Hennekam R, de Klein A, Caron H. Structural genome variations in individuals with childhood cancer and tumour predisposition syndromes. Eur J Cancer. 2013;49(9):2170–8.
6. Malkin D, Nichols KE, Zelley K, Schiffman JD. Predisposition to pediatric and hematologic cancers: a moving target. Am Soc Clin Oncol Educ Book. 2014;34:e44–55.
7. Plon SE, Wheeler DA, Strong LC, Tomlinson GE, Pirics M, Meng Q, Cheung HC, Begin PR, Muzny DM, Lewis L, Biegel JA, Gibbs RA. Identification of genetic susceptibility to childhood cancer through analysis of genes in parallel. Cancer Genet. 2011;204(1):19–25.
8. Custódio G, Parise GA, Kiesel Filho N, Komechen H, Sabbaga CC, Rosati R, Grisa L, Parise IZ, Pianovski MA, Fiori CM, Ledesma JA, Barbosa JR, Figueiredo FR, Sade ER, Ibañez H, Arram SB, Stinghen ST, Mengarelli LR, Figueiredo MM, Carvalho DC, Avilla SG, Woiski TD, Poncio LC, Lima GF, Pontarolo R, Lalli E, Zhou Y, Zambetti GP, Ribeiro RC, Figueiredo BC. Impact of neonatal screening and surveillance for the TP53 R337H mutation on early detection of childhood adrenocortical tumors. J Clin Oncol. 2013;31(20):2619–26.
9. Victor A, Weis E, Messow CM, Marron M, Haaf T, Spix C, Galetzka D. Searching for gene expression differences in primary fibroblasts between patients with one and two neoplasms in childhood. Pediatr Hematol Oncol. 2013;30(1):33–45.
10. deMartel C, Ferlay J, Franceschi S, et al. Global burden of cancers attributable to infections in 2008: a review and synthetic analysis. Lancet Oncol. 2012;13:607–15.
11. Pritchard-Jones K, Pieters R, Reaman G, et al. Sustaining innovation and improvement in the treatment of childhood cancer: lessons from high-income countries. Lancet Oncol. 2013;14(3):e95–e103. doi:10.1016/S1470-2045(13)70010-X.
12. Rushton J, López-Terrada D. Molecular and genetic basis of childhood cancer. Cancer Biomark. 2010;9(1–6):211–34.
13. Davidoff AM. Pediatric oncology. Semin Pediatr Surg. 2010;19(3):225–33.
14. Paugh SW, Stocco G, Evans WE. Pharmacogenomics in pediatric leukemia. Curr Opin Pediatr. 2013;22(6):703–10.
15. Tsimberidou AM, Eggermont AMM, Schilsky RL. Precision cancer medicine: the future is now, only better. Am Soc Clin Oncol Educ Book. 2014;34:61–9.
16. Evans WE, Crews KR, Pui CH. A health-care system perspective on implementing genomic medicine: pediatric acute lymphoblastic leukemia as a paradigm. Clin Pharmacol Ther. 2013; 94(2):224–9.
17. UICC. Childhood cancer: rising to the challenge. Geneva: UICC; 2006.
18. Nyawira G, Kahaki K, Kariuki-Wanyoike M. Survival among retinoblastoma patients at the Kenyatta National Hospital, Kenya. J Ophtholmol East Cent South Afr. 2013;1:16–9.
19. Kazadi Lukusa A, Aloni MN, Kadima-Tshimanga B, Mvitu-Muaka M, Gini Ehungu JL, Ngiyulu R, Ekulu Mfutu P, Budiongo Nzazi A. Retinoblastoma in the democratic Republic of Congo: 20-year review from a tertiary hospital in Kinshasa. J Cancer Epidemiol. 2012;2012, 920468. doi:10.1155/2012/920468.

20. Israels T, Borgstein E, Pidini D, Chagaluka G, de Kraker J, Kamiza S, Molyneux EM. Management of children with a Wilms tumor in Malawi, sub-Saharan Africa. J Pediatr Hematol Oncol. 2012;34(8):606–10.
21. Gray WN, Szulczewski LJ, Regan SMP, Williams JA, Pai ALH. Cultural influences in pediatric cancer from diagnosis to cure/end of life. J Pediatr Oncol Nurs. 2014;31(5):252–71.
22. Ribeiro RC, Steliarova-Foucher E, Magrath I, Lemerle J, Eden T, Forget C, Mortara I, Tabah-Fisch I, Divino JJ, Miklavec T, Howard SC, Cavalli F. Baseline status of paediatric oncology care in ten low-income or mid-income countries receiving my child matters support: a descriptive study. Lancet Oncol. 2008;9(8):721–9.
23. Parkin DM, Whelan SL, Ferlay J, Teppo L, Thomas DB, editors. Cancer incidence in five continents, vol. 8. Lyon: IARC; 2004. IARC Scientific Publication no. 155.
24. Ferlay J, Shin HR, Bray F, Forman D, Mathers C, Parkin DM. GLPBPCAN 2008 v2.0—cancer incidence and mortality worldwide: IARC cancer base N. 10. Lyon: International Agency for Research on Cancer; 2010. http://globocan.iarc.fr. Accessed 29 Nov 2014.
25. Pearce MS, Parker L. Childhood cancer registrations in the developing world: sill more boys than girls. Int J Cancer. 2001;91:402–6.
26. Stiller CA. Epidemiology and genetics of childhood cancer. Oncogene. 2004;23:6429–44.
27. Teplick A, Kowalski M, et al. Screening in cancer predisposition syndromes: guidelines for the general pediatrician. Eur J Pediatr. 2011;170(3):285–94.
28. World Health Organization, Community Genetic Services. Report of a WHO consultation on community genetics in low and middle income countries. Geneva: WHO; 2010. 13–14 Sep 2010.
29. Zimmern RL, Kroese M. The evaluation of genetics tests. J Public Health. 2007;29(3):246–50.
30. Marteau TM, Lerman C. Genetic risk behavioral change. BMJ. 2001;322:1056–9.
31. McClure JB. Are biomarkers useful treatment aids for promoting health behavior change? An empirical review. Am J Prev Med. 2002;22:200–7.
32. Westbrook MT, Legge V, Pennay M. Attitudes towards disability in a multicultural society. Soc Sci Med. 1993;36:615–23.
33. Goss PE, et al. Challenges to effective cancer control in China, India, and Russia. Lancet Oncol. 2014;15(5):489–538.
34. Modell B. Kinship and medical genetics: a clinician's perspective. In: Clarke A, Parsons E, editors. Culture, kinship and genes. London: Macmillan; 1997. p. 27–39.
35. Bredart A. Psycho-social aspects of breast cancer susceptibility testing: a literature review. Eur J Cancer Care. 1998;7:174–90.
36. Rodriguez-Galindo FP, Morrissey L, Frazier L. Global challenges in pediatric oncology. Curr Opin Pediatr. 2013;25:3–15.
37. Wang V, Marsh FH. Ethical principles and cultural integrity in health care delivery: Asian ethnocultural perspectives in genetic services. J Genet Couns. 1992;1:81–92.
38. Dejesus M, Miller EB. Examining breast cancer screening barriers among central American and Mexican immigrant women: fatalistic beliefs or structural factors? Health Care Women In. 2015;36(5):593–607.
39. Beamer L, Linder L, Wu B, Egger J. The impact of genomics on oncology nursing. Nurs Clin North Am. 2013;48(4):585–626.
40. Kingsmore SF, Lantos JD, Dinwiddie DL, et al. Next generation community genetics for low-and middle income countries. Genome Med. 2012;4:25. http://genomemedicine.com/content/4/3/25.
41. Meiser B, et al. Cultural aspects of cancer genetics: setting a research agenda. J Med Genet. 2001;38:425–9.
42. Aspinwall LG, Taber JM, Kohlmann W, Leaf SL, Leachman SA. Unaffected family members report improvements in daily routine sun protection 2 years following melanoma genetic testing. Genet Med. 2014;16(11):846–53. doi:10.1038/gim.2014.37.
43. World Health Organization equity monitoring. http://www.who.int/gho/health_equity/en/
44. Coyne I, O'Mathúna DP, Gibson F, Shields L, Sheaf G. Interventions for promoting participation in shared decision-making for children with cancer. Cochrane Database Syst Rev. 2013;6, CD008970. doi:10.1002/14651858.CD008970.pub2.

45. Hoskins LM, Werner-Lin A. A multi-case report of the pathways to and through genetic testing and cancer risk management for BRCA mutation-positive women aged 18–25. J Genet Couns. 2013;22(1):27–38.
46. Magrath I, Epelman S. Cancer in adolescents and young adults in countries with limited resources. Curr Oncol Rep. 2013;15(4):332–46.
47. Bosch FX, Broker TR, Forman D, Moscicki AB, Gillison ML, Doorbar J, Stern PL, Stanley M, Arbyn M, Poljak M, Cuzick J, Castle PE, Schiller JT, Markowitz LE, Fisher WA, Canfell K, Denny LA, Franco EL, Steben M, Kane MA, Schiffman M, Meijer CJ, Sankaranarayanan R, Castellsagué X, Kim JJ, Brotons M, Alemany L, Albero G, Diaz M, de Sanjosé S. Comprehensive control of human papillomavirus infections and related diseases. ICO monograph 'comprehensive control of HPV infections and related diseases'. Vaccine. 2013;30(S6):G1–31.
48. Kellie SJ, Howard SC. Global child health priorities: what role for paediatric oncologists? Eur J Cancer. 2008;44:2388–96.
49. Pui CH, Ribeiro RC. International collaboration on childhood leukemia. Int J Hematol. 2003; 78(5):383–9.
50. Pui CH, Carroll WL, Meshinchi S, Arceci RJ. Biology, risk stratification, and therapy of pediatric acute leukemias: an update. J Clin Oncol. 2011;29(5):551–65.
51. Pui CH, Robison LL, Thomas LA. Acute lymphoblastic leukaemia. Lancet. 2008;371(9617): 1030–43.
52. Hee YJ. Advancements in the treatment of pediatric acute leukemia and brain tumor—continuous efforts for 100% cure. Korean J Pediatric. 2014;57(10):434–9.
53. Kissoon N. World federation of pediatric intensive care and critical care societies: global sepsis initiative. Pediatr Crit Care Med. 2011;12(5):494–503.
54. Mukherjee D. Disparities in access to pediatric neurooncological surgery in the United States. Pediatrics. 2009;124(4):e688–96.
55. World Health Organization. GLOBOCAN. Cancer incidence and mortality worldwide in 2008. Age specific cancer incidence tables. 2008. http://globocan.iarc.fr.
56. Harding R, Albertyn R, Sherr L, Gwyther L. Pediatric palliative care in sub-Saharan Africa: a systematic review of the evidence for care models, interventions, and outcomes. J Pain Symptom Manage. 2014;47(3):642–51.
57. Delgado E, Barfield RC, Baker JN, et al. Availability of palliative care services for children with cancer in economically diverse regions of the world. Eur J Cancer. 2010;46(12):2260–6.
58. Shad A, Ashraf MS, Hafeez H. Development of palliative-care services in a developing country: Pakistan. J Pediatr Hematol Oncol. 2011;33:S62–3.
59. Ddungu H. Palliative care: what approaches are suitable in developing countries? Br J Haematol. 2011;154:728–35.
60. Wolfe J. Recognizing a global need for high quality pediatric palliative care. Pediatr Blood Cancer. 2011;57:187–8.
61. Uys L. Aspects of the care of people with HIV/AIDS in South Africa. Public Health Nurs. 2003;20(4):271–80.
62. Saad R, Huijer HA, Noureddine S, et al. Bereaved parental evaluation of the quality of a palliative care program in Lebanon. Pediatr Blood Cancer. 2011;57(2):310–6.
63. Laubisch J. Personal communication. 2014.
64. Wiener L, McConnell D, Latella L, Ludi E. Cultural and religious considerations in pediatric palliative care. Palliat Support Care. 2013;11(1):47–67.
65. Perkins HS, Geppert CMA, Gonzales A, et al. Cross-cultural similarities and differences in attitudes about advance care planning. J Gen Intern Med. 2002;17:48–57.
66. Sullivan R, Kowalczyk JR, Agarwal B, Ladenstein R, Fitzgerald E, Barr R, Steliarova-Foucher E, Magrath I, Howard SC, Kruger M, Valsecchi MG, Biondi A, Grundy P, Smith MA, Adamson P, Vassal G, Pritchard-Jones K. New policies to address the global burden of childhood cancers. Lancet Oncol. 2013;14(3):e125–35.

Chapter 30
Cancer Care Among Immigrants to North America

Bahar Javdan and Barrie Cassileth

The chapter begins with an overview of the obstacles immigrants have faced obtaining cancer screening and care in their home countries followed by the issues they face in their effort to seek cancer care in the United States. The cancer-promoting habits they bring with them to the United States as well as their unique cultural beliefs also play an important role and are discussed. Because complementary therapy use is prevalent among ethnic minorities [1] and constitutes an important part of health practice belief systems; it is discussed under a separate subheading. The chapter concludes with descriptions of immigrant acculturation and suggestions for how healthcare practitioners can better educate and deliver culturally appropriate medical care to immigrant patients.

Obstacles to Screening and Cancer Care in Immigrants' Home Countries

The home countries of many immigrants are plagued by an insufficient number of healthcare providers, especially physicians trained to treat complex diseases such as cancer. In China and India, for example, there is a severe shortage of oncologists, especially in rural areas [2]. Immigrant patients who are not accustomed to modern medical care are far less familiar with cancer prevention and modern treatment than are their indigenous, acculturated peers.

In many countries such as China, patients seek medical care only when symptoms arise. Routine or regular health screenings are rarely sought. Chinese patients tend to base their sense of well-being on how they feel day-to-day without

B. Javdan, B.A. • B. Cassileth, Ph.D. (✉)
Integrative Medicine, Memorial Sloan Kettering Cancer Center,
1429 First Avenue, New York, NY, 10021, USA
e-mail: Cassileth@mskcc.org

M. Silbermann (ed.), *Cancer Care in Countries and Societies in Transition*,
DOI 10.1007/978-3-319-22912-6_30

consideration of preventing future disease [3]. Similarly, most cancer centers in China focus on treatment only, rather than on prevention and detection [4]. As with Chinese immigrants, South Asian immigrants are not aware of the concept of screening for asymptomatic diseases in seemingly healthy individuals, and routine screening is not practiced in their home countries [5]. Mammograms are not included in routine breast cancer screening in the public hospitals of many immigrants' home countries. Instead, healthcare providers recommend mammograms only after a lump has been detected [6].

India's highly patriarchal society plays an integral role in the inaccessibility of proper cancer care, as the healthcare problems of men and young family members take precedence over those of women and the elderly [7]. Male partners and elders in the family can block women's access to medical care by not consenting to doctor visits. In a study performed in Karnataka, India, 66.4 % of rural and 37.9 % of urban underprivileged women stated needing the permission of their male spouse or elder for medical testing [8]. In another study, 40 % of noncompliant Indian women stated that their domestic chores and family care responsibilities prevented them from undergoing screening [9]. Therefore, it is not surprising that Indian women are diagnosed with breast cancer at much more advanced stages than are women in developed countries [2]. The same observation has been noted in many Middle Eastern countries [10].

Obstacles to Immigrants' Cancer Care in the United States

The United States and Canada have large and heterogeneous immigrant populations. The largest immigrant groups in the United States come from Mexico, China, and India [11]. The Middle East also represents a substantial and diverse immigrant group in the United States. These areas of the world are the focus of this chapter. The majority of immigrants described here were found to have resided in the United States for 10–20 years.

Ethnic minorities in the United Statesare disproportionately uninsured. In one study, approximately 38 % of Latinos, 24 % of African-Americans, and 22 % of Asian Americans/Pacific Islanders were found to be uninsured, compared to 14 % of non-Latino whites [12]. The absence of access to insurance is a new reality for many immigrants, such as those from Mexico and Columbia, where cancer care and control is a component of health insurance programs throughout the country [13].

Studies show that immigrants, especially those of low–middle income, are less likely to utilize cancer screening, putting themselves at risk of being diagnosed with advanced-stage cancer [14]. In a study investigating breast cancer-screening practices among first-generation immigrant women from South Asia and the Middle East, only 52 % reported having had breast cancer screening in the previous 2 years [6]. This is substantially lower than the national average of 67 % for all women in the United States[15]. Another study reported that only 32 % of non-English-speaking Chinese-American women, compared to 86 % of white American women, had ever had a mammogram [16]. Data from the New York State Cancer Services

Partnership (CSP) reveal low participation in breast and cervical screening among Arab women living in America. In the Queens and Brooklyn Partnerships, less than 1 % of Arab American immigrant women living in the area were screened over a period of 3 years [17].

In addition, several studies demonstrate that cancer disparities continue to exist among immigrants even after controlling for influential confounders such as health care coverage, age, and education [18]. This suggests that immigrants' seemingly lower access to cancer care and screening may be explained by more than socioeconomic differences.

Cancer-Promoting Habits Among Immigrants to the United States

Latino and Asian immigrants have a high incidence of gastric cancer. Typically, this is due to the high rates of *Helicobacter pylori* infection in their countries of origin [19, 20]. Such circumstances stem from immigrants' life conditions in their home countries. Immigrants tend to continue their cancer-promoting habits when they migrate to the United States Arab American tobacco rates (41 % and 38 % among men and women, respectively) are well above the national US average of 23 % [21, 22]. In many Arab immigrants' home countries, tobacco rates are among the highest in the world, and tobacco cessation programs are just beginning to take ground [23].

In South Asia, chewing areca nut (the seed of the areca palm tree) is a popular pastime. In addition to being used for religious purposes areca nut is regarded by many South Asians to have health benefits. It is often used as a traditional Ayurvedic medicine, specifically as a purgative and intoxicant to treat various infections as well as certain gynecologic problems [24]. However, areca nut use has been associated with oral cancer [25].

South Asians are at much greater risk for developing oral cancer due to high rates of tobacco chewing and smoking as well as areca nut consumption [24]. Oral cancer rates among South Asians are much higher than the national average in the United States and the United Kingdom [26, 27]. This is attributed to the continuation of areca nut use among South Asians after migration [28]. In a study investigating paan and gutka (smokeless tobacco combined with areca nut) usage in 138 first-generation Bangladeshi and Indian-Gujarati immigrant adults in the New York metropolitan area, 77 % of Indian-Gujaratis were current users of gutka, and 70 % of Bangladeshis were current users of paan [29].

Immigrant Patients' Health Beliefs

It is essential to understand how cultural beliefs influence patients' understanding and behavior concerning risk assessment and care. Cancer fatalism, the notion that cancer, regardless of stage or specific diagnosis, is a "death sentence," and is prevalent among many ethnic groups. In a study investigating cervical cancer screening among immigrants, cancer fatalism was a shared belief across Middle Eastern, Asian, and Hispanic groups [30]. The belief that death is an inevitable outcome of cancer is a major barrier to cancer screening and treatment.

In China, Ming Dynasty (1368–1644) Taoist beliefs are said to underlie pervasive cancer fatalism. Ming Dynasty beliefs hold that there is an "invisible force," similar to fate, that is responsible for everything in the course of human life, including illness and death [31]. This fatalistic attitude is not conducive to participation in health care interventions, especially preventive efforts and screening.

Among Arab Americans, cancer fatalism is associated with a strong identification of God in the day-to-day happenings of human life. In a study of the cancer beliefs of US Arab immigrants, Arab women were reported to thank God if they received a positive health diagnosis. They perceived cancer diagnosis as "God's punishment," and believed that the course of their cancer was predominantly under God's control as opposed to their own. God was viewed as the "omnipotent protector and healer," thus minimizing the value of prevention or treatment [32].

In addition to cancer fatalism, other cultural beliefs may hinder timely cancer care. In China, for example, there is widespread perception that death after cancer diagnosis is inevitable, and that the final outcome is predestined and unchangeable by medical intervention. In addition to Ming Dynasty notions, Chinese patients are reluctant to speak openly about their cancer before and after diagnosis, believing that "negative thoughts" will lead to worry and to poorer health conditions. Both primary and secondary cancer prevention measures are thought detrimental to a harmonious state of health [2]. Breast and cervical cancers, because they are associated with female sexual organs, are particularly taboo topics in rural China and for that reason are barriers to screening. Chinese women in rural China not only avoid participation in screening for these cancers, but are also reluctant to discuss their health status in their personal lives before and after breast and cervical cancer screening [33].

In India, cancer is a socially stigmatized disease. This prevents patients from seeking treatment until the cancer has progressed to an advanced stage. Patients keep the diagnosis a secret from family and friends, often going to extreme lengths at the expense of a positive outcome with proper treatment [2]. One study showed that Indian women refused colorectal cancer screening because cancer diagnosis was "synonymous with death," and, ironically, that need for a diagnostic biopsy was sufficient justification to avoid attending screening [34].

Cancer fatalism, nihilism, and related beliefs are barriers to cancer screening and to immigrant patients' willingness to participate in clinical trials [35]. A New York City study found that Chinese cultural beliefs were the primary reason that immigrant Chinese patients declined to participate in clinical trials. Some patients were under the impression that merely screening for cancer would ultimately cause cancer [36]. As these data indicate, immigrants' low cancer-screening rates may be largely attributed to their cancer-related beliefs and attitudes, especially among those migrating from low–middle income countries. Having spent the majority of their lives in their home countries and having adopted certain belief systems and ways of life, immigrants bring these beliefs with them when they migrate to the West.

Complementary Therapies and Cancer: What They Can and Cannot Do

In developed countries and elsewhere where evidence-based therapies are the rule, complementary therapies are applied for purposes of symptom control. At Memorial Sloan Kettering Cancer Center (MSK), the home base for the authors of this chapter, and in many other evidence-based practices worldwide, complementary therapies are appropriately applied as adjuncts to mainstream cancer treatment. They are not used to treat cancer because complementary therapies do not treat disease. Rather, they control many physical and emotional symptoms associated with cancer and with modern cancer treatment [37].

Multiple publications in oncology and other medical journals worldwide document the evidence for various complementary therapies to successfully control such symptoms. These manageable symptoms include pain, nausea and vomiting, fatigue, hot flashes, xerostomia (extreme dry mouth), sexual dysfunction, stress, anxiety and depression, neuropathy, insomnia, and possibly lymphedema [38].

Internationally, evidence-based complementary therapies for symptom control include some or all of those practiced at MSK: meditation, yoga, and other mind–body therapies, massage therapy, acupuncture, dietary, nutrition, and herbal remedy counseling, music therapy, and exercise [39]. The importance of exercise and maintaining fitness cannot be overstressed. It is the one complementary therapy that is well documented to produce survival benefits. Overweight and sedentary lifestyles are not healthy, and there is an inverse relationship between level of post-cancer-diagnosis physical activity and risk of cancer recurrence and mortality [40].

What Guides Immigrants to Use Various Therapies

The many ways in which culture and health beliefs impact health-seeking behavior also guide patients' use of complementary therapies. These beliefs also may influence a patient's decision to rely not on modern medicine to treat cancer, but rather on complementary therapies such as acupuncture, meditation, or herbal remedies from their home countries. Many patients seek the typically ancient therapies of their ethnic groups, all of which have rich histories of traditional medicine. For example, Asian Americans use Traditional Chinese Medicine (TCM), which consists of a broad range of medicine practices including acupuncture and herbal remedies [41]. In China, patients mainly rely on TCM to personalize their cancer treatment and to achieve either of the following effects: anticancer activity, chemosensitization, or a yin-yang balance. The underlying principle behind TCM is that mitigating disruptions in the flow of vital energy (qi) in the body through meridian channels is necessary to restore health and "balance." While some patients seek TCM for symptom relief, others hope that TCM will exert a curative effect [42].

Latinos tend to seek healers such as curanderos (folk curer), espiritistas (spiritists), and yerberas (herbalists) [43]. In a study conducted in Mexico, approximately 70 % of the parents of pediatric patients reported using unproven methods. The reasons cited were to mitigate the side effects of conventional treatment (53 %), to fight or cure cancer (32 %), and to achieve both (14 %). Although herbal remedies were most commonly reported (69 %), other products taken orally included rattlesnake, coral calcium, shark cartilage, propolis, royal jelly, opossum, crab, urine therapy, and turkey vulture. Homeopathy also was used (25 %) [44].

India's population also relies largely on traditional medicines to treat cancer, as many patients perceive them as effective as Western medicine. Indian clinicians often integrate popular traditional remedies into their treatments. India has 250,000 homeopathic doctors, and homeopathy is one of the seven recognized national medical systems in that part of the world, despite the absence of data indicating that homeopathy offers any benefit whatsoever [2].

In the Middle East, frequently used natural remedies include honey for the prevention of mucositis in head and neck cancer patients, kefir and yogurt to improve sleep in colorectal cancer patients, and HESA-A (a formulation containing wild celery, cumin, and king prawn) to improve the quality of life in breast and colon cancer patients [45].

Across immigrant groups in the United States, Asian Americans reportedly have higher rates of complementary or alternative therapy use (31.8 %) compared to other ethnic minority groups [46]. In the literature, more studies have been conducted investigating such use for cancer among Chinese immigrants (due to their well-established use of TCM both in their home countries and in the West) followed by Hispanic immigrants. These are the main groups discussed in this section.

Most studies report that the majority of patients in North America, including ethnic minorities, appropriately use complementary modalities as adjuvants rather than as substitutes for mainstream conventional care [47, 48]. In a 2002 national health review survey investigating complementary care among racial and ethnic minority adults, approximately a third of respondents reported using complementary modalities because "it would be interesting to try" and another third responded that "[complementary modalities] with conventional medicine would help." Only 17 % of patients reported seeking complementary care because "conventional treatments would not help." Hispanic respondents were more likely to report complementary care because conventional treatments were too expensive, highlighting the fact that certain underserved populations may use alternative therapies as substitutes for the mainstream conventional treatment they cannot afford [49].

Conversely, studies investigating complementary care in specific immigrant groups find mixed results. While some patients appropriately use complementary therapies for symptom management and overall health maintenance, others use them for curative purposes. For example, a Canadian study investigating Chinese immigrants' perceptions about complementary modalities and cancer found that all respondents believed that mainstream medicine was more effective in curing cancer than is TCM, their complementary therapy of choice. Rather, complementary therapies were used appropriately to mitigate pain and the side effects of chemotherapy and to boost immune function [50]. However, in another study, 66 % of Chinese respondents believed that herbal therapy could cure chronic disease [51].

Disclosure and Nondisclosure of Nonmainstream Therapies

Immigrants in the United States, especially Hispanics, have high rates of nondisclosure of complementary or alternative therapy use to their healthcare providers [52]. This poses major health concerns for two reasons: (1) patients substituting "alternatives" to conventional treatment risk cancer progression, and (2) patients using complementary modalities such as herbal remedies alongside conventional treatment risk negative side effects and adverse reactions. While some herbal remedies may help mitigate chemotherapy and radiation therapy-induced side effects such as diarrhea and poor appetite, others can be harmful [53]. For example, Aristolochia (commonly known as birthwort, pipevine, or Dutchman's pipe) is a popular anti-inflammatory, diuretic, and antibiotic medicinal Chinese plant. However, it has been linked to aristolochic-acid nephropathy and upper-urinary-tract carcinomas [54] and has been classified by WHO as a type 1 carcinogen.

In addition to the harmful effects of some TCMs, herb–drug interactions represent a major concern. A common example of adverse herb–drug reactions include St. John's Wort, a popular herbal remedy for depression, and irinotecan, an important drug used to treat advanced colorectal and lung cancer. Another often-seen adverse interaction is that of the herb ginseng and corticosteroid compounds, which are major cancer treatment regimens [53].

Researchers argue that clinicians should ask about their patients' use of nonmainstream therapies. This is necessary to rule out any potentially harmful effects and to check for possible herb–drug interactions during mainstream cancer treatment. Identifying and characterizing nonmainstream therapy use would help expose the modalities of greatest concern. The source of herb–drug interactions noted above is a free resource of information produced by MSK about the utility and problems associated with herbal and other remedies [53].

The Relationship Between Immigrant Acculturation and Health Practices

A study investigating TCM use among Chinese immigrants found that more than a third of patients used TCM alongside conventional treatment [55]. However, a study performed in Canada found that, compared to highly acculturated Chinese immigrant patients, those with low acculturation were more likely to use TCM [56]. A common proxy measure of acculturation is the number of years lived in the United

States. Acculturation is associated with increased odds of cancer screening for those who have lived in the United States for 10 years or more [57]. Acculturation appears to reduce immigrants' adherence to previous cultural beliefs, and exposure to Western health practices is thought to facilitate the transition to better preventive health behaviors. One study found that compared to Chinese immigrant women with a more "Chinese/Eastern cultural view," those with a Western cultural view were significantly more likely to have regular mammograms. Moreover, English fluency was positively correlated with a greater number of mammograms and clinical breast examinations [58].

A similar trend was observed in other immigrant groups. For example, highly acculturated Latina women were twice as likely to practice correct breast self-examination as were women with low acculturation [59]. Another study assessed the relationship between Hispanic acculturation and participation in colorectal cancer screening. It showed that low acculturation correlated with underutilization of endoscopic colorectal cancer screening [60]. It is also reported that, as Latinos become increasingly acculturated, they become more autonomous in making medical decisions, seek more information, and want to hear a proper diagnosis and prognosis instead of avoiding the truth [61]. Across several related studies, these trends hold true even after controlling for other factors such as age, income, education, and health insurance.

This chapter aims to highlight the importance of delivering viable, modern medicine in the United States and elsewhere. Understanding the cultural factors that underlie immigrants' approaches to cancer care and their high nondisclosure rates suggest the importance of initiating relevant discussions. Guidance about the appropriate use of complementary therapies and avoidance of nonviable "alternative" cancer treatments is important for immigrants to the United States and for patients everywhere. Such understanding will encourage the use of preventive health care and routine screening. The consequent result will be earlier cancer detection, proper treatment, and decreased mortality.

References

1. Mackenzie ER, Taylor L, Bloom BS, Hufford DJ, Johnson JC. Ethnic minority use of complementary and alternative medicine (CAM): a national probability survey of CAM utilizers. Altern Ther Health Med. 2003;9(4):50–6.
2. Goss PE, Strasser-weippl K, Lee-bychkovsky BL, et al. Challenges to effective cancer control in China, India, and Russia. Lancet Oncol. 2014;15(5):489–538.
3. Kwok C, Sullivan G. The concepts of health and preventive health practices of Chinese Australian women in relation to cancer screening. J Transcult Nurs. 2007;18(2):118–26.
4. National Cancer Control Plan. China. http://www.who.int/cancer/modules/China.pdf. Accessed 31 Dec 2014.
5. Pearson N, Croucher R, Marcenes W, O'farrell M. Dental service use and the implications for oral cancer screening in a sample of Bangladeshi adult medical care users living in Tower Hamlets, UK. Br Dent J. 1999;186(10):517–21.
6. Hasnain M, Menon U, Ferrans CE, Szalacha L. Breast cancer screening practices among first-generation immigrant Muslim women. J Womens Health (Larchmt). 2014;23(7):602–12.

7. Broom A, Doron A, Tovey P. The inequalities of medical pluralism: hierarchies of health, the politics of tradition and the economies of care in Indian oncology. Soc Sci Med. 2009;69(5):698–706.
8. Vallikad E, Krishnan, Kumaraswamy S, editors. Studies, strategies, and concepts for women's health in women's hands: a community approach for the control of cancer cervix in Karnataka, India. Bangalore: Kidwai Memorial Institute of Oncology; 1997.
9. Basu P, Sarkar S, Mukherjee S, et al. Women's perceptions and social barriers determine compliance to cervical screening: results from a population based study in India. Cancer Detect Prev. 2006;30(4):369–74.
10. Kawar LN. Barriers to breast cancer screening participation among Jordanian and Palestinian American women. Eur J Oncol Nurs. 2013;17(1):88–94.
11. http://www.cnn.com/2013/11/06/us/immigration-statistics-fast-facts/. Accessed Jan 2015.
12. Brown ER. Public policies to extend health care coverage. In: Andersen RM, Rice TH, Kominski GF, editors. Changing the U.S. health care system: key issues in health services policy and management. 2nd ed. San Francisco: Jossey-Bass; 2001. p. 31–58.
13. Farmer P, Frenk J, Knaul FM, et al. Expansion of cancer care and control in countries of low and middle income: a call to action. Lancet. 2010;376(9747):1186–93.
14. Ghafoor A, Jemal A, Ward E, Cokkinides V, Smith R, Thun M. Trends in breast cancer by race and ethnicity. CA Cancer J Clin. 2003;53(6):342–55.
15. Nunnally JC. Psychometric theory. 2nd ed. New York: McGraw-Hill; 1978. p. 421.
16. Jiang X, Liao Z, Hao J, et al. Palliative care education in China: insight into one medical university. J Pain Symptom Manage. 2011;41(4):796–800.
17. New York State Department of Health. Cancer services program partnerships data: 2004–2006.
18. Zhao X. Cancer information disparities between U.S.- and foreign-born populations. J Health Commun. 2010;15 Suppl 3:5–21.
19. Alexander GA, Brawley OW. Association of Helicobacter pylori infection with gastric cancer. Mil Med. 2000;165:21–7.
20. Wong BC, Lam SK, Wong WM, et al. Helicobacter pylori eradication to prevent gastric cancer in a high-risk region of China: a randomized controlled trial. JAMA. 2004;291:187–94.
21. Rice VH, Kulwicki A. Cigarette use among Arab Americans in the Detroit metropolitan area. Public Health Rep. 1992;107(5):589–94.
22. National Cancer Health Statistics, Center for Disease Control and Prevention. Prevalence of current smoking among adults, aged 18 years and older: United states, 1997–2001. MMWR, 2002. Report No. 50.
23. World Health Organization. Making a difference. Geneva: World Health Organization; 1999.
24. Auluck A, Hislop G, Poh C, Zhang L, Rosin MP. Areca nut and betel quid chewing among South Asian immigrants to Western countries and its implications for oral cancer screening. Rural Remote Health. 2009;9(2):11–8.
25. Jeng JH, Chang MC, Hahn LJ. Role of areca nut in betel quid-associated chemical carcinogenesis: current awareness and future perspectives. Oral Oncol. 2001;37(6):477–92.
26. Liu L, Kumar SK, Sedghizadeh PP, Jayakar AN, Shuler CF. Oral squamous cell carcinoma incidence by subsite among diverse racial and ethnic populations in California. Oral Surg Oral Med Oral Pathol Oral Radiol Endod. 2008;105(4):470–80.
27. Moles DR, Fedele S, Speight PM, dos Santos PSR, Silva I. Oral and pharyngeal cancer in South Asians and non-South Asians in relation to socioeconomic deprivation in South East England. Br J Cancer. 2008;98(3):633–5.
28. Warnakulasuriya S. Areca nut use following migration and its consequences. Addict Biol. 2000;7(1):127–32.
29. Changrani J, Gany FM, Cruz G, Kerr R, Katz R. Paan and gutka use in the United States: a pilot study in Bangladeshi and Indian-Gujarati immigrants in New York City. J Immigr Refug Stud. 2006;4(1):99–110.
30. Johnson CE, Mues KE, Mayne SL, Kiblawi AN. Cervical cancer screening among immigrants and ethnic minorities: a systematic review using the health belief model. J Low Genit Tract Dis. 2008;12(3):232–41.

31. Cheng H, Sit JW, Twinn SF, Cheng KK, Thorne S. Coping with breast cancer survivorship in Chinese women: the role of fatalism or fatalistic voluntarism. Cancer Nurs. 2013;36(3):236–44.
32. Shah SM, Ayash C, Pharaon NA, Gany FM. Arab American immigrants in New York: health care and cancer knowledge, attitudes, and beliefs. J Immigr Minor Health. 2008;10(5):429–36.
33. Zhao L, Li S, Wang T. Cross-sectional study on knowledge, attitude and behavior of breast cancer screening among women in Beijing. Chin J Publ Health. 2008;24:658–9.
34. Basu P, Sarkar S, Mukherjee S, et al. Women's perceptions and social barriers determine compliance to cervical screening: results from a population based study in India. Cancer Detect Prev. 2006;30(4):369–74.
35. Murthy VH, Krumholz HM, Gross CP. Participation in cancer clinical trials: race-, sex-, and age-based disparities. JAMA. 2004;291(22):2720–6.
36. Lin JS, Finlay A, Tu A, Gany FM. Understanding immigrant Chinese Americans' participation in cancer screening and clinical trials. J Community Health. 2005;30:451–66.
37. Deng G, Cassileth BR, Yeung KS. Complementary therapies for cancer-related symptoms. J Support Oncol. 2004;2(5):419–26.
38. Deng G, Cassileth B. Integrative oncology: an overview. Am Soc Clin Oncol Educ Book. 2014;233–42.
39. Cassileth BR. The integrative medicine service at memorial sloan-kettering cancer center. Semin Oncol. 2002;29:585–8.
40. Lemanne D, Cassileth B, Gubili J. The role of physical activity in cancer prevention, treatment, recovery, and survivorship. Oncology (Williston Park). 2013;27(6):580–85.
41. Hsiao AF, Wong MD, Goldstein MS, et al. Variation in complementary and alternative medicine (CAM) use across racial/ethnic groups and the development of ethnic-specific measures of CAM use. J Altern Complement Med. 2006;12(3):281–90.
42. Smith ME, Bauer-Wu S. Traditional Chinese medicine for cancer-related symptoms. Semin Oncol Nurs. 2012;28:64–74.
43. Fishman B, Bobo L, Dosub K, Womeodu RJ. Cultural issues in serving minority populations: emphasis on Mexican Americans and African Americans. Am J Med Sci. 1993;206:160–6.
44. Gomez-martinez R, Tlacuilo-parra A, Garibaldi-covarrubias R. Use of complementary and alternative medicine in children with cancer in occidental, Mexico. Pediatr Blood Cancer. 2007;49(6):820–3.
45. Ben-arye E, Ali-shtayeh MS, Nejmi M, et al. Integrative oncology research in the Middle East: weaving traditional and complementary medicine in supportive care. Support Care Cancer. 2012;20(3):557–64.
46. Su D, Li L. Trends in the use of complementary and alternative medicine in the United States: 2002–2007. J Health Care Poor Underserved. 2011;22(1):296–310.
47. Druss BG, Rosenheck RA. Association between use of unconventional therapies and conventional medical services. JAMA. 1999;282:651–6.
48. Kronenberg F, Cushman LF, Wade CM, et al. Race/ethnicity and women's use of complementary and alternative medicine in the United States: results of a national survey. Am J Public Health. 2006;96:1236–42.
49. Graham RE, Ahn AC, Davis RB, O'connor BB, Eisenberg DM, Phillips RS. Use of complementary and alternative medical therapies among racial and ethnic minority adults: results from the 2002 National Health Interview Survey. J Natl Med Assoc. 2005;97(4):535–45.
50. Watt L, Gulati S, Shaw NT, et al. Perceptions about complementary and alternative medicine use among Chinese immigrant parents of children with cancer. Support Care Cancer. 2012;20(2):253–60.
51. Quan H, Lai D, Johnson D, Verhoef M, Musto R. Complementary and alternative medicine use among Chinese and white Canadians. Can Fam Physician. 2008;54(11):1563–9.

52. Chao MT, Wade C, Kronenberg F. Disclosure of complementary and alternative medicine to conventional medical providers: variation by race/ethnicity and type of CAM. J Natl Med Assoc. 2008;100(11):1341–9.
53. http://www.mskcc.org/cancer-care/integrative-medicine/about-herbs-botanicals-other-products. Accessed Jan 2015.
54. Arlt VM, Stiborova M, Schmeiser HH. Aristolochic acid as a probable human cancer hazard in herbal remedies: a review. Mutagenesis. 2002;17(4):265–77.
55. Leng JC, Gany F. Traditional Chinese medicine use among Chinese immigrant cancer patients. J Cancer Educ. 2014;29(1):56–61.
56. Ferro MA, Leis A, Doll R, Chiu L, Chung M, Barroetavena MC. The impact of acculturation on the use of traditional Chinese medicine in newly diagnosed Chinese cancer patients. Support Care Cancer. 2007;15(8):985–92.
57. Misra R, Menon U, Vadaparampil ST, Belue R. Age- and sex-specific cancer prevention and screening practices among Asian Indian immigrants in the United States. J Investig Med. 2011;59(5):787–92.
58. Liang W, Wang J, Chen MY, Feng S, Yi B, Mandelblatt JS. Cultural views, language ability, and mammography use in Chinese American women. Health Educ Behav. 2009;36(6):1012–25.
59. Peragallo NP, Fox PG, Alba ML. Acculturation and breast self-examination among immigrant Latina women in the USA. Int Nurs Rev. 2000;47(1):38–345.
60. Shah M, Zhu K, Potter J. Hispanic acculturation and utilization of colorectal cancer screening in the United States. Cancer Detect Prev. 2006;30(3):306–12.
61. Costas-muniz R, Sen R, Leng J, Aragones A, Ramirez J, Gany F. Cancer stage knowledge and desire for information: mismatch in Latino cancer patients? J Cancer Educ. 2013;28(3):458–65.

Chapter 31
Promoting Cancer Nursing Education, Training, and Research in Countries in Transition

Lisa Kennedy Sheldon, Jeannine Brant, Kate Shaughnessy Hankle, Stella Bialous, and Barbara Lubejko

> *"Health systems can only operate with a health workforce. Achieving universal health coverage, with priority given to vulnerable groups, depends on the availability, accessibility, acceptability, and quality of health workers."*
> *A Universal Truth: No Health Without a Workforce*
>
> Global Health Workforce Alliance & WHO, 2013 [1]

The Nursing Profession Globally

With growing incidence in cancer globally, there is a great need to address the critical, unmet health needs of populations. This is especially true in countries in transition since the majority of the world's cancers (56.8 %) and cancer deaths (64.9 %) occur in less developed countries [2]. In oncology settings, workforce issues such as insufficient personnel and lack of specialty training impacted initiatives to prevent, diagnosis, and treat cancer, and provide supportive and palliative care to reduce the burden of this disease. Since nurses provide the majority of health care globally,

L.K. Sheldon, Ph.D., A.P.R.N., A.O.C.N.P. (✉)
College of Nursing and Health Sciences, University of Massachusetts-Boston, 100 Morrissey Blvd., Boston, MA, 02125, USA
e-mail: lisa.kennedysheldon@umb.edu

J. Brant, Ph.D., A.P.R.N., A.O.C.N., F.A.A.N.
Department of Nursing, Billings Clinic, 2800 Tenth Avenue North, Billings, MT, 59101, USA
e-mail: jbrant@BillingsClinic.org

K.S. Hankle, M.B.A. • B. Lubejko, R.N., M.S.
Oncology Nursing Society, 125 Enterprise Drive, Pittsburgh, PA, 15275, USA
e-mail: kes202@hotmail.com; blubejko@ons.org

S. Bialous, R.N., Dr.Ph.H., F.A.A.N.
Social and Behavioral Sciences, School of Nursing, University of California, San Francisco, 3333 California Street, Suite 340, Box 0646, San Francisco, CA 94118, USA
e-mail: stella@bialous.com

M. Silbermann (ed.), *Cancer Care in Countries and Societies in Transition*,
DOI 10.1007/978-3-319-22912-6_31

they are the major workforce contributing to world health. The World Health Organization (WHO) estimates that there are approximately 21.2 million nursing personnel globally [3]. This includes nurses, nursing auxiliaries, and midwives with wide disparities by region (Fig. 31.1) and by countries' level of economic development (Fig. 31.2).

While the nursing shortage is a global concern, in some low- and middle-income countries (LMICs) it has reached a critical level that may threaten the progress in improving health outcomes. Political will is essential in ensuring that the health workforce, including nurses and midwives, is adequate to meet the population needs and that its growth is commensurate with the growth and aging of the population

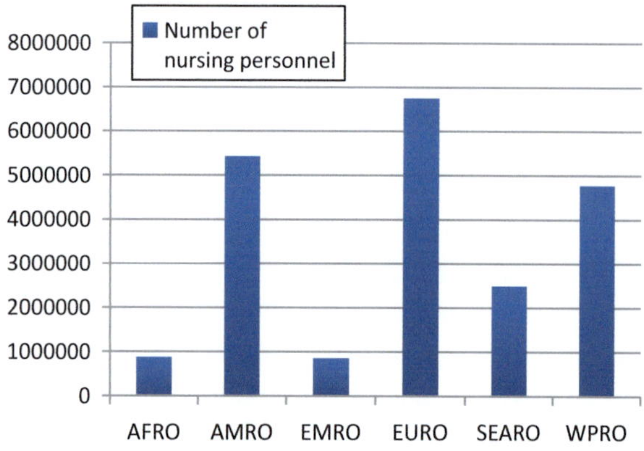

Fig. 31.1 Number of nursing personnel by WHO region. *Source*: The 2013 update, Global Health Workforce Statistics, World Health Organization, Geneva (http://www.who.int/hrh/statistics/hwfstats/). *Note*: AMRO figures include 3.25 million nursing personnel from Canada and the United States, 59 % of the total for the region

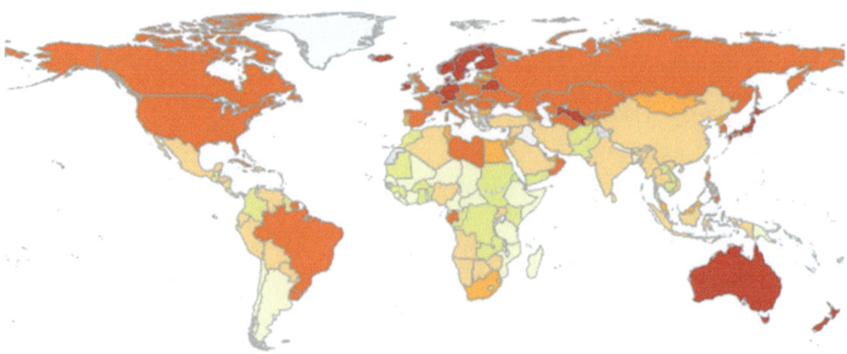

Fig. 31.2 WHO map: density of nursing and midwifery personnel (total number per 1000 population, latest available year). *Note*: AMRO figures include 3.25 million nursing personnel from Canada and the United States, 59 % of the total for the region

[1]. In fact, WHO estimates that the *world currently has four million fewer health workers than are needed*, largely because many countries lack a minimum number of personnel to meet their needs [4]. Less than 2 % of total health expenditures, globally, are spent on health workforce education. A mix of public and private mechanisms is recommended to support education, targeting the most cost-effective methods and mix of healthcare professionals. In LMICs, it is usually more cost-effective to invest in the education of nurses when compared to physicians [5, 6].

Oncology Nursing

No specific data sets exist to evaluate the workforce needs related to cancer nurses. It is known that the cancer care workforce and resources in LMIC and many countries in transition are, at best, inadequate with large disparities between high- and low-income countries [7]. The vast majority of patients with cancer in LMICs receive treatment in general hospitals, making it more difficult to estimate the actual number of oncology nurses globally. Cancer prevention, screening, and early detection are often addressed by generalist nurses working in public health systems who may or may not identify themselves as oncology specialists. The International Society of Nurses in Cancer Care (ISNCC) has 44 full members that are national cancer nursing associations, representing approximately 90,000 oncology nurses worldwide. The European Oncology Nursing Society (EONS) represents 22,000 oncology nurses and the Asian Oncology Nursing Society (AONS) represents over 30,000 nurses. Even if the actual number of nurses in oncology were 3 times higher than those represented by these member organizations, the needs of cancer patients globally would still not be met. In fact, the American Cancer Society estimated that 60 % of the 14 million yearly new cancer diagnoses occur in Africa, Asia, Central and South America [8]. Thus, efforts need to be scaled up significantly in order to meet the needs of patients with cancer as well as to meet the United Nations and Noncommunicable Disease (NCD) Alliance goal of reducing premature deaths by 25 % [9] and WHO Global Action Plan [10].

Despite some progress, patients in many LMICs still tend to receive a diagnosis of cancer at a late stage of the disease, and treatment options are scarce [7]. The emphasis in many of these countries has focused on prevention, early detection and, on the other end of the continuum, palliative care. There has been some progress in promoting prevention and early detection of cancer in LMICs [7, 11], and nurses have played key roles in ensuring that policies on cancer prevention are implemented. Evidence from nursing research has demonstrated the positive impact nurses have in improving access to services and information, but a need exists for a higher level of investment in nursing education [12].

The healthcare workforce in LMIC has also been affected by migration issues. Within LMIC, workers may leave rural settings for urban settings, where jobs are highest paying. Trained healthcare workers such as nurses may leave their home country for better paying jobs in other countries [4]. This migration is especially true in countries with conflict where personal and family safety is an additional concern, and nurses may leave to seek safer lifestyle as well as higher pay [13]. While the International Council of Nurses [14] has called upon governments to ensure the duty to care of nurses and other healthcare workers, there remains a significant safety concern for nurses caring for populations in these settings. This outward migration impacts the destination country, where education and training of nurses may differ and standards of care need to be met in the new job setting [15]. Language issues and variations in healthcare system may impact the safety of care delivery [16]. This is especially true in specialty care such as in oncology settings, where concurrent treatment regimens and complex medical issues make accurate communication essential to patient care and safety.

Vast documentation exists demonstrating a positive correlation between nursing care and patients outcomes in oncology in the outcome of patients in high-income countries [17, 18]. Furthermore, there is a growing body of evidence to demonstrate positive impact of nursing interventions on patient outcomes in LMICs [12]. In addition to improving clinical care, there is emerging evidence to suggest that evidence-based nursing care could lead to enhanced advocacy and policy development to improve cancer care delivery models and systems. For example, in Panama, nursing leadership and advocacy for improved palliative care and access to pain medication spearheaded a movement that resulted in a national palliative care program, one of the first in the region. Nurses play a significant role implementing this successful program [19]. This led Panama to propose a resolution to the World Health Assembly—the governing body of the World Health Organization—to ensure that palliative care is integrated into every national health services program, globally. The resolution was approved at the 67th Session of the World Health Assembly in May, 2014 [20] WHA, and also the Pioneros en Cuidados Paliativos de Panamá en la Organización Mundial de la Salud: Entrevista con el Dr. Gaspar Da Costa [21]. Importantly, a new White Paper is calling for strengthening the oncology nurse workforce in LMIC through education, research, policy, and evidence-based practice (EBP) [22].

Oncology Nursing Specialization

The Role of Oncology Nursing Across the Cancer Trajectory

The cancer trajectory includes many phases with unique experiences and needs along the way. Oncology nurses play an important role in cancer care throughout this disease trajectory, from prevention to early detection, diagnosis to treatment, and survivorship to palliation and end-of-life care. Nurses are often called upon to guide patients throughout each phase of the disease, providing support and resources along the way. The most significant problems along the trajectory are discussed below, and the role of nursing globally in these areas is highlighted in Table 31.1. The Scope and Standards of Oncology Nursing Practice can guide nurses who care for patients with cancer, keeping in mind that scope of practice can vary between

Table 31.1 Nursing roles throughout the cancer trajectory

Phase of the cancer trajectory	Nursing roles
Cancer prevention	Maintain and role model a healthy lifestyle
	Promote tobacco cessation
	• Support the implementation of the WHO framework convention on tobacco control
	• Inclusion of smoking cessation and cancer prevention content in nursing curricula
	• Engage in political activities that will end illicit trade of tobacco
	Provide education about healthy eating and weight maintenance that can prevent cancer
	• Diet rich in fruits, vegetables, and fiber
	• Maintenance of ideal body weight
	• Promote exercise
	Sun protection
	Encourage vaccination of HPV and HBV where resources are available
	Promote safe sexual behaviors
Early detection	Assess personal risk factors and cultural/religious beliefs about cancer
	Encourage adherence to the WHO guidelines for cancer screening within availability of resources per country
	Provide education about breast self-examination and testicular self-examination and the need to report any changes
	Teach about cancer screening and early detection of cancer in nursing curricula
	Organize community screening events and health fairs that encourage higher screening rates
	Engage in political and advocacy activities that will increase funding for cancer screening
Diagnosis	Provide emotional support for those newly diagnosed with cancer and their families
	Provide navigation for patients within the cancer system—for appointments, procedures, and other activities
	Provide education about the specific type of cancer including treatment options as recommended by the physician and possible side effects of each treatment option
Cancer treatment	Provide education about the cancer treatment employed including the following:
	Goals of treatment
	How the treatment works as appropriate to the patient's educational, literacy level
	Potential side effects of treatment—physical and emotional
	How to prevent and manage side effects of cancer treatment
	Assess for side effects of treatment and intervene early to prevent morbidity
	Provide the patient with written information (if literate) on health promotion during treatment, management of side effects, and guidelines for contacting the healthcare team
	Offer classes that educate patients on cancer treatment and side effect management such as I Can Cope

(continued)

Table 31.1 (continued)

Phase of the cancer trajectory	Nursing roles
Survivorship	Provide a survivorship care plan for patients who have completed cancer treatment, highlighting the following:
	Treatment summary
	Follow-up visits
	When to call the healthcare team
	Managing long-term side effects
	Identify persistent symptoms and manage as able to promote optimal quality of life
	Assure patients and families that uncertainty and fear of recurrence are common after completing treatment
	Offer survivorship classes that inform patients about wellness and long-term side effects and surveillance
	Encourage long-term cancer survivors to become advocates for cancer care in their individual countries, helping to distill fatalism that commonly exists
Palliation	Provide emotional support for patients and families
	Diligently assess and manage symptoms throughout the disease trajectory to decrease symptom burden
	Promote holistic care inclusive of physical, emotional, and spiritual aspects of care
	Support implementation of World Health Assembly resolution on palliative care
End-of-Life Care	Encourage patient and family to participate in end-of-life decision making
	Assess and manage deleterious symptoms that compromise quality of life
	Inform family of the impending signs of death
	Incorporate meaningful religious and spiritual practices into end-of-life care
	Development bereavement programs to support families during grieving

countries [23, 24]. The goals from the United Nations meeting on noncommunicable diseases (NCDs) concluded with a declaration to decrease the global cancer incidence by 25 % [25] and, for example, increasing screening for cervical cancer has been recommended by WHO as one of the "best buys," i.e., cost-effective measures, to tackle the global burden of cancer [26]. The World Health Organization also provides resources to assist with cancer care along these major phases of care [27]. Finally, the global goals to reduce NCDs, including cancer, by 2025 identify target initiatives from the NCD Alliance are certainly part of oncology nursing practice and include reducing tobacco use and reducing physical inactivity [9].

Cancer Prevention. Tobacco is the leading preventable cause of cancer death worldwide, causing more than five million deaths per year. Smoking is on the rise, and current trends reveal that tobacco will cause more than eight million deaths by the year 2030 with nearly 80 % of tobacco users globally living in LMICs. Tobacco use accounts for over 20 % of global cancer deaths and about 70 % of global lung cancer deaths [28]. Viruses such as hepatitis B virus (HBV) and human papilloma virus (HPV) cause up to 20 % of cancers in low-income countries [28, 29]. Cancer vaccines, such as Gardisil® to protect against HPV infection, are playing an increasing role in preventing these viral cancers. Currently, vaccination against HPV is recommended for the prevention of cervical and oropharyngeal cancers [30]. Diet and physical activity are also instrumental in preventing cancer.

Early Detection. Cancer screening guidelines exist for some cancers such as cervical, breast, colorectal, and prostate cancers. Screening guidelines for lung cancer are also being investigated in high-risk populations. Screening for these highly prevalent cancers can allow for early detection and higher cure rates. Survival of cancer is directly related to early detection. For example, breast cancer survival in developed countries approaches 90 %, whereas survival is only 39 % in parts of Africa [31]. Unfortunately, cancer is detected at advanced stages in most areas around the world [32].

Diagnosis. The diagnosis of cancer is a vulnerable time for patients. Diagnosis can be made via blood tests, bone marrow biopsies, tissue biopsies, radiographic exams, and surgery. Once spoken, the word cancer may commonly be associated with a perception of death due to the prevalence of late-stage diagnosis within the country. Fear of pain and suffering is also common.

Treatment. Cancer treatment is complex and often multimodal, involving surgery, various types of radiation therapy, chemotherapy, biotherapy, and targeted therapy. It is essential that patients have an understanding of the treatment employed and the possible side effects that exist with each treatment so that self-care strategies can be employed to prevent and manage symptoms throughout treatment.

Survivorship. Early detection and advances in cancer treatment have resulted in increased cancer survival rates in developed countries, but low survival of cancer continues to be a concern in less developed countries. For those who survive cancer, ongoing needs exist for surveillance of recurrence and management of long-term toxicities that can occur post-treatment [33, 34].

Palliative Care. Palliative care occurs throughout the disease trajectory to ameliorate deleterious symptoms that can occur along the way. While palliative care includes end-of-life care, it encompasses much more. Palliative care focuses on quality of life, symptom management, compassion, and human dignity that is essential to nursing care [35]. Excellence in pain management is an essential component of palliative care.

End of Life. Unfortunately, end-of-life care is the most common type of care provided around the world due to late diagnosis of cancer in many countries especially LMIC. Physical, emotional, and spiritual suffering often ensues, requiring diligent assessment of each individual patient and aggressive management of symptoms according to the resources available in each country.

Evidence-Based Practice and Nursing Research

Nursing care quality is of utmost importance to ensure optimal patient outcomes. The Quality and Safety Education for Nurses (QSEN) Project recently developed competencies to prepare nurses around the globe for the care they provide within the current dynamic healthcare environment. The competencies include patient-centered care, teamwork and collaboration, EBP, quality, safety, and informatics [36]. While discussion of all of these topics is beyond the scope of this chapter, EBP is essential as it relates to integrating evidence from research to best practices in nursing and advancing nursing knowledge and practice around the globe.

Evidence-based practice (EBP) is applying the best available research along with patient preferences to make decisions about health care. EBP has been shown to improve healthcare quality, reliability, and patient outcomes. The process of EBP includes five A's: Ask, Acquire, Appraise, Apply, and Audit. Cultivating a spirit of inquiry and dissemination of results are two additional steps proposed by some authors [37] (see Table 31.2). Asking a question in a PICO (Population, Intervention, Control, Outcome) format is most helpful to focus the topic of interest and the literature review. International competencies on EBP have been developed for nurses and for those nurses in advanced practice roles and include essential elements of knowledge and skill among the seven steps. EBP should be used by nurses around the globe and within all healthcare settings including home health, ambulatory care, and inpatient care.

Unfortunately, evidence is often lacking for many nursing care practices. These gaps in knowledge provide opportunities for nursing research, which is the discovery of new knowledge that will enhance practice and patient outcomes. Oncology nurses can contribute to research by identifying gaps in knowledge which require investigation, collecting data for research studies, critiquing existing research for practice relevance, and integrating research into practice [23]. For nurses with

Table 31.2 Seven steps of evidence-based practice

Developing a spirit of inquiry	Involves building a culture of excellence
	Nurses should question practices on a daily basis, keeping in mind the evidence in which they perform tasks and patient care activities
	Organizational activities should support this inquiry such as journal clubs, nursing grand rounds, and discussions about best evidence
Ask	Ask a question about a patient, population, or community
	Frame the question specifically to reflect the following:
	P—Population—who is the patient, population, or community of interest?
	I—Intervention—what intervention is questioned?
	C—Comparison—what is the intervention compared to?
	O—Outcome—what should the intervention improve or affect?
Acquire	Acquire the best evidence on the topic through a comprehensive literature review
Appraise	Appraise or critique the literature
	Is the current literature valid and applicable for the question?
	Be informed of the various levels of evidence
Apply	Apply or translate the information into practice
	Consider contextual factors, values, and preferences of the individual patient.
Assess	Assess the outcome or results of the application
Disseminate	Disseminate the practice change throughout the organization
	Consider presenting or publishing the success along with lessons learned along the way

research degrees, designing and conducting oncology nursing research and adding new knowledge to the field is a primary responsibility.

With the vast amount of gaps in knowledge that exist, determining a direction for research may be challenging. Fortunately, organizations throughout the world have developed research agendas and priorities that can help guide nurse scientists in order to improve cancer care globally [38–43]. Crosscutting themes among some of the world's leading oncology nursing organizations include pain and symptom management and end-of-life and palliative care. These priorities reinforce the gaps in knowledge needed to optimize supportive care. Priorities also communicate strongly about the role of the nurse in supportive cancer care. Table 31.3 includes research priorities and goals for some of the world's cancer nursing organizations.

Table 31.3 Global research priorities and activities for oncology nursing

Organization	Research priorities and activities
Asian Oncology Nursing Society (AONS)	Organization newly established in 2014
European Oncology Nursing Society (EONS)	Symptom management
	End-of-life care
	Survivorship
	Cancer nursing roles
	Psychosocial care
	Nursing aspects of delivering cancer therapy
	Nursing aspects surrounding the cancer diagnosis
International Society for Nurses in Cancer Care (ISNCC)	Pain and symptom management
	Palliative care
Israeli Oncology Nursing Society	Collaborates with the European Oncology Nursing Society
	Focus on multisite research
	Oral adherence
	Symptom clusters
	Complementary and alternative medicine
Japanese Oncology Nursing Society	Diagnosis and treatment
	Nursing education
	Outpatient nursing
	Supportive and palliative care
	Prevention and early detection
Korean Oncology Nursing Society	Symptoms: pain, depression
	Psychosocial topics: quality of life, family adjustment to cancer, self-care, self-management, communication, coping, family functioning, and self-efficacy
	Health promotion: stress management, diet/nutrition, and screening/early detection
	Survivorship and Palliative Care: survivorship, palliative care, rehabilitation, cancer recurrence, and survivor wellness
	Healthcare systems: quality improvement and continuum of care

(continued)

Table 31.3 (continued)

Organization	Research priorities and activities
Oncology Nursing Society (ONS)	Four crosscutting themes
	• Bioinformatics
	• Biomarkers
	• Comparative effectiveness research
	• Dissemination and implementation science
	Content areas and priority topics
	• Symptoms: fatigue, pain, sleep, symptom clusters, chemotherapy-induced peripheral neuropathy, psychological distress
	• Late effects
	• Palliative and end-of-life care
	• Self-management
	• Aging
	• Family and caregivers
	• Improving healthcare systems
	• Risk reduction

Training and Education Initiatives

Globally, nurses are at the forefront of patient care providing the majority of health care especially in LMIC and resource-challenged settings, and to the most disadvantaged. They assess, educate, and provide treatment, improve continuity of care among the members of the interdisciplinary team, and coordinate the majority of family care and interdisciplinary communication. Nurses are also on the forefront of patient advocacy and play an integral role in delivering and ensuring quality care to people with cancer and their families from diagnosis through survivorship and bereavement.

Education and training of nurses varies by country and levels of licensure. Globally, nurses have different levels of educational preparation as generalists and then specialists [44]. Increasingly, nurses are practicing and obtaining specialization to work with a specific patient population such as in cancer care. For example, in Rwanda, students have 6 years primary education, then 3 years of secondary education followed by different levels of training as a nurse. Nurses have three levels: A0, A1, and A2 (from highest-most training to lowest-least training). The first level is an A2 nurse with approximately 3 years of basic training after secondary education and is similar to a technical nurse in other countries. The next level, an A1 requires an additional 3 years of education. The highest level, an A0, requires yet again 3 years of education and would be considered the same as a baccalaureate degree in more developed countries. However, since there was no specialty education in oncology nursing, the Rwandan government Ministry of Health (MOH) developed an ambitious plan (Human Resources for Health [HRH]) to increase capacity of healthcare workforce (nurses, midwives, and physicians) through a partnership with eight medical schools and six schools of nursing from the United States [45]. They contacted Partners in Health (PIH) and Dana-Farber Cancer Institute (DFCI), both in Boston, Massachusetts, USA, to develop specific training for nurses in oncology care. In a unique model nurse fellows from DFCI served three-month rotations in Rwanda. Using DFCI nurse fellows, they were able to develop a sustainable, growing program to build capacity in country [46]. Now in its third year, this ongoing partnership continues to build on previous initiatives to increase knowledge about cancer, increase safety of chemotherapy, and develop documentation and leadership abilities in Rwandan nurses.

The scope of practice also varies with some nurses working in advanced practice roles to meet the needs of the population in settings, where there are a few doctors. For example, in Cameroon, nurses have been working at Baptist Convention Health Services (CBCHS) in the Women's Health Programs (WHP) to improve health care for women. CBCHS provides health care to over 20 % of the population in Cameroon in 5 hospital, 24 integrated health centers, and 50 primary health centers [47]. In the six WHP clinics in Southwest Cameroon, the nurses provide numerous services including cervical cancer screening and treatment of precancerous lesions. In six WHP clinics that cover four of the ten regions of Cameroon, nurses provide numerous services including implementation of HPV vaccination programs, screening for cervical cancer, provision of treatment of precancerous lesions, and referral of women with invasive cancers for radical surgery and/or radio/chemotherapy, and provide follow-up care. In addition, the nurses train new nurses to work in the WHP clinics or in other organizations. In fact, between 2007 and 2013, nurses in the WHP have screened over 34,000 women in stationary CBCHS facilities and mobile clinics to reach remote villages across Cameroon [48]. The WHP nurses screen for cervical cancer using Digital Cervicography (DC) instead of colposcopy and PAP smears because it is less costly than using pathological examination and not dependent on stable, electrical current. DC is an adjunct to visual inspection with acetic acid (VIA) and visual inspection with Lugol's iodine (VILI). In DC, a handheld camera fitted with a macro-convention lens is used to project real time highly magnified cervical images onto a TV monitor through a connecting cord. The image is available to the woman and the clinician and then captured with a digital image. Precancerous changes are treated with cryotherapy or cautery. Nurses biopsy suspicious lesions for pathological examination and follow-up with the women. While this work would be considered advanced practice in more developed countries, these nurses complete 2–3 years of nursing education and then pursue 1 year of specialty training from nurses in the Women's Health Program.

Online resources for oncology nurse education and training are available for viewing and download at numerous international sites. For example, the ISNCC has online trainings on tobacco cessation interventions and other topics and maintains a webinar library on a wide range of topics relate to cancer care and nursing [49]. The International Agency for Research in Cancer (IARC), the specialized cancer agency of the WHO, has online resources for training in screening for both oral and cervical precancerous and cancerous lesions, treatment of cervical precancerous lesions, and breast self-examination [50].

Other initiatives to develop cancer education and training programs arise from volunteer work by healthcare providers from more developed countries. These volunteers often travel to countries deemed “safe” or conflict-free—a significant handicap for the development of programs with in-person training in countries in transition. For example, the American Society of Clinical Oncology (ASCO) developed the International Cancer Corps (ICC, http://www.asco.org/international-programs/international-cancer-corps) and partnered with Health Volunteers Overseas (HVO) to strengthen cancer care programs in low resource countries [51]. ICC works with in-country partners to identify educational and training needs and then creates teams of oncology clinicians from the United States to travel for 2–4 weeks to resource-challenged settings. In Honduras, ICC has returned twice to deliver the first cancer nursing conferences in the country. Training has specifically targeted development and implementation of chemotherapy guidelines, provided presentations on cancer care including palliative/end-of-life care, and other specific topics such as breast and cervical cancer and psychosocial care [52].

It is clear that standardization of the roles and contributions requires standardization. The International Council of Nurses has called for an International Classification for Nursing Practice (ICNP®) to provide a formal terminology for general nursing practice [53]. The ISNCC has urged oncology nurses to create national organizations and develop national standards for oncology nursing. In some LMIC, nurses practice in expanded roles that would be considered advanced practice or nurse practitioner roles in the United States and other high-income countries. While this situation often arises due to scarcity of doctors in these settings, it highlights the country-specific scope of nursing practice. One way to increase capacity in LMIC and countries in transition is to develop the advanced practice role to address cancer control initiatives [54]. In addition, partnerships for education and training also spur mutual learning across borders and reverse innovation including more cost-effective interventions [55]. In conclusion, training and education opportunities stem from partnerships with identified goals and standards of care. Technology has great potential to extend these initiatives across borders for mutual learning and better care outcomes for people with cancer.

International Partnerships to Promote Excellence in Cancer Care

It is essential that partnerships be established between countries and organizations to address disparities in cancer outcomes caused by limited resources, unequal disease burden, insufficient nursing personnel, and limited specialty education. These partnerships between organizations, governments, ministries of health, and academic institutions identify priorities for cancer care and strategically connect key players. They can also promote excellence in education and training to meet designated outcomes and advocate for resources. The ISNCC Training and Education Initiatives are moving to a model of distance learning or e-learning combined with educational opportunities at conferences ISNCC engages in partnerships with several other international cancer organizations with common interests and goals, as well as those focused on oncology nursing. In addition to formal partnerships with the AONS, the EONS, the International Psycho-Oncology Nursing Society, and Multinational Association of Supportive Care in Cancer (MASCC), ISNCC also develops joint project with member associations (see Table 31.3). These activities range from joint symposia or seminars at conferences to engaging in joint research projects. For example, ISNCC partnered with the Oncology Nursing group of the Chinese Nurses Association to develop a distance education program to build capacity among Chinese nurses to provide evidence-based smoking cessation interventions for patients.

A few of the members of ISNCC, such as the Oncology Nursing Societies of the United States, Canada, and Australia (to mention a few), have their own international portfolio. However, a model of close collaboration and synergy building was established to ensure that advocacy for oncology nursing has one voice. This model of collaboration ensures that the interest of nurses and patients in LMICs is prioritized over individual organization's interests. Additionally, through this extensive network, ISNCC can serve as a resource to groups that are working in LMICs, linking organizations with oncology nursing societies or individual nurses, thus enhancing nurses profile in the international health context.

The Oncology Nursing Society (ONS) is a professional organization of more than 35,000 registered nurses and other healthcare providers from around the world who are dedicated to excellence in patient care, education, research, and administration in cancer care. ONS provides information and education to nurses around the world and plays an active role in advocacy activities at the local, state, national, and international levels. The mission of ONS is to promote excellence in oncology nursing and quality cancer care.

Within ONS's four strategic pillars—Knowledge, Technology, Leadership, and Quality—both the Knowledge and Leadership pillars specifically articulate the commitment to disseminate knowledge and educate nurse leaders outside the United States to promote evidence-based cancer care [56]. The needs, challenges, and resource limitations and cultural differences of countries in transition are integral considerations when applying the EBP recommendations that ONS provides. Collaborative partnerships are key to the success of this implementation, and all international education and training initiatives are conducted with local or regional partners. These partners are essential to ensure training programs are culturally relevant, resource sensitive, and meaningful in the setting. When a country is experiencing political or economic challenges and numerous cultural factors must be addressed when preparing and delivering information. Localized content, usage of discussion groups, and trainers with a high level of emotional intelligence and cultural awareness are needed to effectively conduct education and training within these countries.

The Middle East is an area of the world where ONS has a long-standing involvement in education and training, equipping nurses and other healthcare professionals to build clinical capacity and develop leaders. The healthcare landscape is such that governments, advocacy groups, educators, administrators, and physicians recognize the tremendous value of nurses as members of the interdisciplinary team and have identified the need for nursing education and clinical training. Late-stage diagnosis is common in the Middle East, and nurses play a key role in the provision and coordination of palliative care to those with life-threatening illnesses such as cancer. The Gulf Cooperation Council (GCC) countries (Bahrain, Kuwait, Oman, Qatar, Saudi Arabia, and the United Arab Emirates) "will face an unparalleled and unprecedented rise in demand for health care over the course of the next two decades… with the simultaneous need to realign its healthcare systems to be able to treat the disorders of affluence" [57]. This is one reason for the strong emphasis among each state's government agendas to promote the employment of nationals within the private sector [58]. These factors are significant contributors to the strong desire and growing need to increase the capacity of national healthcare teams, within which the nurse plays a vital role, through training and education.

Instilling the idea that each nurse, within his/her cultural context, is a leader and essential to the sustainability of this education and training. ONS's partnership with the Middle East Cancer Consortium (MECC) began with a leadership development workshop for nurses from MECC countries. One of the key strategies to effect real change and to increase the quality of patient care is to equip nurses in a culturally conscientious manner to change agents within their institutions and communities. Sustainable leadership is accomplished by incorporating leadership training into clinical content. Since the first leadership workshop in Israel in December 2007, MECC and ONS have partnered with local organizations and ministries of health to conduct more than six conferences and educational programs covering topics such as symptom management, pain control, spiritual care, and many other nursing-sensitive aspects of cancer care.

Developing these educational programs in the Middle East required evaluation of typical program planning procedures with a focus on meeting the unique cultural perspectives of nurses practicing in this region. MECC and ONS staff worked closely with nurses and other healthcare professionals in the Middle East to clearly identify the knowledge and skills needed by those who would be attending the program. Information used to plan these programs included not just the perceived need, but also detail about the educational background, amount of experience, and current practice settings of the projected attendees. And since nurses attending the MECC-ONS programs have come from countries and communities that are very different from that of most ONS faculty, it was essential to learn as much as possible about the cultural context within which projected attendees live and practice. Faculty was then chosen based not just on their content expertise but also on their interest and experience in teaching and collaborating with nurses in other countries.

The educational approaches utilized in the MECC-ONS programs have changed over time to provide more opportunities for faculty and attendees to explore the program content and learn together. This has led to a carefully planned balance of didactic presentation and interactive activities. Recent programs have relied much more heavily on large and small group activities, such as integrated learning assessments, role play, analysis of case studies, and development of plans for change. The use of Liberating Structures, case study discussions, and breakout groups have also been very helpful in encouraging participation by all group members and creating a safe environment for sharing of opinions and ideas. Additionally, they provide the opportunity for nurses to present small group findings to the larger group, which also supports the development of rising leaders. Often, participants are identified in advance to develop and present a topic related to the conference from their own practice setting.

One of the key lessons learned by faculty conducting ONS programs internationally is that we all have much to learn from each other. While each country and region may have different access to education and patient care resources, all nurses have the same focus—the highest quality care and the best outcomes for their patients. The most important role that ONS can play in the Middle East and among other countries experiencing transition is to support quality cancer care through sharing of knowledge and development of skills needed to facilitate change to current practice.

The contribution of nurses in providing clinical care and research has been extensive throughout the history of the profession and continues to be a growing role in the Middle East. ONS educational programs have sought to develop leadership skills and clinical capacity in nurses across the region by having course participants identify practice and policy improvement strategies in their institutions and communities. It is essential that nurses embrace the initiative to take the problems and solutions discussed during these programs to their professional peers, leaders, policy makers, and the public. It is the hope of ONS that nurses globally will continue their quest to provide comprehensive and compassionate care to patients and families with cancer through their clinical practice and to pursue focused projects, leadership skills, coordination of care, advanced education, and research. It has been, and continues to be, an honor for ONS to be a part of the multilateral education and development of nurse leaders around the world.

Globalization of Oncology Nursing Care

Globalization, a borderless world with international movement of people, services, goods, and knowledge, may provide some answers to the specialty of oncology nursing. The process of globalization has led to greater interdependency among countries with increased mobility of populations and the nursing workforce. Organizational partnerships may increase information sharing and improve training opportunities (see Table 31.4). Standards of oncology nursing practice can also be globalized by international organizations such as ISNCC and ICN. For example, personal protective equipment (PPE) is widely recognized, especially since the Ebola epidemic, as promoting the health and safety for health workers. PPE is also a standard of administering chemotherapy in most countries. The Pan-American

Table 31.4 Examples of international partner organizations to promote cancer nursing training and education initiatives

Organizations	Partners	Initiatives	Countries
International Society of Nurses in Cancer Care (ISNCC)	44 Member organizations		
Oncology Nursing Society (ONS)	Middle East Cancer Consortium (MECC)	Oncology nursing education, palliative care, pain management, leadership development, spiritual care	Cyprus
			Egypt
			Lebanon
			Pakistan
			Saudi Arabia
			Qatar
			Yemen
			United Arab Emirates
			Oman
			Turkey
			Israel
			Palestine
			Jordan
			Iraq
			Iran
International Council of Nurses	134 National nursing organizations		
ASCO International Cancer Corps (ICC)	Health Volunteers Overseas (HVO)	Nursing education	Bhutan, Honduras, Vietnam, Paraguay
http://www.asco.org/international-programs/international-cancer-corps/			
Partners in Health	Human Resources for Health—Rwanda		Rwanda
http://www.pih.org/country/rwanda/			Haiti
			Malawi
Global Nursing Caucus		Nursing advocacy and mentoring	Over 30 countries
http://www.globalnursingcaucus.org/			
Sigma Theta Tau International			
http://www.nursingsociety.org/aboutus/mission/Pages/factsheet.aspx			
European Oncology Nursing Society			33 European Union countries
http://www.cancernurse.eu/			

(continued)

Table 31.4 (continued)

Organizations	Partners	Initiatives	Countries
Multinational Association of Supportive Care in Cancer (MASCC)			Over 60 countries
http://www.cancernurse.eu/membership/ourpartnerships.html			
Union for International Cancer Control	800 Organizations		155 Countries
http://www.uicc.org/			
International Agency for Research in Cancer			
http://www.uicc.org/			

health Organization published a "Safe Handling of Hazardous Chemotherapy Drugs in Limited-Resource Settings" [59]. With international standardization of practice, training programs for PPE were implemented in Rwanda in 2012 to ensure the safety of oncology nurses and could be scaled up to other settings. In fact, training programs that exploit technology are one viable mechanism for bringing educational programs into LMIC, conflict areas, and geographically isolated nurses. Internet-based distance learning approaches, both live (synchronous) and recorded lectures (asynchronous), may be available depending on internet access and bandwidth. Issues related to differing language across borders will limit generalizability and utility of some web-based resources, but newer translation software is improving shared knowledge. Additionally, mobile health devices such as cell phones and tablets have experienced rapid growth in LIMC providing yet another technological mechanism to reach nurses and people at risk for cancer for screening or caring for people after a diagnosis of cancer.

Globalization of oncology nursing can impact health and cancer outcomes for populations. However, it requires the active presence of nurse leaders in national and international organizations. Currently, the Chief Nurse Scientist position has been vacant at the World Health Organization since 2010 and the percent of nurses in professional and leadership positions at WHO has fallen from 2.6 % in 2000 to 0.6 % in 2012 [60, 61]. Other international organizations to reduce the global cancer burden such as WHO's Union for International Cancer Control (UICC) and the Global Task Force on Expanded Access to Cancer Care and Control (GTFEACCC) still lack nurses as members of their boards [62, 63]. Yet, these international organizations have called for government leaders to address issues related to the healthcare workforce to reduce cancer burden, promote equity, and improve outcomes—initiatives that require the world's largest healthcare workforce—nurses.

Conclusion

The UICC, in the *World Cancer Declaration 2025*, set nine Targets for 2025 [64]. Target 9 addresses innovative training and education of all healthcare disciplines in cancer care and control, particularly in LMIC (UICC, 2013). Oncology nurse educators can create innovative programs and exploit technology to increase reach and decrease cancer burden in LMIC. Expert oncology clinicians are needed to collaborate across borders and develop standards of care and best practices based on current evidence. Oncology nurse researchers are desperately needed to participate in translational projects and bring new technologies and treatments to LMIC. Finally, oncology nurse leaders must play key roles in local, regional, national, and international boards to direct policy development and promote the contributions of oncology nursing especially in resource-challenged settings and countries in transition.

References

1. Global Health Workforce Alliance (GHWA) Secretariat, The World Health Organization (WHO). A universal truth: no health without a workforce. Geneva: WHO; 2014. http://www.who.int/workforcealliance/knowledge/resources/GHWA-a_universal_truth_report.pdf?ua=1.
2. International Agency for Research on Cancer (IARC). Latest world cancer statistics: global cancer burden rises 14.1 million new cases 2012: marked increase in breast cancers must be addressed. Press release no. 233. 2013. http://www.iarc.fr/en/media-centre/pr/2013/pdfs/pr223_E.pdf. Accessed 12 Dec 2013.
3. World Health Organization. The 2013 update, global health workforce statistics. Geneva: WHO; 2013. http://www.who.int/hrh/statistics/hwfstats/.
4. World Health Organization. The world health report 2006—working together for health. http://www.who.int/whr/2006/chapter1/en/
5. World Health Organization. Nursing and midwifery services: strategic directions. Geneva: WHO; 2010. http://whqlibdoc.who.int/hq/2010/WHO_HRH_HPN_10.1_eng.pdf4.
6. World Health Organization. Transforming and scaling up health professional education and training. Policy brief on financing education of health professionals. Geneva: WHO; 2013. http://whoeducationguidelines.org/sites/default/files/uploads/whoeduguidelines_PolicyBrief_Financing.pdf. ISBN 9789241506380.
7. CanTreat International. Scaling up cancer diagnosis and treatment in developing countries: what can we learn from the HIV/AIDS epidemic? Ann Oncol. 2010;21(4):680–2. doi:10.1093/annonc/mdq055.
8. American Cancer Society. Global cancer: facts and figures. 2nd ed. Lyon: IARC; 2014. http://www.cancer.org/acs/groups/content/@epidemiologysurveilance/documents/document/acspc-027766.pdf.
9. Noncommunicable disease (NCD) alliance. Global NCD targets. http://www.ncdalliance.org/targets.
10. World Health Organization. Global action plan for the prevention and control of noncommunicable diseases 2013–2020. 2013. http://apps.who.int/iris/bitstream/10665/94384/1/9789241506236_eng.pdf
11. Stewart BW, Wild CP, editors. World cancer report 2014. The cancer atlas. American Cancer Society. 2nd ed. Lyon: IARC; 2014. http://canceratlas.cancer.org. ISBN 978-92-832-0429-9.
12. World Health Organization. Enhancing nursing and midwifery capacity to contribute to the prevention, treatment and management if noncommunicable diseases. Human Resources for

Health Observer No. 12. Geneva: World Health Organization; 2012. http://www.who.int/hrh/resources/observer12.pdf.
13. Kingma M. Nurses on the move: migration and the global health economy. Ithaca: Cornell University Press; 2006.
14. International Council of Nurses. Position statement. Armed conflict: nursing's perspective. 2012. http://www.icn.ch/images/stories/documents/publications/position_statements/E01_Armed_Conflict.pdf
15. Nichols BL, Davis CR, Richardson DR. An integrative review of global nursing workforce issues. Annu Rev Nur Res. 2011;28:113–32.
16. Davis CR, Kritek PB. Foreign nurses in the US workforce: healthy work environments: foreign nurse recruitment for best practices. Washington, DC: American Organization of Nurse Executives; 2005. p. 201.
17. Aiken LA, Sermeus W, Van den Heeded K, Sloane DM, Busse R, McKee M, et al. Patient safety, satisfaction, and quality of hospital care: cross-sectional surveys of nurses in 12 countries in Europe and the United States. BMJ. 2012;344:e1717. doi:10.1136/bmj.e1717.
18. Cheung RB, Aiken LA, Clarke SP, Sloane DM. Nursing care and patient outcomes: international evidence. Enferm Clin. 2008;18(1):35–40.
19. Sheldon LK. International cancer care: what is the role of oncology nursing? Clin J Oncol Nurs. 2010;14(5):539–41.
20. Strengthening of palliative care as a component of integrated treatment within the continuum of care. World Health Assembly. 2014. http://apps.who.int/gb/ebwha/pdf_files/EB134/B134_R7-en.pdf
21. Pioneros en Cuidados Paliativos de Panamá en la Organización Mundial de la Salud: Entrevista con el Dr. Gaspar Da Costa.
22. Al-Ruzzieh MA, Ayala de Calvo LE, Bigirimana JB, Burg A, Buswell L, Challinor J, et al. Strengthening the oncology nurse workforce in low- and middle-income countries via education. International Society for Nurses in Cancer Care. 2015. http://www.isncc.org/?page=Resources
23. Brant J, Wickman R, editors. Standards of oncology nursing practice. Pittsburgh: Oncology Nursing Society; 2013.
24. Tariman JD, Doorenbos A, Schepp KG, Singhal S, Berry DL. Information needs priorities in patients diagnosed with cancer: a systematic review. J Adv Pract Oncol. 2014;2014(5):115–22.
25. United Nations Goals. Millennium development goals and beyond 2015. UN; 2015. http://www.un.org/millenniumgoals/global.shtml
26. World Health Organization. Reducing the economic impact of NCDs in low- and middle-income countries. Executive summary. Geneva: WHO; 2011. http://www.who.int/nmh/publications/best_buys_summary/en/.
27. World Health Organization. Cancer: national cancer control programmes. Geneva: WHO; 2014. http://www.who.int/cancer/nccp/en/. Accessed 31 Dec 2014.
28. World Health Organization. Tobacco free initiative. Geneva: WHO; 2014. http://www.who.int/tobacco/en/. Accessed 31 Dec 2014.
29. American Cancer Society. Cancer facts and figures. 2014. http://www.cancer.org/acs/groups/content/@research/documents/webcontent/acspc-042151.pdf
30. Markowitz LE, Dunne EF, Saraiya M, Chesson HW, Curtis CR, Gee J, et al. Human papillomavirus vaccination: recommendations of the Advisory Committee on Immunization Practices (ACIP). MMWR Recomm Rep. 2014;63(RR-05):1–30.
31. American Cancer Society (Producer). Global cancer facts and figures, 2nd ed. 2008. http://www.cancer.org/acs/groups/content/@epidemiologysurveilance/documents/document/acspc-027766.pdf. Accessed 31 Dec 2014.
32. Jemal A, Bray F, Center MM, Ferlay J, Ward E, Forman D. Global cancer statistics. CA Cancer J Clin. 2011;61(2):69–90. doi:10.3322/caac.20107.
33. Kvale E, Urba SG. NCCN guidelines for survivorship expanded to address two common conditions. J Natl Compr Canc Netw. 2014;12(5 Suppl):825–7.

34. Mayer DK, Birken SA, Check DK, Chen RC. Summing it up: an integrative review of studies of cancer survivorship care plans (2006–2013). Cancer. 2015;121(7):978–96. doi:10.1002/cncr.28884.
35. Brant JM. Palliative care for adults across the cancer trajectory: from diagnosis to end of life. Semin Oncol Nurs. 2010;26(4):222–30. doi:10.1016/j.soncn.2010.08.002.
36. QSEN Institute. Competencies. 2014. http://qsen.org/. Accessed 31 Dec 2014
37. Melnyk BM, Gallagher-Ford L, Long LE, Fineout-Overholt E. The establishment of evidence-based practice competencies for practicing registered nurses and advanced practice nurses in real-world clinical settings: proficiencies to improve healthcare quality, reliability, patient outcomes, and costs. Worldviews Evid Based Nurs. 2014;11(1):5–15. doi:10.1111/wvn.12021.
38. Donovan HS, Nolte S, Edwards RP, Wenzel L. Nursing research in the gynecologic oncology group. Semin Oncol Nurs. 2014;30(1):44–52. doi:10.1016/j.soncn.2013.12.008.
39. Given BA. 2009–2013 Oncology Nursing Society research agenda: why is it important? Oncol Nurs Forum. 2009;36(5):487–8. doi:10.1188/09.onf.487-488.
40. Knobf MT (2014). Oncology Nursing Society research agenda 2014–2018 draft. https://www.ons.org/sites/default/files/Draft%20ONS%20Research%20Agenda.pdf. Accessed 31 Dec 2014
41. Lee E, Chung BY, Chun N, Cho S. Prioritization of research topics of Korean oncology nurses. Asian Oncol Nurs. 2013;13(4):295–303. doi:10.5388/aon.2013.13.4.295.
42. LoBiondo-Wood G, Brown CG, Knobf MT, Lyon D, Mallory G, Mitchell SA, et al. Priorities for oncology nursing research: the 2013 national survey. Oncol Nurs Forum. 2014;41(1):67–76. doi:10.1188/14.onf.67-76.
43. Shaha M, Schmid-Buchi S, Abt J, Mathis-Jaggi F, Holdener E, Riederer E, et al. The contribution of oncology nursing to the Swiss Research Agenda for Nursing—SRAN. Pflege. 2008;21(6):385–403. doi:10.1024/1012-5302.21.6.385.
44. Currie EJ, Carr-Hill RA. What is a nurse? Is there an international consensus? Int Nurs Rev. 2013;60(1):67–74.
45. Bingawaho A, Kyamanywa P, Farmer PE, Nuthulagabnti T, Umubyeyi B, Nyemazi JP, et al. The human resources for health program in Rwanda—a new partnership. N Engl J Med. 2013;368(21):2054–9.
46. Virchick B. If you build it, they will come: cancer care in Rwanda. News and insight from Dana-Farber;2012.http://blog.dana-farber.org/insight/2012/11/if-you-build-it-they-will-come-cancer-care-in-rwanda/
47. Cameroon Baptist Convention Health Services (CBCHS). http://www.cbchealthservices.org/
48. Sheldon LK. Nurse-led cervical cancer prevention and screening programs: innovative models in Cameroon. Year of Advocacy Blog, Global Nursing Caucus. 2014. http://www.globalnursingcaucus.org/blog/nurse-led-cervical-cancer-prevention-screening-programs-innovative-models-cameroon-lisa-kennedy-sheldon/
49. International Society for Nurses in Cancer Care (ISNCC). http://www.isncc.org/
50. International Agency for Research on Cancer (IARC). Training materials. http://screening.iarc.fr/training.php?lang=1
51. American Society of Clinical Oncology (ASCO) International Cancer Corps (ICC). http://www.asco.org/international-programs/international-cancer-corps
52. Sheldon LK, Wise B, Dowds C, Carlson J, Sarchet V, Sanchez J. Development of a longitudinal cancer nursing education program in Honduras. J Cancer Educ. 2013;28(4):669–75. doi:10.1007/s13187-013-0497-6.
53. International Council of Nurses. International Classification for Nursing Practice (ICNP®). http://www.icn.ch/images/stories/documents/pillars/Practice/icnp/ICNP_FAQs.pdf
54. Woodgate RL. International nursing partnerships for global cancer control. Cancer Nurs. 2014;37(5):319.
55. Crisp LN. Mutual learning and reverse innovation—where next? Global Health. 2014;10:14. http://www.globalizationandhealth.com/content/10/1/14.
56. Oncology Nursing Society. Strategic plan 2012–2016. 2012. https://www.ons.org/about/strategic-plan. Accessed 14 Jan 2014.

57. Mourshed M, Hediger V, Lambert T. Gulf cooperation council health care: challenges and opportunities. In: Global competitiveness reports. 2008. http://www.weforum.org/pdf/Global_Competitiveness_Reports/Reports/chapters/2_1.pdf
58. Khoja S. Can GCC workforce nationalization succeed? 2013. http://www.zawya.com/story/Can_GCC_workforce_nationalization_succeed-ZAWYA20130429085608
59. Safe handling of hazardous chemotherapy drugs in limited-resource settings. Washington, DC: Pan-American Health Organization; 2013. http://www.paho.org/hq/index.php?option=com_content&view=article&id=9504&Itemid=2&lang=pt
60. International Council of Nurses. CNR communique. 2013. http://www.icn.ch/images/stories/documents/news/advocacy/Nurse_staffing_WHO/CNR_Communique.pdf
61. International Council of Nurses. Going, going, gone: the nursing presence in the World Health Organization: a fact sheet for national nurses associations. 2013. http://www.icn.ch/images/stories/documents/publications/fact_sheets/7b_FS-Does_Nursing_Matter_within_WHO.pdf
62. Union for International Cancer Care (UICC). http://www.uicc.org/
63. Global Task Force on Expanded Access to Cancer Care and Control (GTFEACCC). http://gtfccc.harvard.edu/icb/icb.do?keyword=k69586&pageid=icb.page474203
64. Union for International Cancer Care (UICC). World cancer declaration 2013. http://uicc.org/sites/main/files/atoms/files/131119_UICC_WorldCancerDeclaration_2013_1.pdf

Index

M. Silbermann (ed.), *Cancer Care in Countries and Societies in Transition: Individualized Care in Focus*, DOI 10.1007/978-3-319-22912-6

L

M

MIX
Papier aus verantwortungsvollen Quellen
Paper from responsible sources
FSC® C105338

If you have any concerns about our products,
you can contact us on
ProductSafety@springernature.com

In case Publisher is established outside the EU,
the EU authorized representative is:
Springer Nature Customer Service Center GmbH
Europaplatz 3, 69115 Heidelberg, Germany

Printed by Libri Plureos GmbH
in Hamburg, Germany